Operative Techniques in
Pediatric Plastic
and Reconstructive
Surgery

Operative Techniques in Pediatric Plastic and Reconstructive Surgery

Arun K. Gosain, MD

EDITOR

Children's Service Board Professor and Chief, Pediatric Plastic Surgery
Anne and Robert Lurie Children's Hospital
Feinberg School of Medicine
Northwestern University
Chicago, Illinois

Kevin C. Chung, MD, MS

EDITOR-IN-CHIEF

Chief of Hand Surgery, Michigan Medicine
Director, University of Michigan Comprehensive Hand Center
Charles B. G. de Nancrede Professor of Surgery
Professor of Plastic Surgery and Orthopaedic Surgery
Assistant Dean for Faculty Affairs
Associate Director of Global REACH
University of Michigan Medical School
Ann Arbor, Michigan

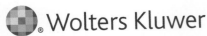

Philadelphia • Baltimore • New York • London
Buenos Aires • Hong Kong • Sydney • Tokyo

Executive Editor: Brian Brown
Development Editor: Ashley Fischer
Editorial Coordinator: John Larkin
Marketing Manager: Julie Sikora
Senior Production Project Manager: Alicia Jackson
Senior Designer: Joan Wendt
Artist/Illustrator: Body Scientific International
Senior Manufacturing Coordinator: Beth Welsh
Prepress Vendor: SPi Global

Printed in China

Cataloging-in-Publication Data available on request from the Publisher.
ISBN 978-1-9751-2720-6

shop.lww.com

To my teachers for giving me the background to contribute to this text and to my family for allowing me the time to do so.
—AKG

To Chin-Yin and William.
—KCC

Contributors

Fizan Abdullah, MD, PhD
Vice-Chair, Department of Surgery
Head, Division of Pediatric Surgery
Program Director, Fellowship in
  Pediatric Surgery
Orvar Swenson Founders' Board Chair
  in Pediatric Surgery
Ann & Robert H. Lurie Children's
  Hospital of Chicago
Professor of Surgery
Northwestern University
Chicago, Illinois

Joshua M. Adkinson, MD
Chief of Hand Surgery
Assistant Professor of Surgery
Division of Plastic Surgery
Indiana University School of Medicine
Indianapolis, Indiana

N. Scott Adzick, MD
Surgeon-in-Chief
Children's Hospital of Philadelphia
C. Everett Koop Endowed Chair of
  Pediatric Surgery
Perelman School of Medicine at the
  University of Pennsylvania
Philadelphia, Pennsylvania

Nicholas J. Ahn, MD
Research Fellow
Children's Hospital of Philadelphia
Center for Fetal Research
Philadelphia, Pennsylvania
Surgical Resident
Albany Medical Center
Department of Surgery
Albany, New York

Asim Ali, MD, FRCSC
Ophthalmologist-in-Chief and Mira
  Godard Chair in Vision Research
Department of Ophthalmology
The Hospital for Sick Children
University of Toronto
Toronto, Ontario, Canada

Lee W. T. Alkureishi, MBChB
Clinical Assistant Professor
Plastic and Reconstructive Surgery
University of Illinois Health
Pediatric Plastic and Craniofacial Surgeon
Plastic Surgery
Shriners Hospitals for Children
Chicago, Illinois

**Jugpal S. Arneja, MD, MBA, FAAP,
FACS, FRCSC**
Professor (Clinical), Surgery
Division of Plastic Surgery
University of British Columbia
Associate Member
Sauder School of Business
University of British Columbia
Associate Chief, Surgery
British Columbia Children's Hospital
Attending Plastic Surgeon
British Columbia Children's Hospital
Vancouver, British Columbia, Canada

Samer Attar, MD
Associate Professor of Orthopaedic
  Surgery
Northwestern Medicine
Chicago, Illinois

Scott P. Bartlett, MD
Mary Downs Endowed Chair in
  Craniofacial Treatment and
  Research
The Children's Hospital of
  Philadelphia
Professor of Surgery
The Perelman School of Medicine
University of Pennsylvania
Philadelphia, Pennsylvania

Bruce S. Bauer, MD, FACS, FAAP
Director of Pediatric Plastic
  Surgery
NorthShore University HealthSystem
Clinical Professor of Surgery
University of Chicago
Pritzker School of Medicine
Highland Park Hospital
Northbrook, Illinois

Maureen Beederman, MD
Resident
Section of Plastic and Reconstructive
  Surgery
Department of Surgery
The University of Chicago Medicine
Chicago, Illinois

Bryce R. Bell, MD
Hand and Upper Extremity Surgery
Department of Orthopaedic
  Surgery
Texas Children's Hospital
Conroe, Texas

David A. Billmire, MD
Chief of Plastic Surgery
Cincinnati Shriners Hospital
Cincinnati, Ohio

Kim A. Bjorklund, MD, MEd
Director of Brachial Plexus Program
Department of Plastic, Reconstructive
  & Hand Surgery
Nationwide Children's Hospital
Assistant Professor
The Ohio State University College of
  Medicine
Columbus, Ohio

Gregory H. Borschel, MD, FAAP, FACS
Associate Professor and Research
  Director
Division of Plastic and Reconstructive
  Surgery
University of Toronto
Associate Professor
Institute of Biomaterials and
  Biomedical Engineering
Associate Scientist, SickKids Research
  Institute
The Hospital for Sick Children
Toronto, Ontario, Canada

Patrick J. Buchanan, MD
Director of Hand Surgery
Plastic and Reconstructive
  Surgeon
Georgia Institute for Plastic
  Surgery
Savannah, Georgia

Charles E. Butler, MD, FACS
Professor and Chairman
Department of Plastic Surgery
The University of Texas MD Anderson
  Cancer Center
Houston, Texas

Michael R. Bykowski, MD, MS
Chief Resident
Department of Plastic Surgery
University of Pittsburgh
Pittsburgh, Pennsylvania

Joseph Catapano, BHSc, MD
Division of Plastic and Reconstructive
  Surgery
Department of Surgery
University of Toronto
Toronto, Ontario, Canada

Paul S. Cederna, MD
Chief
Section of Plastic Surgery
Michigan Medicine
Robert Oneal Professor of Plastic
    Surgery
Professor, Department of Biomedical
    Engineering
University of Michigan
Ann Arbor, Michigan

**Niel K. Chadha, MBChB(Hons),
MPHe BSc(Hons), FRCS**
Associate Clinical Professor
Division of Otolaryngology–Head and
    Neck Surgery
University of British Columbia
Pediatric Otolaryngology Surgeon
Division of Pediatric Otolaryngology–
    Head and Neck Surgery
British Columbia Children's
    Hospital
Vancouver, British Columbia, Canada

Christopher B. Chambers, MD
Associate Professor of Ophthalmology
Associate Professor of Plastic
    Surgery
Department of Surgery
Oculoplastic and Orbital Surgery
    Fellowship Director
Associate Residency Program
    Director
University of Washington School of
    Medicine
Seattle, Washington

Philip Kuo-Ting Chen, MD
Director, Craniofacial Center
Taipei Medical University Hospital
Professor of Surgery
Taipei Medical University
Taipei, Taiwan

Earl Y. Cheng, MD
Division Head of Pediatric Urology
Founder's Board Chair of Pediatric
    Urology
Ann and Robert H. Lurie Children's
    Hospital of Chicago
Professor of Urology
Feinberg School of Medicine
Northwestern University
Chicago, Illinois

Gerald J. Cho, MD
Assistant Professor, Plastic Surgery
Washington University in St. Louis
St. Louis, Missouri

David K. Chong, MBBS, FRACS
Cleft/Craniofacial Surgeon
Department of Plastic and
    Maxillofacial Surgery
Royal Children's Hospital
Melbourne, Australia

Julia Corcoran, MD, FACS, FAAP
Associate (Adjunct) Professor of
    Surgery & Medical Education
Feinberg School of Medicine
Northwestern University
Attending Surgeon
Shriners Hospital for Children
Chicago, Illinois

Gregory A. Dumanian, MD
Lucille and Orion Stuteville Professor
    of Surgery
Chief of Plastic Surgery
Feinberg School of Medicine
Northwestern University
Chicago, Illinois

**Mark Felton, BSc, MBChB, MSc, MD,
FRCS(Eng)**
Consultant Paediatric Otolaryngologist
Evelina London Children's Hospital
Guy's and St. Thomas' NHS
    Foundation Trust
London, United Kingdom

Roberto L. Flores, MD
Joseph G. McCarthy Associate
Professor of Reconstructive Plastic
    Surgery
Director of Cleft Lip and Palate
Hansjörg Wyss Department of Plastic
    Surgery
NYU Langone Health
New York, New York

Brad M. Gandolfi, MD
Craniofacial Plastic and Reconstructive
    Surgeon
Paramus, New Jersey

Benjamin C. Garden, MD
Department of Dermatology
University of Illinois at Chicago
Chicago, Illinois

Jerome M. Garden, MD
Professor of Clinical Dermatology
Northwestern University Feinberg
    School of Medicine
Chicago, Illinois

Catharine B. Garland, MD
Director, Cleft and Craniofacial
    Anomalies Clinic
American Family Children's Hospital
Assistant Professor of Surgery
Division of Plastic and Reconstructive
    Surgery
University of Wisconsin School of
    Medicine and Public Health
Madison, Wisconsin

Patrick A. Gerety, MD
Assistant Professor of Surgery
Division of Plastic Surgery
Indiana University and Riley Hospital
    for Children
Indianapolis, Indiana

Jesse Goldstein, MD, FAAP, FACS
Assistant Professor
Department of Plastic Surgery
Children's Hospital of Pittsburgh
University of Pittsburgh Medical
    Center
Pittsburgh, Pennsylvania

Arun K. Gosain, MD
Children's Service Board Professor and
    Chief, Pediatric Plastic Surgery
Anne and Robert Lurie Children's
    Hospital
Feinberg School of Medicine
Northwestern University
Chicago, Illinois

Jeremy Goss, MD
Research Fellow
Department of Plastic and Oral
    Surgery
Boston Children's Hospital
Harvard Medical School
Boston, Massachusetts

Lawrence J. Gottlieb, MD, FACS
Professor of Surgery
Director of Burn & Complex Wound
    Center
Section of Plastic and Reconstructive
    Surgery
The University of Chicago Medicine &
    Biological Sciences
Chicago, Illinois

Arin K. Greene, MD, MMSc
Department of Plastic and Oral Surgery
Boston Children's Hospital
Professor of Surgery
Harvard Medical School
Boston, Massachusetts

Lorelei Grunwaldt, MD, FACS, FAAP
Associate Professor of Plastic
    Surgery
Children's Hospital of Pittsburgh
Pittsburgh, Pennsylvania

Dennis C. Hammond, MD
Clinical Assistant Professor
Department of Surgery
Michigan State University College of
    Human Medicine
East Lansing, Michigan
Associate Program Director
Plastic and Reconstructive Surgery
Grand Rapids Medical Education
    Partners
Private Practice
Partners in Plastic Surgery of West
    Michigan
Grand Rapids, Michigan

Jamie C. Harris, MD
General Surgery Resident
Rush University Medical Center
Chicago, Illinois

Gregory G. Heuer, MD, PhD
Assistant Professor of Neurosurgery
Department of Neurosurgery
University of Pennsylvania
Division of Neurosurgery
Children's Hospital of Philadelphia
Philadelphia, Pennsylvania

C. Scott Hultman, MD, MBA, FACS
Director of Johns Hopkins Burn
  Center
Professor of Plastic Surgery (PAR)
Johns Hopkins University School of
  Medicine
Vice Chair for Strategic Development
Department of Plastic and
  Reconstructive Surgery
Vice President of Academic Affairs
American Society of Plastic Surgeons
Member, ACGME Review Committee
  for Plastic Surgery
Associate Editor
Annals of Plastic Surgery
Baltimore, Maryland

Kathryn V. Isaac, MD, FRCSC
Clinical Fellow
Department of Plastic and Oral
  Surgery
Boston Children's Hospital
Boston, Massachusetts

Sarah M. Jacobs, MD, MEd
Assistant Professor
Department of Ophthalmology
University of Alabama
Ophthalmic Plastic and Reconstructive
  Surgeon
Department of Ophthalmology
Callahan Eye Hospital
Birmingham, Alabama

Deborah L. Jacobson, MD
Fellow of Pediatric Urology
Department of Urology
Northwestern University
Division of Pediatric Urology
Lurie Children's Hospital
Chicago, Illinois

Michael J. A. Klebuc, MD
Associate Clinical Professor of Plastic
  and Neurosurgery
Weill Medical College
Cornell University
Director Center for Facial Reanimation
  and Functional Restoration
Houston Methodist Hospital
Houston, Texas

Terence Kwan-Wong, MD, FRCSC
Staff Surgeon
Pediatric Plastic Surgery
The Hospital for Sick Children
Toronto, Ontario, Canada

Eric Yu Kit Li, MD
Private Practice
Plastic and Reconstructive Surgery
  Associates
San Jose, California

Jan Lilja, MD, PhD, DDS
Associate Professor
Department of Plastic Surgery
Sahlgrenska University Hospital
Gothenburg, Sweden

Yuen-Jong Liu, MD
Plastic and Hand Surgeon
Aesthetic Surgery Center
Darien, Connecticut

Joseph E. Losee, MD, FACS, FAAP
Dr. Ross H. Musgrave Endowed Chair
  in Pediatric Plastic Surgery
Associate Dean for Faculty Affairs
University of Pittsburgh School of
  Medicine
Professor and Executive Vice Chair
Department of Plastic Surgery
Division Chief
Pediatric Plastic Surgery
Children's Hospital of Pittsburgh of
  UPMC
Pittsburgh, Pennsylvania

Jeffrey R. Marcus, MD, FAAP, FACS
Professor and Chief
Director, Duke Cleft and Craniofacial
  Center
Division of Plastic, Reconstructive,
  Maxillofacial and Oral Surgery
Duke University
Durham, North Carolina

Andre P. Marshall, MD, MPH
Plastic Surgeon
Aesthetic Plastic Surgical Institute
Laguna Beach, California

Hani Matloub, MD
Professor, Department of Plastic Surgery
Program Director, Hand Surgery
  Fellowship
Department of Plastic Surgery
Medical College of Wisconsin
Milwaukee, Wisconsin

Jennifer L. McGrath, MD
Division of Plastic and Reconstructive
  Surgery
Feinberg School of Medicine
Northwestern University
Ann and Robert H. Lurie Children's
  Hospital of Chicago
Chicago, Illinois

McKay Mckinnon, MD
Attending Plastic Surgeon
Ann and Robert Lurie Children's Hospital
Chicago, Illinois

Alexander F. Mericli, MD
Assistant Professor
Department of Plastic Surgery
MD Anderson Cancer Center
University of Texas
Houston, Texas

Christopher D. Morrison, MD
Chief Resident
Department of Urology
Feinberg School of Medicine
Northwestern University
Chicago, Illinois

Vikram S. Pandit, MDS
Oral and Maxillofacial Surgeon
Consultant Oral and Maxillofacial
  Surgeon
Pandit Clinic
Pune, India

Christina Marie Pasick, MD
Resident
Division of Plastic Surgery
Department of Surgery
Icahn School of Medicine at Mount Sinai
New York, New York

Pravin K. Patel, MD, FACS
Professor of Surgery
University of Illinois at Chicago
Chief of Pediatric and Craniofacial
  Surgery
Division of Plastic and Reconstructive
  Surgery
The Craniofacial Center
Chicago, Illinois

Terrance Peabody, MD
Edwin Ryerson
Professor and Chair
Department of Orthopaedic Surgery
Feinberg School of Medicine
Northwestern University
Chicago, Illinois

Gregory D. Pearson, MD
Associate Professor Clinical
Director, Center for Complex
  Craniofacial Disorders
Nationwide Children's Hospital
Columbus, Ohio

William H. Peranteau, MD
Assistant Professor of Surgery
Division of General, Thoracic, and
  Fetal Surgery
Department of Surgery
The Children's Hospital of Philadelphia
Philadelphia, Pennsylvania

Chad A. Purnell, MD
Resident Physician
Division of Plastic Surgery
Feinberg School of Medicine
Northwestern University
Chicago, Illinois

Whitney Laurel Quong, MD
Resident Physician
Division of Plastic & Reconstructive
  Surgery
University of Toronto
Burnaby, British of Columbia, Canada

Kenneth E. Salyer, MD, FACS, FAAP
Founder and Chairman of the Board
World Craniofacial Foundation
Clinical Professor
Department of Biomedical Sciences
Baylor College of Dentistry
Texas A&M University Dallas
Dallas, Texas

Rosemary Seelaus, MAMS
Senior Anaplastologist
Division of Plastic & Reconstructive
  Surgery
University of Illinois at Chicago
Chicago, Illinois

Ji H. Son, MD, MS
Resident Physician
Department of Plastic and
  Reconstructive Surgery
Case Western School of Medicine
Cleveland, Ohio

Robert J. Steffner, MD
Assistant Clinical Professor
Musculoskeletal Tumor Surgery
Department of Orthopaedic Surgery
School of Medicine
Stanford University
Redwood City, California

Adam R. Sweeney, MD
Fellow, Oculoplastic and Facial
  Reconstructive Surgery
Department of Ophthalmology
Baylor College of Medicine
Houston, Texas

Peter J. Taub, MD, FACS, FAAP
Professor, Surgery, Pediatrics, Dentistry,
  and Neurosurgery
Professor, Medical Education
Division of Plastic and Reconstructive
  Surgery
Residency Program Director
Chief, Craniomaxillofacial Surgery
Icahn School of Medicine at Mount Sinai
Chief, Pediatric Plastic Surgery
Director, Mount Sinai Cleft and
  Craniofacial Center
Director, Mount Sinai Vascular
  Anomalies Program
Kravis Children's Hospital at Mount Sinai
New York, New York

Jesse A. Taylor, MD, FACS, FAAP
Peter Randall Endowed Chair
  and Chief
Division of Plastic Surgery
Children's Hospital of Philadelphia
The University of Pennsylvania
Philadelphia, Pennsylvania

**T. Guy Thorburn, BMBS, BMedSci,
MA, FRCS(Plastic Surgery)**
Consultant Cleft and Plastic
  Surgeon
Spires Regional Cleft Centre
Oxford University Hospitals NHSFT
Oxford, United Kingdom

Charles H. Thorne, MD
Chairman
Department of Plastic Surgery
Lenox Hill Hospital
New York, New York

Ali Totonchi, MD
Associate Professor
Case Western Reserve University
Associate Director of the Plastic
  Surgery Residency Program
MetroHealth Medical Center
Cleveland, Ohio

Sergey Y. Turin, MD
Resident Physician
Division of Plastic and Reconstructive
  Surgery
Feinberg School of Medicine
Northwestern University
Chicago, Illinois

John van Aalst, MD, MA, FACS, FAAP
Professor and Director
Division of Pediatric and Craniofacial
  Plastic Surgery
Cincinnati Children's Hospital Medical
  Center
Cincinnati, Ohio

Akira Yamada, MD, PhD
Professor of Surgery
Feinberg School of Medicine
Northwestern University
Department of Plastic Surgery
Ann & Robert H. Lurie Children's
  Hospital of Chicago
Chicago, Illinois

Ji-Geng Yan, MD, PhD
Department of Plastic Surgery
The Medical College of
  Wisconsin
Milwaukee, Wisconsin

Elizabeth B. Yerkes, MD
Associate Professor
Department of Urology
Feinberg School of Medicine at
  Northwestern University
Attending Pediatric Urologist
Division of Pediatric Urology
Department of Surgery
Ann and Robert H. Lurie Children's
  Hospital of Chicago
Chicago, Illinois

Michael R. Zenn, MD, MBA, FACS
Zenn Plastic Surgery
Raleigh, North California
Adjunct Professor of Plastic
  Surgery
University of North Carolina at Chapel
  Hill
Chapel Hill, North Carolina

Emily M. Zepeda, MD
Pediatric Ophthalmology and Adult
  Strabismus Fellow
Kellogg Eye Center
University of Michigan School of
  Medicine
Ann Arbor, Michigan

**Ronald Zuker, MD, FRCSC, FACS,
FRCSEd(Hon)**
Staff Surgeon
Division of Plastic and Reconstructive
  Surgery
The Hospital for Sick
  Children
University of Toronto
Toronto, Ontario, Canada

Preface

Having a pediatric practice is a cherished component of a surgeon's contribution. We often comment that children are not like small adults because they have unique needs, and their growth produces a great deal of unpredictability in outcomes of our surgical reconstruction. Under the outstanding leadership of Dr. Gosain, we have solicited the contributions of all the experts on pediatric plastic surgery to make this an authoritative textbook, which creatively leverages illustrative procedural concepts to provide efficient delivery of educational content. The chapters were written in a clear and sequential fashion so that you can follow each step of the surgical procedures to impact confidence in the myriad of surgical conditions in children.

This textbook is a collaboration among many specialties caring for children. Some of the procedures such as cleft lip and palate have standard approaches; however, many other operations require a multispecialty team to apply various viewpoints to arrive at a comprehensive plan. I am sure you will find this book a constant companion in your care of children whose conditions and diseases require the knowledge of senior surgeons' rich experience. I am grateful for the contributions of the authors and for your recognition of our dedication by adding this book to your collection.

Kevin C. Chung, MD, MS
Chief of Hand Surgery, Michigan Medicine
Director, University of Michigan Comprehensive Hand Center
Charles B. G. de Nancrede Professor of Surgery
Professor of Plastic Surgery and Orthopaedic Surgery
Assistant Dean for Faculty Affairs
Associate Director of Global REACH
University of Michigan Medical School
Ann Arbor, Michigan

Contents

Contributors vi
Preface x

SECTION I CLEFT LIP

1 Anatomical Subunit Repair of Unilateral Cleft Lip 2
   David K. Chong and Kathryn V. Isaac

2 Unilateral Cleft Lip Repair: Millard/Mohler Modifications 12
   Roberto L. Flores and Gerald J. Cho

3 Salyer Unilateral Cleft Lip/Nose Repair 22
   Kenneth E. Salyer

SECTION II CLEFT PALATE REPAIR

4 Lip Adhesion 35
   Catharine B. Garland, Jesse Goldstein, and Joseph E. Losee

5 Bilateral Cleft Lip Repair 43
   John A. van Aalst

6 Secondary Deformities 50
   Catharine B. Garland, Jesse Goldstein, and Joseph E. Losee

7 Delayed Hard Palate Repair in UCLP Patients 64
   Jan Lilja

8 Furlow Palatoplasty 68
   T. Guy Thorburn

9 von Langenbeck Palatoplasty 74
   Kathryn V. Isaac and David K. Chong

10 Sommerlad Palatoplasty 81
    T. Guy Thorburn

11 Two-Flap Palatoplasty 89
    David K. Chong, Kathryn V. Isaac, and Kenneth E. Salyer

12 Tongue-Lip Adhesion/Floor of Mouth Muscle Release for Pierre Robin Sequence 96
    Chad A. Purnell and Arun K. Gosain

13 Palatal Fistula 102
    Gregory D. Pearson

14 Velopharyngeal Insufficiency 112
    Jennifer L. McGrath and Arun K. Gosain

SECTION III CLEFT RHINOPLASTY

15 Secondary Cleft Rhinoplasty 120
    Ali Totonchi and Ji H. Son

SECTION IV ATYPICAL CLEFTS-SOFT TISSUE COMPONENT

16 Tessier 3 and 4 Clefts (Nasal-Cheek Region) 125
    Philip Kuo-Ting Chen and Vikram S. Pandit

17 Tessier 7—Macrostomia Repair 135
    Patrick A. Gerety and Scott P. Bartlett

SECTION V CUTANEOUS LESIONS

18 Tissue Expansion for Congenital Nevi 141
    Lee W. T. Alkureishi and Bruce S. Bauer

19 Surgical Treatment of Congenital Midline Nasal Mass 150
    Patrick A. Gerety and Scott P. Bartlett

SECTION VI SOFT TISSUE MASSES

20 Surgery of Neurofibromatosis in the Pediatric Patient 158
    McKay McKinnon

21 Vascular Anomalies 165
    Arin K. Greene and Jeremy Goss

SECTION VII PEDIATRIC BURNS AND WOUNDS

22 Functional Burn Reconstruction 171
    David A. Billmire and Kim A. Bjorklund

23 Harvesting a Skin Graft 175
    David A. Billmire and Kim A. Bjorklund

24 Burned Hand Reconstruction 178
    David A. Billmire and Kim A. Bjorklund

25 Reconstruction of Burned Eyelids 183
    David A. Billmire and Kim A. Bjorklund

26 Burn Neck Contracture Release   186
    David A. Billmire and Kim A. Bjorklund

27 Adolescent Burned Breast Reconstruction   189
    David A. Billmire and Kim A. Bjorklund

28 Pressure Injuries (Sacral and Pelvic Region,
    Columella—From CPAP)   192
    David A. Billmire and Kim A. Bjorklund

29 Pressure Injuries   196
    Lawrence J. Gottlieb and Maureen Beederman

30 Vascular Lesions   204
    Benjamin C. Garden and Jerome M. Garden

31 Laser Burn Scar Revision   211
    C. Scott Hultman and Yuen-Jong Liu

32 Fat Grafting for Nerve Entrapment Within Burn
    Scars   216
    C. Scott Hultman and Yuen-Jong Liu

SECTION VIII **EAR RECONSTRUCTION**

33 Auricular Reconstruction for Microtia and
    Post-traumatic Deformities   221
    Charles H. Thorne

34 Stahl Ear   227
    Akira Yamada and Arun K. Gosain

35 Constricted Ear   232
    Akira Yamada and Julia Corcoran

36 Cryptotia   238
    Akira Yamada and Arun K. Gosain

37 Prominent Ear   242
    Akira Yamada and Arun K. Gosain

SECTION IX **EYELID RECONSTRUCTION**

38 Eyelid Coloboma   248
    Adam R. Sweeney and Christopher B. Chambers

39 Congenital Ptosis   255
    Adam R. Sweeney and Christopher B. Chambers

40 Epiblepharon   263
    Adam R. Sweeney and Christopher B. Chambers

41 Canthopexy   269
    Adam R. Sweeney and Christopher B. Chambers

42 Nasolacrimal Duct Obstruction   276
    **Emily M. Zepeda, Sarah M. Jacobs, and
    Christopher B. Chambers**

43 Management of the Microphthalmic or
    Anophthalmic Orbit   283
    Sarah M. Jacobs and Christopher B. Chambers

SECTION X **NASAL RECONSTRUCTION**

44 Nasal Tip Hemangioma   293
    Terence Kwan-Wong and Jugpal S. Arneja

45 Nasal Septal Hematoma   299
    Whitney Laurel Quong and Jugpal S. Arneja

SECTION XI **PEDIATRIC NECK MASSES**

46 Branchial Cleft Sinuses and Cysts   304
    Mark Felton, Jugpal S. Arneja, and Neil K. Chadha

47 Thyroglossal Duct Cysts   311
    Mark Felton, Jugpal S. Arneja, and Neil K. Chadha

SECTION XII **FACIAL REANIMATION**

48 Sural Nerve Harvest   317
    **Andre P. Marshall, Jeffrey R. Marcus, and
    Michael R. Zenn**

49 Cross Face Nerve Graft   319
    Michael J. A. Klebuc

50 Motor Branch of Masseter for Innervation of
    Free Muscle Flap   325
    Michael J. A. Klebuc

51 Masseter-to-Facial Nerve Transfer   330
    Michael J. A. Klebuc

52 Pediatric Facial Reanimation Using a Functional
    Gracilis Muscle Transfer   338
    **Brad M. Gandolfi, Jeffrey R. Marcus, and
    Michael R. Zenn**

53 Corneal Neurotization   348
    **Joseph Catapano, Ronald Zuker, Asim Ali, and
    Gregory H. Borschel**

SECTION XIII **BRACHIAL PLEXUS
(OBSTETRICAL INJURY)**

54 Primary Treatment of Neonatal Brachial
    Plexus Palsy   354
    Bryce R. Bell, Ji-Geng Yan, and Hani Matloub

55 Secondary Neonatal Brachial Plexus Palsy
    Reconstruction   364
    Joshua M. Adkinson

SECTION XIV LOWER EXTREMITY

56 Rotationplasty of the Lower Extremity 376
Samer Attar, Robert J. Steffner, and
Terrance Peabody

SECTION XV BREAST

57 Poland Syndrome 383
Patrick J. Buchanan and Paul S. Cederna

58 Gynecomastia 389
Dennis C. Hammond and Eric Yu Kit Li

59 Juvenile Hypertrophy 398
Dennis C. Hammond and Eric Yu Kit Li

60 Pectus Excavatum and Pectus Carinatum 407
Jamie C. Harris and Fizan Abdullah

SECTION XVI THORAX AND BACK

61 Myelomeningocele: Postnatal Repair 413
Gregory G. Heuer and Jesse A. Taylor

62 Myelomeningocele, Prenatal (Fetal) Repair 418
Gregory G. Heuer and N. Scott Adzick

63 Sacrococcygeal Teratoma 423
Nicholas J. Ahn and William H. Peranteau

SECTION XVII ABDOMEN

64 Prune Belly 428
Jamie C. Harris and Fizan Abdullah

65 Gastroschisis and Omphalocele 432
Jamie C. Harris and Fizan Abdullah

66 Management of the Open Abdomen 436
Alexander F. Mericli and Charles E. Butler

67 Umbilicoplasty 443
Sergey Y. Turin, Chad A. Purnell, and
Gregory A. Dumanian

SECTION XVIII PERINEUM

68 Hypospadias Repair 447
Christopher D. Morrison and Earl Y. Cheng

69 Vaginal and Vulvar Reconstruction 458
Elizabeth B. Yerkes and Julia Corcoran

70 Ambiguous Genitalia 468
Deborah L. Jacobson and Elizabeth B. Yerkes

SECTION XIX EMERGENCY DEPARTMENT LACERATIONS

71 Facial Laceration Emergency Room Closure
Techniques 480
Christina Marie Pasick and Peter J. Taub

SECTION XX CRANIOFACIAL PROSTHETICS

72 Craniofacial Anaplastology: Prosthetic
Osseointegration 490
Chad A. Purnell, Rosemary Seelaus, and
Pravin K. Patel

SECTION XXI CONJOINED TWINS

73 Conjoined Twin Separation 498
Michael R. Bykowski, Joseph E. Losee, and
Lorelei Grunwaldt

Index 509

Video Clips

Chapter 12 Tongue-Lip Adhesion
Chapter 21 Vascular Anomalies
Chapter 31 Fractional Carbon Dioxide Laser
            Pulsed Dye Laser
Chapter 32 Puregraft
            Lipovage
Chapter 48 Sural Nerve Harvest

Chapter 51 Masseter-to-Facial Nerve Transfer
Chapter 52 Facial Reanimation
Chapter 55 PT Release
            FCU to ERCB Tendon Transfer for Wrist
            Extension
Chapter 67 Umbilicoplasty

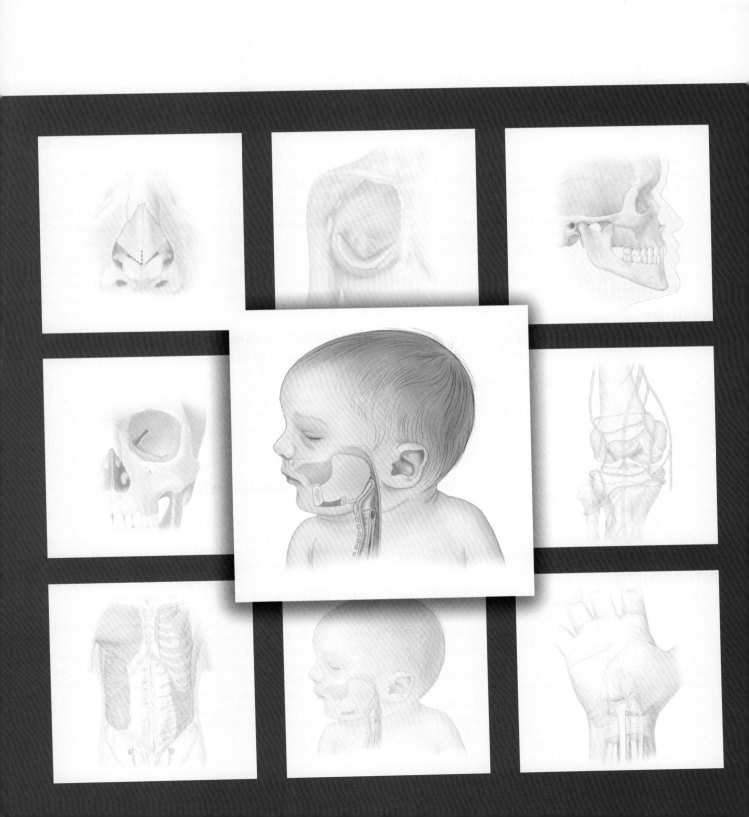

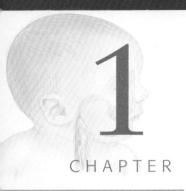

Section I: Cleft Lip

Anatomical Subunit Repair of Unilateral Cleft Lip

David K. Chong and Kathryn V. Isaac

DEFINITION

- Cleft lip is a congenital malformation in embryonic development leading to discontinuity of the upper lip. The cleft may be:
  - Complete or incomplete
  - Bilateral or unilateral
- Cleft lip may occur in isolation or in combination with a cleft palate. It may occur as part of a syndrome or in the absence of associated anomalies.
- A cleft lip has an associated cleft nasal deformity with characteristic features varying in severity depending on the type of cleft lip, width of the cleft, and presence of associated cleft palate.
  - The cleft lip nasal deformity affects the skeletal, cartilaginous, and muscular framework.

ANATOMY

- During the 5th to 7th weeks of gestation, cleft lip occurs as a failure of complete union of the medial nasal process and the maxillary prominence.
- Clefting occurs through the skin, muscle, and mucosa of the labial and nasal structures.
- The cleft of the lip distorts and/or disrupts several important anatomic structures.
  - Muscles
    - Orbicularis oris (pars marginalis and pars peripheralis)
    - Pars alaris, depressor alae nasi
  - Upper lip
    - Cutaneous lip: philtral columns, central dimple, cutaneous roll
    - Red lip: Cupid's bow, vermillion, mucosa
  - Nose
    - Nasal floor, alar base, nasal cartilages, septum, columella

PATHOGENESIS

- The etiology of cleft lip is genetically complex and is due to multiple genetic and environmental risk factors.
  - Most cases are sporadic, but some are familial, X-linked, or autosomal dominant. Familial history of clefting is an important risk factor.
- Cleft lip and cleft lip with cleft palate are considered variants of an entity that differ in severity.
  - The environmental risk factors associated with clefting include maternal smoking, infection, poor nutrition, teratogen exposure (alcohol, phenytoin, valproic acid, retinoic acid), and advanced paternal age.

PATIENT HISTORY AND PHYSICAL FINDINGS

- Diagnosis of a cleft lip is made by prenatal ultrasonography, by MRI, or by physical examination at birth. Detailed assessment is made of the child's breathing, feeding, growth, and development.
- Assessment of growth and weight is key to identify and monitor feeding difficulty and use of feeding aids (Haberman/Pigeon teat).
- The plastic surgeon should define the cleft lip type according to the anatomic structures involved, laterality, width of the cleft, and presence/absence of a cleft palate.
- Also, the child should be assessed for associated anomalies suggestive of a syndrome—craniofacial dysmorphism, airway compromise, cardiac defects, ocular and auricular abnormalities, and musculoskeletal anomalies. A genetics referral is suggested if suspicious of a syndromic etiology.

DIFFERENTIAL DIAGNOSIS

- Syndromic cleft lip with or without cleft palate
  - Van der Woude syndrome
  - Gorlin syndrome
  - CHARGE syndrome
  - Ectrodactyly-ectodermal dysplasia-clefting
  - Brachio-oculofacial syndrome
  - Kabuki syndrome
  - Kallmann syndrome

SURGICAL MANAGEMENT

- Cleft lip repair is ideally performed at age 6 months because the landmarks are larger and easier to identify.
- The principles of the anatomical subunit repair enable the surgeon to formulate a plan for the predictable and successful closure of any type of cleft lip.[1]
- The labial cleft closure is designed, measured, and determined prior to skin incision. The operation is the execution of a formulated plan. This eliminates the potential of compromising landmarks and removes the fear of underrotation, as well as lip height or length discrepancies.
- With this repair, the most visible part of the scar lies along the anatomical subunits, and the labial elements are perfectly matched in length to create an optimal continuity of vermilion, cutaneous lip, and alar-labial junction.
- Rotation of the labial elements is achieved by:
  - Skin triangle above the cutaneous roll
  - Muscle repair
  - Mucosal release

- Risks of the procedure are scar deformity, nasolabial asymmetry and/or deformity, wound dehiscence, and infection.
- The main objectives of the cleft lip repair are to (1) separate the nasal and oral cavities; (2) restore lip continuity and continence; (3) reconstruct a functional labial sphincter for facial expression, speech, and feeding; (4) and restore aesthetics of the labial and nasal subunits.
- The main steps of the procedures are as follows:
  - Marking key landmarks and designing closure of labial elements based on pre-incision measurements
  - Medial lip element release of skin, muscle, and mucosa to adequately balance the Cupid's bow, then composite elevation of lateral lip elements to insert into the created "jigsaw"
  - Restoration of muscle continuity
  - Closure of the mucosa
  - Closure of the nasal floor
  - Skin and vermilion closure
  - Nasal correction with suture techniques
- In discussing this repair, the language used in Millard's description of the rotation-advancement cleft lip repair will be used.[2] The application of this language will help to clarify and describe this technique for surgeons who have adopted the Millard technique or modifications of it.

Preoperative Planning

- If the child has a cleft lip and cleft palate, dentofacial orthopedics are utilized for aligning the cleft maxillary arches and improving the nasal deformity (lower lateral cartilage shape and position and septal cartilage alignment). The device is discontinued prior to the cleft lip repair.

Positioning

- The patient is positioned supine with the neck neutral and head stabilized in a head ring.

- The surgeon must have the ability to freely examine the face from all angles throughout the procedure to ensure that three-dimensional balance is achieved. Corneas are protected with transparent tape to use the plane and position of the eyes in the surgical field as an aid to assessing labial and nasal symmetry. The transparent tape should still allow the cheek to move freely.
- Loupe magnification is helpful for accurate identification of anatomical landmarks, for precise tissue dissection, and for perfect approximation.

Approach

- Successful application of this cleft lip repair is facilitated by highlighting conceptual differences between the rotation-advancement repair and anatomic subunit repair.
- Important landmarks are marked out, never compromised, and incisions are made for closure that follows anatomical subunits.
  - Paradigm shift: Spend more time marking before any incisions are made and the surgeon is committed to the plan.
- Calipers are used to measure incisions for perfect length match.
  - Paradigm shift: The artistic "eye" is supplemented by precise measurements.
- Foundation of repair is in the muscle.
  - Paradigm shift: Extension of skin incision outside of the proposed philtrum to achieve rotation is not required.
- Inferior triangle is placed above the cutaneous roll. This location restores the cutaneous roll without interruption and achieves any additional lip lengthening required for the skin.
  - Paradigm shift: Triangle is premeasured. Most measure 1 to 2 mm because the muscle repair and mucosal M flap both contribute to lip lengthening.

■ Planning the Repair: Medial Nasolabial Element

- Markings are made with methylene blue dye after the patient is prepped and draped.
  - Markings of landmarks and anatomic contours are made with dots at the landmarks listed below and along the line of interest for measurement, incision, or alignment of elements.
  - Tattoo all points to prevent loss of landmarks.

Vermilion, Cupid's Bow, and Nose

- Mark the junction of the vermilion and mucosa along both medial and lateral lip elements (TECH FIG 1A).
  - This helps determine the vermilion height discrepancy and points of closure and ensures a continuous natural curve is achieved.
- The following marks are placed on the *medial lip element* (TECH FIG 1B):

- Mark the peak of Cupid's bow on the noncleft side with one point above and below the cutaneous roll.
- Mark the trough of Cupid's bow.
- Mark the peak of Cupid's bow on the cleft side with one point above and below the cutaneous roll. The point above the cutaneous roll guides the placement of the opening incision for insertion of the triangular cutaneous flap, if required. Choose this point just medial to the actual peak of the Cupid's bow because it is difficult to surgically create a curve. It is preferable to use the existing curve on the lateral lip element.
- Mark the columellar points: one central and two adjacent that are symmetrically distanced from the center and lie at the superior end of the philtrum.
  - The noncleft side of the medial lip element will guide you to pick the superior extent of the philtrum, and you can mirror this onto the anticipated created philtrum on the cleft side of the medial lip element (TECH FIG 1C).

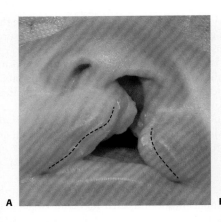
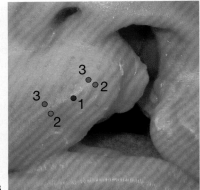
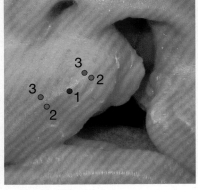

1: ● Trough of Cupid's bow
2: ● Peak of Cupid's bow*—
    vermilion edge of cutaneous
    roll
3: ● Peak of Cupid's bow*—
    skin edge of cutaneous roll

4: ● Midline columellar base
5: ● Lateral columella*
6: ● Nasal floor closure*(Nx)—
    skin edge of cutaneous roll

*Paired elements that are marked bilaterally

TECH FIG 1 • Medial lip markings. **A.** Vermilion. The border between the vermilion and the mucosa is marked. **B.** Cupid's bow. **C.** Nose. (Copyright © David Chong.)

- Remember that the apparent curve of the noncleft side philtral column is due to the unopposed action of the unrepaired orbicularis oris and is almost always a straight line in the Caucasian population once repaired.
  - In the noncleft nasal sill, mark the point where the medial footplate of the medial crus meets the nasal floor (Nx). This point is used to guide the nasal sill closure on the cleft side.

Measurements and Interpositional Triangle

- Measure the distance on the *noncleft side* from the superior extent of the philtrum to the peak of Cupid's bow above the cutaneous roll (**TECH FIG 2A**).
  - This is the total height of the philtrum (*a*) on the noncleft side that you need to recreate on the cleft side philtrum.
- Measure the distance on the *cleft side* from the superior extent of the philtrum to the peak of Cupid's bow above the cutaneous roll with tissue unfurled to mimic repair (**TECH FIG 2B**). This is the height of the cleft philtrum (*b*). It is key to unfurl the convex surface of the medial lip during this measurement; this maneuver aims to mimic the lengthening achieved with muscle dissection and repositioning with mucosal release.
- Perform a simple calculation to decide the need for an opening triangle: subtract the distances between the

philtrum of the noncleft side and the cleft side ($a - b - 1$) (**TECH FIG 2C**).
  - Note that 1 mm of length will be achieved by the Rose-Thompson effect (**TECH FIG 2D,E**). If greater than 1 mm of difference remains between the philtral lengths, a cutaneous triangle from the lateral lip element will be required, with its base equal to the distance deficit remaining.
  - Most cutaneous triangles have a base width of 1 mm (70% of cases), 1.5 mm (20% of cases), or no triangle (10%) depending on whether the cleft is complete or incomplete.
- Place a reference point in the nasal sill at the junction of the skin and mucosa on the cleft side of the medial lip. This point (N_m) will guide you to place the alar base at the correct vertical position. Ideally, this point is placed in mirror image to the contralateral side, where the medial footplate of the medial crura meets the nasal floor (N_x). Practically, you would like to maximize the amount of skin available for nasal closure when learning to perform this lip repair. Therefore, this reference point should be placed at the vermilion cutaneous junction. In the initial learning phase of this repair, there is a certain amount of "cut as you go" during closure of the nasal sill, as permitted by the laxity of the skin in this region.
- Tattoo all points listed above to prevent loss of landmarks.

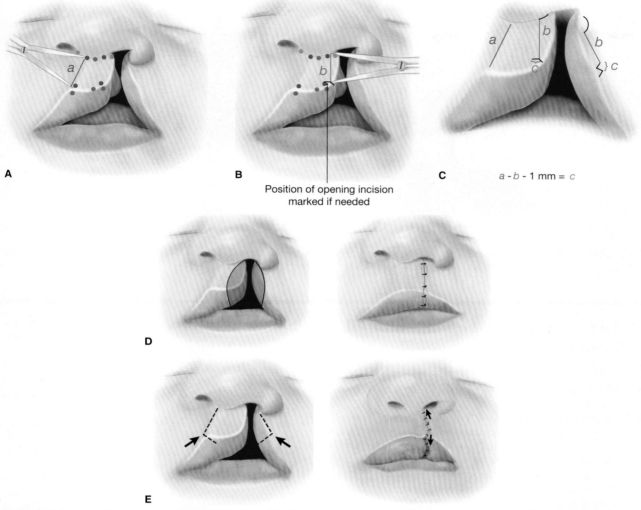

A

B

Position of opening incision
marked if needed

C $a - b - 1\ mm = c$

D

E

TECH FIG 2 • Medial lip measurements. **A.** Noncleft philtral column length is measured (a). **B.** Length of the cleft philtrum is measured while placing gentle downward traction (b). **C.** To determine whether an interpositional triangle is needed, the difference between the philtral heights of the cleft and noncleft sides is calculated by subtraction ($a - b - 1 = c$ [height of equilateral triangle]). **D.** Rose-Thompson effect. Original description of lip lengthening with biconcave excision closure by Rose in 1879. **E.** Rose-Thompson effect applied to the anatomic subunit repair.

■ Elevate the Lateral Lip Element

- Before placing the lateral lip markings, release the gingivobuccal sulcus and lateral nose at the level of piriform aperture to facilitate marking the nasal closure in complete clefts. Incise along the gingivobuccal sulcus beginning at the junction point in the nasal floor between the vestibular mucosa, oral mucosa, and nasal skin.
  - Continue the incision laterally and superiorly into the nasal cavity (**TECH FIG 3A**).
- Dissect the lateral lip element and alar base off of the maxilla in a supraperiosteal plane (**TECH FIG 3B**).

- Place one digit along the inferior orbital rim to help control the extent of dissection needed and to prevent inadvertent entry into the orbit, as the maxilla is vertically short in this age group.
  - Blunt dissection will prevent infraorbital nerve injury.
- Dissect all attachments off the lateral and inferior portions of the piriform aperture to ensure that the aberrant connection between the lower lateral cartilage and the maxilla is released.
- Release is complete once the lateral lip element and alar base are sufficiently mobile to allow tension-free repositioning of the alar base, permitting visualization of the repair and symmetrical nasal closure.

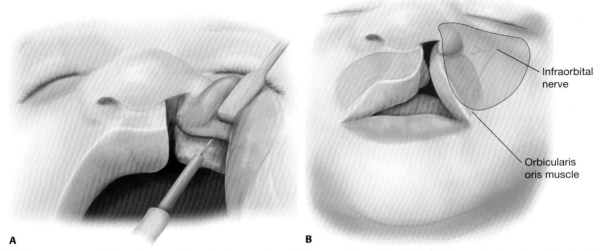

TECH FIG 3 • **A.** Lateral labial element release. **B.** Supraperiosteal dissection of lateral lip element. The shaded area is undermined in the supraperiosteal plane to allow mobilization and medial advancement of the muscle.

■ Planning the Repair: Lateral Nasolabial Element

Nordhoff's Point

- With the lateral lip element and alar base mobilized, you may now predictably mark the lateral lip:
- Mark the point of lip closure "Nordhoff's point" with a point above and below the cutaneous roll[3] (**TECH FIG 4**). Parameters used to select this point include the following:
  - Quality and shape of the cutaneous roll
  - The thickest portion of the red lip (vermilion)
  - The most anterior projecting point (need to assess from head of table)
  - The authors do not use the distance from commissure to the peak of Cupid's bow for determining the point of lip closure. It is unreliable due to the variable extent of contraction that may be present from the orbicularis oris muscle.

Nasal Sill

- Mark the point for the nasal sill closure (Nl).
  - It is helpful to have an assistant to simultaneously assess the symmetric positioning of the alar base in all planes.
  - Looking from the head of the bed, mimic nasal closure by moving the lateral lip element to the medial lip element and position the alar base on the cleft side at the same vertical height as the noncleft side.
  - From the submental view, the assistant should use forceps to elevate the slump of the alar rim and recreate an oval nostril shape with a symmetric diameter.
  - When the correct diameter of the nostril and the correct alar base position are determined compared to the noncleft side, place a point (Nl) on the lateral lip skin to mark closure to the equivalent point on the medial lip (Nm) (**TECH FIG 5**).

- When these two points meet (Nm and Nl), the nostril should be of equal diameter, and the vertical position of the alar bases should be the same.
- The alar base vertical position (in the cephalad-caudal dimension) is most difficult to correct postoperatively if it is placed too low or too high relative to the noncleft side.
- In practice, you will find that minor adjustments in the width of the nasal floor are achievable so err on the side of placing Nl more medial during the initial application of this repair. This can then be adjusted by excising excess tissue during nasal closure. As you begin to use this repair with increasing confidence, you will trust the point you mark, minimizing the need to cut as you go.

Matching Nasolabial Lengths

- Now, you have two points of closure: one on each side of the lip to match the vermilion and white lip and one on each side of the nasal sill to match and achieve the right vertical height for the alar base and symmetrical diameter of the nostril opening (**TECH FIG 6A**).
- Finally, you must mark the following on the lateral lip:
  - The dimensions of the inferior triangular skin flap
  - The labial and nasal sill incisions within the confines of the two fixed points of Nordhoff and nostril sill closure (**TECH FIG 6B**)
- Set the caliper equal to the distance of the noncleft philtral height (*b*). Orient the caliper to determine the inclination of the line b on the lateral lip.
  - Select the ideal orientation to account for the caliper distance (b), the inferior triangle size (t), and nasal floor distance (d) to tailor the "advancement flap" for precise lip and nasal closure (**TECH FIG 6C**).
- Mark the advancement triangle in the vermillion as required by the discrepancy in the vermilion height and volume between the cleft and noncleft sides. The red lip advancement flap includes mucosa.

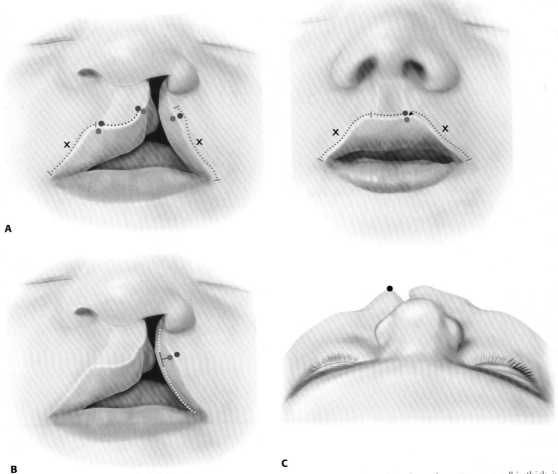

TECH FIG 4 • Selection of Nordhoff's point. **A.** This point is selected along the vermilion border where the cutaneous roll is thick, just starting to flatten, and beginning to converge with the red line (*arrowhead*). The distances marked by x should be equal at the end of surgery but are not measured when marking as they are hard to determine prior to repair. **B.** When marking Nordhoff's point, it is important to always mark at 90 degrees to the cutaneous roll. With appropriate positioning of Nordhoff's point, closure of the labial elements should result in mirror-image symmetry of the cutaneous roll and red line of Cupid's bow. **C.** The most anterior projecting point on the lateral lip.

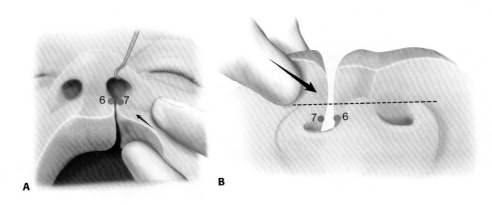

6: ● Medial nasal sill point = Nm
7: ● Lateral nasal sill point = Nl

TECH FIG 5 • Selection of nasal sill points of closure. **A.** The lateral point of the nasal sill is determined by lifting the cleft ala medially. Use the noncleft side nasal sill point (Nx) to help select the cleft side nasal sill points of closure (Nm and Nl). **B.** Alar bases are leveled.

TECHNIQUES

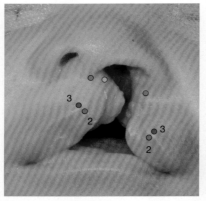

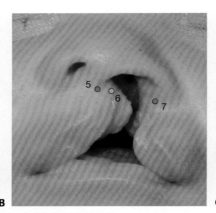

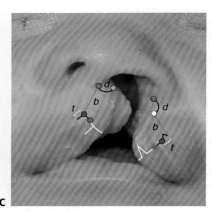

A

B

C

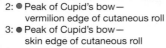

2: ● Peak of Cupid's bow—
        vermilion edge of cutaneous roll
3: ● Peak of Cupid's bow—
        skin edge of cutaneous roll

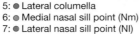

5: ● Lateral columella
6: ● Medial nasal sill point (Nm)
7: ● Lateral nasal sill point (Nl)

TECH FIG 6 • Lateral lip markings. Lip (**A**) and nasal (**B**) points of closure are marked, and then limbs are drawn between those points (**C**). Like an articulated ruler, with the two end points fixed, the two intermediate points are selected by establishing best fit with known measurements. (Copyright © David Chong.)

- By planning the repair, one recognizes the variability of unilateral cleft lip presentations and individualizes the repair to the presenting deformity, much like a tailor would measure a suit for an individual. With this approach, you will achieve a balanced lip with:
    - The correct thickness of vermilion and mucosa of the red lip

- A continuous cutaneous roll
- A symmetric Cupid's bow
- A length-matched closure of the lip incision that reflects the philtral column position
- A nasal sill closure with the appropriate orientation, position, and diameter to match the contralateral naris

■ Dissection

Medial Labial Element

- Incise the medial lip element first (**TECH FIG 7**). This allows you to verify that prior to cutting the lateral lip element, you are able to achieve the necessary rotation to create a vertically balanced lip and ensure no adjustments are required to the size of the triangle.
- Use a no. 11 blade to incise along the medial lip markings. It is critical to precisely cut perpendicular to the cutaneous roll. If a triangle is planned, make the opening incision above the cutaneous roll as your final cut to level Cupid's bow and ensure its size is appropriate.
- Incise along the markings of the vermilion and continue the incision onto the mucosa and release the maxillary frenulum.
- Release the aberrant muscular insertions to the anterior nasal spine. Perform minimal dissection of the muscle from the skin and mucosa.
- Elevate the skin along the vermilion-cutaneous junction (analogous to C-Flap elevation) to facilitate nasal sill closure and allow access to the nasal septum.
- Elevate the mucosa (analogous to M-flap elevation) off the medial cleft edge to inset at the site of the maxillary frenulum release and elongate the medial lip mucosa.

Nasal Structures

- Expose the caudal septum on the noncleft side with elevation of the mucoperiosteal flaps for direct visualization of the cartilage. Reposition the caudal septum with gentle traction toward the cleft side.

- The amount of lower lateral cartilage dissection varies according to surgical preference.[4-7]
    - If nasal degloving is to be performed, place scissors carefully in the plane between the skin and medial crura. Gently dissect in this plane between the skin and the cartilage from the medial crus toward the lateral crus.
    - Opponents of nasal cartilage degloving consider the risk of cartilage injury, tissue destruction, subsequent scarring, and impaired growth to far outweigh the

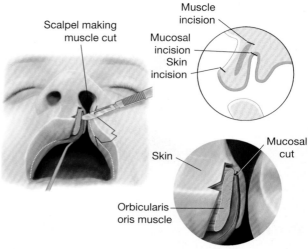

TECH FIG 7 • Medial labial incisions and dissection of the skin, muscle, and mucosa.

minimal benefit achieved with this degloving. In primary nasal correction without cartilage degloving, the correction is achieved with release of abnormal ligamentous attachments at the piriform and suture techniques, avoiding the risks listed above.

- The muscle release, repositioning, and approximation are the foundation of the lip repair.
- Verify the muscle is sufficiently released by measuring the lip length. Once committed to the opening incision, make the cut perpendicular to the philtral incision and above the cutaneous roll with a beaver blade.
- By incising and committing to the medial lip plan first, you can then adjust the lateral lip markings if the planned triangle size was incorrect. This is particularly helpful in the learning stages of this technique (the planned triangle may not be necessary or the wrong size).

Lateral Nasolabial Element

- Use a no. 11 blade to incise the lateral lip and a beaver blade to make the fine incisions around the triangle.
- Release the muscle from the alar base. Continue dissection laterally for a 2-cm distance dividing the muscle to allow for its advancement and to create a muscle of symmetric height for repair.
- Perform dissection between skin and muscle, especially along the superior portion of the lateral lip to allow for advancement. Perform minimal release of the muscle from the underlying mucosa.
- Elevate the nasal floor off the nasal vestibule to allow for repositioning in a horizontal plane for nasal floor closure.
- If cartilage degloving is being performed for primary nasal correction, complete the degloving in the plane between the skin and cartilage joining the previously dissected pocket.

■ Closure of the Lip

Muscle Repair

- The muscle repair sets the foundation for the lip repair. To correctly position the muscle elements for repair, have

an assistant use a skin hook to lengthen the medial lip element to balance the Cupid's bow (taking care not to excessively elongate) and another skin hook to hold the lateral lip element at the ideal position for a lip closure (**TECH FIG 8A**).

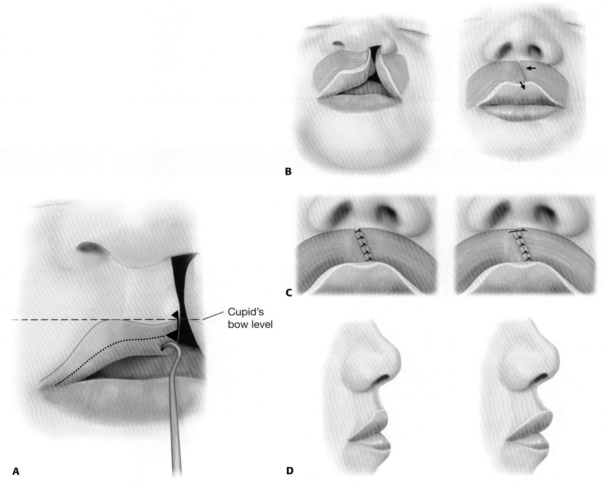

Cupid's bow level

TECH FIG 8 • A. Level Cupid's bow to position the muscle elements for repair. **B.** A. In repair of a cleft lip, it is essential to release the aberrant orbicularis oris muscle insertions and reposition the muscle fibers to restore continuity. After release, repositioning, and repair of the orbicularis oris muscle, a superior gathering suture is placed (**C, right**) to improve the shape of the lip on profile view (**D**).

TECHNIQUES

- With the setup outlined above, repair the muscle beginning superiorly. Place the initial stitch superiorly to set the lip length and set the alar base in a symmetrical vertical position. To ensure the cutaneous roll points of closure are perfectly matched, check the alignment of the points of closure after each successive muscle stitch.
- After repairing the length of the muscle, consider placing a plication suture at the superior end of the muscle repair at the base of the columella. This accentuates the pout of the repaired lip (**TECH FIG 8B–D**).
- Repair the mucosal incision with eversion of the mucosal edges. Ensure correct approximation of the mucosal lengths and excise excess length at the cephalad margin as required.

Cutaneous Approximation

- Suture the labial skin and the vermilion without any cutaneous excision or alteration of the labial incisions. A perfectly approximated closure of the labial elements should be achieved based on the planned markings.
- The only "cut as you go" occurs at the nasal sill where some adaptation is often required to ensure the right diameter and shape of the nostril opening.

■ Primary Nasal Correction: Suture Techniques

- Suture techniques detailed below necessitate that the alar base and aberrant nasal attachments to the piriform and underling maxilla are completely released.
    - The alar bases must be symmetrically repositioned and the caudal septum must be centralized.
- If cartilage degloving was performed:
    - Place an alar shaping suture as an interdomal suture between the genua of the lower lateral cartilages (LLC).
    - Place a lower lateral hitching suture with an absorbable suture to secure the dome of the LLC to the contralateral nasal bone periosteum. This elevates the slumped LLC. Beginning from inside the nasal vestibule on the cleft side, pierce the suture through the nasal mucosa, capture the dome of the slumped LLC, exit the nasal skin with grasped nasal bone periosteum, and back through the same cutaneous needle puncture to return to the nasal vestibule through the same tissues.
- If cartilage degloving was not performed:
    - Place an internal nasal valve plication suture in the vestibule between the upper and LLC to recreate the scroll area.
    - Place an alar transfixion suture to lateralize the vestibular web. Beginning from inside the vestibule, pierce through the nasal mucosa just below the caudal LLC and exit the skin at the alar-facial junction. Re-enter the same cutaneous puncture hole but exit more posteriorly in the nasal mucosa. Tying the knot will lateralize the nasal mucosa.

PEARLS AND PITFALLS

Planning	■ Important landmarks are marked and never compromised. ■ There should be no "cut as you go" on the lip. The labial closure should be precisely measured and tailored fitted because compromise in the lip closure point is unforgiving. ■ Spend more time marking before any incisions are made and commit to a plan. ■ It may be disconcerting initially as a lot more tissue seems to be discarded than when "hedging your bets" by unnecessary preservation of tissue.
Markings	■ Choose the cleft side of Cupid's bow point just medial to the actual peak of the Cupids bow as it is difficult to surgically create a curve. Pick a slightly more lateral point on the lateral lip element (which has the curve). ■ The triangular cutaneous flap is smaller than anticipated for two main reasons: 　■ The skin is elastic and rests in a concave contour due to the aberrant insertion of the muscle. It will lengthen with release of the muscle and dissection between these layers. 　■ Rotation of the medial lip is also achieved by the muscle repair and the mucosal release.
Measurements	■ Use calipers for measurements. This results in length-matched incisions and precise alignment.
Muscle repair	■ The muscle is detached from its abnormal insertion, and the lateral lip muscle is advanced into the gap superiorly as the muscle released medially is drawn caudally to achieve lip length. This allows planning the skin incision to mimic the philtral column position rather than the misguided intention that it achieves rotation.
Inferior triangle above the cutaneous roll	■ Creates a continuous cutaneous roll without interruption. Insert any required triangle in the shadow of the roll, that is, just above the roll. ■ Achieves any additional lip lengthening required. ■ Work out the precise size of triangle and confirm measurement by cutting medial lip element first.

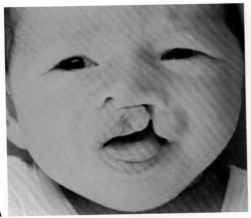 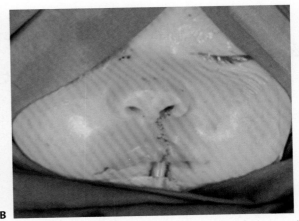

A **B**

FIG 1 • Preoperative and postoperative images of an infant with cleft lip and palate following repair with anatomical subunit technique. (Copyright © David Chong.)

POSTOPERATIVE CARE

- Prevent crusting along the suture line with incision care.
- Apply saline as required to prevent scab and then emollient.
- Sutures are removed after 5 days.
- Nasal stents are kept for up to 6 weeks.

OUTCOMES

- Since 2008, Dr. Chong has performed 200 consecutive cleft lip repairs using the technique described (**FIG 1**).
  - Nasolabial revisions were required in three cases (1.5%), one for alar repositioning and two for retained permanent suture.
  - There have been no revisions required for a shortened lip.

COMPLICATIONS

- Infection
- Hemorrhage
- Lip or nasal revision required for asymmetry
- Poor scarring
- Nasal airway obstruction

REFERENCES

1. Fisher DM. Unilateral cleft lip repair: An anatomical subunit approximation technique. *Plast Reconstr Surg*. 2005;116:61-71.
2. Millard DR. Complete unilateral clefts of the lip. *Plast Reconstr Surg*. 1960;25:595-605.
3. Nordhoff MS, Chen Y, Chen K, Hong K, Lo L. The surgical technique for the complete unilateral cleft-lip nasal deformity. *Oper Tech Plast Reconstr Surg*. 1995;2:167-174.
4. McComb H. Primary correction of unilateral cleft lip nasal deformity: A 10-year review. *Plast Reconstr Surg*. 1985;75:791-799.
5. Salyer KE. Primary correction of the unilateral cleft lip nose: A 15-year experience. *Plast Reconstr Surg*. 1986;77:558-568.
6. Salyer KE. Early and late treatment of unilateral cleft nasal deformity. *Cleft Palate Craniofac J*. 1992;29:556-569.
7. Fisher MD, Fisher DM, Marcus JR. Correction of the cleft nasal deformity: from infancy to maturity. *Clin Plast Surg*. 2014;41:283-299.

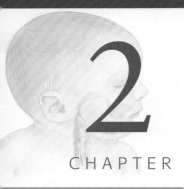

2 CHAPTER

Unilateral Cleft Lip Repair: Millard/Mohler Modifications

Roberto L. Flores and Gerald J. Cho

DEFINITION

- A unilateral cleft lip is a congenital separation of the upper lip. The degree of clefting can be microform, minor form, incomplete, or complete.
  - Microform
    - Discontinuity of the vermilion-cutaneous junction
    - Cupid's bow symmetrical
    - Slight notching of mucosal free border
    - Variable nostril deformity and alveolar defect
  - Minor form
    - Vermilion notch greater than 3 mm above the level of Cupid's bow on the noncleft side
    - Discontinuity of orbicularis oris
    - Nasal deformity
    - Alveolar cleft present
  - Incomplete
    - Complete full-thickness separation of upper lip with intact nasal sill or a Simonart band along the nasal floor
  - Complete
    - Complete full-thickness separation of upper lip

ANATOMY

- Both the soft (upper lip and nose) and hard tissues (maxilla, septum, lower lateral cartilages of nose) are affected (**FIG 1**).
- Upper lip—The deformities in this area can be categorized into those affecting the medial and lateral lip elements.
  - In the medial lip element, Cupid's bow is preserved but with vertical deficiency of the vermilion. The columella and philtral column are shortened on the cleft side. The orbicularis oris has an abnormal and unilateral insertion at the nasal base, and its disruption results in vertical shortening of the medial upper lip, superior rotation of the Cupids bow, and vertical shortening of the vermilion.
  - In the lateral lip element, the height and transverse length are shortened. Medially, there is a distinct point where the white cutaneous roll and junction of the wet and dry vermilion start to converge medially (Nordhoff point). The pars superficialis on the lateral lip alters the direction of this muscle to run almost vertically in the area below the ala, leading to aberrant attachments to the nostril and periosteum of the piriform aperture. This leads to a vertically foreshortened lateral lip, sometimes producing a bulge in this area.
- Nose—The alar base on the cleft side sits on the piriform margin of the maxilla, which is laterally and posteriorly displaced. The malposition of the bony foundation combined with separation of the orbicularis oris causes unopposed action of the ipsilateral zygomaticous major. This results in

widening of the nostril, depression of the alar dome, and canting of the columella toward the cleft side (see **FIG 1**). Unilateral attachment of the orbicularis oris to the medial crura footplates, anterior nasal spine, and caudal septum on the noncleft side exacerbates the columellar tilt and contributes to deviation of the caudal septum toward the noncleft side. Internally, the caudal portion of the ala has a vestibular web. The underlying cartilaginous structures are also malformed. On the cleft side, the medial crus of the lower lateral cartilages is shortened, and the lateral crus is elongated and inferiorly displaced. The septum is dislocated out of the vomer and bows toward the cleft side.
- Maxilla—The underlying skeleton forms the platform upon which the soft tissues rest. Thus, the skeletal abnormalities of the maxilla can explain many of the soft tissue abnormalities seen, particularly in the nose. The greater segment of the alveolus is anteriorly rotated due to the fetal protrusion of the tongue. The lesser segment of the alveolus rotates posteriorly. The medial buttress of the maxilla can be hypoplastic and posteriorly displaced.

PATIENT HISTORY AND PHYSICAL FINDINGS

- The preoperative assessment of a patient with a unilateral cleft lip includes complete physical exam with assessment for other comorbidities. Facial exam includes the side (left vs right vs midline), the degree of clefting (microform, minor form, incomplete, or complete), and the extent of nasal deformity.

IMAGING

- Typically not needed unless within the context of a midline or facial cleft

SURGICAL MANAGEMENT

- This surgery is often the first step in the larger multidisciplinary treatment plan for cleft care.
- The quality of the primary repair establishes the initial function and appearance for the patient and has great bearing on their future quality of life.
- Nasoalveolar molding (NAM) is strongly recommended for patients with a complete cleft or a significant nasal deformity.
- Microform clefts can be repaired with less extensive methods than a full rotation advancement.
- Minor forms can be repaired with a modified rotation-advancement–type repair with complete primary nasal reconstruction.
- Incomplete and complete clefts can be repaired with a full rotation-advancement–type repair.
- Initial lip and nose repairs are performed at approximately 3 months of age.

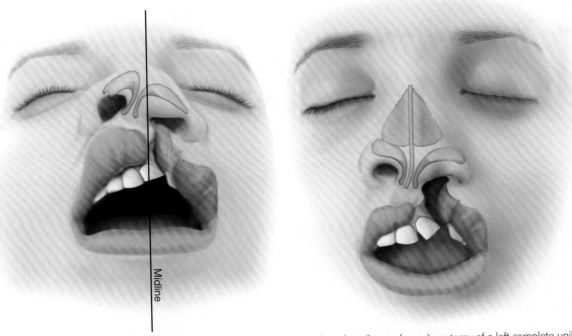

FIG 1 • The soft (upper lip and nose) and hard tissue (maxilla, septum, lower lateral cartilages of nose) anatomy of a left complete unilateral cleft lip.

Preoperative Planning

■ The authors use NAM in patients with a complete cleft or a significant nasal deformity. As mentioned above, a cleft through the maxilla not only disrupts the platform upon which the soft tissues sit but also interrupts the dental arch. NAM can help correct the outwardly rotated greater segment and posterolaterally displaced lesser segment. The correction of the skeletal platform into an anatomic position helps place the lip and nose into a more favorable alignment. Furthermore, when the alveolar segments are aligned within 1 mm, a gingivoperiosteoplasty can be performed, which can avoid a secondary bone grafting procedure in 60% to 73% of patients without detriment to midface growth by midterm follow-up. For these reasons, we feel that NAM provides a more predictable lip and nose repair and potentially decreases the overall number of surgical procedures for the child.

■ NAM typically commences 2 weeks after birth and is completed after 10 weeks of therapy in patients with a unilateral cleft.

Positioning

■ Supine with gentle neck extension from a shoulder roll

Approach

■ There are many techniques to repair a unilateral cleft lip, each with its own advantages and disadvantages. In this chapter, we will present Cutting's modification of the extended Mohler repair.

■ In this approach, there are eight main steps to the operation: markings, incisions, medial lip dissection, lateral lip dissection, mucosa closure, nasal dissection, lip closure, and nasal refinement.

■ Millard/Mohler Modifications for Unilateral Cleft Lip Repair

Markings (TECH FIG 1A–D)

■ Medial and lateral lip elements (**TECH FIG 1A**)
  ■ Medial lip element: The depth (point 1) and height of the noncleft side (point 2) are identified and marked. The distance between these two points is used to mark the height of the Cupid's bow on the cleft side (point 3). The white roll usually starts to disappear at this point. If Cupid's bow is wide or indistinct, the marks can be placed more narrowly so that less downward rotation is required.
  ■ Lateral lip element:

• The height of the lip from the alar base to the height of the Cupid's bow on the noncleft side is measured with a caliper, and the vertical distance is used to locate the corresponding white roll point on the lateral lip element (point 4). Some surgeons use the widest point of the vermilion (Nordhoff point) to determine point 4. However, in patients with a wide cleft, Nordhoff point will commonly result in a vertically foreshortened lip. Using the vertical height of the contralateral upper lip can sacrifice horizontal lip length for preservation of vertical lip height. The horizontal lip discrepancy will correct over time; however, a vertically shortened upper lip will remain.

- Mohler Back Cut (**TECH FIG 1B**)
  - The apex of the back cut is critical to the success of the design (see Pearls below). This point (point 5) is placed approximately 1.5 mm superior to the base of the columella and just over halfway (four-sevenths) across the noncleft side.
  - A line is drawn connecting point 5 to a point just lateral to point 3. This line should be bowed out to the same degree as the philtral column of the unaffected side to recreate the subtle curve.
  - A straight line is drawn from the apex of the Mohler backcut (point 5) to the height of the philtrum on the noncleft side but no farther (point 6). The angle formed by these two lines and length of the backcut will affect the degree of downward rotation of the Cupid's bow.

- C flap and M flap on the medial lip element (**TECH FIG 1C**)
  - C flap: A line is drawn along the skin/mucosa junction lateral to point 3. Care is taken to incorporate as much white lip into the C flap as possible while avoiding the mucosa (see Pearls below).
  - M flap: The medial/inferior border of the M flap is drawn as a straight line starting from point 3 and perpendicular to the white roll. A second line is drawn on the vermilion of the medial lip element as an oblique line starting at a point 1 mm inferior to the white roll, traveling laterally and inferiorly to the red line. This is the receiving incision for the Nordhoff triangular flap.
- Alar base and L flap on the lateral lip element (**TECH FIG 1D**)

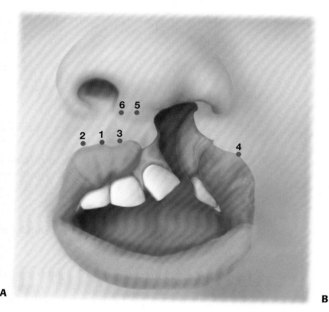

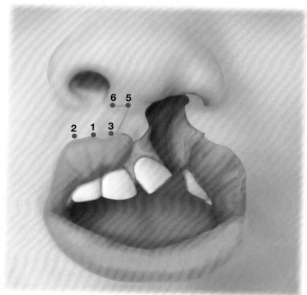

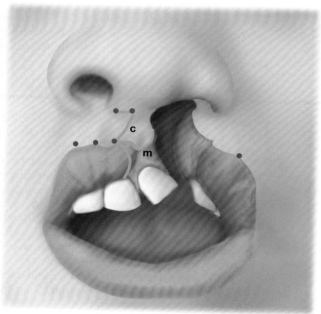

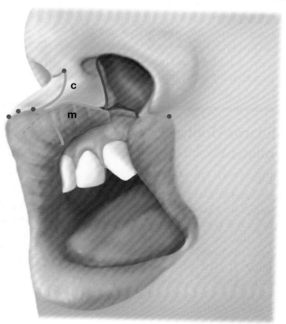

TECH FIG 1 • Markings. **A.** Key tattoo points. **B.** Mohler back cut. **C.** C flap and M flap. Dashed blue line represents the receiving incision for a vermilion triangular flap if used. The dashed red line represents the intranasal incisions on the septum and vomer made during nasal floor closure.

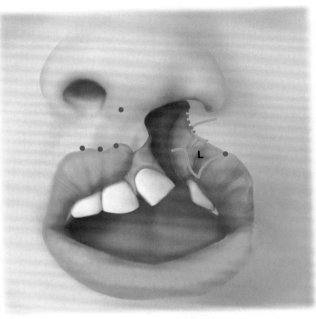
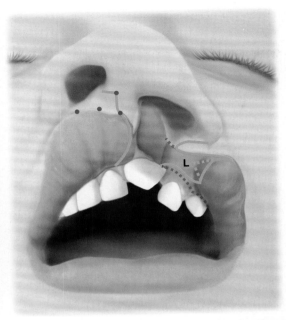

D

TECH FIG 1 (Continued) • **D.** Alar base and L flap (L) outlined in *blue*. The *dashed blue line* is the triangular flap as described by Nordhoff. *Dashed green line* is the intranasal incision at the piriform aperture, and the *dashed red line* is the gingivobuccal sulcus incision, which will be made at the time of the lateral lip dissection.

- Alar base: A small incision is marked along the alar crease on the cleft side with care not to extend this incision around the alar base.
- L flap: The border of the L flap is then marked by first marking an incision 1.0 mm inferior to the white roll on the lateral lip element. This mark then transects the white roll perpendicularly and then curves swiftly and softly to meet the medial edge of the previously made mark on the alar crease. The remainder of the L flap can then be made with or without the addition of a vermilion triangular flap, as described by Nordhoff. When marking the L flap, care is taken to extend the mark just superior to the alveolus. This will base the L flap off of the lateral nasal wall and not the alveolus, as originally described by Millard.
- Points 1 to 6 are tattooed. The lip and nose are infiltrated with 0.5% lidocaine with 1:200 000 epinephrine.

Incisions

- All premarked incisions are made through skin and mucosa.

Medial Lip Dissection (**TECH FIG 2A,B**)

- M flap is elevated in a submucosal plane (**TECH FIG 2A**).
- C flap is elevated in the subcutaneous plane with care to preserve the underlying orbicularis oris (see **TECH FIG 2A**).
- Mohler back cut (**TECH FIG 2B**).
  - A transverse incision is made across the full-thickness orbicularis oris muscle where it abnormally inserts at the nasal base. This incision is made at the base, not the apex, of the Mohler back cut. If this incision is made at the apex of the back cut, the medial crura will be transected. Care should also be taken to avoid going through the underlying mucosa during this incision.

- Complete full-thickness transection of the muscle should be confirmed by placing a small single hook into the medial lip element and pulling the lip down. The lip should rotate downward with no tension.
  - If additional downward rotation is still required, the labial frenulum is horizontally transected. This defect may be filled by the mucosa of the lateral lip element.
- Medial lip element preparation: The philtral skin is dissected free from the muscle in a subcutaneous plane up to but not past the philtral dimple.

Lateral Lip Dissection (**TECH FIG 3**)

- L flap elevation:
  - The L flap is carefully elevated from the orbicularis oris in the subcutaneous and submucosal plane. As one approaches the area of the piriform aperture, the dissection plane changes from a submucosal to a subperiosteal plane.
  - A Woodson elevator is then used to create a subperiosteal pocket in the interior/lateral aspect of the piriform aperture. A horizontal incision is made at the exact border of the lateral nasal wall with the nasal floor. An incision is made at the base of the vomer, and a vomer flap is elevated with the periosteal elevator. The lateral nasal wall flap and vomer flap will be used to close the anterior nasal floor later in the surgery.
- Piriform aperture incision:
  - A vertical intranasal incision is made at the border of the nasal mucosa and squamous skin to meet the superior border of the L-Flap. Sharp dissection is performed to reach the bone of the piriform aperture.
  - Subperiosteal dissection will complete the elevation of the L flap posteriorly until it is based off the lateral nasal wall.

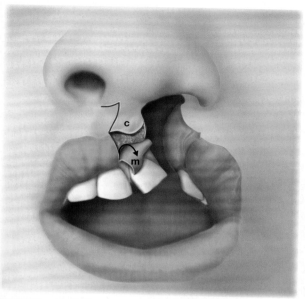

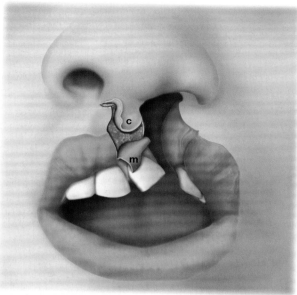

A   **B**

TECH FIG 2 • Medial lip dissection. **A.** M flap (m) elevated in a submucosal plane and turned down. C flap elevated in the subcutaneous plane. **B.** Mohler back cut. *Dashed yellow line* represents a transverse incision made across the full-thickness orbicularis oris muscle where it abnormally inserts at the nasal base. Complete full-thickness transection of the muscle should be checked by placing a small single hook into the medial lip element and pulling the lip down. The lip should rotate downward with no tension. The philtral skin is dissected free from the muscle in a subcutaneous plane up to but not past the philtral dimple.

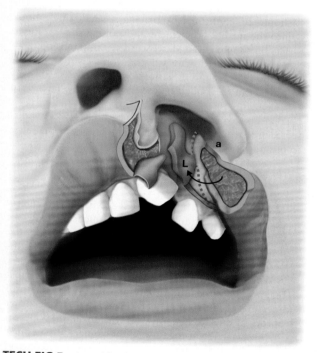

TECH FIG 3 • Lateral lip dissection. L flap (*L*) elevated in a submucosal plane and shown retracted medially. The stippled area represents the L flap that will be trimmed before inset into the lateral nasal wall. As one approaches the area of the piriform aperture (*dashed green line*), the dissection plane changes from a submucosal to a subperiosteal plane. A gingivobuccal sulcus incision (*dashed red line*) is made in continuity with the piriform aperture incision, with care to preserve the L flap. A supraperiosteal dissection is made across the maxilla to fully mobilize the alar base and lateral lip element. The alar base skin (*a*) should be elevated as a thick split-thickness skin graft so that a layer of dermis is present on the underlying dermal-muscular pennant flap.

- Gingivobuccal sulcus incision:
  - A gingivobuccal sulcus incision is made in continuity with the piriform aperture incision, with care to preserve the L flap. A supraperiosteal dissection is made across the maxilla to fully mobilize the alar base and lateral lip element. In cases where presurgical orthopedics is not used, this dissection may continue widely across the face in the maxilla.
  - Tension-free translation of the alar base flap to the anterior nasal spine will demonstrate adequate dissection.
- Alar base flap:
  - The alar base skin should be elevated in a thick split-thickness skin graft plane so that a layer of dermis is present on the underlying muscular flap. The dermal-muscular pennant will be used to relocate the alar base.
- Lateral lip element preparation:
  - The lateral lip skin is mobilized from the orbicular oris as far lateral as the alar base incision.

Mucosa closure: If gingivoperiosteoplasty is to be performed, it should be completed before the mucosa is closed.

- L flap inset (**TECH FIG 4A**)
  - The L flap is sutured under tension to the base of the piriform aperture incision. Excess L flap is trimmed, and the remainder of the L flap is sutured into the defect created by the piriform aperture incision.
- Nasal floor closure (**TECH FIG 4B**)
  - The lateral nasal wall flap/L flap is sutured to the vomer flap using several absorbable sutures. The sutures are placed first in a simple fashion and then in a horizontal mattress fashion to create a watertight closure of the nasal floor. Closing the anterior nasal floor will facilitate successful gingivoperiosteoplasty and/or alveolar bone graft.

- Oral mucosa (**TECH FIG 4C**):
  - The gingivobuccal sulcus incision is closed using several oblique oriented sutures. This will relieve tension from the midline of the mucosal reconstruction. The mucosa of the upper lip is then closed with simple sutures, with care not to incorporate muscle in the mucosal reconstruction.

Nasal Dissection (**TECH FIG 5**)

- The rhinoplasty portion of this procedure will elongate the columella and elevate the depressed lower lateral cartilage.
- A hemimembranous septum incision is first made on the cleft side.

- Through the apex of the Mohler backcut, blunt dissection is performed to create a dissection pocket between the medial crura. This dissection pocket is then connected with the hemimembranous incision in the septum, and this dissection is continued superiorly toward the septal angle.
- Dissection scissors are then inserted through this pocket and over the upper and lower lateral cartilages on the cleft and noncleft side.
- Careful blunt dissection will create a subcutaneous pocket over the upper and lower lateral cartilages in preparation for rhinoplasty. Care is taken not to close the dissection scissors in the dissection pocket, as it can lead to damage to the lower lateral cartilages.

TECHNIQUES

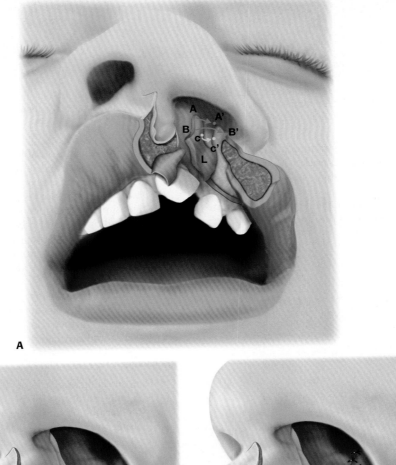

A

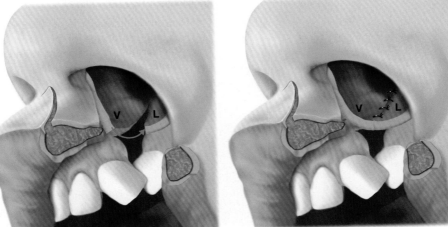

B

TECH FIG 4 • Closure. **A.** Excess L flap (*L*) is trimmed, and the remainder of the L flap is sutured into the defect created by the piriform aperture incision (A to A′, B to B′, C to C′). **B.** The L flap is then sutured to the vomer flap (*V*) to close the nasal floor.

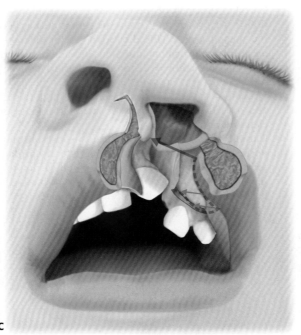 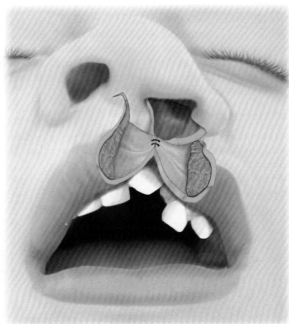

C

TECH FIG 4 (Continued) • **C.** The gingivobuccal sulcus incision is closed using several oblique oriented sutures (*blue arrows*); this will relieve tension from the midline of the mucosal reconstruction (*green arrow*). The mucosa of the upper lip is then closed with simple sutures, with care not to incorporate the musculature in the mucosal reconstruction.

- If no NAM is performed, an additional nostril rim incision is made and a dissection pocket created to connect the rim incision to the subcutaneous pocket underneath the nasal tip.
- A retractor is used to elevate the depressed lower lateral cartilage in a supercorrected position.

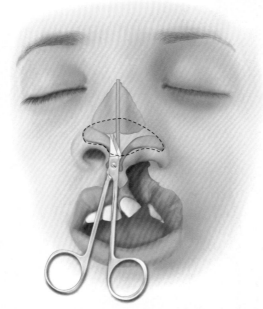

TECH FIG 5 • Nasal dissection. Blunt-tipped scissors are inserted through the apex of the Mohler back cut and at the intranasal incision made at the septal angle. Blunt dissection frees the underlying lower lateral cartilages.

- A long-lasting absorbable suture is then placed as a horizontal mattress to affix the medial crus on the cleft side in its newly elevated position. Several such sutures are placed from superior to inferior to affix the medial crus in its superior location and help shape the columella.
- An additional row of horizontal mattress sutures is then placed using transfixion sutures to affix the medial crura to the cartilaginous septum. Elongation of the columella should be appreciable at the end of this point of the procedure.
- If a nostril rim incision is used, a suture is placed from the cleft side lower lateral cartilage to the upper lateral cartilage to further reinforce the elevated position of the lower lateral cartilage.

Lip Closure (TECH FIG 6A,B)

- Repositioning of alar base (**TECH FIG 6A**)
  - A long-lasting absorbable suture is first placed through the dermomuscular pennant underneath the alar base. Using this suture as a leash, the location of the caudal septum is sighted and then placed through this area and the medial crus on the noncleft side. Tying the suture down will set the alar base in an anatomic position, medialize the columella, and straighten the anterior septum.
  - A second such suture is placed to reinforce the first.
- Muscle (see **TECH FIG 6A**)
  - The orbicularis oris is then reconstructed from superior to inferior using several buried sutures. Prior to reconstruction, excess orbicularis oris is carefully trimmed so that the skin edges are perfectly opposing at the completion of the muscular reconstruction. The superior suture may be attached to the anterior and nasal spine to prevent elongation at the upper lip.

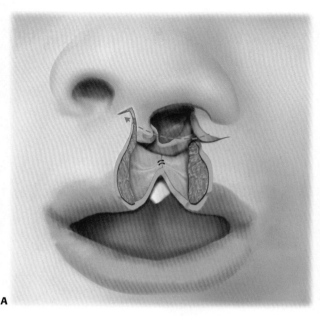
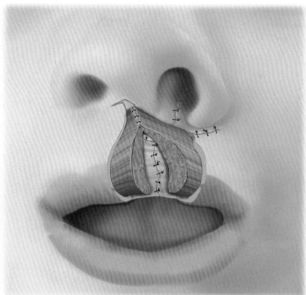

A

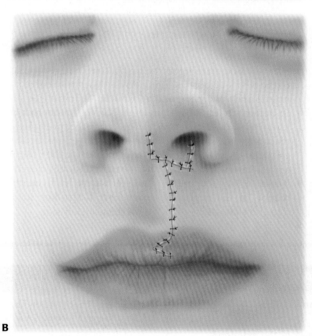

B

TECH FIG 6 • Closure. **A.** The dermal-muscular flap at the alar base is sutured to the area of the anterior nasal spine and the medial crus on the noncleft side (*dashed light blue arrow*). The orbicularis oris is then reconstructed from superior to inferior. **B.** The white roll point is first reconstructed, and the remainder of the upper lip is meticulously closed using several fine permanent sutures. The vermilion is also inset at this time. If a triangular flap is used, this is trimmed and inset.

- Upper lip skin (**TECH FIG 6B**)
  - The white roll point is first reconstructed, and the remainder of the upper lip is meticulously closed using several fine permanent sutures. The vermilion is also inset at this time. If a triangular flap is used, this is trimmed and inset.
- C-Flap inset (see **TECH FIG 6B**)
  - In the extended Mohler repair, the C flap is used to fill the defect created by the downward rotation of the Cupid's bow. The C flap is carefully scored and cut. The C flap is then inset into this defect, and the columellar incision is also closed with several simple sutures. The alar base incision is also closed at this time. Excess C flap and alar skin are also trimmed, and the nostril floor is closed.

- Nostril floor (see **TECH FIG 6B**)
  - Care is taken to close the nostril floor and the philtral incision in a stair-step fashion to avoid a confluence of four corners at the nostril floor incision.

Nasal Refinement

- Nostril apex elevation (**TECH FIG 7**)
  - If NAM was used, the nostril apex overhang is addressed using a long-lasting absorbable suture that is placed just behind the nostril rim, through the depressed lower lateral cartilage on the cleft side, underneath the skin of the nasal tip, and out the nostril on the opposite side. The trajectory of this suture is oblique, directed laterally and posteriorly. The suture is then returned 2 mm behind the exit suture hole in the

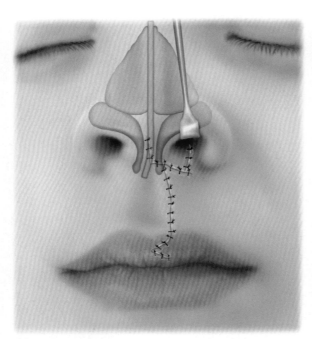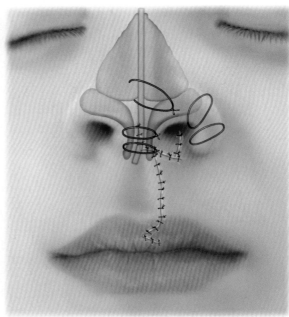

TECH FIG 7 • Nostril apex elevation (*red*) and vestibular web obliterating sutures (*blue*).

noncleft side, parallel to the first suture, and returning to the cleft side nostril. Tying down this suture corrects nostril apex overhang and adds to tip definition.
- In patients who did not undergo NAM, the depressed lower lateral cartilage is elevated by the previously placed suture from the lower lateral to upper lateral cartilage. A small rim of overhanging skin at the nostril apex is carefully trimmed and the rim incision is closed.
- Regardless of technique, there should be an overcorrection of the depressed lower lateral cartilage such that the cleft side is higher than the noncleft side.

- Vestibular web obliterating suture (**TECH FIG 7**)
  - The vestibular web can be addressed by placing a long-lasting absorbable suture behind the web out of the nasal facial groove; the suture can then be returned through the same cutaneous hole and back into the nostril anterior to the vestibular web. Tying this suture down will obliterate the vestibular web and accentuate the nasal facial groove. Multiple sutures may be required to achieve the full effect.

PEARLS AND PITFALLS

Anatomy	▪ It is critical that the surgeon has a thorough understanding and ability to identify the pathologic soft and hard tissue deformities and individualize the surgery as needed.
The apex of the extended Mohler back cut	▪ It should be high enough onto the columella to allow for full downward rotation of the Cupid's bow. If point 5 is too low, it will result in inadequate downward rotation. ▪ If point 5 is too close to the cleft side, the C flap will be too narrow and inadequately fill the defect created by the downward rotation of the Cupid's bow. ▪ Placing point 5 too far toward, the noncleft side will result in a narrow philtral column at the superior aspect of the upper lip.
C flap	▪ In wide clefts where presurgical orthopedics (NAM) was not used, it is important to incorporate as much white lip into the C flap as possible because the C flap may be used in its entirety to fill the defect created by the downward rotation of the Cupid's bow. ▪ Care must be taken to avoid incorporating mucosa, which will result in the transposition of mucosal tissue onto the nose and upper lip.
Tension-free closure essential for optimal wound healing	▪ Medial lip element: Adequate release of the orbicularis oris muscle where it abnormally inserts at the nasal base to allow for full rotation downward ▪ Lateral lip element: Supraperiosteal dissection is made across the maxilla to fully mobilize the alar base and lateral lip element. ▪ Adequate release of abnormal attachment of cleft-side lower lateral cartilage from piriform rim
Multidisciplinary care	▪ Essential for optimal outcomes

POSTOPERATIVE CARE

- Children are placed in elbow restraints for 5 to 7 days.
- A syringe feeder or cleft feeding nipple (ie, Haberman nipple) is used for feeding.
- Sutures are removed after 5 days and the lip taped in compression for 5 weeks.

OUTCOMES

- In experienced hands, primary cleft lip and nasal repair can achieve lasting symmetry to the lip and nose while camouflaging scars within the subunit borders of the face.

COMPLICATIONS

- Relapse of the nasal deformity
- Scar contracture/widening
- Inadequate multidisciplinary care and follow-up during growth
- Maxillary growth inhibition

SUGGESTED READINGS

Cutting CB, Dayan JH. Lip height and lip width after extended Mohler unilateral cleft lip repair. *Plast Reconstr Surg.* 2003;111(1):17-23.

Grayson BH, Garfinkle JS. Early cleft management: the case for nasoalveolar molding. *Am J Orthod Dentofacial Orthop.* 2014;145(2):134-142.

McComb H. Primary correction of unilateral cleft lip nasal deformity: a 10-year review. *Plast Reconstr Surg.* 1985;75(6):791-799.

Millard DR, Jr. Discussion: unilateral cleft lip repair. *Plast Reconstr Surg.* 1987;80(4):517.

Mohler LR. Unilateral cleft lip repair. *Plast Reconstr Surg.* 1987;80(4): 511-516.

Mulliken JB, LaBrie RA. Fourth-dimensional changes in nasolabial dimensions following rotation-advancement repair of unilateral cleft lip. *Plast Reconstr Surg.* 2012;129(2):491-498.

Noordhoff MS. Reconstruction of vermilion in unilateral and bilateral cleft lips. *Plast Reconstr Surg.* 1984;73(1):52-61.

Salyer KE. Primary correction of the unilateral cleft lip nose: a 15-year experience. *Plast Reconstr Surg.* 1986;77(4):558–568.

Yuzuriha S, Mulliken JB. Minor-form, microform, and mini-microform cleft lip: anatomical features, operative techniques, and revisions. *Plast Reconstr Surg.* 2008;122(5):1485-1493.

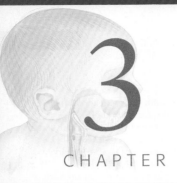

3
CHAPTER

Salyer Unilateral Cleft Lip/Nose Repair

Kenneth E. Salyer

DEFINITION

- Cleft lip/nose deformity occurs during embryonic development when there is lack of normal migration and proliferation of neural crest cells leading to failure of the facial prominences to fuse.

ANATOMY

Normal Upper Lip Anatomy

- The foundation of the face is the facial skeleton. The upper lip is supported by the underlying maxillary and mandibular framework, with its teeth and alveolar bone. Alveolar bone develops and matures with primary and secondary tooth eruption.
- The orbicularis oris muscle consists of two well-defined and functional components: the pars superficialis and the deep pars marginalis.
  - The pars superficialis is located under the skin of the lip and is related to other facial muscles of expression (levator labii superioris, alaeque nasi, and zygomaticus minor), and these retract the upper lip as a group. The pars superficialis consists of an upper and lower bundle.
    - The upper bundle represents the common insertion of the muscles of facial expression and itself inserts onto the anterior nasal spine, septopremaxillary ligament, and the nostril sill, passing deep to the alar base.

- The lower bundle derives its fibers from the depressor anguli oris muscle on each side and decussates in the midline, inserting in the skin and forming the philtral ridges of the contralateral side.

- The deep portion of the pars marginalis muscle is responsible for sphincteric action of the mouth and runs under the vermilion from one modiolus to the other.
- The two portions of the orbicularis oris muscle thus correspond to the double function of the upper lip. The deep pars marginalis, extending from one modiolus to the other, seals the extrinsic facial muscles to open the mouth as a retractor.
- Contraction of the deep pars marginalis, when the mouth is pursed, thickens the vermilion and lengthens the upper lip height. Simultaneous relaxation of the pars superficialis produces perioral fine wrinkles and accentuates the philtral columns while flattening the nasolabial folds.
- In contrast, when the mouth is opened, the contraction of the pars superficialis leads to flattening of the perioral wrinkles and philtral columns and accentuates the nasolabial fold. In addition, the upper lip height shortens. Simultaneous relaxation of the deep pars marginalis decreases the thickness of the vermilion.

Abnormal Cleft Lip/Nose Anatomy (FIG 1)

- Varying degrees of cleft dysmorphogenesis of the lip, alveolus, and palate result in skin, soft tissue, muscle, and skeletal deficiencies with functional and aesthetic imbalance.

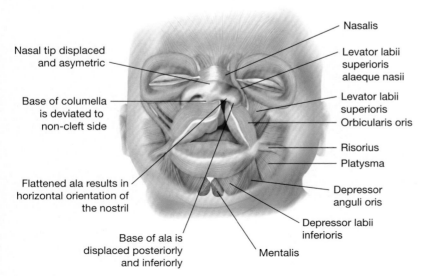

Nasal tip displaced and asymmetric

Base of columella is deviated to non-cleft side

Flattened ala results in horizontal orientation of the nostril

Base of ala is displaced posteriorly and inferiorly

Mentalis

Nasalis

Levator labii superioris alaeque nasii

Levator labii superioris

Orbicularis oris

Risorius

Platysma

Depressor anguli oris

Depressor labii inferioris

FIG 1 • Three-month-old with left unilateral complete cleft lip/nose and palate.

- This affects nasal symmetry in both complete and incomplete unilateral cleft lip/nose deformity by distorting the position of the ala base and shape of the nostril.
- With an interruption of the orbicularis oris muscle in the unilateral cleft lip/nose, the other attached facial muscles pull the ala base more laterally compared to the noncleft side. The existing muscle imbalance also changes the position of the alar cartilage, as well as the orientation of the nostril from an oblique to a horizontal orientation.
- When the muscle inserted on the base of the septum and columella is contracted on the noncleft side, the septum and columella is pulled toward that side. Thus, the severity of the cleft nasal deformity depends on the degree of separation of the orbicularis.
- Hypoplasia of the lesser segment, or base, of the cleft nose results in the displacement of the lower lateral cartilage laterally and inferiorly on the cleft side. The nasal dome is flattened and slumped in a downward position.
- The alar cartilage on the cleft side is flat, giving it the false appearance of having greater length when compared to the contralateral alar cartilage, which also is abnormally displaced to the noncleft side.
  - The relationship of the lower lateral cartilage to the septum is normal; however, the septum itself is deformed, thereby tilting the base of the nose toward the noncleft side and the tip of the nose toward the cleft side.
- The following summarizes a list of characteristics typical of a unilateral cleft lip/nose deformity. The degree and severity of the deformities vary, and not all of them are present in each patient.
  - The columella is shorter on the cleft side with its footplate displaced and tethered inferiorly.
  - The base of columella is deviated to the noncleft side.
  - The medial crus of the alar cartilage is shorter on the cleft side.
  - The lateral crus of the alar cartilage on the cleft side is longer and, together with the adherent skin, is drawn to an S-shaped fold.
  - The alar cartilage on the cleft side is displaced in the backward and downward planes.

- The nasal tip is displaced and asymmetric, with loss of the defining point on the cleft side.
- The dome on the cleft side is obtuse.
- The flattened ala results in horizontal orientation of the nostril on the cleft side, and it is usually larger than the opposite side.
- The entire nostril is retropositioned.
- The base of the ala is displaced posterior and inferiorly where it is tethered to the displaced underlying bone on the cleft side.
- The nasal floor is lower or absent on the cleft side.
- The caudal septum and anterior nasal spine are deflected to the noncleft vestibule (**FIG 2**).
- Septal deviation of varying degrees leads to posterior nasal obstruction on the cleft side due to the deviation of the septum and, often, the narrowing of the internal nasal valve.
- The lower turbinate on the cleft side is hypertrophic.
- Nasolabial fistula may be present.
- The lesser maxillary segment is hypoplastic and displaced on the cleft side.
- The nasal pyramid is asymmetric.

PATHOGENESIS

- Three major factors influence the nasal deformity in both complete and incomplete unilateral clefts:
  - Muscle imbalance
  - Tissue hypoplasia
  - Asymmetry of the skeletal base

NATURAL HISTORY

- Orofacial clefting is the most common craniofacial birth defect, occurring in 1:500 to 1:750 live births worldwide.
- The incidence of cleft lip in combination with cleft palate is estimated at 1:1000 with a gender ratio of 2:1 (male to female) with reverse gender ratio for cleft palate only.
- In the population of children with cleft lip and/or cleft palate (CL +/– P), approximately 50% have CLP, 30% to 35% CP, and 15% to 20% CL.
- Approximately 15% of CLP patients will have a syndrome, whereas 40% of CP patients are part of a syndrome.

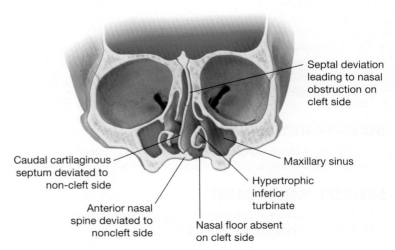

Septal deviation leading to nasal obstruction on cleft side

Maxillary sinus

Hypertrophic inferior turbinate

Nasal floor absent on cleft side

Anterior nasal spine deviated to noncleft side

Caudal cartilaginous septum deviated to non-cleft side

FIG 2 • Anterior nasal spine deviated to the right and noncleft side.

PATIENT HISTORY AND PHYSICAL FINDINGS

- The diagnosis of a cleft lip and/or palate is made by prenatal ultrasonography or by physical examination at birth and in early infancy. A detailed assessment is made of the child's breathing, feeding, growth, and development.
- Airway assessment must exclude the presence of sleep apnea and micro-/retrognathia.
- Assessment of growth and weight is key to identify and monitor feeding difficulty, gastroesophageal reflux, and use of feeding aids (Haberman/Pigeon teat).
- Hearing and middle ear function must be assessed and treated early by an otolaryngologist when associated with cleft palate.
- The plastic surgeon should define in detail the cleft lip type according to the anatomic structures involved, ie, complete or incomplete, unilateral with or without a Simonart band or bilateral, and presence or absence of a cleft palate.
- The child should also be assessed for associated anomalies suggestive of a syndrome, including craniofacial dysmorphia, airway compromise, cardiac defects, ocular and auricular abnormalities, and musculoskeletal anomalies. A genetics referral is suggested if syndromic cleft palate is suspected.

IMAGING

- At 16 weeks gestational age or older, 3D, 4D, and HD in utero ultrasound provide early diagnosis readily available in the developed and, in certain places, in the developing world. Parents may seek consultation with experienced surgeons, genetics experts, and other team members for education and decision-making about treatment.

DIFFERENTIAL DIAGNOSIS

- One of the main questions to determine in the presence of a cleft lip or cleft lip and palate is, "Does the patient have an isolated, or syndromic, cleft, which plays a major role in prognosis of treatment and genetic inheritance?" Van der Woude syndrome is a prime example, diagnosed with the presence of lip pits and means 50% subsequent inheritance.
- If cleft lip and palate are present, then 15% will be syndromic.

Syndromic Cleft Lip and Palate

- Stickler syndrome
- Robin sequence
- 22q11.2 deletion syndrome
- Treacher Collins syndrome
- Nager syndrome
- Ectrodactyly-ectodermal dysplasia
- Klippel-Feil syndrome
- Others

NONOPERATIVE MANAGEMENT

- All cleft lip patients should be treated surgically unless in extreme cases where anesthetic risk for surgery is high.

SURGICAL MANAGEMENT

- Cleft lip repair is ideally performed at 3 months of age, with the infant weighing greater than 5 kg.

- Risks of the procedure are based on the risk of the anesthetic, which is minimal.
- Main objectives of the procedure:
  - Separate the oral and nasal communication
  - Completely release and restore orbicularis oris function
  - Reconstruct the lip and nose to restore normal oral and nasal function
  - Provide an aesthetic result, which is accepted by the society and the patient
- Main steps of the procedure:
  - Mark the lip.
  - Dissect, release, and mobilize all abnormally displaced structures of the lip and nose simultaneously: muscles of the lip and base of the nose with other abnormal soft tissue attachments including alar and septal cartilage of the nose.
  - A complete tension-free closure must be achieved, or further dissection is necessary.
  - Focus on creating 3D aesthetic balance and functional harmony of the lip and nose.
- Muscle repair:
  - The muscle alignment is more important than the design of skin incision in achieving an excellent result.
  - Repositioning the muscle is one of the keys to achieving a good and stable result whether sub- or supraperiosteal, as this provides the foundation and support of the repair, maintaining alar base and nasal tip projection and symmetry.
  - To achieve complete mobilization and reconstruction, the complete release of the abnormal attachments of the muscle, and proper alignment, is key. The muscle should be vigilantly aligned.
    - Any under- or over-rotation of a carefully planned repair is usually due to a malaligned muscle repair.
- Nose repair: Correction of the nasal cleft deformity is a necessary and integral part of the primary surgery.

Preoperative Planning

- Perioperative orthopedics
  - Preoperative passive appliance: Hotz of Zurich introduced the use of an appliance placed preoperatively to control the greater and lesser segments, providing guidance for positioning the segments after lip/nose closure. This is left in place to prevent arch collapse until palatoplasty is performed.
    - Definitive scientific proof that this improves the end result is lacking. Thirty years of experience in Dallas improves the dental skeletal result, maxillary deformity, septal deviation, and other related deformities.
  - Preoperative active appliance: Nasoalveolar molding (NAM) with active preoperative segmental positioning has become internationally popular and used by many centers and teams. It provides better positioning of the maxillary segments while expanding and positioning the nasal soft tissues. It makes the surgery easier, particularly for the inexperienced surgeon.
  - Latham's earlier techniques using active forces were proven to be detrimental to maxillary growth and alignment. Adverse effects on growth need further scientific investigation before the final outcome of all active techniques is known.

- In my experience, excellent results can consistently be obtained without adding nasoalveolar molding in the unilateral cleft lip and palate patient. The technique can be labor intensive requiring family compliance and frequent visits to the orthodontist.
- With NAM, the molding of the nose must be done carefully to prevent creating a mega nostril through the potential tissue expansion effect, rather than just the desired reshaping of the nostril.
- Skin incision.
  - After three decades of cleft surgery, we believe that the skin incision is not very important in and of itself. The final aesthetic and functional outcome is determined by the extended dissection that allows the surgeon to free all the anatomic elements of the lip and nose that were displaced by the cleft in order to achieve complete repositioning of these elements.
  - The concept of the Salyer lip/nose repair is one of totally freeing all elements of the lip and nose in a plane above the periosteum, so they are floating free above the abnormal skeletal base.[1]
  - The lip and nose elements are then placed in the proper position, visualizing the 3D reconstruction and attempting to make form and function as normal as possible. The aesthetic result always remains foremost.
  - Repositioning the muscle is one of the keys to achieving a good and stable result, as this provides the foundation and support of the repair, maintaining alar base and nasal tip projection and symmetry. Lining up the muscle is the single most important maneuver in the repair, and it should be vigilantly aligned.
  - Various techniques today put emphasis on exact preoperative markings, which commits the surgeon. The repair should be fluid, allowing for improvisation and artistry by the surgeon, especially with respect to the nose.
  - For the first 20 years, I believed that an incision around the alar base was necessary to reshape the ala; however, today, this incision has been entirely eliminated, and we feel it only adds an unnecessary scar.[2]

Positioning

- The infant's head is stabilized on a small donut-shaped gel headrest placed at the edge of the head of the table.
  - The surgeon sits at the head of the table operating upside down with the infant's head almost in the surgeon's sterile lap slightly hyperextended to provide complete visualization of the infant's face.
- The patient is orally intubated by the anesthesiologist with a prebent tube fixed in the midline providing no distortion to the face or lip with minimal protrusion so as not to interfere with the procedure but provide safe control of the airway.

Approach

- Delaire described a subperiosteal approach with a wide dissection and incisional release of the periosteum with anatomic muscle closure.
- Supraperiosteal dissection is preferred by most plastic surgeons. We believe that the dissection above the periosteum is less detrimental to growth. Whether this philosophy is totally valid needs to be established.
- Preperiosteal dissection offers the advantage of allowing the tissue to move more easily, which is especially important in wider clefts. The analogy can be drawn to a scalp flap, which mobilizes with greater freedom when raised in a preperiosteal (ie, subgaleal) plane vs a subperiosteal plane.

■ Salyer Unilateral Lip/Nose Repair

- Key identifiable points are marked on the lip and nose (TECH FIG 1A).
- The base of each ala is identified and marked using methylene blue or appropriate marking pen. The alar base on the cleft side is usually elongated and distorted compared to the normal side.
- The peak of the Cupid's bow is identified and marked on the normal side. The height of the lip, from the alar base to the peak of the Cupid's bow at rest and without tension on the noncleft side, is measured using a caliper or is just estimated.
- The height to be achieved on the cleft side is usually 6 to 11 mm and averages 7 mm in the 3-month-old.
- The midline nadir, or lowest point, of the Cupid's bow is identified and marked. An equal distance, from the height of Cupid's bow on the noncleft side to the midline of Cupid's bow, is used to identify the peak of the new Cupid's bow on the cleft side and is marked on the vermilion-cutaneous junction.
- The exact point may have to be altered a millimeter in order to have a lip that is long enough. The lip height needs to be equal to the normal side when completely dissected and placed on tension with a skin hook.

- The wet line is marked with dots along its course on the vermilion on both sides of the cleft. Identification of this line provides symmetry and improved color match of the vermilion.
- The peak of the Cupid's bow and height of the lip on the lateral lip segment are determined by the height of the lip on the normal side, based on the initial measurement. The distance along the vermilion and down the lateral lip segment may be altered according to the height of the lip desired.
- It may be necessary to go along the vermilion-cutaneous border, down the lateral lip segment, a few millimeters more in order to create a lip, which is equal to the normal side. This may result in a shorter distance from the new peak of the Cupid's bow on the medial cleft side to the commissure of the lateral lip segment, as compared to the peak of the Cupid's bow to the commissure on the normal side.
- The proposed operation is marked with methylene blue, shown in the illustration as dots forming broken lines (TECH FIG 1B). The incision is marked from the peak of the Cupid's bow on the cleft side on the medial lip element and extends up and below the columella, across

TECHNIQUES

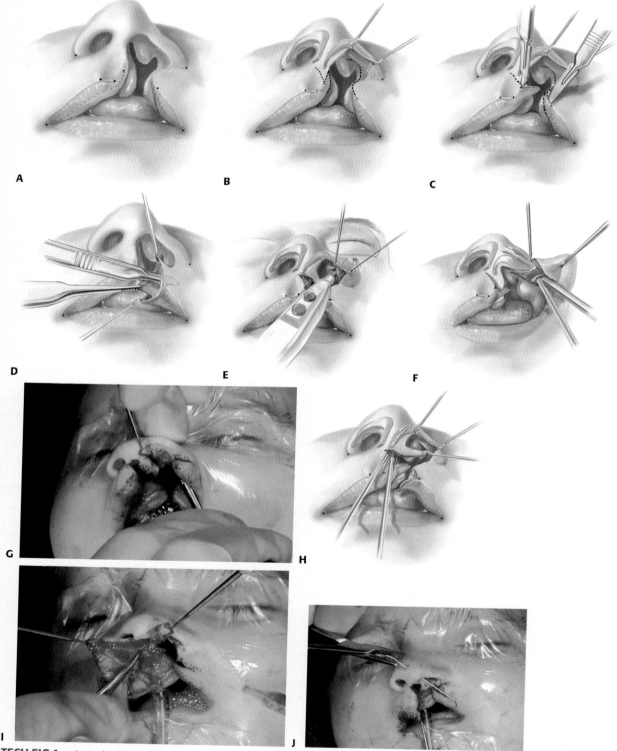

TECH FIG 1 • A. Key landmarks identified on the unilateral cleft lip/nose. **B.** Cleft lip incisions marked with *dotted lines*. An alternative technique does not extend the incision into the nose above the inferior turbinate. **C.** Initial performance of the medial and lateral lip element incisions for Salyer lip/nose procedure. **D.** Skin of lateral lip element is undermined over the orbicularis oris muscle for a maximum of 4 to 5 mm, thereby holding and freeing the orbicularis oris muscle. **E.** Preperiosteal dissection of the lateral lip element up to the infraorbital nerve using a Colorado needle. **F.** Alar base approach for dissection and release of the lateral crus of the alar cartilage and muscles of the lip from their abnormal attachment to the alar base along with freeing the nasal skin envelope to shift the cartilage, reshaping and projecting the nasal tip. **G.** Intraoperative view showing the dissection demonstrating the technique. **H.** Medial incision approach for the subcutaneous dissection of the nasal tip skin and releasing the abnormal attachment of the medial crus of the alar cartilage so the entire alar lcartilage can be shifted without exposure to create nasal tip projection. **I.** Intraoperative view demonstrating the dissection and technique of the medial approach. **J.** Intraoperative view of a Keith needle with Prolene with Dacron pledget to shape and reposition the alar cartilage and secure it while it heals. Sutures can alternately be used.

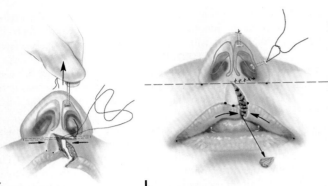
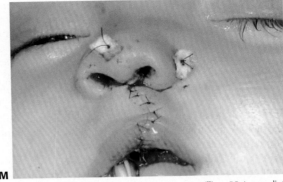

TECH FIG 1 (Continued) • **K.** Alar base cinch and alar cartilage tip sutures. **L.** Suturing of the muscle and trimming excess vermillion. **M.** Immediate postoperative view showing use of Dacron pledges (other materials may be used) for nasal reshaping with lip sutures.

the base of the columella, toward the opposite normal philtrum edge, but stops just short of this landmark.

- The surgeon should pull the lip down with a single skin hook and hold the lip in its new position while marking. If the incision is carried past the philtral ridge on the normal side, there is a risk that over-rotation of the lip may occur and a long lip may be created.

- The lateral lip element is marked along the cleft margin down to the newly marked peak of the new Cupid's bow (**TECH FIG 1C**). The design of the lip repair is the Salyer modification of the rotation-advancement procedure and is noted by the dotted lines. The classic incision around the alar base is not necessary and only adds scar to the final result.

- The incision on the lateral lip element continues from the vermilion-cutaneous border, and enters the nasal cavity, onto the lateral nasal wall above the inferior turbinate at the level of the piriform aperture extending to the nasal bones as necessary.

- Through this incision, the displaced and abnormally attached soft tissues of the alar base are freed from the underlying abnormal skeletal base. The incision made on the medial lip element attempts to simulate the normal philtrum, creating a normal symmetric shield-shaped Cupid's bow. The incision can be made with a no. 15 or no. 11 standard type blade, or a no. 65 or no. 67 beaver blade, which is our preference.

- The medial incision is cut through and through, including the skin and muscle; while along the vestibule of the lip, the mucosa is released and partially separated from the muscle. The medial lip element is dissected and mobilized so that it can be gently pulled down, with a skin hook, to rest at the same height as the normal side, leveling the Cupid's bow.

- The excess vermilion, containing a small amount of muscle, is left attached to the medial lip element. The lateral lip element is likewise incised, leaving an excess vermilion-muscle flap attached to it.

- These two vermilion-muscle flaps are tailored as the lip is closed and used to produce a full pouting vermilion of the lip. This helps eliminate vermilion notching of the lip at the suture line.

- The incision of the lateral lip element is carried along the free border of the lip.

- The muscle of the lateral lip element, overlying the lesser segment, is completely freed and released above the periosteum, so the muscle can be mobilized and sutured, creating a normal anatomic muscle with nice pout to the lip (**TECH FIG 1D**). In the incomplete cleft lip, there is usually more muscle available than in the complete cleft lip.

- The orbicularis oris muscle is pulled with pickups, and the dermis is undermined 4 to 5 mm, releasing it from the underlying muscle on the lateral lip element. The operation is estimated by an experienced surgeon.

- Laterally, the point corresponding to the new peak of the Cupid's bow is marked on the border of the vermilion-cutaneous junction, along the cleft margin, at a distance equal to the future height of the lip.

- This measurement should begin superiorly on the lip, however, not in the nose, so that the skin designated for the floor of the nose is not compromised. This is an important step in achieving an adequately reconstructed nose.

- The incision on the medial lip element begins at the newly marked peak of the Cupid's bow and continues up to, but not through, the philtral column on the non-cleft side.

- If the incision is continued past the philtral column on the normal side, it has the potential to create an overly rotated philtrum and abnormally lengthen the cleft side, creating disproportion to the lip as well as an obviously abnormally placed scar that no longer mimics the philtral column.

- The vermilion and muscle on each side of the lip are cut and maintained until closure of the vermilion. Excess vermilion is tailored to create fullness of the vermilion, preventing notching.

- The incision on the medial lip element is made with a no. 15 standard blade but may be performed with a no. 67 beaver blade or a no. 11 standard blade, as shown on the lateral lip element in the image.

- This incision should be made perpendicular to the skin and include the muscle, creating the C-flap, or columellar flap. This flap is used as dictated by each case when all the elements are totally freed.

- The incision on the lateral lip segment is carried through and through along the vermilion-cutaneous border, dissecting a vermilion flap for orbicularis marginalis reconstruction. How the surgeon holds and cuts the lip determines the amount of muscle left in the vermilion.

- This lateral lip incision extends inferiorly, at least to where an adequate white roll begins, but may be continued down the lateral lip element as lip length is needed.

- The freshly cut orbicularis marginalis muscle is pulled with pickups, and the skin of the lateral lip segment is undermined from the underlying muscle for a distance of 4 to 5 mm from the edge of the incision.

- The medial lip segment is rotated downward and pulled with a skin hook until its height matches that of the non-cleft side.

- The medial lip is freed from the underlying skeleton in a preperiosteal plane, using scissors. Additional dissection may be necessary to achieve adequate rotation of the philtrum and lengthening of the lip.

- Again, an opening incision above the white roll is used if additional rotation is required, and then a triangle is incorporated into the lateral lip markings. This is why the medial skin incision is always cut first.

- A Colorado needle (Stryker-Leibinger) is used to create the incision through the nasal lining just above the inferior turbinate (**TECH FIG 1E**). This provides a bloodless field for the dissection.

- Through this intranasal incision, as well as a vestibular buccal sulcus incision beneath the lateral lip element, the Colorado needle is used to dissect above the periosteum to the level of the infraorbital nerve.

- This maneuver provides for a bloodless dissection and the appropriate release of the abnormally displaced orbicularis oris muscle to provide symmetric closure. Complete preperiosteal release of the muscles facilitates complete reconstruction of the muscle of the lip.

- The beginning surgeon should be aware that the vertical height of an infant maxilla is short, and a guiding finger at skin level will ensure that inadvertent entry into the orbit is avoided as well as transection of the infraorbital nerve.

- Small curved tenotomy scissors with a round tip are inserted through the incision of the cleft-side alar base to dissect the skin from the lateral crus of the lower lateral cartilage (**TECH FIG 1F**).

- The nasal lining, if distorted, is dissected as well from the lower lateral cartilage as necessary. The nasal lining is left attached and never dissected at the region of the genu.

- The scissors are carried over the alar dome and into the subcutaneous pocket to be created from the medial nasal approach over the tip of the nose (**TECH FIG 1G**). The intraoperative view shows the placement of the surgeon's finger as the tenotomy scissors dissect above the alar cartilage freeing the entire skin of the nasal tip on the cleft side.

- Attention is now turned to the nasal tip from the medial approach. Tenotomy scissors are placed through the medial lip incision and used to subcutaneously dissect the nasal dome (**TECH FIG 1H**).

- The scissors are inserted subcutaneously and between the medial crura, separating the skin of the nasal tip from the alar cartilage, and carried over to the nasal dome.

- The skin over the noncleft side alar cartilage is likewise freed in order to shift the nose and gain equal projection of the ala cartilages at the tip (**TECH FIG 1I**). The intraoperative photographic view shows this maneuver.

- Once all the elements of the lip and nose are totally freed, a Keith needle with Prolene suture and a Dacron pledget is used to shift the alar cartilage within the skin envelope without exposure of the cartilage to project and create a new symmetric nasal tip (**TECH FIG 1J**).

- The alar cartilage is shifted into its new position held by a surgical assistant as the surgeon places a key suture shifting the lateral orbicularis muscle.

- This may have to be repeated until the desired symmetry is achieved. It is a very important step.

- Simultaneously, a 4-0 Monocryl suture (Ethicon Inc., Somerville, NJ) is placed from below into each alar base to achieve symmetry shown by the dotted line (**TECH FIG 1K**).

- At the completion of the muscle repair with 3-0 and 4-0 chromic sutures, the orbicularis oris and pars marginalis have been positioned to provide symmetry of the lip as well as maintain projection of the nasal tip (**TECH FIG 1L**).

- The vermilion excess is trimmed until the proper volume to obtain a full lip remains, preventing notching of the free margin of the lip.

- An additional suture of nylon over Dacron pledgets is placed through the lateral ala, correcting intranasal webbing and providing additional contouring and projection of the nasal tip. Initiation of skin closure is begun with the nasal sill.

- The subdermis is closed with interrupted 6-0 PDS (Ethicon, Inc., Somerville, New Jersey).

- Mucosal closure is performed with a 4-0 chromic suture, and 6-0 nylon is used for the skin closure. Intraoperative view at completion of the Salyer lip/nose repair (**TECH FIG 1M**).

- To diminish scarring, we utilize lip taping over the scar for 3 months postoperatively, and we educate parents on how to massage the upper lip in hopes of preventing hypertrophic scarring and diminishing postoperative redness.

- Preoperative frontal view of a left unilateral complete cleft lip/nose and palate patient (**TECH FIG 2A**). Postoperative frontal view 1 year postoperative following Salyer lip/nose repair (**TECH FIG 2B**).

- Preoperative submental vertex view of the same patient (**TECH FIG 2C**). Postoperative submental vertex view 1 year postoperative of the patient (**TECH FIG 2D**).

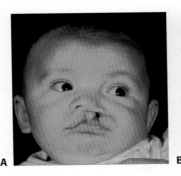
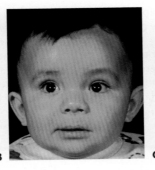
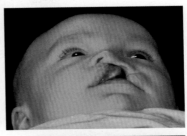
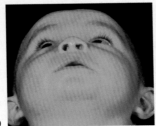

TECH FIG 2 • A. Preoperative frontal view of a 3-month-old patient. **B.** Postoperative view of the same patient 1 year following Salyer lip/nose repair. **C.** Preoperative submental vertex view. **D.** Postoperative 1-year submental vertex view.

■ Triangular Skin Flap for Lengthening the Lip

- At the time of closure, when the peak of Cupid's bow on the cleft side is too high (or short), an additional technique that provides lengthening of the lip can be performed.
- This can be executed at the time of lip closure when the peak of the Cupid's bow on the cleft side is not balanced and is short by 1 or 2 mm. The dotted lines demonstrate the design of the incisions (**TECH FIG 3A**). By placing an incision 2 to 3 mm in length in the lateral lip element at a 45-degree angle

3 to 4 mm above the vermillion, a flap is created that can be advanced into an incision in the medial lip. This opens to receive the flap, which becomes triangular in shape when sutured in place. This provides 1 to 2 mm lowering of the peak of the Cupid's bow on the cleft side. This is only needed in about 30% of the time in my experience. Fisher's repair designs a triangular flap as part of the lip repair.

- The medial lip incision opens to receive the insertion of the lateral lip triangular flap, and this lengthens the lip on the cleft side (**TECH FIG 3B**). The triangular flap should be designed 3 to 4 mm above the white roll, and

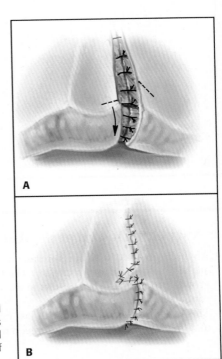

TECH FIG 3 • A. The design of the triangular flap is shown by dotted straight lines as marked when determined at the time of closure that the peak of the Cupid's bow on the cleft side is too high (30%). **B.** The incisions create a lateral triangular flap that is advanced into the medial lip incision lengthening the peak of the Cupid's bow on the cleft side to match the height of the normal side.

should not be confused with the white roll flap, which I have found to be inadequate compared to the technique described.

- We use this technique on innumerable occasions finding it to be quite helpful. Variations of this, first described by Bardach and now Fisher, are planned at the time of the initial marking and utilize a larger triangular flap. This is needed in my estimation in 35% of cases and is unnecessary the rest of the time.

- The triangular flap is almost always used by Fisher and Chong and incorporated into the original planning. This provides a nicer lip with better anatomic proportions in their experience. (See Chapter 1: Anatomical Subunit Repair of Unilateral Cleft Lip.)

Noordhoff's Vermilion Flap Technique

- Another useful technique for matching the wet and dry vermilion at the time of lip closure is Noordhoff's vermilion flap.[3]

- This is designed along the line where the color change in the vermilion occurs between the wet and dry vermilion. Frequently, the vermilion on the medial lip element cannot be adequately matched to maintain the width of both the wet and dry vermilion at the level of the peak of the Cupid's bow, because the height of the dry vermilion on the medial lip element is inadequate.

- To correct this mismatch, a triangular flap of dry vermilion is designed from the lateral lip element and sutured into an opening created in the medial vermilion along the wet line (**TECH FIG 4A**, upper).

- This eliminates the vermilion color mismatch that occurs in the vermilion border that acts as an obvious visual indicator of an abnormal lip (**TECH FIG 4B**, lower).

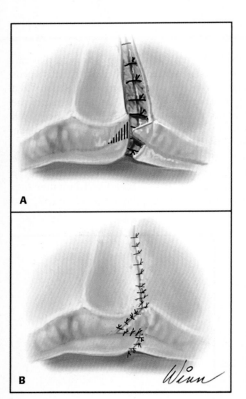

TECH FIG 4 • A. An incision along the *red line* in the medial lip vermillion receives a triangular flap created from the lateral lip wet vermillion when the excess vermillion is trimmed. This provides a uniform *red line* and vermillion. **B.** Suture closure of the lip using vermillion flap of Noordhoff to increase the height of the vermillion matching the red line.

Abyholm Closure of the Anterior Palate

- Abyholm in Oslo used an anterior vomer flap closure at the time of primary lip closure. The results regarding growth produced the best results in the Eurocleft studies conducted by Semb and Shaw.[4,5]

- This provides a simple and much less invasive approach that I highly recommend every surgeon to consider using.

I use this in mission surgery where this is a good and simple technique to add to the Salyer lip/nose or whatever your preference for the lip closure.

- The technique is shown in combination with the lip closure in **TECH FIGS 5 TO 7**.

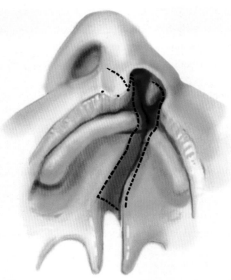

TECH FIG 5 • *Dotted line* shows lip closure with anterior vomer flap in combination with closure of floor of nose, alveolus, and anterior palate. Performing this while the lip is open facilitates closure of the anterior palate in one simple procedure, which is minimally detrimental to growth.

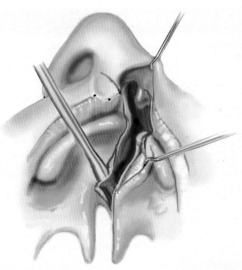

TECH FIG 6 • Incisions are made in the lip showing elevation of the vomer flap in the subperiosteal plane and opening of the palatal subperiosteal mucosa flap to receive it.

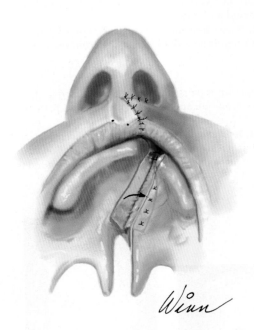

TECH FIG 7 • The lip is closed with sutures and the palate closed showing single layer closure of the anterior palate by fixing the mucosal or raw surface of the vomer flap below the elevated oral mucoperiosteal edge of the lesser segment creating a pocket to insert the vomer flap.

PEARLS AND PITFALLS

Age at operation	■ Development of structures occurs by 3 mo or older, which is the best time to perform the operation.
Overview	■ Surgeon must view the deformity as a lip/nose complex and repair both at the time of the primary repair. Technical skill and 3D visualization are important.
Dissection	■ All displaced and abnormally tethered structures must be completely released including the skin, cartilage, muscle, and mucosa.
3D puzzle	■ Float all structures freely in space 3D so they can be reconstructed. The biggest mistake seen repeatedly is inadequate release of the abnormal attachments of the alar base and alar cartilage medially and laterally resulting in relapse, which is really inadequate release of all the structures.
Nasal lining	■ Inadequate closure of the floor of the nose. Develop septal mucosa flap and lateral mucosa closing floor of nose as far back as possible.
Cleft nose	■ If technically capable, perform submucosal dissection of the septal cartilage, to straighten the caudal septum. ■ Create adequate skin pocket and totally free the alar cartilage so it can be translocated, shaped, and fixed.
Closure	■ Completely tension-free. The muscle is the key to the lip and nose and must be dissected, mobilized, and sutured into position setting up the lip and nose three-dimensionally.
Muscle alignment	■ Any under- or over-rotation of a carefully planned repair is usually due to a misaligned muscle repair.

POSTOPERATIVE CARE

■ Routine suture line care is important. Keep the suture line clean from blood and other fluids.

■ A liquid diet is recommended without the use of a nipple. Keep patient's hands and all objects away from the repair.

OUTCOMES

■ Unless a simple lip repair, all cases require multiple procedures to achieve excellence, as illustrated by the patient in **FIGS 3** to **10.**[6]

　■ The patient underwent left unilateral cleft lip repair and primary cleft nasal repair at age 3 months, followed by palatoplasty at age 9 months. Very minor secondary

lip/nose revision was required before 5 years of age. Orthodontic treatment with palate expansion was performed following eruption of the permanent first molars. This was followed by alveolar bone graft with cancellous bone at the time of eruption of the lateral canine tooth into the cleft.

■ In addition to good surgical technique, a coordinated team approach is critical to achieving excellence.[7]

COMPLICATIONS

■ There should be no dehiscence of any closure. Tension-free closure is important.

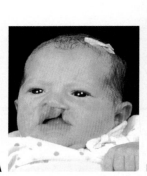
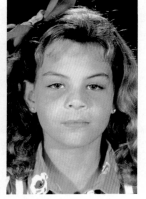

FIG 3 • A. Preoperative frontal view of a 3-month-old girl with a left unilateral complete cleft lip and palate. **B.** Postoperative view after primary stage 1 Salyer lip/nose repair demonstrates a slightly larger nostril on the cleft side performed so as not to constrict the nostril, anticipating a minor secondary procedure when the patient is older. The primary lip/nose repair at age 3 months corrected the major deformity at the time of the primary operation.

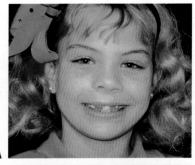
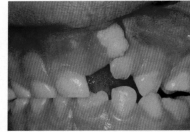

FIG 4 • A. Orthodontic treatment during mixed dentation stage. **B.** Demonstrates occlusion with mixed dentition before bone grafting.

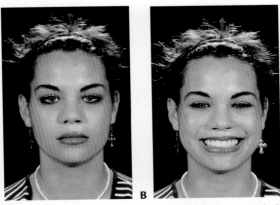

FIG 5 • A. Frontal view after secondary cleft lip/nose repair. Stage 2. Cleft lip/nose. Stage 3. Palatoplasty. Stage 4. Cancellous bone graft. **B.** Smiling view after completion of treatment.

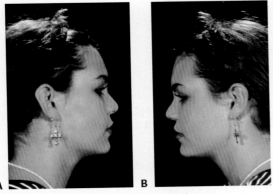

FIG 6 • A. Right lateral view. **B.** Left lateral view.

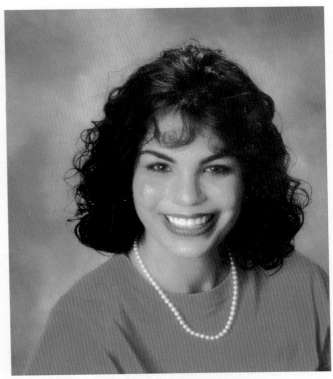

FIG 7 • Popular photographic view (nonclinical).

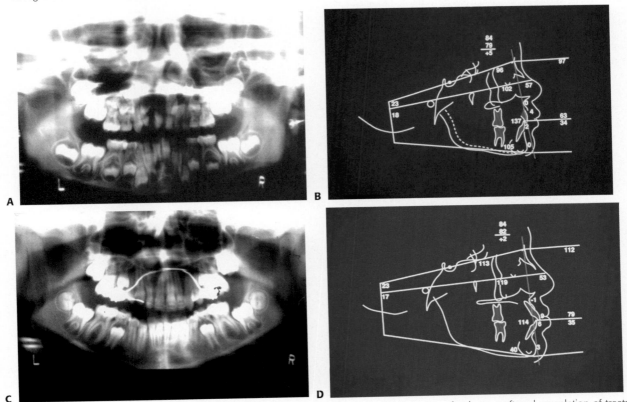

FIG 8 • A. Panoview before bone graph mixed dentition. **B.** Cephalometric view, age 6. **C.** Panoview after bone graft and completion of treatment. **D.** Cephalometric view, age 12, after completion of treatment.

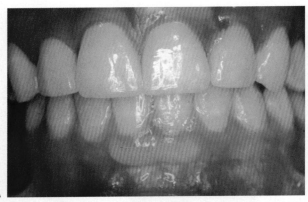
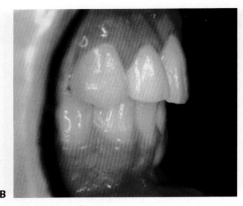

FIG 9 • Frontal view of occlusion of teeth showing also small anterior lower gingival graft below central incisors.

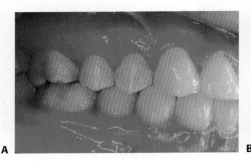
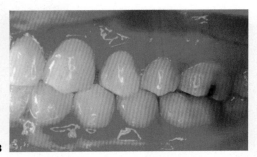

FIG 10 • **A.** Right lateral occlusion.
B. Left lateral occlusion.

REFERENCES

1. Salyer KE. Primary correction of unilateral cleft lip-nose: a 15-year experience. *Plast Reconstr Surg.* 1986;77:558-568.
2. Salyer KE. Excellence in cleft lip and palate treatment. *J Craniofac Surg.* 2001;12(1):2-5.
3. Noordhoff M.S. Reconstruction of vermillion in unilateral and bilateral cleft lip. *Plast Reconstr Surg.* 1984;73:52-61.
4. William SC, Erik D, Asher-McDade C, et al. A six-center international study of treatment outcome in patients with clefts of the lip and palate. Part 5. General discussion and conclusions. *Cleft Palate Craniofac J.* 1992;29(5).
5. Nollet PJPM, Katsaros C, van't Hof MA, et al. Treatment outcome after two-stage palatal closure in unilateral cleft lip and palate: a comparison with Eurocleft. *Cleft Palate Craniofac J.* 2005;42(5):512-516.
6. Salyer KE. A passion for excellence. *J Craniofac Surg.* 2009;20(Suppl 2):1632-1634.
7. Salyer KE, Genecov E, Genecov DG. Unilateral cleft lip-nose repair long-term outcome. *Clin Plast Surg.* 2004;31(2):191-208.

Lip Adhesion

4

CHAPTER

Catharine B. Garland, Jesse Goldstein, and Joseph E. Losee

DEFINITION

- For infants with complete unilateral or bilateral cleft lip, lip adhesion is an alternative to presurgical infant orthopedics (PSIO).
- Any child with a wide complete cleft lip may be a good candidate for some form of presurgical intervention to reduce tension and optimize symmetry prior to repair.
- Presurgical interventions include the following:
  - Lip adhesion surgery, which converts a complete cleft lip into an incomplete cleft lip
  - Presurgical orthopedics such as nasoalveolar molding (passive)[1] or use of a Latham device (active)[2]
- Lip adhesion decreases the tension on the final repair, improves symmetry of the nasal alar bases, and restores compressive forces on the alveolar segments to assist with alignment.[3] In the wide unilateral or bilateral cleft lip, this may ultimately improve the final surgical outcome.[4]

ANATOMY

- A complete cleft lip distorts both the lip and nose anatomy.
- In the unilateral complete cleft lip (**FIG 1**):
  - The orbicularis oris muscle is not in continuity. In the lateral lip element, the orbicularis oris muscle inserts vertically into the alar base and piriform.
  - The alar base on the cleft side is typically positioned laterally, inferiorly, and posteriorly on the collapsed minor alveolar arch.
  - The caudal septum and columella are deviated to the non-cleft side. The medial component of the orbicularis oris muscle inserts on these structures.

- In the bilateral complete cleft lip (**FIG 2**):
  - The premaxilla is often displaced anteriorly and may be twisted or locked out of the transversely collapsed lateral maxillary segments.
  - The lateral maxillary segments are relatively retropositioned and often collapsed.
  - The orbicularis oris muscle is widely separated, inserting into the alar bases at the piriform bilaterally.
  - The alar bases are laterally displaced and often asymmetric.
  - The columella is shortened.
- Normalizing some of this anatomy prior to definitive lip repair may improve the outcomes of surgery with regards to lip and nose symmetry.

PATIENT HISTORY AND PHYSICAL FINDINGS

- The sequence of surgical intervention for a complete cleft lip depends on individual patient and family characteristics and the surgeon and cleft center experience. This determines whether a patient undergoes a single-stage lip repair, lip adhesion prior to formal lip repair, or PSIO prior to lip repair.
- On physical examination, the width of the cleft, the presence of nostril sill tissue (a Simonart band), the relationship of the major and minor alveolar segments in the unilateral cleft lip, or the size and position of the premaxilla in the bilateral cleft lip are all evaluated carefully.
- Patient history must include an assessment of the infant's feeding and growth and identification of any medical comorbidities that may alter treatment.
- Family characteristics that factor into decision-making include financial, geographic, or other constraints. These may influence the parents' ability to frequently travel for PSIO or to be compliant with the daily care required.

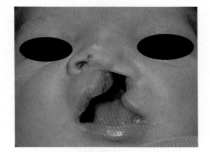

FIG 1 • Unilateral complete cleft lip and nose. Note inferior, lateral, and posterior positioning of cleft side alar base and deviation of columella. (Reprinted from Kirschner RE, Adetayo OA, Losee JE. Lip adhesion. In: *Comprehensive Cleft Care*. 2nd ed. Vol 2, Chapter 41. Boca Raton, FL: CRC Press; 2016:781-791, www.thieme.com, with permission.)

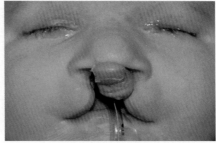

FIG 2 • Bilateral complete cleft lip and nose. Note wide alar bases, short columella, and the anterior displacement of the premaxilla relative to the lateral maxillary arches.

- Determining whether an infant is a good candidate for a lip adhesion includes weighing the advantages and disadvantages with the family:
  - Lip adhesion will convert the complete cleft lip to an incomplete cleft lip and reduce the alveolar gap as well as tension on the final repair.[5]
  - Compared with nonoperative PSIO, which requires frequent office visits, lip adhesion can reduce the burden of care on the family.[6]
  - In the bilateral complete cleft lip, labial adhesion may retract the prominent premaxilla and help to lengthen the columella.[7]
  - Lip adhesion incurs the additional costs of a second operation[6] and risks of an additional general anesthetic for the infant.

IMAGING

- None needed

NONOPERATIVE MANAGEMENT

- PSIO
  - Nasoalveolar molding (NAM)[1]: NAM is a passive technique that aligns the maxillary arches, narrows the alveolar gap, and molds the nasal cartilage. It is typically initiated within the first several weeks after birth. The infant must wear the device daily, and the orthodontist adjusts it weekly.
  - Latham device[2,5]: For the protruding premaxilla, the Latham device employs active lateral movement of the maxillary alveolar segments and retraction of the premaxilla posteriorly to realign the arch form.[7] This is a more rapid repositioning than nasoalveolar molding but does require a general anesthetic for placement of the Latham device.
- Single-stage cleft lip repair: Some authors argue that lip adhesion is an unnecessary procedure, despite the width of the cleft, and that equivalent results can be obtained in a single-stage repair.

SURGICAL MANAGEMENT

- Indications for lip adhesion include patients with wide complete clefts who are unable to undergo nonsurgical PSIO.
- Risks of surgery include infection, dehiscence, and scarring.

- In the bilateral cleft lip and palate patient with a protuberant premaxilla, lip adhesion may be combined with a premaxillary setback to optimize alignment of the premaxilla. This is typically reserved for older patients whose tissues (ie, premaxilla) are unlikely to mold under the compression of the lip adhesion alone.

Preoperative Planning

- All infants with a cleft must undergo full physical examination to rule out any concomitant cardiopulmonary disease or airway abnormalities. If additional medical problems are identified, genetic evaluation may be warranted.
- After birth, feeding evaluation is performed by instructing parents in the use of specialized bottles as needed. Weight gain is monitored weekly to ensure that nutrition is adequate.
- A complete blood count can be performed before surgery to evaluate for anemia of infancy. After birth, hemoglobin typically reaches a nadir between 8 and 12 weeks of life in healthy term infants. In premature infants, the nadir is more profound and occurs earlier.

Positioning

- General anesthesia is induced, and the patient is intubated with an oral Rae tube, which is taped in the midline of the chin to prevent any distortion of the upper lip.
- The patient is positioned supine with the head on a small gel donut.
- Lubrication ointment is placed in the eyes.
- The face is prepared with Betadine, and sterile drapes are applied.

Approach

- Loupe magnification is used to optimize precision of the procedure.
- The markings for a formal cleft lip repair are performed, as they would be at the time of definitive repair. Key points are tattooed with methylene blue.
- Importantly, the alar bases and alar-facial grooves are marked, so that the adhesion will lead to both vertical and horizontal symmetry of these features.
- The markings for the lip adhesion are then made within the tissues that would be discarded at the time of the formal repair or within the "L" and "M" flaps.
- Some surgeons perform primary nasal repair at the time of lip adhesion, while others defer this until the time of the formal lip repair.

■ Unilateral Cleft Lip Adhesion

Markings

- The unilateral cleft lip repair is marked and key points are tattooed. The alar bases and alar-facial grooves are marked (**TECH FIG 1A**).
- Incisions for the labial adhesion are marked within the area of the vermillion that is normally discarded on both the medial and lateral lip element. The incisions are around 10 to 15 mm in length and symmetric (**TECH FIG 1B,C**). The inferior half of the incision is performed on the upper lip, and, the superior half is performed on the nasal floor—truly making this a "lip-nose adhesion." On the medial lip element, the midpoint of the incision is centered at the columellar-lip junction. On the lateral lip element, the alar base denotes the midpoint of the incision. The position of these incisions is critical for alignment of the alar base. *The alar base must be symmetric with the contralateral side in both the horizontal and vertical plane*, or an asymmetric adhesion and repair will be performed and will make the subsequent definitive cleft lip and nose repair more challenging.
- The lateral buccal sulcus incision is marked to mobilize medially of the lateral lip element and ultimately a tension-free adhesion. This incision is carried up around the piriform aperture to just above the inferior turbinate (**TECH FIG 1D**).

Incision and Dissection

- Epinephrine is infiltrated into the incisions.
- Incisions are made using a number 15 blade or ophthalmic knife.
- The buccal sulcus incision is dissected in a supraperiosteal plane. The alar base is released from the piriform rim

and the lateral lip element is widely mobilized to reduce tension on the adhesion.

- During this mobilization, some surgeons may continue their lateral dissection up and over the lower lateral cartilage if they plan to perform primary nasal repair at the time of adhesion.
- The adhesion incisions on the medial and lateral lip elements are then made. The skin and mucosa are dissected to expose the orbicularis oris muscle.
- In the medial lip element, the dissection is carried toward the anterior nasal spine. Here the quadrangular cartilage is found displaced away from the cleft (**TECH FIG 2A**). The caudal septum may be repositioned now, rather than at the time of definitive lip repair. The quadrangular cartilage is released from the anterior vomer at the anterior nasal spine (for about 1 cm). This allows the caudal septum to be repositioned to the cleft side of the anterior nasal spine (**TECH FIG 2B**).

Suturing

- The septum is brought back to the midline, and it is sutured into place using a 4-0 Monocryl suture.
- A 2-0 Prolene horizontal mattress retention suture (single armed on a large needle) is placed in the orbicularis oris muscle. This stitch begins at the inferior end of the lateral lip incision (**TECH FIG 3A**). It is passed in a subcutaneous plane laterally into the cheek, then deep through muscle, and exits in the buccal sulcus laterally (**TECH FIG 3B**). The Prolene suture is then passed back through the same exit site and is passed in the submucosal plane out through the superior end of the lateral lip incision (**TECH FIG 3C**). Care is taken to ensure that the skin does not dimple with this stitch. The process is repeated on the medial lip element, from superior to inferior (**TECH FIG 3D,E**).

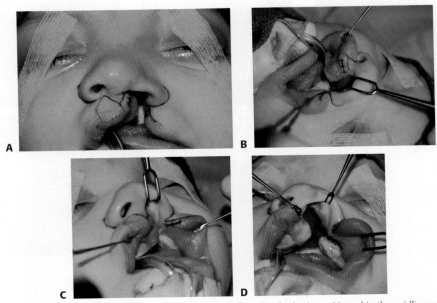

A **B** **C** **D**

TECH FIG 1 • A. Preparation for a unilateral lip adhesion. An oral Rae endotracheal tube is positioned in the midline and taped into place. The markings for a unilateral cleft lip and nose repair are marked and tattooed, including the alar bases. The lip adhesion incisions are made within the tissue that would normally be discarded. Design of the lip adhesion incisions on the **(B)** medial and **(C)** lateral lip elements. **D.** An upper buccal sulcus incision is carried up around the piriform aperture over the inferior turbinate. (Reprinted from Kirschner RE, Adetayo OA, Losee JE. Lip adhesion. In: *Comprehensive Cleft Care*. 2nd ed. Vol 2, Chapter 41. Boca Raton, FL: CRC Press; 2016:781-791, www.thieme.com, with permission.)

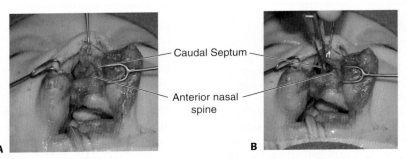

TECH FIG 2 • Repositioning the caudal septum. **A.** The anterior nasal spine and caudal septum are deviated away from the cleft in the native position. **B.** After the caudal septum is separated from the anterior nasal spine, it may be repositioned (forceps are mobilizing the septal cartilage).

The stitches exit on the inferior aspect of the lip adhesion incisions on both sides (**TECH FIG 3F**). As much of the orbicularis oris muscle is captured in the loops of the sutures as possible (**TECH FIG 3G**). This allows the medial and lateral lip elements to be approximated through the orbicularis muscle (**TECH FIG 3H**). The ends of the suture are clamped and tied later.

- As the lateral lip element is advanced, the buccal sulcus incision back cut is closed with interrupted 4-0 chromic sutures.
- The deep/posterior edge of the mucosal incision is then closed using interrupted 5-0 Vicryl sutures. Half of this suture line makes up the floor of the nose, and half makes up the superior lip.

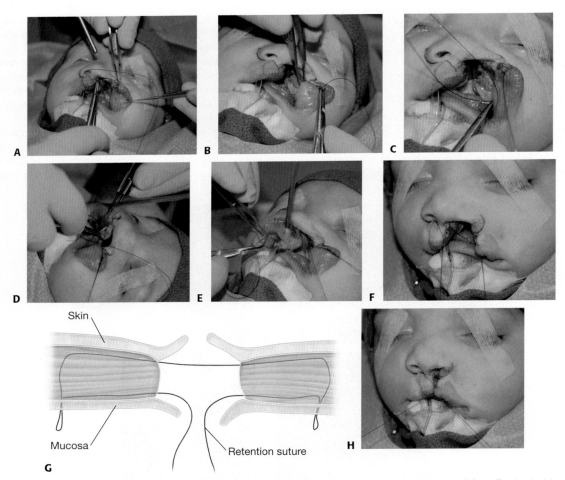

TECH FIG 3 • Placement of the internal retention suture. **A.** The suture is passed through the inferior aspect of the adhesion incision. **B.** After capturing the muscle, it exits laterally through the oral mucosa. **C.** The needle is placed back through the same exit site to exit through the superior part of the adhesion incision. **D,E.** The process is repeated on the medial lip element. **F,G.** The orbicularis oris muscle is captured in the loop of suture on both sides of the cleft. **H.** The ends of the suture are pulled together. The tension placed on a wide swath of orbicularis oris muscle reapproximates the lip and nose. (Reprinted from Kirschner RE, Adetayo OA, Losee JE. Lip adhesion. In: *Comprehensive Cleft Care*. 2nd ed. Vol 2, Chapter 41. Boca Raton, FL: CRC Press; 2016:781-791, www.thieme.com, with permission.)

- The Prolene suture is tied down, and care is taken to bury it into the muscle.
- The edges of the orbicularis oris muscle are approximated with three 4-0 Monocryl sutures.

Completion

- The anterior edge of the adhesion incision is closed last with interrupted 5-0 fast-absorbing plain gut sutures (**TECH FIG 4A**)
- If nasal repair is planned with the lip adhesion, this is performed now. The senior author, however, uses post-adhesion nasal stents to mold the nose during the healing process and *defers* the rhinoplasty to the time of

definitive cleft lip-nose repair. At that time, our preferred technique is open primary rhinoplasty through rim incisions to expose and reposition the lower lateral cartilage.[8,9] A Tajima, inverted-U rim incision is utilized on the cleft side of the nose.
- Duoderm is placed on the cheeks bilaterally. While bringing the cheeks together, a Steri-Strip is placed across the lip to additionally take tension off the repair.
- Our practice is to use nasal conformers postoperatively to optimize nasal symmetry. These conformers are sized in the operating room (**TECH FIG 4B**) and subsequently taped into place (never sewn) and used daily by the parents at home in the months between lip adhesion and definitive lip repair (**TECH FIG 4C**).

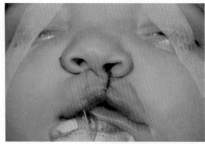 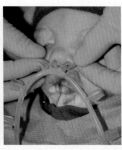 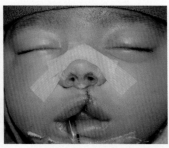

TECH FIG 4 • A. Completion of unilateral cleft lip adhesion and **(B)** sizing of nostril conformers. **C.** The nostril conformers are taped into place and worn daily in the postoperative period after both the lip adhesion surgery and after definitive lip and nose repair, as shown here. (Reprinted from Kirschner RE, Adetayo OA, Losee JE. Lip adhesion. In: *Comprehensive Cleft Care*. 2nd ed. Vol 2, Chapter 41. Boca Raton, FL: CRC Press; 2016:781-791, www.thieme.com, with permission.)

■ Bilateral Cleft Lip Adhesion

- The bilateral cleft lip repair is marked and key points are tattooed (**TECH FIG 5A**).
- The incision for the adhesion is marked on both sides of the prolabium at the junction of the skin and mucosa, approximately 10 to 15 mm in length (**TECH FIG 5B**). The incision is centered at the junction of the columella and prolabium, such that half of the incision is on the prolabial lip element and half is intranasal.
- The lateral lip incisions are marked in the part of the vermilion that would normally be discarded or used as a "C" flap. These are also centered at the alar base, such that half of the incision is on the lip vermilion and the

superior half is within the nose. The incisions are drawn so that the alar bases will be positioned symmetrically when the lip-nose adhesion is completed (**TECH FIG 5C**).
- Epinephrine is infiltrated into the incisions and these are made with a number 15 blade or ophthalmic knife. The orbicularis oris muscle is exposed in the lateral lip element bilaterally.
- The buccal sulcus incision on both lateral lip elements is marked and carried into the nose, around the piriform rim, and above the inferior turbinate. Supraperiosteal dissection is performed to completely release the lateral lip and alar base from the maxilla and piriform rim so that they may be advanced to reach the premaxilla.

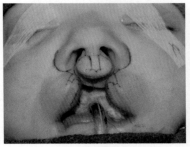 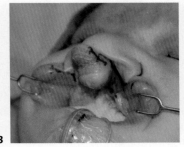 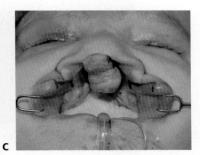

TECH FIG 5 • A. Preparation for bilateral cleft lip adhesion begins with marking the bilateral cleft lip repair. Bilateral lip adhesion markings on the **(B)** prolabium and **(C)** lateral lip elements.

TECHNIQUES

- A 2-0 Prolene retention suture is placed in the orbicularis oris muscle. This is performed similar to the unilateral case (see **TECH FIG 3**). The stitch begins at the inferior end of the lateral incision on the left side. It is passed in a subcutaneous plane laterally into the cheek then deep through muscle and exits in the buccal sulcus laterally. It is then passed back through the same exit site in the submucosal plane to exit the incision at the level of the nasal sill. Care is taken to ensure that the skin does not dimple with this stitch. After capturing the orbicularis muscle on one side, the suture is passed deep across the premaxilla in a preperiosteal plane, at the level of the nasal sill. This exits through the contralateral prolabial incision at the level of the nasal sill. The process is repeated on the right side, with the suture capturing the right orbicularis muscle, entering through the lateral incision at the level of the nasal sill, and exiting at the inferior margin. The suture is again passed deep across the prolabium through the inferior margins of the prolabial incisions. Once positioned, the ends of the suture

- are clamped. With tension through the orbicularis oris muscle, this suture brings the lateral lip elements to meet the prolabium.
- The posterior edge of the mucosa is closed with 5-0 Vicryl suture from the superior/nasal end of the incision down toward the inferior/labial end on both sides.
- The 2-0 Prolene suture is tied down and the knot is buried in the lateral muscle.
- Additional 4-0 Monocryl sutures are placed to secure the orbicularis oris muscle to the prolabium on each side.
- The anterior skin incisions are then closed using interrupted 5-0 fast-absorbing plain gut sutures.
- At the completion of the closure, the markings for the C flap and nasal sill on both sides should be perfectly lined up such that the alar bases are symmetric in both the vertical and horizontal planes (**TECH FIG 6**).
- Duoderm is placed on each cheek. While bringing the cheeks together, a long Steri-Strip is placed across the labial adhesion to reduce tension on the repair.

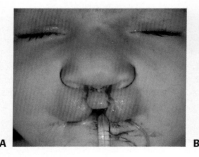 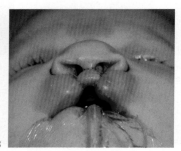

TECH FIG 6 • Bilateral complete cleft lip after premaxillary setback and lip adhesion **(A)** anteroposterior and **(B)** worm's-eye views.

■ Premaxillary Setback

- In the infant who is older than 6 months, the vomer is likely to be ossified. In these cases, a protuberant premaxilla will be unlikely to move when subjected to the forces of lip adhesion alone. In these cases, we will typically perform a premaxillary setback at the time of lip adhesion.

- A 10 mm vertical incision is marked along the anterior vomer, just posterior to the premaxillary segment (**TECH FIG 7A**).
- The periosteum is elevated off the vomer bilaterally to the level of the quadrangular cartilage.
- A closing wedge osteotomy is designed behind the premaxilla, and a small rongeur is used to remove this

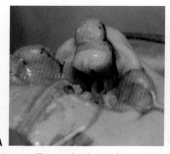 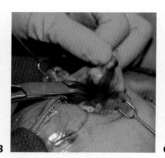 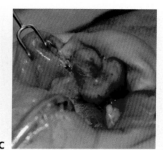

TECH FIG 7 • Premaxillary setback. **A.** The incision is marked on the vomer just behind the premaxilla. **B.** After dissecting in a subperiosteal plane, rongeurs are used to create a closing wedge osteotomy. **C.** The premaxilla is repositioned in alignment with the lateral maxillary arches and affixed with 4-0 PDS sutures.

bone (**TECH FIG 7B**). No cartilage is removed. The closing wedge osteotomy is noted to be sufficient when the premaxilla can be repositioned posteriorly and in good alignment with the lateral alveolar segments (**TECH FIG 7C**).

- A 4-0 PDS is sufficient to fixate the premaxilla into its new position, promoting bone-to-bone contact. This is secured from the premaxilla to the posterior vomer. Additionally, on each side, a 4-0 PDS suture can be passed directly through the mucosa of the lateral premaxillary alveolus and through the medial edge of the lateral arch alveolus (as an external stitch). When tied, this will secure the repositioned premaxilla to the lateral segments during healing.

- The vomer incision is closed using a running 5-0 Chromic gut suture.

- Combining a premaxillary setback and bilateral lip adhesion, as described herein, will not compromise the perfusion of the premaxillae. The authors do not perform a premaxillary setback and complete bilateral cleft lip and nose repair, rather stage the late presenting patient with: stage 1: premaxillary setback and lip adhesion. Stage 2: complete cleft palate repair. Stage 3: complete cleft lip and nose repair.

PEARLS AND PITFALLS

Timing	▪ Optimal timing is at 2 months of age.
Incisions	▪ Incisions must be placed in tissue that will be discarded at the time of definitive lip repair. ▪ Therefore, the markings for a definitive lip repair are performed first.
Permanent retention suture	▪ A permanent suture is placed through the orbicularis oris muscle on both sides of the cleft. ▪ It must capture a large swath of orbicularis oris muscle on both sides in order to reduce tension on the lip adhesion and decrease the risk of dehiscence.
Alar base positioning	▪ Symmetrical placement of the alar bases during the lip adhesion is critical. ▪ Alar bases must be symmetric in both the horizontal and vertical planes. ▪ If the alar bases are asymmetric at the completion of lip adhesion, this deformity will be more difficult to correct at the time of definitive cleft lip repair.
Nasal stents and conformers	▪ The use of nasal conformers after lip adhesion helps to lengthen the columella and mold the lower lateral cartilages to optimize nasal form prior to definitive lip repair.

POSTOPERATIVE CARE

- The patient is admitted postoperatively for monitoring and typically discharged home the following day if oral intake is adequate to maintain hydration.
- Patients may return to their usual bottle-feeding.
- Elbow splints are typically used to prevent inadvertent injury to the repair.
- Steri-Strips are utilized and can be replaced for 2 weeks following surgery to take tension off of the repair.
- Nasal conformers are used postoperatively. The parents are taught how to clean and replace the stents daily. If the adhesion was performed under more tension than desired, or if there is a tenuous soft tissue closure, nasal stenting can be started in 1 to 2 weeks after adequate healing has occurred.
- The nasal conformers are increased in size as the infant grows over the next 3 to 4 months.
- Definitive cleft lip and nose repair is then performed in 3 to 4 months, at approximately 6 months of age. At the time of the repair, the adhesion scar is excised and the permanent retention suture is removed.

OUTCOMES

- Labial adhesion has been shown to increase the vertical height of the medial and lateral lip elements in unilateral cleft lip[10] and increase the bulk of orbicularis oris muscle tissue for closure and reconstruction of the philtral ridge.[11]

- The adhesion of the orbicularis oris muscle molds the alveolar segments and reduces a wide alveolar gap by approximately 60% in both unilateral and bilateral cleft lips.[3,12] If gingivoperiosteoplasty is planned, however, passive alveolar molding may still be required to align the maxillary segments.

COMPLICATIONS

- Dehiscence: Either partial or total dehiscence occurs between 4% and 17% of the time.[6,10,12] Dehiscence is more common in the bilateral than the unilateral complete cleft lip, because the bilateral lip (without premaxillary setback) is often under more tension. Partial dehiscence may not require operative intervention if some of the alignment is maintained.

- Scarring: Scarring of the lip can occur, and some authors report that it can interfere with the final repair. When the incisions are planned carefully, however, the scarring will only occur in tissues that would normally be discarded at the time of definitive lip repair.

REFERENCES

1. Grayson BH, Santiago PE, Brecht LE, et al. Presurgical nasoalveolar molding in infants with cleft lip and palate. *J Craniomaxillofac Surg.* 1992;20:99-110.
2. Latham RA. Orthopedic advancement of the cleft maxillary segment: a preliminary report. *Cleft Palate J.* 1980;17:227-233.
3. Meijer R. Lip adhesion and its effect on the maxillofacial complex in complete unilateral clefts of the lip and palate. *Cleft Palate J.* 1978;15:39-43.
4. Randall P. A lip adhesion operation in cleft lip surgery. *Plast Reconstr Surg.* 1965;35:371-376.
5. Millard DR, Latham R, Huifen X, et al. Cleft lip and palate treated by presurgical orthopedics, gingivoperiosteoplasty, and lip adhesion (POPLA) compared with previous lip adhesion method: a preliminary study of serial dental casts. *Plast Reconstr Surg.* 1999;102:1630-1644.
6. Shay PL, Goldstein JA, Paliga JT, et al. Comparative cost analysis of cleft lip adhesion and nasoalveolar molding before formal cleft lip repair. *Plast Reconstr Surg.* 2015;136:1264-1271.
7. Bitter K. Repair of bilateral clefts of lip, alveolus and palate. Part 1: A refined method for the lip-adhesion in bilateral cleft lip and palate patients. *J Craniomaxillofac Surg.* 2001;29:39-43.
8. Lu TC, Lam WL, Chang CS, Chen PK. Primary correction of nasal deformity in unilateral incomplete cleft lip: a comparative study of three techniques. *J Plast Reconstr Aesthet Surg.* 2012;65:456-463.
9. Monson LA, Kirschner RE, Losee JE. Primary repair of cleft lip and nasal deformity. *Plast Reconstr Surg.* 2013;132:1040e-1053e.
10. Van der Woude DL, Mulliken JB. Effect of lip adhesion on labial height in two-stage repair of unilateral complete cleft lip. *Plast Reconstr Surg.* 1997;100:552-557.
11. Ridgway EB, Estroff JA, Mulliken JB. Thickness of orbicularis oris muscle in unilateral cleft lip: before and after labial adhesion. *J Craniofac Surg.* 2011;22:1822-1826.
12. Gatti GL, Lazzeri D, Romeo G, et al. Effect of lip adhesion on maxillary arch alignment and reduction of a cleft's width before definitive cheilognathoplasty in unilateral and bilateral complete cleft lip. *Scand J Plast Reconstr Surg Hand Surg.* 2010;44:88-95.

Bilateral Cleft Lip Repair

John A. van Aalst

DEFINITION

- A cleft of the lip occurs when the maxillary prominence fails to fuse, first with the lateral nasal prominence and then the medial nasal prominence; when this failure of fusion occurs bilaterally, a bilateral cleft deformity is the result.[1]
- Cleft lip occurs most commonly in patients from Southeast Asia and the southwestern United States (1/250 to 1/400 live births), is less common in Caucasians (1/1000), and is least common among African Americans (1/2000).[1]

ANATOMY

- Bilateral clefts of the lip involve the tissues of the primary palate. This includes the skin, muscle, and mucosa of the lip and the alveolus, extending posteriorly to the incisive foramen.
- The premaxillary segment contains the central alveolus (maxilla) with the tooth buds of the central incisors; this bone is attached to the vomer, the bony underside of the septum.
- The premaxillary segment presents with variable anterior flaring, which may have variable presentation: it may be very anteriorly positioned or may be correctly positioned within the maxillary arch.
  - A complete bilateral cleft is likely to have significant anterior flaring, whereas the premaxillary segment of an incomplete cleft is likely to be positioned correctly between the lateral segments of the maxilla.
- Gingiva and mucosa cover the bone of the premaxillary segment and then transition to skin; this segment does not contain true lip vermilion. The skin is generally circular in shape and is without a true white roll. No muscle is present in this region (except in incomplete clefts, where the muscle is in continuity with the lateral lip elements).
- Lateral segments of a bilateral cleft lip have all of the elements of the lip present lateral to the nasal ala (wet vermilion, dry vermilion, white roll, skin, and muscle); moving medially, the

fullness of each of these components diminishes as the lip structures narrow and ascends toward the cleft of the nose.

PATHOGENESIS

- Lip fusion occurs on day 42 of gestation.
- Fusion may be interrupted secondary to genetic causes (MSX1 gene anomaly), environmental causes (including medications—steroid, anticonvulsants, retinoic acid—alcohol, tobacco use), or a combination of the two (alcohol consumption and cigarette use in the face of an MSX1 genetic anomaly).[1]
- The medial migration of the maxillary prominence is arrested, leading to failure of fusion with the medial and lateral nasal prominences; failure of fusion of these latter two leads to clefting of the nostril floor.

PATIENT HISTORY AND PHYSICAL FINDINGS

- Many children with bilateral cleft lip will be diagnosed in utero, prompting a prenatal visit with cleft team members, including the surgeon. The cleft team member describes the concept of team care to the family, the needs of the child immediately following birth, and the surgical preparation for cleft lip repair at approximately 3 months of age.
- Patient history should include the presence of family members with clefting; maternal exposure risks: cigarette and alcohol use; medications, including anticonvulsants and steroids; and folic acid supplementation during early pregnancy.[1]
- Following delivery, the first visit to the surgeon is generally within the 1st week of life.
- In addition to a full physical examination, the tailored examination of the face detects whether the cleft is complete or incomplete, whether there is asymmetry between the two sides, and whether the premaxilla is proclined (**FIG 1**). In addition, the presence of clefts of the alveolus and of the palate must be documented.

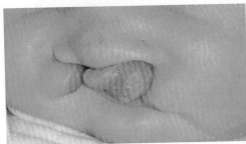
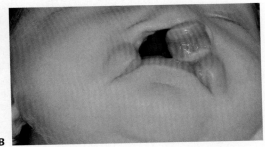

A **B**

FIG 1 • Infant with bilateral cleft lip. Figure **A** demonstrates a frontal view of an infant with a bilateral complete cleft lip and palate; the premaxilla is anteriorly positioned (proclined). Figure **B** is a worm's eye view of the same infant, demonstrating the asymmetry of the cleft, with the premaxilla positioned more to the patient's left. As can be noted more clearly in this figure, the patient also has a cleft of the alveolus and palate.

IMAGING AND OTHER DIAGNOSTIC STUDIES

- No routine imaging studies are required for children with bilateral cleft lip prior to surgical repair.
- Because these children may have other congenital anomalies, additional findings on physical examination will dictate the need for additional diagnostic studies.
- If the child has evidence of breathing difficulties, or sleep apnea, a sleep study may be warranted. If there is any evidence of feeding/swallowing difficulties with concerns about aspiration, a swallow study may be warranted; if other cranial abnormalities are present, a craniomaxillofacial computed tomography scan may be warranted.

NONOPERATIVE MANAGEMENT

- Although nonsurgical management of the bilateral cleft lip is not appropriate, presurgical management for control of the proclined maxilla is recommended.
- The proclined maxilla can be treated with a simple taping regimen (**FIG 2**), with nasoalveolar molding[2,3] or actively with a Latham device[4,5] to direct position of the alveolar segments prior to surgical repair.

SURGICAL MANAGEMENT

- Children are judged ready for surgery using the rule of 10s: approximately 10 lb (4.5 Kg), 10 week of age, and a hemoglobin count of 10.[6–8]
- If there are any other symptomatic comorbidities or concerns about appropriate weight gain, delay in surgery is warranted.

Positioning

- At the time of surgery, the child is positioned in the supine position and intubated with an oral Ring-Adair-Elwyn (RAE) tube (**FIG 3A**).
- A shoulder roll is placed to obtain gentle extension of the neck.
- The entire face is prepped and draped, and a throat pack is placed.
- Markings are made for lip repair with tattooing of key landmarks (**TECH FIG 1**).
- Local anesthetic with epinephrine is injected following the markings.

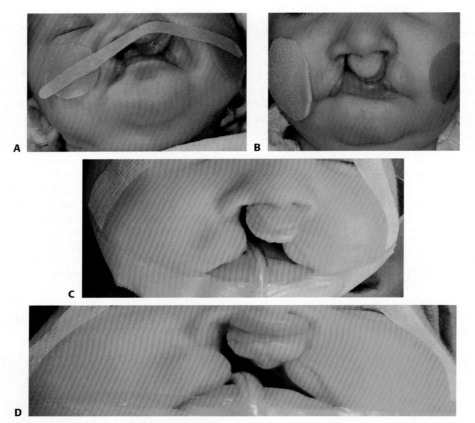

FIG 2 • Preoperative preparation of the patient in **FIG 1** with a taping regimen. This taping regimen needs to start shortly after birth to maximize the effect on premaxillary segment retroclining (an early start is also true for other forms of presurgical orthopedics, including nasoalveolar molding). **A.** During the taping regimen. **B.** At completion of the taping regimen. **C,D.** Immediate preoperative photographs demonstrate an improved position of the premaxilla in a more symmetrical position after taping regimen.

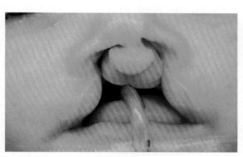
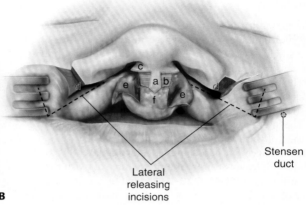

FIG 3 • A. The patient is positioned supine and intubated with an oral RAE tube, with taping on the chin so that the upper lip is not distorted. **B.** Landmarks. The central philtral column with skin (*a*) is 2 mm wide at the waist and 2 mm from low to high point of Cupid's bow. The lateral flanking de-epithelialized regions (*b*) are also 2 mm wide. The remnant skin and mucosa of the premaxillary segment have been incised into three parts. These areas are labeled (*e*) bilaterally and (*f*) centrally and inferiorly. At the superior philtral column (*b-a-b*) are extensions of skin (*c*) that will be eventually be used to close the floor of the nose. The central flap (*f*) is used to reconstruct the central upper buccal sulcus; the two lateral flaps (*e*) are turned out laterally and used to reconstruct the anterior surface of both alveolar clefts. Bilateral upper buccal sulcus incisions (*d*) allow medialization of cheek tissue to minimize tension at final closure. The vertical component of the incision is made medial to Stensen duct (the greater the height of this incision, the greater the capacity to medialize cheek tissue). The horizontal incision is made at the junction of the gingiva and oral mucosa to the base of the L flap (without injuring the L flap). A Freer elevator is used to lift the periosteum from the maxillary surface, exposing the infraorbital nerve. The region of the nerve is the most significant area of tethering, which prevents medial movement of cheek tissue. The periosteum medial and lateral to the nerve is cut vertically, avoiding injury to the nerve and releasing the tethering effect of the periosteum.

■ Markings

- The two most commonly used techniques to repair the bilateral cleft lip are the Millard technique[6] and the Mulliken technique.[7-10]
- Based on modifications of the Mulliken technique, markings for the neophiltrum include the following:
  - 2 mm at the waist (at the junction of the columella with the premaxillary skin; **TECH FIG 1**)
  - 2 mm between the low and high points of Cupid bow
  - Flanking de-epithelialized regions, each 2 mm wide and the same height as the philtral column
- The three-part division of the premaxillary mucosa is marked.
- The bilateral advancement flaps are marked, with 2 mm of intact white roll retained with the vermilion component on both sides, with as much as possible skin conserved, but avoiding vermilion (see **TECH FIG 1**).
- Bilateral upper sulcus-releasing incisions are marked:
  - The vertical component is medial to Stensen duct.
  - The horizontal component is marked at the junction of the gingiva and upper buccal sulcus mucosa, extending medially to the edge of the L flap.

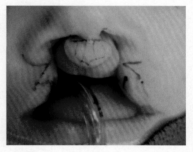

TECH FIG 1 • Attention to detail in the markings is key to an aesthetic outcome. Before making the marks, take note of the asymmetries present. Markings are made before injection of local anesthetic, and the points are tattooed into tissue with a 30-gauge insulin needle using either Bonnie blue or methylene blue. The high and low points of Cupid's bow are 2 mm wide; the waist of the philtral column is also 2 mm wide. The flanking regions that will be de-epithelialized on either side of the philtral column skin are also 2 mm in width. At the superior lateral position of the two areas marked for de-epithelialization, there should be a horizontal extension along the skin, which will be used for eventual closure of the nostril floor. The lateral lip markings begin with the medial marking for the white roll. This point should be marked at the medial-most position of full (complete) white roll (moving further medial from this position, the white roll tapers); a second point is marked 2 mm lateral to the first point. The medially curved line on the vermilion has its furthest medial extension at the junction of dry and wet vermilion; the 2 mm of white roll will remain with the vermilion and be used to reconstruct the white roll under the philtral column (also 2 mm in width). The upper buccal sulcus—releasing incisions are also tattooed so the marks continue to be visible despite oral secretions or bleeding (shown in **FIG 3B**).

◼ Incisions

- The neophiltrum is incised with de-epithelialization of the two flanking regions. These three regions are lifted as a single unit (**TECH FIG 2A**), improving blood supply to the philtral skin.
  - The three parts of the premaxillary mucosa are incised (see **TECH FIG 2A**). The central portion is used to reconstruct the upper buccal sulcus (**TECH FIG 2B**).
  - The lateral two flaps are used to provide coverage over each of the alveolar clefts (**TECH FIG 2C,D**).
- The advancement flap is incised, starting laterally, at the white roll, leaving 2 mm of intact white roll with the dry vermilion (see **TECH FIG 2B–D**), extending along the junction of skin and vermilion (carefully avoiding inclusion of vermilion with the skin flap).
  - The incision is then extended inferior to the nose, then laterally, along the crease between the nose and lip, but not extending beyond the alar margin (see **TECH FIG 2C,D**).
- The lateral vermilion flap (L flap) is incised, leaving excess dry and wet vermilion for lip reconstruction (this helps to create a pout of the central lip).
  - The inferior part of the incision is continued on the mucosal side toward the alveolus in a line parallel to the advancement flap incision.

- At the superior-medial incision of the advancement flap, the L flap incision is extended into the nose at the junction of skin and mucosa, extending toward the inferior turbinate.
- The skin margin of the advancement flap is then separated for 3 to 4 mm from the orbicularis oris muscle (during reconstruction, this separation will allow approximation of the muscle as a separate layer; see **TECH FIG 2D**).
- Next, the lateral releasing incision is made in the upper buccal sulcus: the vertical component is made 1 cm medial to the Stensen duct, extending down to the junction of the oral mucosa and gingiva; the horizontal component is then incised along the junction of the oral mucosa and gingiva, to the base of the L flap (see **FIG 3B**).
- Using the lateral releasing incision, maxillary tissue is dissected from the maxilla in a subperiosteal plane with a Freer elevator. The infraorbital nerve is identified.
  - The periosteum is incised medial and lateral to the nerve, allowing medialization of cheek tissue.
  - The right angle of the releasing incision can now be extended medially to decrease tissue tension during closure.

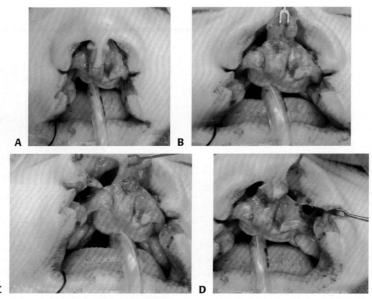

TECH FIG 2 • **A.** Incisions for bilateral cleft lip. A beaver blade is used to make all incisions. At the skin markings, part of the tattooed mark is maintained on the retained flap in order to clarify positioning of the flaps at final closure. **B.** Lifting of the philtral flap with flanking de-epithelialized regions. Note the inset of the central premaxillary mucosal flap to the periosteum of the premaxillary segment with a central stitch; this reconstructs the central upper buccal sulcus. Closure of the right nostril floor with the L flap and the right turnover flap from the premaxilla. These two flaps are sutured to each other, simultaneously closing the nostril floor and the anterior surface of the alveolar cleft (**(C)** on the **left**, **(D)** on the **right**). Note that the nostril orifice is maintained despite approximation of these flaps.

◼ Reconstruction

- The L flap is inset into the floor of the nose using 5-0 chromic with the intact mucosa facing down toward the oral cavity and raw surface up toward the lip (see **TECH FIG 2B–D**).

- The lateral premaxillary flaps are turned over (intact surface down) and sutured with 5-0 chromic to the periosteum of the maxilla at the lateral base of the L flap.
  - The two flaps are then sutured to each other, to close the floor of the nose.

- A 4-0 PDS is used as an alar cinch suture (**TECH FIG 3A**), setting the alar margins at the medial canthi bilaterally (**TECH FIG 3B**).
- Oral mucosa is reapproximated at the medial-most extension of the releasing incision (medializing tissue that was at a right angle into a straight line) using 4-0 and 5-0 chromic interrupted sutures.
- Muscle is approximated using 4-0 PDS interrupted sutures with buried knots (**TECH FIG 3C**).
- The dry vermilion and white roll are approximated with 5-0 plain interrupted sutures (**TECH FIG 3D**).

- The neophiltrum is inset with 6-0 Monocryl deep dermal suture at the lateral margins of the flap, which correspond to the high points of Cupid's bow, followed by 6-0 plain suture at the skin.
- 6-0 plain sutures are placed from philtrum to vermilion between the high and low points of Cupid's bow. 6-0 Monocryl is used for deep dermal closure along the philtral column.
- 7-0 PDS subcuticular stitch is used to close the skin. The nostril floor is closed using 5-0 chromic suture (**TECH FIG 3E**).
- Dermabond or Steri-Strips are applied to the lip incisions.

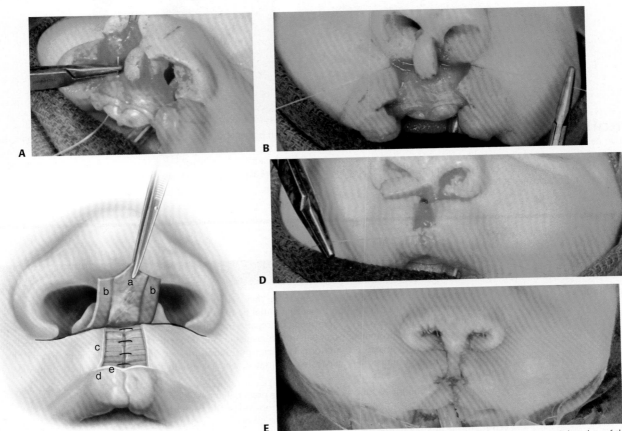

TECH FIG 3 • The alar cinch suture (which sets the lateral ala at the medial canthus bilaterally) is placed on the underside of the alae of the nose **(A)** and is used to set the lateral alae at the medial canthi bilaterally **(B)**. Importantly for the lip repair, positioning the base of the nose begins the process of medializing tissue to close the lip. **C.** Muscle closure is performed using 4-0 PDS interrupted buried sutures. Reapproximation of muscle must be accomplished throughout the full extent of the lip. The philtral tissue is visualized from the underside ((*a*) with skin and bilateral (*b*) regions that are de-epithelialized). The de-epithelialized regions will be placed under the skin advancement flaps (*c*) and will provide fullness in the lateral philtral column bilaterally. The philtral flap will be inset at (*d*) bilaterally for final closure. Note the white roll (*e*) at the medial superior area of vermilion. The areas of white roll (*e*) will be approximated to each other. **D.** Reapproximation of the white roll with dry vermilion prepares for inset of the philtral column. **E.** Final closure of the lip.

■ Variations in the Technique

- The same technique can be used in older patients requiring correction of a wide philtrum (**TECH FIG 4**).
- Though the author's preferred sutures are delineated in this chapter, multiple sutures can be substituted during various junctures of the repair. For example, 4-0 Vicryl can be substituted for 4-0 PDS for reapproximation of the muscle.

- Although the width of philtral column skin flap in a 3-month old patient is recommended as 2 mm from low to high point of Cupid's bow, and 2 mm at the philtral waist (abutting the nasolabial junction), surgeons may choose to incorporate the flanking de-epithelialized regions (also approximately 2 mm wide) into the actual skin-based philtral flap, thereby increasing the width of the skin.

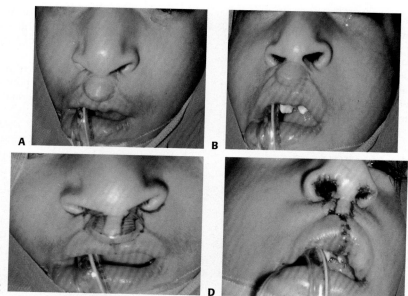

TECH FIG 4 • A 9-year-old with previous bilateral cleft lip repair. **A,B.** The high points of Cupid's bow are elevated bilaterally because the entire skin paddle of the premaxillary segment was used for lip repair. Retained mucosa of the premaxillary segment is present; the patient has a wide philtrum due to use of the central maxillary skin and mucosa as a vermilion substitute. The white roll remains laterally displaced. **C.** Markings have been made for repair of the cleft lip with central philtral column, flanking de-epithelialized regions, scar excision, and premaxillary segment mucosa excision. **D.** Final closure at revision surgery.

PEARLS AND PITFALLS

Physical findings	▪ Be cognizant of asymmetries on initial examination; they may be correctable by presurgical molding techniques; if not, they must be accounted for during initial lip markings. ▪ Retroclining the premaxilla is key to improving lip repair outcomes. ▪ Failure to retrocline the prominent premaxilla often results in lateral maxillary arch collapse, thereby "locking out" the premaxillary segment in its abnormal anterior position. If this occurs, the premaxilla cannot be positioned properly until maxillary expansion is initiated, which is usually done during the phase of mixed dentition.
Markings	▪ Make the philtral column as long as possible on the premaxillary skin. ▪ An appropriately narrow philtral column avoids a too-wide philtrum with continued facial growth. ▪ Borrowing white roll from the lateral lip segments is crucial because true white roll does not exist at the skin margin of the premaxillary segment. ▪ Provide extra fullness in the central vermilion to avoid a whistler's deformity.
Incisions	▪ Avoid the mistake of making the incisions on the lateral lip elements too medial. This will make the height of the lip incongruent with the philtral column height.
Closure	▪ Closure with tension is the primary cause of muscle dehiscence and scar widening. ▪ Releasing incisions in the upper buccal sulcus provide tension-free closure. ▪ If tension persists, re-examine the releasing incisions for further release in areas of periosteal banding. ▪ Muscle closure should be performed along the full height of the lip.
Postoperative care	▪ No change in feeding regimen is needed after surgery. ▪ Scar massage at 1 mo

POSTOPERATIVE CARE

▪ Postoperative in-hospital stay is optional.
▪ Arm restraints should be considered.
▪ Gentle narcotic use for pain is recommended.
  ▪ Undertreatment of pain may hinder the child's ability to feed.
  ▪ Overtreatment can lead to constipation.

▪ Breast or bottle feeding is initiated in the recovery room following completion of surgery.

OUTCOMES

▪ Ideally, primary repair of the bilateral cleft lip should result in a symmetrical, aesthetically pleasing repair that does not require revision (**FIG 4**).

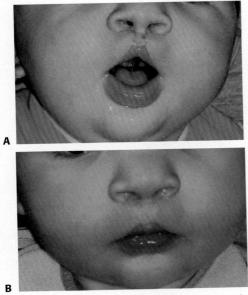

FIG 4 • The child in **FIGS 1** and **2** is shown at 1 month **(A)** and 4 months **(B)** after surgery.

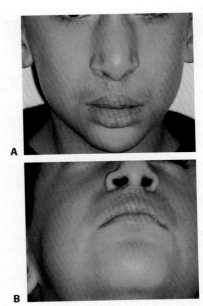

FIG 5 • Postoperative results of the lip revision shown in **TECH FIG 4**. The patient is seen in a frontal view **(A)** and a worm's eye view **(B)**. Note that the patient has improved philtral width, Cupid's bow, and wet with dry vermilion balance.

- However, the reality is that revisions are often needed (**TECH FIG 4** and **FIG 5**).
- Timing for revision is controversial. Times for possible lip revision:
  - 5 years of age, on entry into kindergarten
  - Life changes, including transfer to a new school
  - Timed with other surgeries, such as speech surgery or bone grafting
  - After skeletal maturity following orthognathic surgery

COMPLICATIONS

- Early
  - Bleeding
  - Dehiscence of the repair, either partially or totally
  - Loss of the neophiltral column
  - Stitch spitting/abscess
  - Rarely, infection
- Late
  - Scar widening, including the philtrum becoming too wide in proportion to the overall size of the lip
  - Asymmetry: the most noticeable asymmetries are of the Cupid's bow, with one high point being higher than the other
  - Poor animation because of muscle dehiscence or heavy scar burden

REFERENCES

1. Watkins SE, Meyer RE, Strauss RP, Aylsworth AS. Classification, epidemiology, and genetics of orofacial clefts. *Clin Plast Surg.* 2014;41(2):149-163.
2. Dec W, Shetye PR, Davidson EH, et al. Presurgical nasoalveolar molding and primary gingivoperiosteoplasty reduce the need for bone grafting in patients with bilateral clefts. *J Craniofac Surg.* 2013;24(1):186-190.
3. Grayson BH, Santiago PE, Brecht LE, Cutting CB. Presurgical nasoalveolar molding in infants with cleft lip and palate. *Cleft Palate Craniofac J.* 1999;36(6):486-498.
4. Millard DR, Latham R, Huifen X, et al. Cleft lip and palate treated by presurgical orthopedics, gingivoperiosteoplasty, and lip adhesion (POPLA) compared with previous lip adhesion method: a preliminary study of serial dental casts. *Plast Reconstr Surg.* 1999;103(6):1630-1644.
5. Cruz C. Presurgical orthopedics appliance: the Latham technique. *Oral Maxillofac Surg Clin North Am.* 2016;28(2):161-168.
6. Millard DR. Bilateral cleft lip and a primary forked flap: a preliminary report. *Plast Reconstr Surg.* 1967;39(1):59-65.
7. Mulliken JB. Principles and techniques of bilateral complete cleft lip repair. *Plast Reconstr Surg.* 1985;75(4):477-487.
8. Mulliken JB. Primary repair of bilateral cleft lip and nasal deformity. *Plast Reconstr Surg.* 2001;108(1):181-194.
9. Mulliken JB, Wu JK, Padwa BL. Repair of bilateral cleft lip: review, revisions, and reflections. *J Craniofac Surg.* 2003;14(5):609-620.
10. Yuzuriha S, Oh AK, Mulliken JB. Asymmetrical bilateral cleft lip: complete or incomplete and contralateral lesser defect (minor-form, microform, or mini-microform). *Plast Reconstr Surg.* 2008;122(5):1494-1504.

CHAPTER 6

Secondary Deformities

Catharine B. Garland, Jesse Goldstein, and Joseph E. Losee

DEFINITION

- After cleft lip and nose reconstruction, secondary deformities of the lip and nose are common. The actual incidence of deformity is difficult to quantify because of individual variability in assessing what constitutes a deformity. For example, the incidence of revisionary surgery ranges from 0% to 100%.[1]
- Asymmetries leading to deformity can be encountered anywhere along the lip-nose complex. These are caused by inadequate tissue in some cases and excessive tissue in others.
- This chapter focuses on addressing secondary cleft lip deformities rather than secondary cleft rhinoplasty. Correcting asymmetries of the alar bases, however, is often an important component of secondary lip revision surgery.

ANATOMY

- The ideal lip and nose complex is composed of the following features:
  - A symmetric nostril shape, with symmetric nostril sills and alar base position
  - A balanced Cupid's bow with a smooth curve to the vermilion border
  - Symmetric philtral columns with a well-defined philtral dimple[2]
  - Smooth contour and balance of the mucosa
  - A central pouting tubercle in the vermilion
  - A functional orbicularis oris muscle sling that leads to symmetry with animation
  - Appropriate tooth show at rest

PATHOGENESIS

- Some secondary deformities are intrinsic, such as the nasal deformity characterized by a hypoplastic and flattened lower lateral cartilage.
- Other deformities are iatrogenic from the primary cleft repair. These include deformities caused by scarring, inadequate correction, an unbalanced reconstruction, or altered growth and development.

PATIENT HISTORY AND PHYSICAL FINDINGS

- The most important part of the history is to ascertain what bothers the patient and the family. This may not always be congruent with what the surgeon sees as the most significant deformity. Realistic expectations of operative intervention must be discussed preoperatively.
- The physical examination must include a careful analysis of the deformity. The reconstruction is then tailored to address the specific anatomic abnormality.

- Are the alar bases symmetric in shape and position? They must be symmetric in the vertical, transverse, and sagittal plane.
- What is the nature of the cutaneous scar? Assess whether the scar is hypertrophic, atrophic, or pigmented. This helps to inform the surgeon about the patient's innate healing response.
- Is the philtrum well defined and symmetric?
- Is Cupid's bow balanced or is there a discrepancy in height on the cleft side? Are the vermilion border and white roll congruous structures?
- Is the red line, wet-dry junction, in alignment? An excess of wet mucosa in a region that should be composed of dry vermilion often causes persistent chapping of the lip in that area.
- Is there adequate lip length and appropriate tooth show? Is the buccal mucosa scarred and tethered?
- Is the mucosa symmetric? Is there excess mucosa on the cleft side or deficient mucosa at the central tubercle? Is there a notch in the mucosa at the site of repair?
- Is the lip symmetric in animation? Bunching of the lip may suggest dehiscence of the orbicularis oris muscle.

SURGICAL MANAGEMENT

Preoperative Planning

- Preoperative workup is per hospital routine.
- Under anesthesia, a careful analysis of the lip and nose is again performed to characterize the asymmetries.
- For more severe deformities, consideration must be given to a complete revision of the primary cleft lip and nose repair.[3,4]

Positioning

- Supine
- We typically use an oral RAE endotracheal tube. This minimizes any asymmetry caused by taping a standard endotracheal tube in the corner of the mouth.
- The table is turned according to surgeon preference.
- The face is prepped with Betadine, and sterile drapes are applied. A head wrap or four towels may be used for draping according to surgeon preference.

Approach

- Markings: Mark all the key anatomical landmarks of the lip and nose (eg, alar bases, columella, peak and nadir of Cupid's bow, white roll, and wet-dry junction). Tattoo the key points with methylene blue.
- Measure: Measure both the normal and cleft sides with calipers to determine the exact discrepancy of height and/or width in the lip and nose that requires correction.

- Epinephrine: Consider whether epinephrine is needed for your surgery. The hemostatic benefit is helpful in many cases. However, for subtle contour abnormalities, epinephrine infiltration may obscure your ability to assess the result on the table. In these cases, pinch the lip between the thumb and index finger to occlude the labial artery while you are incising the tissues and use Bovie electrocautery sparingly.
- Skin repair: Although hypertrophic scarring may be inherent to the patient, all precautions are taken to minimize this risk. Care is taken to ensure a tension-free closure. The skin is approximated with 5-0 or 6-0 Monocryl buried dermal sutures. When these are placed precisely, additional cutaneous sutures may not be required. When cutaneous sutures are needed, we use strategically placed 6-0 fast-absorbing plain gut or 6-0 nylon sutures in the epidermis to align the skin edge. These are removed 4 to 5 days after surgery.

- Muscle repair: Muscular dehiscence may be suspected in patients who have a muscle bulge laterally with facial animation. In addition, muscular dehiscence can contribute to a shortened lip, notching of the mucosa, or widening of the cutaneous scar. When these are noted, reconstruction of the orbicularis oris musculature must also be performed with the repair. The orbicularis oris muscle is dissected free from the skin and mucosa. When the muscle is found dehisced, it is reapproximated or overlapped. Some surgeons describe a benefit to tightening the orbicularis oris muscle with horizontal mattress sutures to evert the muscle and accentuate the philtral column.
- Mucosa repair: After the planned local tissue rearrangement or excision, the mucosa is typically repaired with 5-0 chromic gut sutures. These can be placed as everting horizontal mattress sutures to prevent a notch in the vermilion and mucosa.

■ Deformities of Cupid's Bow

Small Vermilion Mismatch (Less Than 1 mm) or a Widened Scar at the Cutaneous-Vermilion Border

- This can be managed by a diamond or curved excision of the scar, similar to the classically described Rose-Thompson straight line repair (**TECH FIG 1A**).
- The Cupid's bow nadir and high points are marked (**TECH FIG 1B**). An equal distance from high point to nadir is transposed to the cleft side, and this is typically positioned on the medial side of the scar. The vermilion border is marked medially and laterally to the scar that is to

be excised. These points will come together to create the new high point of Cupid's bow on the cleft side.
- The white roll is marked, as is the red line wet-dry junction. The diamond excision is marked to excise the scar or mismatch and allow realignment of the vermilion border and white roll.
- The critical points are tattooed with methylene blue.
- Epinephrine-containing solution is infiltrated into the tissues for hemostasis.
- Using an ophthalmic knife, the diamond is excised through the skin down to muscle. If the muscle repair is adequate, superficial scar is excised, but the muscle is left intact.

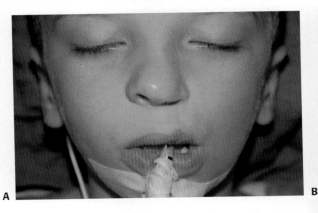
A

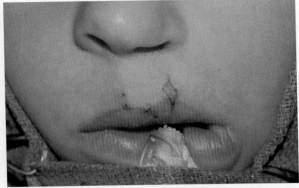
B

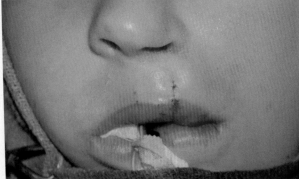
C

TECH FIG 1 • A. Hypertrophic scar at the vermilion border with slight shortening of Cupid's bow on the cleft side preoperatively. The remainder of the cutaneous scar is well healed. **B.** The peak and nadir of Cupid's bow are marked on the noncleft side and transposed to the cleft side. The white roll is marked and these points are tattooed. A diamond excision of the scar is marked at the vermilion border. **C.** The diamond excision realigns the vermilion border and white roll and provides adequate additional length to balance Cupid's bow.

T E C H N I Q U E S

- 5-0 Monocryl is used to realign the vermilion border with a deep dermal suture (**TECH FIG 1C**). Additional deep dermal sutures are used to realign the wound margins precisely.
- 5-0 Chromic is used to reapproximate the mucosa with everting sutures. To prevent a standing cone or "dog ear," excess mucosa is excised as needed in this process.

Cupid's Bow Mismatch of 1 to 2 mm

- For a Cupid's bow mismatch of 1 to 2 mm (**TECH FIG 2A**), a small triangular flap is inserted at the cutaneous border.
- This excision and reconstruction are often similar to the microform cleft repair described by Mulliken.[4]
- The cutaneous-vermilion border, white roll, Cupid's bow peak on the normal side, low point, and peak on the cleft side are marked and tattooed (**TECH FIG 2B**).
- Using calipers, the distance from subnasale to the normal Cupid's bow peak is measured, and the equal distance from subnasale is marked on the cleft side.

- A laterally based cutaneous equilateral triangular flap is marked on the lip above the white roll, with the base of this triangle being the difference in the distance between subnasale and height of Cupid's bow peak on each side.
- An incision of equal length is marked on the medial lip element above the white roll.
- The length of vertical excision is long enough to excise any abnormal scar tissue or to prevent formation of a "dog ear."
- If there is a deficiency of central tubercle vermilion, a laterally based triangle of vermilion may be designed as well.[3] If there is an excess of lateral mucosa, a mucosal excision may be included (**TECH FIG 2C**).
- The tissue is infiltrated with epinephrine. It is excised with an ophthalmic knife or no. 15 blade.
- The scar tissue is excised and the skin flaps are separated from the underlying orbicularis oris muscle.
- The muscle is reconstructed if needed, and skin and mucosa repair proceeds as previously described (**TECH FIG 2D,E**).

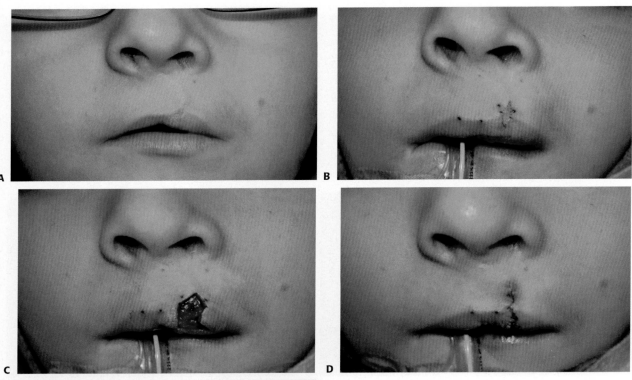

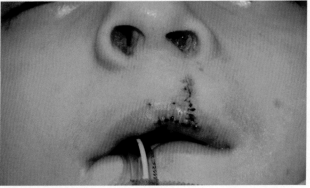

TECH FIG 2 • A. Lip deformity characterized by both shortening of Cupid's bow on the cleft side and lateral mucosal fullness. **B.** The peak and nadir of Cupid's bow are marked on the noncleft side, and the peak of Cupid's bow is marked symmetrically on the cleft side. The excision is designed with a laterally based triangular flap at the white roll. In addition, the lateral mucosal fullness is addressed with an excision planned along the red line or junction of wet and dry mucosa. **C.** After excision of the tissues, prior to repair. Mucosa is being excised in both the transverse and vertical planes. **D.** Closure includes the inset of a laterally based triangular flap above the white roll to increase the length of the lip on the cleft side. This realigns and balances Cupid's bow. **E.** After excision of excess mucosa, the mucosa is more symmetric. The scar is hidden along the red line and closed with 5-0 chromic sutures.

Cupid's Bow Asymmetry More Than 2 mm High

- For a larger asymmetry, a complete revision of the cutaneous scar is performed (**TECH FIG 3**).
- Many primary lip repair techniques may be adapted to achieve the necessary goals in these more complex deformities.
- The vermilion discrepancy may be addressed by rerotation of the medial lip element as in a classic Millard repair (**TECH FIG 3C**).

- Use of a triangular flap above the white roll in the manner first described by Tennison and Randall and subsequently modified by Fisher[5] is also an option for a complete revision of the lip repair to address a major deformity.
- The orbicularis oris muscle may need to be reconstructed fully or in part to achieve adequate repair.
- In the bilateral cleft lip, complete revision is used for patients with a wide philtrum, significant philtral scarring, or a severe deficiency of vermilion in the midline (**TECH FIG 4**).

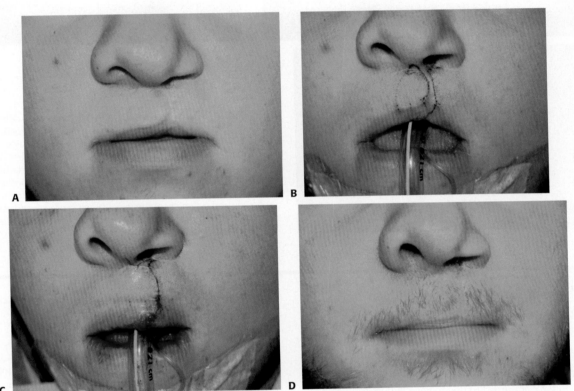

TECH FIG 3 • A. Shortening of the unilateral lip with mild widening of the cutaneous scar. **B.** A complete excision of the cutaneous scar is planned. A backcut is designed to allow secondary rotation of the medial lip element. **C.** After rotation of the medial lip element, Cupid's bow is now more symmetric. **D.** The improvement in the symmetry of Cupid's bow is maintained at 18 months postoperatively.

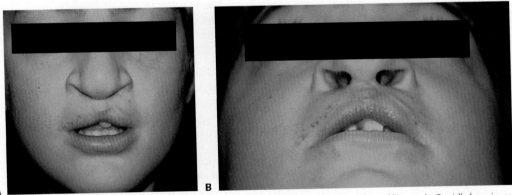

TECH FIG 4 • A,B. A 12-year-old boy with significant residual cleft lip and nasal deformity after bilateral lip repair. Cupid's bow is unbalanced, and there is a paucity of mucosa in the central tubercle. He has had no correction of his cleft nasal deformity with lateral displacement of the alar bases.

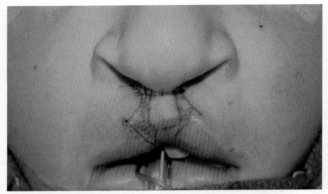

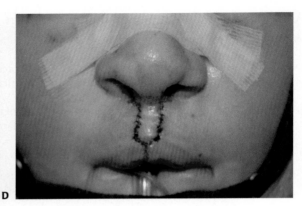

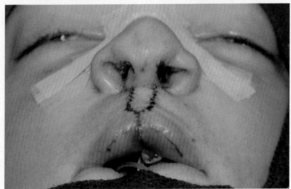

TECH FIG 4 (Continued) • **C.** With this degree of deformity, a complete bilateral lip and nose repair is planned and marked as if this were a primary incomplete bilateral lip repair. The peak of Cupid's bow is marked at Noordhoff point on the lateral lip element. The skin and mucosa between this and his existing scar are planned for excision. **D,E.** The bilateral lip and nose are completely reconstructed to restore balance to Cupid's bow and the vermilion. Note the improved positioning and symmetry of the lower lateral cartilages and alar bases after open reconstruction with inverted-U rim incisions to address the lower lateral cartilages.

■ Abnormalities of the Vermilion and Mucosa

- Minor notches in the vermilion, asymmetries of the mucosa, incongruity of the red line, or asymmetry of the dry vermilion may all be managed with small elliptical excisions or local tissue rearrangement.
- Incisions are confined to the mucosa and vermilion unless a cutaneous deformity must also be addressed.
- Each problem discussed here has a slightly different solution, but our typical step-by-step approach is as follows:
  - Assess the deformity and design the excision or flap for reconstruction.
  - Mark the red line for accurate realignment later. Tattoo this with methylene blue if needed.
  - We typically do not infiltrate the tissues with epinephrine-containing solution when addressing a mucosal defect. The infiltration will distort the tissues and prevent accurate intraoperative assessment. We find it is easier to determine if adequate tissue has been excised or rearranged without infiltration.
  - Rather than using epinephrine, the labial artery is pinched between two fingers while making an incision in the tissues with a no. 15 blade.
  - Electrocautery is used for hemostasis as needed.
  - Mucosal flaps are elevated from the underlying orbicularis oris muscle.
  - The orbicularis oris muscle is reconstructed as needed with 4-0 Monocryl mattress sutures.
  - The mucosa is redraped to assess contour of the lip. Additional excision, augmentation, or dissection is performed as needed to optimize the contour.
  - Closure of the mucosa is performed with interrupted 5-0 chromic sutures.

Malalignment of the Red Line

- This may lead to a notch in the border or an area of chapped mucosa interposed between dry vermilion.
- A notch caused by inadequate dry vermilion at the central tubercle can be addressed by advancing lateral vermilion excess. A small laterally based triangular flap of vermilion is raised above the muscle. An incision is made along the red line medially. After any necessary muscle repair, the lateral triangular flap is inset into the medial incision.
- Alternatively, when wet mucosa is interposed in the vermilion, this may be excised with a vertical ellipse of this tissue. The mucosa is elevated on both sides to reduce tension. After muscle reconstruction or reinforcement, the mucosa is closed with the red line now in precise alignment.

Lateral Mucosa Fullness

- This is common after unilateral cleft lip repair. It can often be corrected by excising an ellipse of tissue from the mucosa.
- A transversely oriented ellipse addresses excess in the anteroposterior direction. This may be placed along the red line if there is an excess of both dry vermilion and mucosa (**TECH FIG 5**), or it may be hidden in the labial buccal sulcus if the excess is composed only of wet mucosa.
- Festooning of the lip suggests excess mucosa in the transverse direction. This should be addressed with a vertical ellipse of mucosa along the cleft scar.
- We find that often both ellipses are needed (**TECH FIG 6**). In these cases, both are marked and the closure is usually in the shape of a "T."

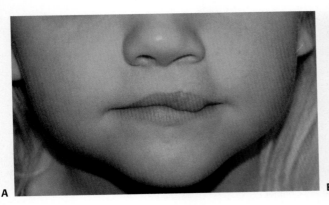

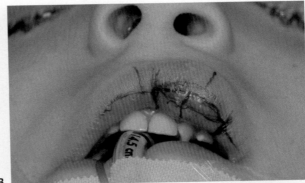

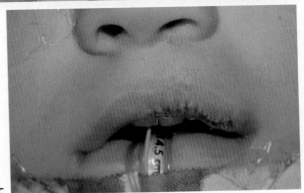

TECH FIG 5 • A. Lateral mucosal fullness is noted after unilateral cleft lip repair. **B.** The excess was primarily in the anteroposterior dimension. A transverse ellipse, centered on the red line, is marked for excision to address the region of excess. **C.** After excision and closure, the contour of the lip margin is improved.

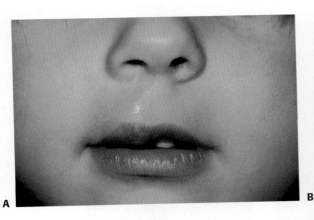

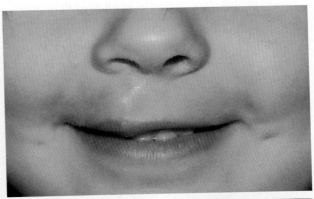

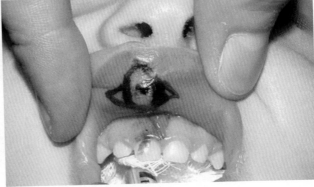

TECH FIG 6 • A. This child has lateral mucosa excess at rest and **(B)** with animation after unilateral cleft lip repair. **C.** On closer evaluation, the mucosal excess was felt to be in both the transverse direction and anteroposterior direction. For this reason, both a transverse ellipse and vertical ellipse were marked. The final closure will be in a "T" configuration along the cleft lip scar and in the buccal sulcus.

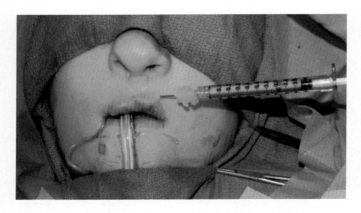

TECH FIG 7 • After fat is harvested from the lower abdomen, it is placed in 1-mL syringes for injection. This is typically injected via a fine fat grafting cannula or 18-gauge needle under the vermilion border.

Hypoplastic Medial or Lateral Lip Element

- In this case, soft tissue augmentation is required. Autograft, allograft, and synthetic tissue fillers have all been described. When possible, our preference is to use autograft either as a structural fat graft or dermal fat graft.
- Structural fat grafting may be used for secondary lip augmentation.
  - Autologous fat is harvested in the standard fashion from the lower abdomen and prepared according to the Coleman technique.
  - This can then be injected under the vermilion border using a very small cannula (**TECH FIG 7**).
  - Structural fat grafting is versatile. In addition to augmenting the vermilion, it may also be used to augment a deficient philtral column or nostril base.[6] Limitations with fat grafting include unpredictable resorption and

survival, as well as the risk of asymmetric hypertrophy with added weight gain over time.

- Autologous dermal fat graft is used when a larger augmentation is needed (**TECH FIG 8**).
  - The requisite size graft is typically harvested from the groin and de-epithelialized.
  - The graft is ideally positioned between the mucosa and muscle under the vermilion border and dry vermilion.
  - Two small counterincisions in the mucosa can be made to create a tunnel for the graft, which is passed with a tendon passer (**TECH FIG 8D**). Chromic sutures are placed on both ends of the graft prior to passing it through the tunnel. These are then used to anchor the graft into the appropriate location.
  - If a Z-plasty or V-Y advancement of the buccal sulcus tissue is planned in addition to augmentation, this

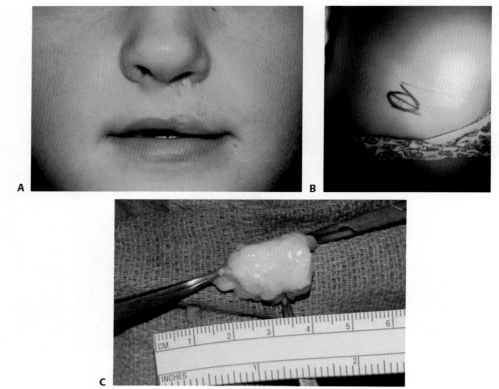

TECH FIG 8 • **A.** After unilateral cleft lip repair, this patient has an asymmetric free margin of the lip. She has mucosal excess on the left, with a relatively hypoplastic lip on the right side. Given the thin lip on the right side, augmentation with an autologous dermal fat graft was planned. **B.** Harvest from the right hip was planned, with the incision in a favorable location. **C.** The graft is de-epithelialized and thinned to the necessary size.

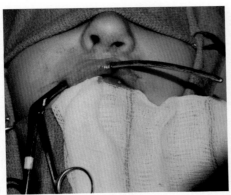
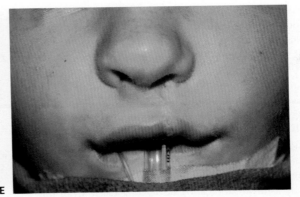

TECH FIG 8 (Continued) • **D.** In this case, a tunnel was made from the lateral commissure to the central lip. A tendon passer is used to introduce the graft into the planned location along the right lip. **E.** After graft inset, the lip thickness is more uniform across the upper lip.

flap is raised and the dermal fat graft may be placed directly and sutured into place (**TECH FIG 9**). We commonly use this strategy to augment the central tubercle in the bilateral cleft lip.

- Dermal allograft is an alternative to autologous tissue and may be used in a similar manner to a dermal fat graft.[7]

Notch in the Free Edge of the Lip or Whistle Deformity

- This may be caused by inadequate tissue, dehiscence of the orbicularis oris muscle, or scarring of the mucosa that leads to tethering or shortening of the lip.

- When scarring is present, the buccal mucosa may be lengthened by local tissue rearrangements or grafts, such as:
  - Mucosa Z-plasty
  - V-to-Y advancement of the buccal sulcus tissue
  - Transposition of a buccal mucosa flap[8]
  - Interposition of a buccal mucosal graft harvested from inside the lateral cheek
- When the cause is a deficiency of tissue rather than scarring, augmentation with autologous fat may be adequate.
  - For a mild deficiency, structural fat grafting may be used.
  - Elevation of a buccal flap and augmentation with dermal fat graft are used for a moderate-size defect (see **TECH FIG 9**).

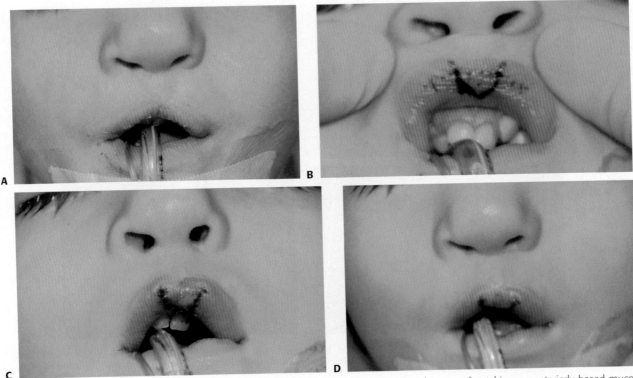

TECH FIG 9 • **A.** Persistent central vermilion deficiency after bilateral cleft lip repair. **B.** In the area of notching, an anteriorly based mucosa flap is designed. The flap and surrounding mucosa are elevated from the orbicularis muscle, and a dermal fat graft is positioned in the region of deficiency. **C,D.** After augmentation with a dermal fat graft, the fullness of the central tubercle fullness is improved.

- In more significant cases, or when vermilion deficiency is associated with a widened philtrum and nasal base, complete revision of the repair may be performed to recruit additional lateral mucosa into the defect (see **TECH FIG 4**).

- In severe cases, usually after bilateral cleft lip repair, the whistle deformity may require reconstruction with an Abbe flap (see below).
- The orbicularis oris muscle must be reconstructed in all cases.

■ Abbe Flap

- The bilateral cleft lip often is accompanied by a deficiency of mucosa as well as a shortened philtrum. Furthermore, horizontal lip deficiency may limit the ability to reconstruct the central tubercle by borrowing tissue from the lateral lip elements.
- For these severe whistle deformities (**TECH FIG 10A**), an Abbe flap may provide the best option for reconstruction of the entire philtral unit.[9,10]
- The patient is nasally intubated in preparation for surgery (**TECH FIG 10B**).
- If the patient is in braces, tight elastics are placed to prevent full mouth opening after surgery. Alternatively, intermaxillary fixation screws may be placed with tight elastics or wires.
- The flap is designed in the midline of the lower lip (**TECH FIG 10C**). The length and width of the new philtrum are designed and drawn onto the lower lip. The flap tapers slightly toward midline as it approaches the labiomental crease. Darts are made at the labiomental crease to address the donor site "dog ear" at closure.

- The vermilion border and white roll are marked and tattooed on the lower lip.
- The flap is incised full-thickness through the skin, muscle, and mucosa on one side (**TECH FIG 10D**). During this dissection, the location of the labial artery is noted, so that this area is well preserved on the contralateral side. A Doppler may be used to confirm the pedicle location if there is prior scarring in the area.
- The remainder of the flap is dissected with preservation of the labial artery. A small muscular cuff is preserved around the artery. The composite flap is then able to be rotated a full 180 degrees.
- The lower lip incision is closed in layers. The mucosa is repaired with 4-0 chromic gut, the lower lip orbicularis oris muscle is repaired with 3-0 Monocryl sutures, and the skin is closed with 5-0 Monocryl sutures in the dermis and 6-0 nylon in the skin.
- The critical points of the upper lip are marked. The columella, vermilion border, and white roll are marked and tattooed. The scarred prolabium is marked for excision.

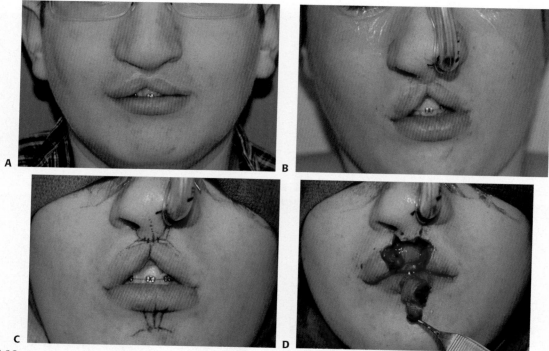

TECH FIG 10 • A. Bilateral cleft lip with significant whistle deformity composed of deficiency of mucosa, vermilion, and philtrum. On worm's-eye view, the patient also has a severely shortened columella. **B.** Preparation for Abbe flap includes nasal intubation. This patient's braces were used for intermaxillary fixation with heavy elastics. **C.** The Abbe flap is planned and marked in the midline of the lower lip. The flap is measured to the desired length and width of the new philtrum. The length is limited by the location of the labiomental crease, but this crease is used to accommodate any dog ear at closure. The columella, scarred philtrum, and new high points of Cupid's bow are marked. The high points of Cupids bow are marked to match the length and fullness of the lower lip flap. **D.** The central upper lip defect is created and the orbicularis oris muscle is dissected out for repair. The lower lip Abbe flap is cut full thickness through skin, muscle, and mucosa. One side remains pedicled on the labial artery.

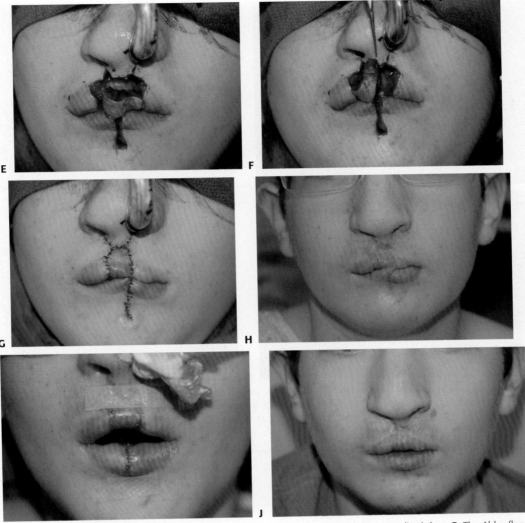

TECH FIG 10 (Continued) • **E,F.** The Abbe flap is able to be rotated a full 180 degrees into the upper lip defect. **G.** The Abbe flap is inset with care taken to align Cupid's bow and the lower lip vermilion border. **H.** After 10 to 14 days, the flap is well healed and ready for division. The lip pedicle may be compressed to ensure there has been adequate vascular ingrowth. **I.** The mucosal bridge is divided, and the mucosa is repaired. Silicone tape is applied to the cutaneous portions of the scars to optimize healing. **J.** Several months after surgery, the patient has improved lip contour and increased philtral length.

- The new high point of Cupid's bow is selected. This is ideally at a height that matches the new philtral column created by the Abbe flap. Furthermore, this point is selected such that the thickness of the upper lip mucosa matches the lower lip tissue bulk to achieve a smooth mucosal contour.
- Prior to incising the upper lip, 0.25% bupivacaine is infiltrated as bilateral infraorbital nerve blocks. Epinephrine may be infiltrated into the upper lip tissues.
- The cutaneous incisions are made with a no. 15 blade, and the prolabial scarring is excised. The upper lip is divided at 90 degrees to the white roll and vermilion. The orbicularis oris muscle is dissected and preserved.
- Buccal mucosal incisions are made bilaterally to advance the lateral lip medially toward the new philtrum. The lateral lip is advanced and the buccal mucosa backcut is closed with 4-0 chromic gut suture.
- After the defect has been created, the Abbe flap is rotated to fill the defect (**TECH FIG 10E,F**). The mucosa is inset with 4-0 chromic gut to the lateral lip elements.

- The orbicularis oris muscle of the upper lip is then repaired to the muscle of the Abbe flap.
- The vermilion and white roll are aligned at the previously tattooed points, and the remainder of the skin and mucosa is inset (**TECH FIG 10G**).
- During the inset, the color of the Abbe flap is monitored to ensure the flap remains adequately perfused. If perfusion is compromised, routine maneuvers for flap ischemia are taken, such as release of tension, replacement of flap to donor site, hyperbaric oxygen, etc.
- Flap division is performed 10 to 14 days later (**TECH FIG 10H–J**). After division, the mucosa of the upper and lower lip is closed with 5-0 chromic gut sutures.
- The vermilion Abbe flap may be modified from this pattern to address a severe defect of the mucosa only (**TECH FIG 11**). This eliminates the need for cutaneous scarring while augmenting a severe deficiency of tissue at the central tubercle.

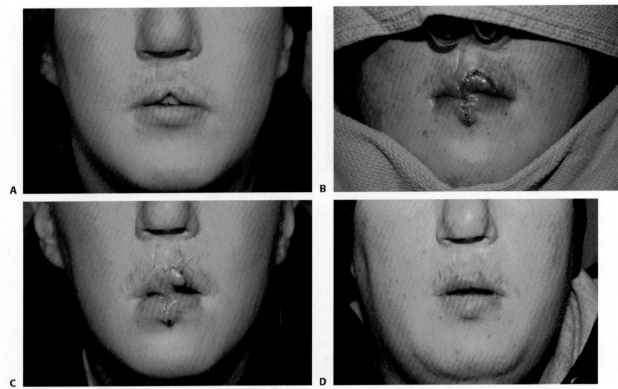

TECH FIG 11 • A. In some cases, the philtral length is adequate, but the deficiency of vermilion is so severe that Abbe flap is considered. **B.** In this case, however, the Abbe flap is designed to stay within the mucosa and does not cross the vermilion on either the upper or lower lip. **C.** Two weeks later, the flap is ready for division. **D.** After several months, the mucosa is well healed with a significant improvement in upper lip contour.

■ Lip Pits

- Lip pits are commonly associated with cleft lip and palate in van der Woude syndrome. Most lip pits occur on the lower lip as paired structures lateral to midline; however, midline pits on the upper or lower lip are also possible. They can range from slight depressions to deep tracts lined with epithelium.[11]
- The tracts are associated with serous or mucous glands along their course and track toward the labiogingival sulcus.
- Excision must include management of the mucosal deformity as well as removal of the entirety of the tract.
- The orbicularis oris muscle may need to be reconstructed after excision of the tract.
- A lacrimal probe is used to assess the course and depth of the tract. Methylene blue is then injected into the tract with an angiocatheter to mark the tract.
- The mucosal excision is planned to optimize contour. Authors have described multiple different approaches to address the concerns with mucosal contour.

Simple Transverse Elliptical Excision of the Pit and Tract

- In this technique, a transverse ellipse is designed around each pit (**TECH FIG 12A,B**).

- Dissection is carried down around the tract until it is completely excised, using the lacrimal probe to guide the excision.
- The orbicularis oris muscle is reconstructed with 4-0 Vicryl sutures.
- The mucosa is closed using interrupted 5-0 chromic gut sutures (**TECH FIG 12C**).
- Simple excision may be adequate when a single lip pit is present or when lip pits are small and shallow.
  - Multiple deep pits may result in contour abnormalities of the lower lip.

Vertical Elliptical Wedge Excision

- A full-thickness vertical elliptical wedge of the lower lip is designed. This wedge extends to the mucosa internally and crosses the vermilion border onto the skin externally (**TECH FIG 13**).
- The lacrimal probe is used to verify that the sinus tract is contained within the wedge. The wedge is excised full thickness.
- The orbicularis oris muscle is repaired.
- The mucosa, vermilion border, and skin are closed.
- Though this technique may lead to a smoother contour of the lower lip, the scarring on the skin of the lower lip is a major drawback.

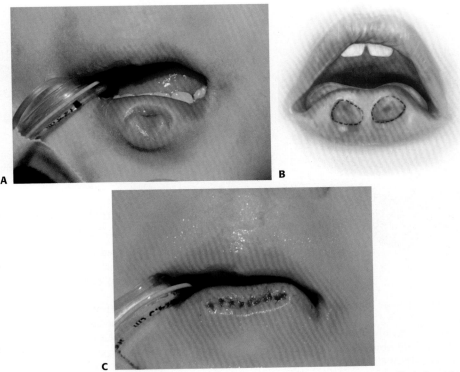

TECH FIG 12 • A. Central lower lip pit in a child with van der Woude syndrome. **B.** Simple transverse elliptical excision. **C.** After simple transverse elliptical excision of the lip pit.

Split Lip Advancement Technique (SLAT)[12]

- In SLAT, the pits and tracts are excised in a central wedge of tissue from the vermilion border to the gingivobuccal sulcus.
- The lip is then split from the central incision to a point near the commissure.
- An incision is made along the vermilion border through the pars marginalis. This incision is then carried vertically and inferiorly in a plane between the orbicularis oris muscle and the submucosa (**TECH FIG 14**).
  - The labial artery is preserved within this posterior mucosa flap with the pars marginalis, whereas the skin

and majority of the orbicularis oris muscle are maintained in the anterior flap.
- The posterior mucosa flap is advanced toward the midline, and the orbicularis oris muscle is reconstructed.
- Skin and mucosa closure is in a T from the midline along the vermilion border anteriorly.

Inverted-T Excision[13]

- The lip pits are both included in a large transverse ellipse. The outer edge of this ellipse is parallel to the white roll, which helps to maintain a constant thickness of vermilion.

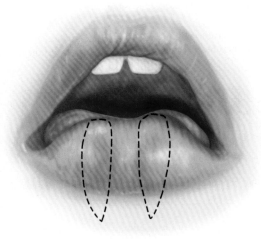

TECH FIG 13 • Vertical wedge excision of lower lip pits.

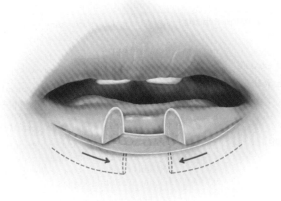

TECH FIG 14 • SLAT technique for lower lip pits.

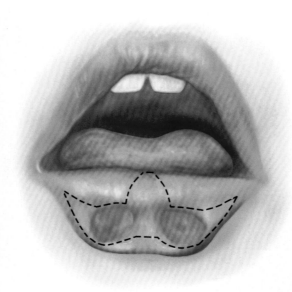

TECH FIG 15 • Inverted-T excision of lower lip pits.

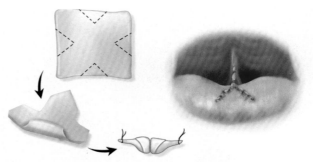

TECH FIG 16 • V-Y mucosal flap with use of dermal allograft for augmentation.

- Centrally, the ellipse meets a vertical inferior wedge that extends from the lip pits laterally toward the midline of the lower labiobuccal sulcus (**TECH FIG 15**).
- Using the lacrimal probe to identify the sinus tracts, these are fully excised within the vertical wedge of tissue.
- The vertical wedge is excised, and the orbicularis oris muscle is reconstructed.
- The transverse wedge is closed with chromic gut sutures.

Excision and Reconstruction of Lower Lip Fullness With Acellular Dermal Allograft[14]

- A large central V-shaped mucosal flap is designed with the apex in the midline of the inferior gingivobuccal sulcus. The lateral arms of the flap include ellipses that excise the lip pits.
- The pits and tracts are fully excised, and the orbicularis oris muscle is reconstructed.
- To restore fullness to the lower lip, an acellular dermal allograft, structural fat grafting, or autogenous dermal fat grafts are utilized to create a natural shape for augmentation (**TECH FIG 16**).
  - This is placed under the V-shaped mucosal flap and sutured into place with 4-0 Vicryl sutures at each commissure.
- The mucosa is closed as a V-to-Y advancement flap with chromic sutures.

PEARLS AND PITFALLS

Etiology of deformities	■ Some secondary cleft lip deformities are intrinsic to the disease. ■ Others are iatrogenic from the primary repair. Care must be taken to create a balanced lip and nose with release and repositioning of the lower lateral cartilage on the cleft side and complete reconstruction of the orbicularis oris muscle sling at the *first* operation to minimize the risk of iatrogenic deformities.
Analysis	■ Accuracy in analyzing the problem is essential. One must identify the underlying anatomic cause of the deformity in order to accurately reconstruct it. ■ Assess the entire lip/nose complex in planning your reconstruction. ■ Assessment must include all tissues from the underlying bony skeleton, mucosa, muscle, skin, cartilage, and soft tissue.
The repair must match the deformity.	■ Minor deformities may be addressed with minor scar revisions and insertion of triangular flaps. ■ A more complex deformity involving multiple elements is best treated by a complete revision of the lip and nose repair.
Mucosa excess	■ This may often be resolved by direct excision.
Mucosa deficiency	■ A minor deficiency of the central tubercle may be addressed by creation of a laterally based vermilion triangular flap, which can be inset in the central tubercle medially. ■ A larger deficiency of lip soft tissue can be treated by various techniques including autologous structural fat grafting, autologous dermal fat graft, or allograft.
Abbe flap	■ An Abbe flap is best used to reconstruct a deficiency of all tissues of the central lip unit—philtral skin, vermilion, muscle, and mucosa. ■ This treats the most severe forms of lip notching that cannot be addressed adequately by local flaps and augmentation alone.
Lip pits	■ The entire pit and epithelialized tract must be excised. ■ Reconstruction requires repair of the orbicularis oris muscle and reconstruction of the mucosa to achieve a natural lower lip contour.

POSTOPERATIVE CARE

- Antibiotic ointment is typically applied to the incision until it is healed.
- Patients often may resume their usual diet.
- With young children, elbow restraints may be used to keep the child from putting the hands in the mouth or traumatizing the incision.
- Special care is taken to optimize cutaneous scar healing after surgery.
  - When cutaneous absorbable sutures are used, we ensure that they have absorbed by 4 to 5 days postoperatively. We apply diluted hydrogen peroxide to them several times daily to speed this process along to avoid track marks from the sutures.
  - Permanent sutures are removed within 5 days after surgery to avoid scarring.
  - Once the wound margins have healed, silicone tape is applied to the scar. It is changed every few days and used continuously for approximately 3 months.
  - Patients and families are educated on techniques in scar massage and avoidance of sun exposure for the first year after surgery.
  - If hypertrophy is noted in the early postoperative period, consideration is given to applying steroid-impregnated tape or performing steroid injections with triamcinolone.

OUTCOMES

- Outcomes after correction of secondary deformity are usually good.
- Depending on the severity of the deformity, asymmetry or contour abnormalities can be persistent.
- The degree of residual deformity and patient level of concern typically dictate whether additional revision surgeries are recommended.

COMPLICATIONS

- Inadequate correction of the deformity may be caused by an incorrect diagnosis and treatment plan, such as performing a minimal excision when a complete revision is necessary.
- Hypertrophic scarring is possible, and attempts are made to minimize it as described.
- Wound dehiscence and infection are rare.
- Intraoperative complications such as bleeding or anesthesia concerns are rare.

REFERENCES

1. Sitzman TJ, Coyne SM, Britto MT. The burden of care for children with unilateral cleft lip: a systematic review of revision surgery. *Cleft Palate Craniofac J.* 2016;53:84-94.
2. Rogers CR, Meara JG, Mulliken JB. The philtrum in cleft lip: review of anatomy and techniques for construction. *J Craniofac Surg.* 2014;25:9-13.
3. Li W, Steinbacher DM. Unilateral cleft lip revision with conversion to the modified inferior triangle. *Plast Reconstr Surg.* 2015;136:353e-361e.
4. Mulliken JB. Double unilimb Z-plastic repair of microform cleft lip. *Plast Reconstr Surg.* 2005;116:1623-1632.
5. Fisher DM. Unilateral cleft lip repair: an anatomical subunit approximation technique. *Plast Reconstr Surg.* 2005;116:61-71.
6. Jones CM, Morrow BT, Albright WB, et al. Structural fat grafting to improve reconstructive outcomes in secondary cleft lip deformity. *Cleft Palate Craniofac J.* 2017;54(1):70-74.
7. Attar BM, Haghighat A, Naghdi N, et al. Acellular dermal graft in secondary cleft lip deficiencies: assessment of results with a reproducible quantitative technique. *J Craniofac Surg.* 2016;27:313-316.
8. Lee SW, Kim MH, Baek RM. Correction of secondary vermilion notching deformity in unilateral cleft lip patients: complete revision of two errors. *J Craniomaxillofac Surg.* 2011;39:326-329.
9. Cannon B, Murray JE. Further observations on the use of the split vermilion bordered flap. *Plast Reconstr Surg.* 1953;11:497-501.
10. Cutting CB, Warren SM. Extended Abbe flap for secondary correction of the bilateral cleft lip. *J Craniofac Surg.* 2013;24:75-78.
11. Van der Woude A. Fistula labii inferioris congenital and its association with cleft lip and palate. *Am J Hum Genet.* 1954;6:244-256.
12. Mutaf M, Sensoz O, Ustuner ET. The split-lip advancement technique (SLAT) for the treatment of congenital sinuses of the lower lip. *Plast Reconstr Surg.* 1993;92:615-620.
13. Chen CH, Liao HT, Shyu VB, Chen PK. Inverted-T lip reduction for lower lip repair in Van der Woude syndrome: a review and comparison of aesthetic results. *Int J Oral Maxillofac Surg.* 2013;42:198-203.
14. Bozkurt M, Kulahci Y, Zor F, et al. Reconstruction of the lower lip in Van der Woude syndrome. *Ann Plast Surg.* 2009;62:451-455.

7

CHAPTER

Delayed Hard Palate Repair in UCLP Patients

Jan Lilja

DEFINITION

- In UCLP patients, the cleft palate will lead to speech difficulties.
- Poor ventilation of the Eustachian tubes results in a high incidence of hearing problems due to middle ear infection.
- Early surgery on the palate may result in reduced maxillary growth.
- Late surgery on the palate may result in aberrant speech.

ANATOMY

- The palate can be thought of as an anterior bony part limited by the dental arch and a posterior mobile part where muscles, oral mucosa, and nasal mucosa are important functional structures.
- The anterior palate (hard palate) is a horseshoe-formed bony structure concave toward the mouth and convex toward the nose where it forms the nasal floor. Both sides are covered by mucosal epithelium.
- The muscles in the posterior part (soft palate) will act on the soft palate and produce tension, lifting, or lowering of the soft palate. Lifting of the soft palate is most important and is accomplished by the levator veli palatini muscles. In speech, the soft palate should be lifted as far back as the posterior pharyngeal wall and be able to stop airflow through the nose in order to produce distinct pronunciation of certain sounds.

PATHOGENESIS

- In a complete cleft of a unilateral cleft lip and palate, a cleft separates the lip, the alveolar bone, and the hard and soft palate. The lateral incisor on the cleft side is usually missing in both deciduous and permanent dentition. The cleft separates the hard palate lateral to the vomer, establishing a cleft side and a noncleft side in the hard palate where the vomer is attached to the noncleft side. The soft palate is separated in the midline, but the cleft side is usually smaller.
- Feeding is often difficult for the child because there is an opening between the oral and nasal cavity. Food may pass into the nasal cavity and sucking is compromised because adequate negative pressure cannot be achieved during breast-feeding.
- In the soft palate, the muscles are not attached to each other; the muscles follow an anteroposterior direction along the cleft edges. Some of the muscles are attached to the posterior edge of the hard palate on both sides of the cleft.
  - This morphological aberration impairs development of speech and hinders ventilation of the Eustachian tube.

IMAGING AND OTHER DIAGNOSTIC STUDIES

- The diagnosis of a patient with complete unilateral cleft lip and palate is usually made by clinical examination.
- Photographs taken from anterior, lateral, and inferior views can be taken to document the condition.
- In some centers, plaster casts are made from both upper and lower jaws.
- Postoperatively, the patients are followed on a regular basis with photos, speech evaluation, cephalometric assessment, and plaster casts.
- When needed for evaluation of velopharyngeal incompetence (VPI), nasendoscopy and videofluoroscopy can be used.

SURGICAL MANAGEMENT

- There are numerous protocols for operating on the palatal cleft in patients with complete cleft lip and palate. These protocols differ in procedure and timing.
  - Early surgery of the soft palate is a prerequisite for good speech, but combined with closure of the hard palate, it will produce reduction of maxillary growth.
  - Closure of the whole palate at an older age will give less problems with maxillary growth but may give more problems with impaired speech.
- When delayed hard palate repair is performed in UCLP patients, soft palate closure is performed early to promote speech, and hard palate closure is delayed until 2 years of age to promote growth. The palatal closure is continued over to the oral side, where a pushback procedure can be done within the soft palate.
- Closure of the soft palate with a posteriorly based vomer flap will result in anchorage of the anterior part of the soft palate to the base of the vomer flap.
  - This part of vomer is situated at the insertion of the vomer to the cranial base. The direction of the soft palate will therefore be posterior-upward, resulting in reduction of the openings toward the nose.
  - This may explain the favorable speech results in our patients, improving the posterior positioning of the levator muscles and thereby reducing VPI.

Positioning

- The patient is positioned supine on the operating table.
- A shoulder roll is placed, serving to tilt the head backward to facilitate visualization.

Soft Palate Repair

- Incisions begin around the posterior part of the maxillary tuberosities and then follow a zigzag route at the posterior border of the hard palate (**TECH FIG 1A**).
- A posteriorly based vomer flap is dissected, which does not reach the vomero-premaxillary suture anteriorly. The base of the flap lies at the junction of the vomer with the cranial base (**TECH FIG 1B**).
- Mucosal flaps in the soft palate are raised by blunt dissection. The hamulus is identified but not broken (**TECH FIG 1C**).

- The insertions of the velar muscles and the nasal mucosa at the posterior border of the hard palate are cut (**TECH FIG 1D**).
- A flap with the muscles attached to the nasal layer is then dissected free and mobilized.
- The palatal muscles, including the levators, are then reconstructed to a transverse course at the level of the opening of the Eustachian tube (**TECH FIG 1E**).
- The vomer flap is raised, and the nasal layer of velum can be closed anteriorly to the level of the muscular sling by use of the vomer flap. In this way, the vomer bone is connected to the anterior velum (**TECH FIG 1E**).

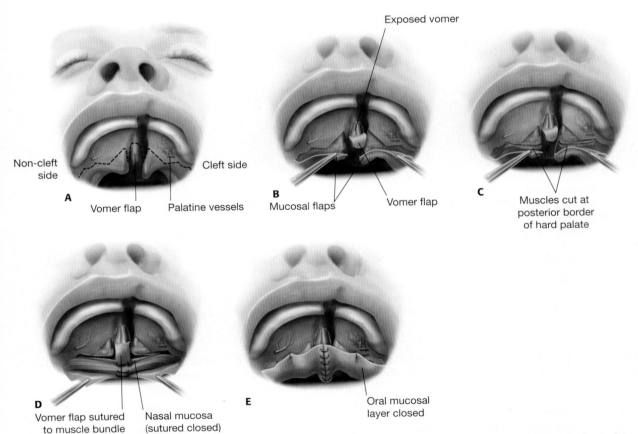

TECH FIG 1 • Soft palate closure. **A.** The incisions follow a zigzag line between the soft and hard palate. A posterior vomer flap is dissected, which has its base at the posterior-cranial part of the vomer. **B.** Both sides of velum are divided into two layers: the oral mucosa and the nasal mucosa. **C.** The muscles including the nasal mucosa are cut at the border of the hard palate. **D.** The muscles are redirected to a transverse course, sutured together medially in a posterior position, and also attached anteriorly to the backward-turned vomer flap. **E.** The muscles and the raw surface of the vomer flap are covered by the oral flaps, which are pushed in a medial-posterior direction.

Hard Palate Repair

- Incision lines are made for a flap on the noncleft side using palatal mucoperiosteum. The flap is based on the vomer (vomer flap). On the cleft side, an incision is made at the cleft border (**TECH FIG 2A**).

- The vomer flap is raised leaving a raw bone surface on the noncleft side (**TECH FIG 2B**).
- Suturing starts on the oral mucosa, going into the pocket between the bone and the mucoperiosteum. The needle catches the vomer flap from the mucosal side, coming out on the raw side, going back to the mucosal side and

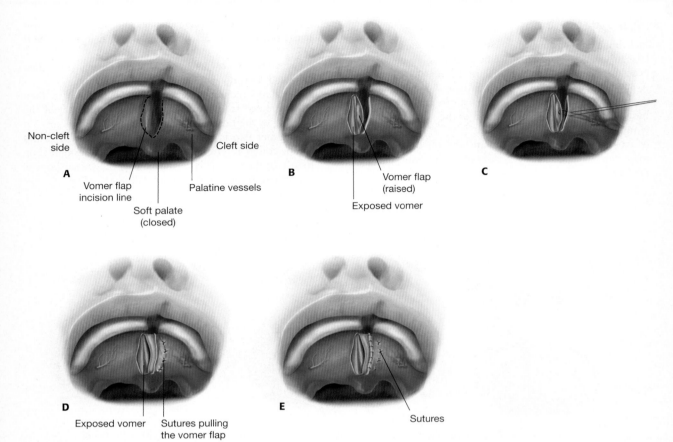

TECH FIG 2 • Repair of a residual cleft in the hard palate. **A.** Incision lines. On the noncleft side, the incision goes into the flat medial part of the palate. On the cleft side, the incision is made at the cleft border between the oral and nasal mucosa. **B.** The vomer flap is raised. It contains some oral mucosa leaving a raw bone surface in the medial part of the palate on the noncleft side. Sutures are put to bring the vomer flap into the incision on the cleft side. **C.** The vomer flap is brought into the pocket between bone and mucoperiosteum on the cleft side. Suturing starts on the oral mucosa going into the pocket between the bone and the mucoperiosteum. The needle catches the vomer flap from the mucosal side, coming out on the raw side and then going back to the mucosal side and thereafter into the pocket and out in the mucosa. Pulling the suture will bring the vomer flap into the pocket between the bone and the mucoperiosteum. Four or five sutures are placed. **D.** The vomer flap sutured in place. **E.** The mucoperiosteum on the cleft side is sutured to the vomer flap in order to ensure good attachment.

thereafter into the pocket and out on the mucosal side. Therefore, the knots are tied on the mucosal side (**TECH FIG 2C**).

■ Four to five such sutures are placed.
■ Pulling the suture will bring the vomer flap into the pocket between the bone and the mucoperiosteum (**TECH FIG 2D**).
■ When the vomer flap is well positioned under the mucoperiosteum of the cleft side, sutures are tied, keeping the

vomer flap in place and also covering the residual cleft with a one layer closure (**TECH FIG 2E**).

■ Additional sutures are put at the border of the cleft, keeping the raw surface of the vomer flap attached to the raw surface of the mucoperiosteum on the cleft side, thereby ensuring good healing (**TECH FIG 2E**).

PEARLS AND PITFALLS

Diagnostic studies	■ Nasendoscopy and videofluoroscopy are reserved postoperatively for cases demonstrating persistent VPI following palate repair.
Rationale for delayed hard palate repair	■ Delayed hard palate repair is done to optimize both speech and palatal growth. ■ Soft palate closure is performed early to promote speech. ■ Hard palate closure is delayed until 2 y of age to promote growth.
Posteriorly based vomer flap for soft palate closure	■ Base of the flap lies at the junction of the vomer with the cranial base and does not extend anteriorly to the vomero-palatine suture. ■ Results in anchorage of the anterior part of the soft palate to the base of the vomer flap ■ Improves the posterior positioning of the levator muscles and thereby reducing VPI
Soft palate repair	■ Insertions of the velar muscles and the nasal mucosa at the posterior border of the hard palate are cut. ■ The nasomuscular flaps are reconstructed to a transverse course at the level of the opening of the Eustachian tube. ■ The nasal layer of the nasomuscular flap is connected anteriorly to the vomer flap.
Hard palate repair	■ Closure is performed with a mucoperiosteal vomer flap raised from the noncleft side and sutured to the mucoperiosteum at medial edge of the cleft side. ■ Lateral mucoperiosteal dissection is avoided to minimize subsequent restriction of maxillary growth.
Outcomes	■ Long-term outcomes for both speech and growth have not been surpassed by any other surgical procedure for palate closure.

OUTCOMES

■ Long-term growth and speech outcome are excellent in patients with two-stage palatoplasty with early soft palate repair and delayed hard palate repair.[1,2]

■ Results from growth studies and speech evaluation have not been surpassed by any other surgical procedure for palate closure.

REFERENCES

1. Friede H, Lilja J, Lohmander A. Long-term, longitudinal follow-up of individuals with UCLP after the Gothenburg primary early veloplasty and delayed hard palate closure protocol: maxillofacial growth outcome. *Cleft Palate Craniofac J.* 2012;49(6 suppl):649-656.
2. Lohmander A, Friede H, Lilja J. Long-term, longitudinal follow-up of individuals with unilateral cleft lip and palate after the Gothenburg primary early veloplasty and delayed hard palate closure protocol: speech outcome. *Cleft Palate Craniofac J.* 2012;49(6 suppl):657-671.

8
CHAPTER

Furlow Palatoplasty

T. Guy Thorburn

DEFINITION

- Furlow Palatoplasty is widely used technique for repair of either cleft palate (CP) or submucous cleft palate (SMCP). It can also be used in revision palate repair. Some surgeons who routinely use a Sommerlad repair for complete CP will instead use a Furlow for SMCP.
- The technique is based on the concept of lengthening the soft palate by use of "Double-opposing Z-plasties." This involves mirror-image Z-plasties to the oral and nasal layers while also retropositioning and reconstructing the levator muscle mechanism by keeping the levator palatini muscle on each side attached to the limb of the Z-plasty that moves posteriorly (**FIG 1**).[1]
- Randall has described a variation for wider CP that involves using Langenbeck-type lateral releasing incisions to relieve the tension on the oral Z-plasty (**FIG 2**).[2]

ANATOMY

- The key functional issue in CP or SMCP is that the levator muscle mechanism is not in continuity on the two sides. In addition, the fibers become tethered to the posterior border of the hard palate. Successful functional palate repair therefore requires repair of the "levator sling" as well as just closure of the tissues across the cleft.
- The tethering to the hard palate seems to be an equal problem in differing types of cleft, whether unilateral or bilateral cleft lip and palate, cleft palate only, or SMCP.
- **Tip:** the oral layer of the soft palate is more elastic than the nasal layer, and the elasticity increases as you move from

the hard palate–soft palate junction toward the uvula. This means that the oral layer Z-plasty will tend to inset better with slightly wider flaps (closer to 80–90 degrees), whereas for the nasal layer, 60 degrees is sufficient. On the oral layer, the tissue elasticity is even greater in the posterior part of the palate, so the posterior limb is best designed slightly wider (around 90 degrees) as it will narrow after incision.

PATIENT HISTORY AND PHYSICAL FINDINGS

- The initial assessment of the newborn with a cleft involving a palate would usually be alongside a pediatrician and will include:
  - Pregnancy and birth history (including information from any antenatal testing), gestation, birth weight, and Apgar scores.
  - Initial assessment of cleft type and any related anomalies, including any airway concerns suggesting Robin sequence.
  - Medical history, drug history, and allergy history.
  - Family history of clefts, other major health problems, or anesthetic problems and any genetic diagnosis.
  - Feeding history including bottle type (eg, squeezy bottle, free flow, Haberman, etc.), current weight, maximum percentage weight loss and number of days to regain birth weight, and volume/duration/frequency of feeds.
  - Physical examination to assess the upper airways, cleft type, cleft width, and how much deficiency there is of surrounding tissues, as well as any related anomalies or

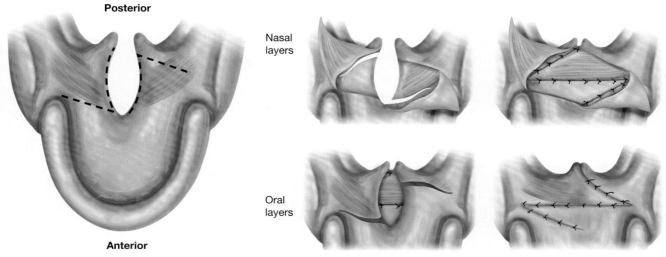

FIG 1 • Schematic diagrams of the Z-plasties of both oral and nasal layers before and after inset.

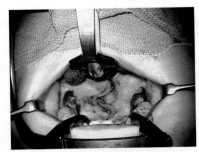

FIG 2 • The variation described by Randall utilizing lateral releasing incisions (von Langenbeck) for wider or more complete cleft palate.

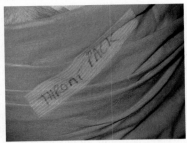

FIG 3 • Applying a sticker across the head drapes as a warning that the throat pack is in place, so that the drapes cannot be removed without first removing the sticker.

dysmorphic features. The pediatrician would then complete a fully newborn examination, looking in particular for related health issues such as cardiac, respiratory, renal, or neurological signs.

IMAGING

- No routine preoperative imaging is required for typical clefts. For older children presenting with SMCP or velopharyngeal incompetence (VPI), assessment with a speech lateral videofluoroscopy helps to assess the position of the levators and relative size of the soft palate to the size of the pharynx.
- Standardized preoperative clinical photos should be taken as these are invaluable when assessing outcomes many years later.

SURGICAL MANAGEMENT

Preoperative Planning

- A key aspect of successful cleft palate repair is in optimizing the patient prior to surgery. A pediatrician is a crucial member of the Cleft team. Although there is much discussion of age at palate repair, different team protocols vary from around 3 months old to 15 months or more. Very young babies will tend to be more susceptible to airway compromise around the time of surgery. Delaying repair until much older and speech has developed has been associated with poorer speech outcomes, particularly related to articulatory errors.
- **Tip:** our team protocol is for palate repair around 8 to 12 months (corrected for prematurity), but our emphasis is much more on ensuring the child is well and thriving in the run-up to surgery. If they are not growing along their expected percentiles (with growth plotted on the appropriate chart for syndromic children), then we would want to address this before surgery. We will also routinely postpone for about 4 weeks if children have upper respiratory tract infections. By following this approach, we have seen a significant reduction in fistulae and concerns with speech function.
- Routine blood tests or cross match samples are not required, unless the child is known to have a specific risk factor.
- For children, with cardiac or respiratory problems, an up-to-date echocardiogram or sleep study may be relevant.

Positioning

- A south-facing Rae uncuffed or microcuffed tube is used. The taping of the tube needs to be secure but avoiding taping the mouth closed or limiting access. Taping in a V shape along the line of the mandible avoids displacing the tapes when the gag is opened.
- The child is placed supine on a warming blanket, with the head at the very end of the operating table. A large horseshoe

gel head ring is placed under the shoulders and around the head to provide support without overextending the neck.

- A head drape is applied, and the face is prepped.
- **Tip:** we use a clear plastic drape [3M Steri-Drape Fluoroscope Drape 90 ×110 cm] over the trunk, which allows the anesthetist to see their endotracheal tube and circuit without disturbing the surgical field. We avoid any adhesive drapes near the endotracheal tube as these have the potential to catch and dislodge the airway.
- The table is tilted to a slight head-up position. An operating microscope is used for the procedure. The height of the table is adjusted once the microscope has been brought in to place (adjusted according to whether the surgeon prefers to sit or stand).
- A modified Dingman mouth gag is placed.
- A throat pack is placed, and a marker sticker put across the drapes as a reminder to ensure it is removed at the end. The sticker is placed so that the drapes cannot be removed without needing to disturb the warning sticker (**FIG 3**). The throat pack is also included in the scrub nurse count as an additional precaution.
- The nose and mouth are rinsed with aqueous chlorhexidine solution.

Approach

- The width of the cleft is measured, and any unusual features are noted.
- The incisions are marked with pen and ink. Depending on tissue condition and tension, the limbs of the oral Z are usually about 8 to 10 mm long. The angles are usually 80 to 90 degrees (slightly wider on the limb in the posterior soft palate) (**FIG 4**).
- **Tip:** for a right-handed surgeon, the oral layer Z is typically marked with the posteriorly based limb (where the muscle remains attached to the flap but has to be dissected from the nasal layer) on the left. This will tend to give the easiest access to the hardest part of the dissection.

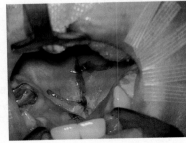

FIG 4 • Oral layer markings for a standard Furlow palatoplasty. Note the angles of the Z are wider than for the skin, approaching 80 to 90 degrees.

TECHNIQUES

■ Hard Palate

- Levobupivacaine or bupivacaine long-acting local anesthetic with adrenaline 1:100 000 is infiltrated and left about 7 to 8 minutes for vasoconstriction (**TECH FIG 1A**). The injection is used to help hydrodissect the hard palate subperiosteal layer.
- **Tip:** Steri-Strips are placed to protect the corners of the mouth from abrasion by instruments (**TECH FIG 1B**).
- The incision is begun along the cleft margin (or in the midline for a SMCP or rerepair).
- For clefts involving the hard palate, incise carefully down to the bone along the margin of the hard palate and 3 to 5 mm past the hard palate–soft palate junction and elevate

subperiosteally with a raspatory or Warwick-James elevator. Be careful approaching the posterior nasal spine as the tissues are more adherent here, and it is easy to tear the oral layer if there is a tethered salivary gland at this point. Switching between 15 blade and raspatory is usually necessary. **Tip:** for incising the margin of the rest of the soft palate and back to the uvula, a 12 blade tends to be easiest.
- Depending on the cleft type, it may be necessary to raise vomer flaps to help close the nasal layer without tension.
- After raising the vomer flaps, elevate the nasal layer off the hard palate (again in a subperiosteal plane) with a raspatory or dental flat plastic.

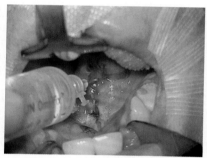
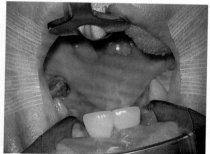

TECH FIG 1 • A. Infiltration of local anesthetic with a Luer-lock syringe, using the infiltration to hydrodissect. **B.** Steri-Strip "cat's whiskers" to protect the oral commissures during the procedure.

■ Oral layer

- A skin hook is placed on the left margin of the cleft, where the incision has been marked to create the posteriorly based flap. Using the skin hook to tension, a 15 blade is used to incise the oral layer and muscle, down to the nasal layer (which is left intact) (**TECH FIG 2A**).
- The muscle is then freed carefully from the nasal layer with the 15 blade and/or dissecting scissors. Keeping tension on the muscle toward the midline (rather than posteriorly or superiorly) makes this dissection easier without buttonholing the nasal layer.

- The muscle is freed off the nasal layer out toward the hamulus, so it is dissected more laterally than the extent of the oral layer incision.
- On the right side, the opposite flap is raised in a similar way but leaving the muscle intact on the nasal layer (**TECH FIG 2B,C**).
- **Tip:** after incising the leading edge of the posteriorly based oral flap and elevating the anteriorly based flap, then applying topical 1:1000 adrenaline on neuro patties provides excellent vasoconstriction and facilitates the subsequent dissection (**TECH FIG 2D,E**).

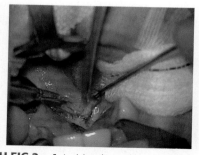
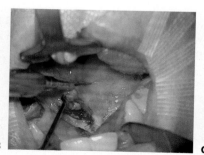
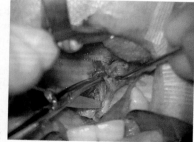

TECH FIG 2 • A. Incising the oral layer posteriorly based flap (the muscle and mucosa flap on the left side of the palate). **B.** Raising the oral layer anteriorly based flap (the mucosa-only flap on the right side of the palate). **C.** Spread dissection with scissors can be very useful for identifying the plane between the muscle and the mucosal flap.

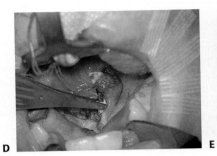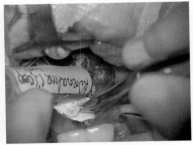

TECH FIG 2 (Continued) • **D,E.** After the initial dissection of the oral layer, topical 1:1000 adrenaline helps with the next stage of dissection by vasoconstricting. First, neurosurgical patties are placed in the wound to keep the solution in the desired area, and then 1 mL of 1:1000 adrenaline solution is dripped onto the patties.

■ Nasal layer

- To make access easier for the stage, a stay suture can be used to hold the oral flaps out of the way if the surgeon prefers, or the assistant can use a dental flat plastic or skin hook to do this (**TECH FIG 3A**).
- The nasal Z-plasty is a similar size to the oral layer. The angles are usually just over 60 degrees.
- On the nasal layer, the Z-plasty is a mirror image of the oral layer Z-plasty. At this stage, the muscle is present and attached to the nasal layer on the right side, while on the left, the nasal layer has already been dissected bare.
- A skin hook in the margin on the right side is used to place tension toward the midline. The posteriorly based flap is then raised by incising the nasal layer and muscle

together with a 15 blade and/or dissecting scissors (**TECH FIG 3B**). The nasal layer is kept adherent to the muscle (**TECH FIG 3C**).

- **Tip:** when incising the muscle/nasal layer on the right, plan to keep a rim of the tensor aponeurosis tissue intact. This makes it much easier to inset the contralateral flap during closure.
- As with the muscle on the oral layer, it is necessary to free the muscle more laterally than the limit of the nasal layer incision.
- Once the posteriorly based flap is fully mobilized, hold it across to the opposite side to check the position of the nasal layer–only flap (**TECH FIG 3D**).
- Then incise the anteriorly based nasal layer flap on the left side (**TECH FIG 3E, F**).

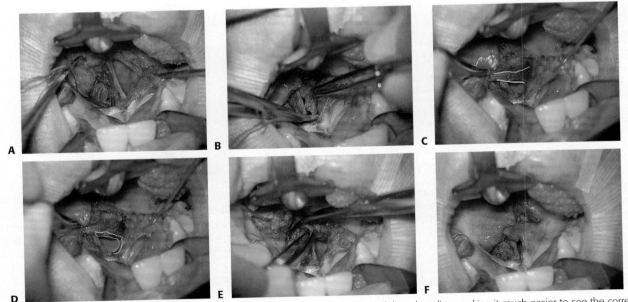

TECH FIG 3 • A. The longitudinal incision in the nasal layer. Note the effectiveness of the adrenaline, making it much easier to see the correct planes. **B.** Incising the posteriorly based nasal layer flap (the muscle and mucosa flap on the right of the palate). Gentle traction of the muscle bulk toward the midline, as opposed to lifting or posteriorly, allows clean incision with either scissors or 15 blade. **C.** As the flap is incised and retropositioned, the levator muscle (*marked*) comes into view on the nasal aspect of the other muscle fibers. **D.** Designing the flap in order to leave a rim of the tensor aponeurosis (*marked*) makes subsequent suturing of the flaps much easier. **E.** After checking the position with the right sided flap, the anteriorly based nasal layer flap is incised (the mucosa-only flap on the left side of the palate). **F.** Position of flaps at rest before inset. Assuming correct design of the flaps, they will tend to want to move toward their new positions, and the palate is already visibly lengthened.

■ Closure

- Start with the inset of the nasal flaps—it is usually easier to begin by insetting the posteriorly based flap. A resorbable monofilament suture is used, preferably with a round or tapercut needle to avoid inadvertent tears of the mucosa. We use 5-0 Monocryl plus on the nasal layer and 4-0 Monocryl on the oral layer (**TECH FIG 4A,B**).
- **Option:** although this technique provides good overlap of the muscle mass on two sides, it is worth noting that the two levator muscles are not directly opposed or joined. Some surgeons therefore choose to directly suture the levators as well. In this situation, first complete inset of the nasal layer. Then a 5-0 nylon suture is placed through the levator muscle which is visible on the

underside of the left oral layer flap. The oral flap is then held out to length to allow placement of the suture to pick up the levator muscle on the right side (**TECH FIG 4C**). This muscle is lying out of direct sight on the deep aspect of the muscle that is attached to the nasal layer on the right side (**TECH FIG 4D**).

- The oral flaps are then inset. McGregor corner sutures combined with Barron sutures to the flap edges allow the avoidance of knots or ischemic areas at the distal ends of the oral mucosal flaps (**TECH FIG 4E**). If the oral flaps appear too tight, they can be inset a little short with a raw area left laterally.
- The local anesthetic is topped up.
- The throat pack is removed.

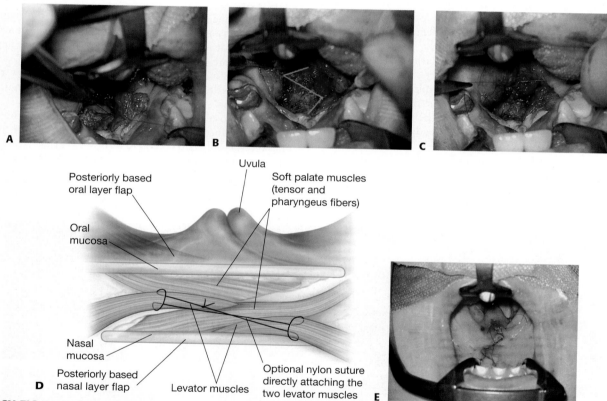

TECH FIG 4 • A. The nasal layer flaps are inset first; the rim of tensor aponeurosis makes suturing the nasal layer easier. **B.** The position of the nasal layer flaps after inset is complete. **C.** With inset of the nasal and oral layer posteriorly based flaps, the levator mechanism has been retropositioned. But in the classic Furlow, the two levator muscles are not directly connected, which can give an asymmetric lift of the palate. Therefore, some surgeons prefer to place permanent nylon mattress sutures directly connecting the two halves of levator. **D.** A schematic diagram of the soft palate in cross section to show the layers of the oral and nasal Z-plasties and the inset of the levator mechanism. **E.** The position of the oral layer flaps after inset is complete.

■ Alternative: Z-Plasty with Intravelar Veloplasty

- It is possible to use a hybrid of a Sommerlad and a Furlow approach. This can be particularly useful in SMCP.
- Preparation, draping, and hard palate are the same as above.

- The oral layer is raised as per a Sommerlad repair but is marked out a Z-plasty as for a Furlow repair.
- Incision and retraction of the Z-plasty flaps can give easier access for the muscle dissection (radical intravelar veloplasty) which is the same as for a Sommerlad repair.

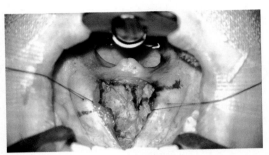

TECH FIG 5 • The marking for the nasal layer Z-plasty at the base of the uvula in the hybrid procedure.

- The muscle is dissected off the nasal layer on both sides.
- A Z-plasty is then made in the posterior 1/3 of the nasal layer (in a mirror image of the oral layer Z-plasty) (**TECH FIG 5**).
- **Tip:** a principle of Z-plasties is that increased length is achieved by redistributing tension in a lateral direction. Therefore, placement of the Z-plasty on the posterior 1/3 of the nasal layer, toward the base of the uvula, means that the lateral tightening achieved by the process of inset-ting the Z-plasty also tightens the velopharyngeal port.
- The muscles on the two sides are sutured with three 5-0 nylon mattress sutures, aiming to pick up both the leva-tor muscle and the tougher tensor aponeurotic tissue with each bite. The knots must be tied very carefully to allow the ends to be cut extremely short.
- The oral layer is then closed with inset of the Z-plasty.

PEARLS AND PITFALLS

Timing of surgery	■ Careful optimization of the baby prior to surgery is important; good growth following percentile lines is a use-ful indicator—a thriving baby at the time of surgery is more important than a specific age.
Shared airway	■ As with all "shared airway" surgery, it is important for the anesthetist and surgeon to communicate well with each other—the WHO checklist and team brief are very useful for this.
Operating microscope	■ The routine use of the operative microscope for palate repair gives excellent lighting and visualization of the operative field. It is also very helpful for giving trainees a better view and involvement, as well as reducing the strain on the surgeon's neck.
Postoperative elevation	■ Nursing the baby "head-up" in the recovery room and on the ward after surgery is helpful for reducing postop-erative swelling—cuddling the baby over the parent's shoulder tends to give ideal positioning.

POSTOPERATIVE CARE

- Topping up the local anesthesia with a long acting agent at the very end of the operation is useful for postoperative comfort and feeding.
- Nurse the baby with head elevated.
- Babies can be offered feeds straight away once they are awake.
- Monitor airway and saturations especially over the first night after surgery.

OUTCOMES

- The main outcome measures for cleft palate repair are fis-tula rate, structural speech problem rate, need for secondary surgery, and impact on maxillary growth.[3]
- There has been a systematic review comparing Furlow with straight-line repairs. This shows considerable variation in outcomes according to the cleft type. The average fistula rate ranged from 2.6% to 11.6% with different cleft types. The hypernasality rate (indicating structural speech problems) ranged from 8.9% to 18.5%, and the secondary surgery for speech rate ranged from 0% to 11.4%. There is a lack of data on the effect of maxillary growth from Furlow repairs, even though that was a starting focus in Furlow original description.[4]

COMPLICATIONS

- Infection, significant bleeding, and transfusion are all rare after palate surgery.
- Airway compromise is a potential risk especially in babies with Robin sequence and in younger/smaller babies.
- Fistula is reported to have a lower incidence than in some other techniques of palate repair in some series, but there is wide variation between series, and the extent and width of the cleft palate play a major factor in the fistula rate.
- Speech problems—whether VPI or "cleft type characteris-tic" articulatory errors.

REFERENCES

1. Furlow LT. Cleft palate repair by double opposing Z-plasty. *Plast Reconstr Surg.* 1986;78(6):724-738.
2. Randall P, LaRossa D, Solomon M, Cohen M. Experience with the furlow double-reversing Z-plasty for cleft palate repair. *Plast Reconstr Surg.* 1986;77(4):569-576.
3. Sitzman TJ, Allori AC, Thorburn G. Measuring outcomes in cleft lip and palate treatment. *Clin Plast Surg.* 2014;41(2):311-319. doi:10.1016/j.cps.2013.12.001.
4. Timbang MR, Gharb BB, Rampazzo A, et al. A systematic review comparing Furlow double-opposing Z-plasty and straight-line intrave-lar veloplasty methods of cleft palate repair. *Plast Reconstr Surg.* 2014;134(5):1014-1022. doi:10.1097/PRS.0000000000000637.

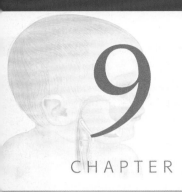

CHAPTER 9

von Langenbeck Palatoplasty

Kathryn V. Isaac and David K. Chong

DEFINITION

- Cleft palate is the failure of fusion of the palatal shelves during embryological development.
- There are many surgical techniques used for cleft palate repair. The repair technique chosen varies depending on the type of cleft palate and beliefs regarding facial growth and speech repercussions[1].

ANATOMY

- Embryologically, the cleft may affect the primary or/and secondary palate.
- Anatomically, the cleft is defined according to the involvement of the hard and soft palates.
- A complete cleft of the palate is defined as a cleft involving both the primary and secondary palates. Hence, a complete cleft involves the soft palate and the hard palate.
- The Veau classification (**FIG 1**) provides a clinically useful description of the cleft type according to the involvement of the alveolus, the hard palate, and the soft palate. It guides selection of the surgical treatment.[2]
- The von Langenbeck palatoplasty is most commonly employed for incomplete cleft palates, where the primary palate is unaffected (ie, soft palate and hard palate to incisive foramen) or where the primary palate was previously repaired (commonly with a superiorly based vomerine flap at the time of lip repair).[1,3]
  - Von Langenbeck palatoplasty is less commonly used to repair isolated clefts of the soft palate (Veau I) and mostly employed to repair clefts of the soft palate and secondary palate [hard palate posterior to the incisive foramen (Veau II)].

- This technique may also be modified for complete clefts and is named a hybrid procedure.[4] This hybrid procedure employs the bipedicled von Langenbeck flap on the greater segment and a unipedicled flap on the lesser segment. It is not used for the treatment of submucous clefts.
- Additionally, the von Langenbeck technique of a bipedicled mucoperiosteal flap may be used for the repair of fistulae located in the hard palate or junction with the soft palate.

PATHOGENESIS

- The etiology of cleft palate is multifactorial: environment, teratogen exposure (alcohol, anticonvulsants, steroids, diazepam), nutrition, maternal infections (rubella, toxoplasmosis), and genetics.
- Cleft palate repair restores anatomical closure between the oral and nasal cavities.
- An unrepaired cleft palate may result in impaired breathing, feeding, speech, and hearing.

NATURAL HISTORY

- Orofacial clefting is the most common craniofacial birth defect, occurring in 1:750 live births.[5]
  - The incidence of cleft palate alone is 1:2000, with a female-to-male ratio of 2:1.
  - The incidence of cleft palate in combination with cleft lip is greater, estimated at 1:1000 with a reverse gender ratio.
- In the population of children with cleft lip and/or cleft palate (CL+/–P), approximately 50% will have CLP, 30% to 35% CP, and 15% to 20% CL.

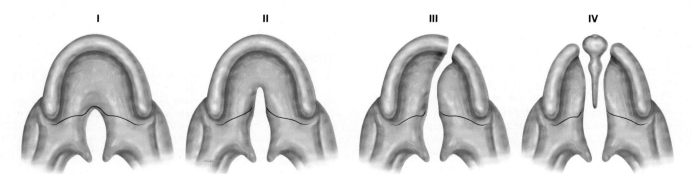

FIG 1 • Veau classification of cleft palate types. **I.** Cleft of soft palate only. **II.** Cleft of secondary hard and soft palates. **III.** Unilateral cleft extending through secondary hard and soft palate, through right or left primary palate, and through the alveolar process. **IV.** Bilateral cleft through secondary hard and soft palate, through bilateral primary palate and bilateral alveolar processes.

- Approximately 40% of CP patients will have a syndrome, and 15% of CLP will have a syndrome.

PATIENT HISTORY AND PHYSICAL FINDINGS

- The diagnosis of a cleft palate is made by prenatal ultrasonography or by physical examination at birth and in early infancy. A detailed assessment is made of the child's breathing, feeding, growth, and development.
- Airway assessment must exclude the presence of sleep apnea and micro-/retrognathia.
- Assessment of growth and weight is key to identify and monitor feeding difficulty, gastroesophageal reflux, and the use of feeding aids (Haberman/Pigeon teat).
- Hearing and middle ear function must be assessed and treated early by an otolaryngologist.
- The plastic surgeon should define the cleft palate type according to the anatomic structures involved, the laterality, width of the palate, and the presence/absence of a cleft lip.
- Also, the child should be assessed for associated anomalies suggestive of a syndrome: craniofacial dysmorphism, airway compromise, cardiac defects, ocular and auricular abnormalities, and musculoskeletal anomalies. A genetics referral is suggested if suspicious for a case of syndromic cleft palate.

DIFFERENTIAL DIAGNOSIS

- Syndromic cleft palate
  - Van der Woude syndrome
  - Stickler syndrome
  - Robin sequence
  - 22q11.2 deletion syndrome
  - Treacher Collins syndrome
  - Nager syndrome
  - Ectrodactyly-ectodermal dysplasia
  - Klippel-Feil syndrome

NONOPERATIVE MANAGEMENT

- It is very uncommon not to repair a cleft palate.
- If the child is unable to undergo surgical treatment secondary to airway concerns or medical fitness, a palatal obturator may be considered.
  - Such patients should be reassessed on a regular basis (at least annually), as they may become sufficiently stable for delayed surgical correction of the cleft palate.

SURGICAL MANAGEMENT

- Cleft palate repair is ideally performed between 9 and 12 months of age, with the infant weighing greater than 8 kg.
- Airway and middle ear disease assessment is performed and treated prior to or simultaneously with cleft palate repair.
- Risks of the procedure are hemorrhage/hematoma, airway compromise, wound dehiscence, infection, oronasal fistula, flap necrosis, velopharyngeal insufficiency, and reduced midfacial growth.
- The main objectives of the cleft palate repair are:
  - To separate the oral and nasal cavities
  - To reposition to the velar musculature for restoration of the velopharyngeal sphincter, in particular the reconstruction of the levator muscular sling
  - To improve Eustachian tube function
  - To minimize detrimental effects on subsequent maxillary growth

- The goals of the palatoplasty are to improve feeding and speech.
- The main steps of the procedure are:
  - Marking and elevation of bipedicled mucoperiosteal flaps off the hard palate
  - Dissection and separation of the nasal mucosa, velar musculature, and oral mucosa
  - Careful dissection of pedicles (greater palatine artery)
  - Tension-free closure of nasal mucosal layer
  - Reconstruction of the velopharyngeal sphincter with repositioning of the levator sling
  - Recreation of the uvula
  - Closure of the oral mucosal layer

Preoperative Planning

- With the patient anesthetized, the width of the cleft is measured at the junction of soft and hard palate. The width of the cleft is important to predict difficulty of the cleft palate repair and anticipated amount of dissection required for closure.
- The von Langenbeck technique provides less flap mobilization relative to other techniques (two-flap palatoplasty). Thus, this technique is best reserved for narrow clefts.

Positioning

- The patient is positioned supine with shoulder roll to allow neck extension. An oral Rae tube, with the circuit directed caudally, is carefully taped centrally. Corneas are protected with eye tapping.
- Access and visualization of the entire palate are very important and cannot be understated. It is especially important to ensure visualization from the uvulae to the anterior extent of the palate.
- It is essential for the surgeon to ensure positioning is correct prior to scrubbing. This will facilitate the procedure.
- The surgeon should have a headlight or lighted instruments for optimizing visualization in the confined space and a skilled attentive assistant.
- It is advantageous to have a bed that has Trendelenburg positioning capability. Some surgeons stand to perform palate surgery from below, but having the baby's head supported with the surgeon seated operating upside down provides the best exposure and is the preferred position by most surgeons.

Approach

- The aim of cleft palate surgery is tension-free closure of the palate oral and nasal mucosal layers and restoration of the velopharyngeal muscular sphincter.
- Difficulties anticipated include:
  - Access
  - Lighting
  - Bleeding obscuring visualization
- Surgical approaches differ with regard to the amount of dissection performed to achieve tension-free closure and muscle repositioning.
- Critical step is adequate exposure and dissection of tissues to provide comfort for the operating surgeon to achieve tension-free closure.
- Oral layer mobilization is largely dependent on careful mobilization of the greater palatine artery from its periosteal sleeve.
- Nasal layer mobilization is largely dependent on careful mobilization of the mucosa as a sheet from its dense bony attachments.

T E C H N I Q U E S

■ Markings

- Carefully insert an intraoral gag and a throat pack (it is the surgeon's responsibility to insert and remove).
- Mark the incision lines:
  - Along the medial edges of the cleft from the uvulae to the anterior extent of the cleft at the primary palate
  - Laterally at the junction of the hard palate and maxillary alveolus, extending from the posterior maxillary tubercle anteriorly to the level of the canine tooth (**TECH FIG 1**).
- Inject local anesthetic with adrenaline into the hard palate and soft palate (average of 8 mL).
  - The vasoconstrictive properties reduce blood loss and enhance visual field.
  - Local anesthetic also facilitates hydrodissection of the mucoperiosteal flaps off of the hard palate and tissue expansion for ease of layer dissection in the soft palate.
- Wait 8 minutes or until injection sites stop bleeding.

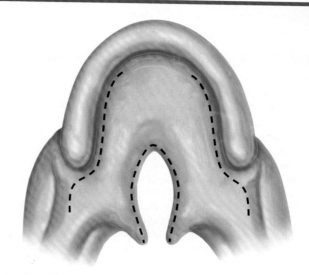

TECH FIG 1 • Incision markings of a von Langenbeck palatoplasty for cleft of the secondary palate.

■ Elevation of Oral Mucoperiosteal Flaps

- Perform incisions with needle tip cautery to reduce bleeding. Use a skin hook on the uvula or stay sutures for countertraction.
- Incisions, flap elevation, and pedicle dissection are done similarly on both the greater and lesser segments.
- Begin with lateral incisions: from the retromolar trigone along the junction of the alveolus and palate with diathermy down to the bone and slightly angled medially so as to avoid injury of developing teeth.
- For the medial incisions, palpate the posteromedial edge of the hard palate before incising to ensure the incision medially will be onto the bone (hard palate) as you can inadvertently cut into the nasal layer and do a "double

cut" that reduces the available tissue for nasal layer closure (**TECH FIG 2A**).
- Oral palatal mucosa is susceptible to tearing so dissect continuously along the entire length of the lateral incision toward the cleft to elevate the mucoperiosteal flaps.
  - Avoid "tunneling" as this can cause tearing of the hard palate mucosa due to dense periosteal attachments.
- Use a periosteal elevator to raise the mucoperiosteal flaps from lateral to medial beginning at the anterior extent of the incision (**TECH FIG 2B**).
- Dissect from anterior to posterior along the hard palate in sweeping motions toward the greater palatine foramina and posterior limit of the hard palate.

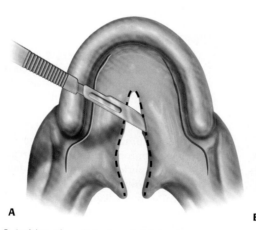

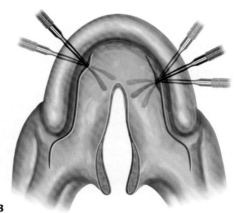

A   **B**

TECH FIG 2 • **A.** Incision of medial edge of cleft beginning at posterior-medial border of the hard palate, separating oral and nasal mucosal layers. **B.** Dissection of oral mucoperiosteal flaps.

■ Isolation of Greater Palatine Vessels

- As you approach the greater palatine artery at the posterolateral edge of the hard palate, the vessel becomes visible on the undersurface of the flap. The visibility of the pedicle is limited with this bipedicled flap technique. Given the difficulty in visualization, the amount of dissection of the pedicle may be limited. Knowledge of the pedicle location will enable you to gently and circumferentially release the dense periosteal attachments around the pedicle.
  - A surface landmark for the pedicle is the dimpling in the mucosa near the posterior edge of the hard palate. This represents the dense periosteal attachments of the pedicle.
- Start laterally, and then work circumferentially around the foramina, staying on the bone and taking care not to dissect into the artery or the leash of veins surrounding it.
  - Staying on the bone during pedicle dissection is very important and rewarding for there are tethering ligaments that insert into the oral mucosa.

- Dissection directly off the bone facilitates the circumferential release of these ligaments, which otherwise make it exceedingly easy to tear the oral mucosa and injure the pedicle.
- Spreading of dissecting scissors parallel to the vascular pedicle will help to release some dense periosteal attachments; this should be done with care not to avulse the vessel.
- Previous hydrodissection during local anesthetic injection will also aid in finding the bloodless plane between the oral layer mucosal glands and the muscular layer.
- Complete circumferential pedicle dissection is achieved once the periosteal sleeve is released behind the greater palatine foramina, and the flaps can be mobilized toward the midline.
- It is critical for the surgeon to anticipate the location of the pedicle and appreciate the careful dissection to be completed with limited visibility, mainly using the lateral approach to perform the release.
- Once sufficiently mobilized, retract the flaps out of the surgical field with stay sutures, and secure to the intra-oral gag/retractor.

■ Dissection and Separation of the Oral Mucosa, Nasal Mucosa, and Muscle

- Oral mucosa dissection: under magnification, dissect in the plane between oral mucosal glands and the muscle layer posteriorly in the soft palate from the edge of the bony palate to the uvula.
- Nasal mucosa dissection:
  - Mobilize the nasal mucoperiosteal layer with care, beginning on the lesser segment of the cleft. This requires the gradual and wide dissection of this continuous sheet of nasal mucosa, which is firmly attached to the hard palate along its medial and posterior edges, along the nasal surface of the bony palate and the medial surface of the medial pterygoid plate.
  - The elevation of the nasal layer anteriorly on the greater segment will necessitate elevation off the vomer.
- The nasal mucosa is even more unforgiving than the oral mucosa. Once a tear occurs, it is easy to propagate. Resist the temptation to tunnel before a whole edge has been liberated.
- To liberate the dense attachments of the medial hard palate, a Mitchell trimmer double-ended elevator or a similar blunt edged instrument is used.
  - The dissection starts at the cleft margin, scraping the oral surface of the bone until the edge of the nasal mucosa starts to be defined.
  - As the edge of the hard palate becomes apparent, elevate the nasal mucoperiosteum widely off the entire extent of the medial aspect of the hard palate.
- The judicious use of needlepoint diathermy on low setting can help to elevate firmly attached areas that are not easily released with the Mitchell trimmer.
- Once the edge of the nasal mucoperiosteal flap is defined, slide the trimmer around the corner of the hard palate

onto the nasal surface of the bone staying right on the bone. If the edge is sufficiently liberated, sweep anteriorly and posteriorly to liberate the entire sheet off the nasal surface.
- If a portion of the edge is still attached, resist further sweeping until releasing the portion that remains tethered to prevent a tear.
- This dissection is continued to the posterior nasal spine.
  - At this juncture, there are always muscle attachments.
  - Release these aberrant velar muscle attachments with needlepoint diathermy.
- Continue dissection along the nasal surface following the posterior edge of the bone cephalad and lateral toward the medial surface of the medial pterygoid plate.
- Release the nasal mucoperiosteum directly off the bony surface of the medial surface of the medial pterygoid plate with careful dissection of the fibrous attachments.
  - Be patient and careful during the release of this densely adherent portion of the nasal mucosa working posteriorly and cephalad along the pterygoid plate and palatine bone.
  - Confirm complete release by directly visualizing the plane of the medial surface of the medial pterygoid plate.
  - If further release is required, the origin of the tensor veli palatini along the medial pterygoid plate may be severed to improve mobilization.
- The sheet of mucosa should now be freely mobile as one continuous sheet posteriorly and along the anterior medial hard palate.
- Attention is then turned to the greater segment.
  - The dissection of the nasal mucoperiosteal flap is identical posteriorly along the hard palate cleft margin.
  - Anteriorly, at the bony junction of the vomer and bony palate, the nasal mucoperiosteum is raised in

continuity with the vomerine periosteum. This vomerine flap is raised cephalad directly off the bone and in continuity with the periosteum of the nasal surface of the hard palate.
- In a cleft of the secondary palate only, the caudal edge of the vomer is located in the midline of the two hard palate shelves.
  - The caudal vomer is incised in the midline and nasal mucoperiosteal flaps raised off each side of the vomer.

- Both vomerine flaps are used for closure of the nasal lining anteriorly; each vomerine flap is secured to the ipsilateral hard palate nasal mucoperiosteal flap.
- As you close the nasal lining from anterior to posterior, you will continue beyond the vomerine flaps and directly approximate nasal lining from the palatal shelves.

■ Closure of Nasal Mucosa

- Nasal layer closure is then commenced once assurance that the repair is tension free by checking that both sides are sufficiently liberated (**TECH FIG 3**).
- Meticulous closure is executed with knots tied on the nasal side.
- Small wedges are excised at the base of the oral surface of the uvula to assist closure.
  - Place eversion sutures during the closure of the uvulae to prevent notching or bifidity.
  - It is helpful to pare the musculus uvulae into a nasal and oral component during dissection so that musculus uvulae can be included in the suture closure of both oral and nasal layers of the uvula to further strengthen the closure.

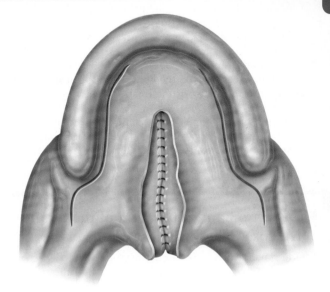

TECH FIG 3 • Closure of nasal mucosal flaps from anterior extent of cleft to the uvula.

■ Dissection of the Muscle and Intravelar Veloplasty

- With the nasal layer completely closed, proceed with the muscle dissection and reconstruction of the velopharyngeal sphincter.
- Three steps are critical for muscle repositioning:
  - Identification and separation of levator veli palatini (LVP)
  - Velar musculature dissection and release from its attachments to the cleft margin and hard palate shelf
  - Velar musculature repositioning and repair
- Deep to the muscles inserted into the back of the bony hard palate, the LVP inserts abnormally at the cleft margin in the anterior half of the velum.
- Using a scalpel, sharply dissect the velar muscle layer off the nasal mucosa along the cleft margin. This is done with a paramedian incision lateral to the nasal mucosal closure line through the muscle until nasal mucosal surface is identified.
- It is easiest to separate the muscle layer once the nasal mucosa has been repaired to give a "trampoline" effect, providing tactile feedback and countertraction during this careful dissection.

- The bulk and breadth of the muscle widen as you dissect laterally. This is analogous to the changing depth of a swimming pool, with a shallow end (paramedian) becoming deeper as one progressively dissects laterally.
- The velar musculature is raised off the nasal mucosa and separated from the tendinous fibers of the tensor veli palatini (TVP). This separation is done laterally along the hard palate shelf at the junction of "salmon pink" velar muscle fibers and tendinous fibers of the TVP.
  - The velar musculature is further dissected until it can be freely mobilized to lie parallel to the posterior hard palate margin and overlying the contralateral velar muscle bundle.
  - You have completed the levator dissection when the "salmon pink"-colored longitudinal fibers of the levator are identified emerging from the skull base and the entire dissected muscle is free to be reoriented to a more functionally effective position in the posterior half of the soft palate.
  - The dissection of the velar musculature is performed on both sides.
- Repair the muscles, and reconstruct the levator muscular sling by suturing the muscles and securing with multiple sutures, knots facing the nasal surface.
- Ensure proper hemostasis is achieved.

■ Closure of the Oral Mucosa

- Close the oral layer beginning with stay sutures placed anteriorly and progressing posteriorly toward the uvulae with horizontal mattress sutures. There is no attempt of push-back of the flaps for lengthening with a V-Y closure (**TECH FIG 4**).
- During oral layer closure, place some full-thickness sutures through both the oral and nasal layers just posterior to the hard palate shelf (anterior to muscle repair) to help obliterate the dead space and position the muscle repair.
- Place interrupted simple sutures between each of the mattress sutures.
- Attempt to minimize raw bone exposure by closing palatal flaps to the alveolus wherever possible.
- Recheck for adequate hemostasis, irrigate, and remove throat pack.
- If concerned for airway during postoperative period, consider nasopharyngeal tube insertion and a tongue stitch. Note that a tongue stitch is rarely used in our practice.

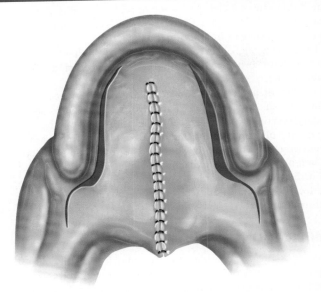

TECH FIG 4 • Closure of oral mucosa after medialization of the bipedicled flaps.

PEARLS AND PITFALLS

Headlight and positioning	■ Good lighting and access to the palate are important
Pedicle dissection	■ Visibility of the greater palatine foramina is limited. The release is accomplished with careful and near-circumferential dissection from the lateral approach. Complete the dissection from the medial approach.
Hemostasis	■ Ensure meticulous hemostasis throughout the case to optimize visualization. ■ Judicious use of needlepoint diathermy. ■ Failure to do so may result in airway compromise, flap necrosis, and wound dehiscence.
Use needlepoint diathermy to make hard palate incisions	■ Controls bleeding and persisting ooze.
Work on broad front	■ Avoid tunneling during dissection.
Patience and precision during dissection especially around palatine foramina	■ Bleeding obscures view, and careless dissection risks injury to pedicle and vascularity of the flap.
Handle tissues with care	■ The nasal mucosa is especially susceptible to tears.
Inset palatal flaps with stay sutures to help control closure	■ Helps to put the most difficult sutures anteriorly with stay sutures to judge closure and maintains good exposure.
Do not attempt closure until all layers are sufficiently mobilized	■ Prevents tearing. ■ If sutures are prematurely placed, further attempts to mobilize tissue are more likely to result in tears. Prematurely suturing may also result in tears if tension is still present.
Oronasal fistula	■ Critical to achieve adequate tissue dissection, perfect approximation, and apposition of tissue layers with meticulous suture technique to prevent fistulae.

POSTOPERATIVE CARE

- Nasopharyngeal tube as required.
- Remove tongue stitch in recovery if used.
- Analgesia to reduce blood pressure and distress (24 hours of intravenous opioids).
- Encourage feeding.
- Postoperative visit in 4 weeks.

OUTCOMES

- Primary von Langenbeck palatoplasty with levator reconstruction provides a reliable repair and good speech outcomes with 89% of patients having acceptable or normal speech.
  - Velopharyngeal insufficiency necessitated surgical correction in 11% of patients.

- The fistula rate of a cleft palate repair with a bipedicled flap technique is 10.2% (95% CI, 6.3% to 15%) according to a systematic review of international data.[6]
  - There was an observed trend toward higher fistula rates with bipedicled compared to unipedicled flap technique.
- The effect of palatoplasty on maxillary facial retrusion is controversial. Inherent maxillary growth deficiency, secondary scarring from palatal flap elevation, and timing of repair are all contributing factors to midfacial retrusion. Deleterious growth has been shown to be greatest in patients treated by Veau push-back technique.[7]
  - Further long-term studies are required to compare the effect of palatal flap technique on maxillary growth restriction.

COMPLICATIONS

- Bleeding is a feared complication as it may lead to an emergency with airway obstruction and respiratory compromise. Additionally, hematoma may lead to compression of the pedicle or flap, with resultant flap necrosis, wound dehiscence, and oronasal fistulae.
  - To prevent this complication, vigilant hemostasis is an absolute necessity, and adequate postoperative analgesia avoids stressing the repairs.
- Airway obstruction may occur in the absence of hemorrhage, and a tongue stitch or nasopharyngeal tube may assist in preventing obstruction in infants at risk.

- Flap necrosis is rare and avoidable with careful dissection and release of the periosteal sleeve of the greater palatine pedicle.
- Infection and wound dehiscence leading to oronasal fistulae are detrimental.
  - A small fistula secondary to delayed wound healing may heal with conservative measures.
  - Failure of closure may necessitate reoperation with re-elevation and closure of oral and nasal flaps, as well as possible augmentation using local flaps and/or biologic adjuncts.

REFERENCES

1. von Langenbeck B. Weitere Erfahrungen im Gebiete der Uranoplastik mittels Ablosung des mucosperiostalen Gaumenuberzuges. *Arch Klin Chir.* 1864;5:1-70.
2. Wallace AF. A history of the repair of cleft lip and palate in Britain before World War II. *Ann Plast Surg.* 1987;19:266-275.
3. Trier WC, Dreyer TM. Primary von Langenbeck palatoplasty with levator reconstruction: rationale and technique. *Cleft Palate J.* 1984;21:254-262.
4. Gillett DA, Clarke HM. The hybrid palatoplasty: a preliminary report. *Can J Plast Surg.* 1996;4(3 suppl):157-160.
5. van Aalst JA, Kolappa KK, Sadove M. CME article: nonsyndromic cleft palate. *Plast Reconstr Surg.* 2008;121(1 suppl):1-14.
6. Hardwicke JT, Landini G, Richard BM. Fistula incidence after primary cleft palate repair: a systematic review of the literature. *Plast Reconstr Surg.* 2014;134:618e-627e.
7. Lee YH, Liao YF. Hard palate repair technique and facial growth in patients with cleft lip and palate: a systematic review. *Br J Oral Maxillofac Surg.* 2013;51:851-857.

Sommerlad Palatoplasty

T. Guy Thorburn

DEFINITION

- Cleft palate repairs can be broadly classified into straight-line repairs (such as the Sommerlad technique) vs Z-plasty repairs (such as the Furlow technique).
- Otto Kriens proposed the intravelar veloplasty based upon his work on the anatomy of the cleft palate.[1]
  - Sommerlad then developed this dissection into a more radical procedure and popularized the technique.
- The underlying principle is identification and retropositioning of the soft palate muscles, before connecting the levator muscle mechanisms from the two sides of the soft palate.

ANATOMY

- The key functional issue in CP or SMCP is that the levator muscle mechanism is not in continuity on the two sides. In addition, the fibers become tethered to the posterior border of the hard palate.
  - Successful functional palate repair therefore requires repair of the "levator sling" as well as closure of the tissues across the cleft.
- The tethering to the hard palate seems to be an equal problem in differing types of cleft: whether unilateral or bilateral cleft lip and palate, cleft palate only, or submucous cleft palate.
- The key functional muscle is the levator palatini, but the surrounding muscle/aponeurotic tissue is kept in continuity to allow more reliable tissue handling and retropositioning and subsequent suturing.
  - Of note, the levator sits on the nasal aspect of the soft palate and so becomes visible only when the dissection is well underway.

PATIENT HISTORY AND PHYSICAL FINDINGS

- The initial assessment of the newborn with a cleft involving a palate would usually be alongside a pediatrician and includes:
  - Pregnancy and birth history (including information from any antenatal testing), gestation, birth weight, and Apgar scores.
  - Initial assessment of cleft type and any related anomalies, including any airway concerns suggesting Robin sequence.
  - Medical, drug, and allergy histories.
  - Family history of clefts, other major health problems, or anesthetic problems and any genetic diagnosis.
  - Feeding history, including bottle type (eg, squeezy bottle, free flow, Haberman), current weight, maximum percentage weight loss and number of days to regain birth weight, and volume/duration/frequency of feeds.
  - Physical examination to assess the upper airways, cleft type, cleft width and how much deficiency there is of surrounding tissues, as well as any related anomalies or dysmorphic features. The pediatrician would then complete a fully newborn examination looking in particular for related health issues such as cardiac, respiratory, renal, or neurological signs.

IMAGING

- No routine preoperative imaging is required for typical clefts. For older children presenting with SMCP or velopharyngeal incompetence (VPI), assessment with a speech lateral videofluoroscopy helps to evaluate the position of the velum during phonation and relative size of the soft palate to the size of the pharynx.
- Standardized preoperative clinical photos should be taken as these are invaluable when assessing outcomes many years later.

SURGICAL MANAGEMENT

Preoperative Planning

- A key aspect of successful cleft palate repair is optimizing the patient prior to surgery. A pediatrician is a crucial member of the cleft team.
- Although there is much discussion of age at palate repair, different team protocols vary from around 3 months old to 15 months or more.
  - Very young babies will tend to be more susceptible to airway compromise around the time of surgery.
  - Delaying repair until much older and speech has developed has been associated with poorer speech outcomes, particularly related to articulatory errors.
- Our team protocol is for palate repair around 8 to 12 months (corrected for prematurity), but our emphasis is much more on ensuring that the child is well and thriving as surgery approaches.
  - If the child is not growing along his or her expected centiles (with growth plotted on the appropriate chart for syndromic children), this should be addressed before surgery.
  - We routinely postpone for about 4 weeks if children have upper respiratory tract infections.
  - By following this approach, we have seen a significant reduction in fistulae and concerns with speech function.

- Routine blood tests or cross match samples are not required, unless the child is known to have a specific risk factor.
- For children with cardiac or respiratory problems, an up-to-date echocardiogram or sleep study may be relevant.

Positioning

- A Rae uncuffed or microcuffed tube is positioned in the midline and secured to the lower face.
  - The taping of the tube needs to be secure but avoiding taping the mouth closed or limiting access. Taping in a V shape along the line of the mandible avoids displacing the tapes when the mouth gag is opened.
- The child is placed supine on a warming blanket, with the head at the very end of the operating table.
- A large horseshoe gel head ring is placed under the shoulders and around the head to provide support without over-extending the neck.
- A head drape is applied, and the face is prepped.
- The table is tilted to a slight head-up position.
- An operating microscope is used for the procedure. The height of the table is adjusted once the microscope has been brought into place (adjusted according to whether the surgeon prefers to sit or stand).
- A modified Dingman mouth gag is placed.
- A throat pack is placed, and a marker sticker put across the drapes as a reminder to ensure it is removed at the end.
  - The sticker is placed so that the drapes cannot be removed without needing to disturb the warning sticker.
  - The throat pack is also included in the scrub nurse count as an additional precaution.
- The nose and mouth are rinsed with aqueous chlorhexidine solution.

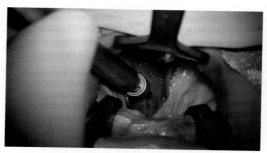

FIG 1 • Marking the incisions at the margin of the cleft.

Approach

- The width of the cleft is measured. The extent of the cleft and any unusual features are noted.
- The incisions are marked with pen and ink (**FIG 1**).
  - Depending on the extent and shape of the anterior edge of the cleft, either a horseshoe shape or a triangular flap can be marked anteriorly.
  - The line of the incision in the soft palate can be identified by the pale line where the nasal mucosa meets the oral mucosa along the margin of the cleft.
- For very wide clefts, lateral von Langenbeck incisions can be marked at the outset, or these can be decided later in the procedure after the closing tension around the hard palate-soft palate junction is apparent.
  - Tension is a factor of the soft tissue cleft width, the width of the lateral shelves of the palate, the elasticity of the tissue, and how vertical the shelves were sitting (which gives a "drawbridge effect").

■ Hard Palate

Incisions and Dissection

- Levobupivacaine or bupivacaine long-acting local anesthetic with adrenaline 1:100 000 is infiltrated and left about 8 minutes for vasoconstriction.
  - The injection is used to help hydrodissect the hard palate subperiosteal layer and the vomer flaps if these are being used (**TECH FIG 1A**)
- The incision is begun along the cleft margin (or in the midline for a SMCP or rerepair).

- For complete clefts of the palate, it is usually easier to start with the posterior two-thirds of the hard palate extending across the hard palate-soft palate junction, then to move on to the very anterior portion of the cleft, and finally to move on to the posterior soft palate and uvula (**TECH FIG 1B**).
- For clefts involving the hard palate, use a no. 15 blade to incise carefully down to the bone along the margin of the hard palate and 3 to 5 mm past the hard palate-soft palate junction and elevate subperiosteally with a periosteal elevator or Warwick-James elevator (**TECH FIG 1C,D**).

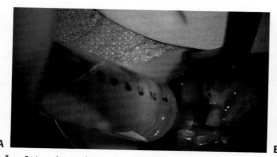

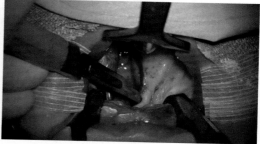

TECH FIG 1 • **A.** Local anesthetic is injected to hydrodissect the oral mucoperiosteal flaps. **B.** A no. 15 blade is used to incise the margin of the cleft, starting with the anterior third of the soft palate up to the posterior two-thirds of the hard palate at this stage.

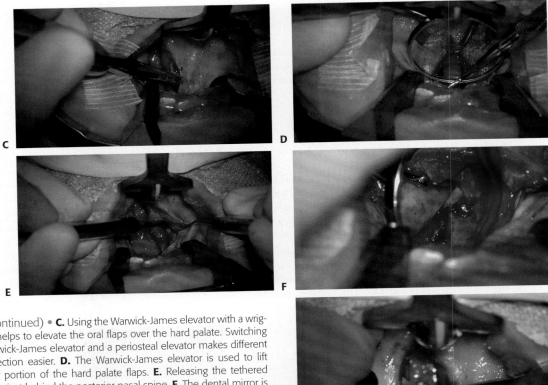

TECH FIG 1 (Continued) • **C.** Using the Warwick-James elevator with a wriggling movement helps to elevate the oral flaps over the hard palate. Switching between the Warwick-James elevator and a periosteal elevator makes different parts of the dissection easier. **D.** The Warwick-James elevator is used to lift the most anterior portion of the hard palate flaps. **E.** Releasing the tethered salivary gland from just behind the posterior nasal spine. **F.** The dental mirror is showing the underside of the oral layer flap to demonstrate the extent of the dissection laterally, including out toward the great palatine artery. **G.** A no. 12 blade is aimed posteriorly to incise the margin of the uvula and posterior third of the soft palate.

- Be careful approaching the posterior nasal spine as the tissues are more adherent here, and it is easy to tear the oral layer if there is a tethered salivary gland at this point. Switching between a no. 15 blade and periosteal elevator is usually necessary (**TECH FIG 1E**).
- For wider clefts, a more radical hard palate dissection is required to reduce the tension when closing.
- The Warwick-James elevators and dental flat plastic can be alternated to lift more laterally and, if needed, to free up the periosteal attachments around the greater palatine artery to improve mobilization (**TECH FIG 1F**).
- For incising the margin of the rest of the soft palate and back to the uvula, a no. 12 blade tends to be easiest (**TECH FIG 1G**).
- Depending on the cleft type, it may be necessary to raise vomer flaps to help close the nasal layer without tension.
- For wide clefts, it may be useful to incorporate a sphenoid flap in the nasal layer closure.
  - This is a flag-shaped extension to one of the vomer flaps, which rotates with insetting to provide additional tissue to the nasal layer around the hard palate-soft palate junction where it is usually tightest.[2]

Elevation of the Nasal Layer

- After raising the vomer flaps, elevate the nasal layer off the hard palate (again in a subperiosteal plane) with a periosteal elevator or dental flat plastic.
- Mobilize the nasal layer off the hard palate bony shelves, taking care not to damage the nasal layer (**TECH FIG 2**).

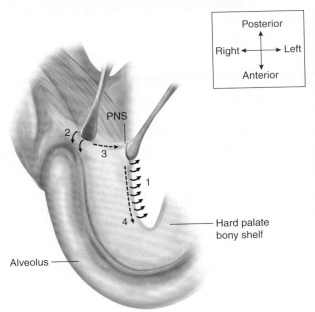

TECH FIG 2 • The stages of dissecting the nasal layer mucoperiosteal flap from the hard palate bony shelf. (1) Using a periosteal elevator with the spoon facing nasally, gently lift the periosteum off the margin of the bone with small movements. (2) Rotate periosteal elevator 180 degrees, so spoon faces orally, and insert it subperiosteally on nasal aspect of posterior edge of the bony shelf of the hard palate. (3) Wiggle and rotate spoon across the postnasal spine, the most adherent point. (Always return to position 2 if the periosteal elevator slips out of place.) (4) Continue to make wiggling and rotating movements with the periosteal elevator from the postnasal spine anteriorly.

- Start by using a periosteal elevator to gently free the periosteum off the margin of the bone and postnasal spine.
- Next, use a periosteal elevator to wriggle beneath the bone shelf in a subperiosteal plane, working from the area of the tensor aponeurosis, around the postnasal spine, and then onto the medial margin.

von Langenbeck–Type Releasing Incisions

- For wide clefts, it may be necessary to use lateral von Langenbeck–type releasing incisions.
    - This decision may be clear at this point in the operation, in which case making early incisions can be efficient.
    - When the decision is less obvious, continue with the rest of the dissection, and the releasing incision can be made immediately prior to oral layer closure.
- When a von Langenbeck–type releasing incision is required, mark out a lazy S incision along the medial aspect of the alveolus and around its posterior limit to overlie the hamulus (**TECH FIG 3A**). The incision is kept

as short as possible while allowing good mobilization of the oral layer flaps.
    - Local anesthetic with adrenaline is injected to help with hydrodissection and vasoconstriction: it is important to have a clear view to reduce the risk of damage to the greater palatine vessels.
- The incision is started in the hard palate with a no. 15 blade, incising down through periosteum at the medial base of the alveolus but ensuring that you stay lateral to the course of the artery.
- The incision is extended more superficially around the tubercle and over the hamulus.
    - A periosteal elevator is used to elevate the flap subperiosteally (**TECH FIG 3B**). It is often easier to have a second periosteal elevator to elevate simultaneously the tissues via the previous incision at the medial aspect of the palate until the two instruments meet.
    - It is then possible to work posteriorly, and one should elevate carefully the tissues around the greater palatine artery until the oral flap is sufficiently mobile to meet the opposite flap in the midline.

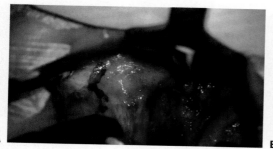 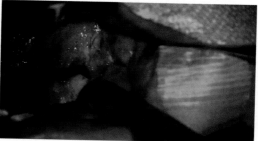

TECH FIG 3 • A. Marking for the incision of lateral releasing incision around the posterior aspect of the alveolus on the left, using a lazy S shape. **B.** Following incision of the mucosa, a periosteal elevator is used to lift under the periosteum and mobilize the flap.

■ Oral Layer

- To separate the oral layer from the muscle layer, the periosteal elevator or a dental flat plastic is swept back from the posterior margin of the palatal bone shelf (**TECH FIG 4**).
    - The plane is easier to develop laterally, near the hamulus, so the process starts here and then moves medially.
- A no. 12 blade is then used to incise posteriorly along the margin of the cleft toward the uvula.

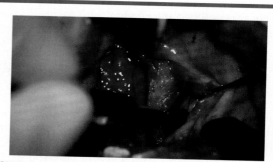

TECH FIG 4 • The periosteal elevator is slid off the back of the hard palate shelf to separate the oral layer off the muscle fibers. Note the tip of the periosteal elevator is just reaching the hamulus, as the plane is easier to develop more laterally.

■ Nasal Layer

- Use interrupted sutures to close the nasal layer, incorporating vomer flaps anteriorly if available and needed.
    - A resorbable monofilament suture is used, preferably with a round or tapercut needle to avoid inadvertent tears of the mucosa. We use 5-0 Monocryl plus on a round-bodied needle for this closure.

- The bites pick up more of the glandular tissue, with only a small amount of nasal mucosa, and knots are laid on the nasal aspect. This helps to evert the edges toward the nasal aspect (**TECH FIG 5**).
- If the nasal layer is too tight for closure around the hard palate-soft palate junction, then leave closure of this section until after the muscle dissection.

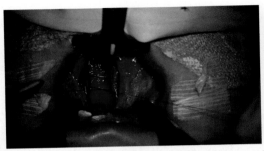
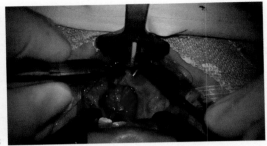

TECH FIG 5 • A. Suturing of the nasal layer, with the knots placed on the nasal aspect. Interrupted sutures are placed, working posteriorly toward the uvula. **B.** Suturing the uvula using horizontal mattress sutures to pick up the fibrous "core" of the uvula, as the mucosa tends to become friable in this area.

■ Muscle Dissection of the Nasal layer

- Applying topical 1:1000 adrenaline on neuro patties for about 5 minutes before beginning the muscle dissection provides excellent vasoconstriction and facilitates the subsequent dissection (**TECH FIG 6A**).
- To make access easier for the next stage, a stay suture can be used to hold the oral flaps out of the way (**TECH FIG 6B**).
- Closure of the nasal layer has now pulled the soft palate muscles out to length, with the resultant tension helping with the next stage of dissection.
  - A fresh no. 15 blade is used for each side of the palate. Alternatively, some surgeons find it easier to use a straight Beaver blade (**TECH FIG 6C**).
- Start on each side by incising the posterior border of the muscles; this will leave behind a triangular block of fibrous/glandular tissue around the base of the uvula (**TECH FIG 6D**).

- Next, incise the medial margin of the muscle (**TECH FIG 6E**).
- Finally, incise the tensor aponeurosis anteriorly (**TECH FIG 6F**), and extend posterolaterally to divide the tendinous material from the hamulus.
  - Bipolar diathermy is then used sparingly to assist with the lateral dissection, but the aim is to preserve as much of the vascular supply to the levator muscle as possible (**TECH FIG 6G**).
- A dental flat plastic is then used to slide between the remaining levator and the nasal layer and particularly to free up any fascial sheath that can sit on the distal aspect of the muscle and restrict its retropositioning (**TECH FIG 6H**).
- When it has been properly dissected, the levator muscle should easily displaced to the posterior end of the soft palate (**TECH FIG 6I,J**).

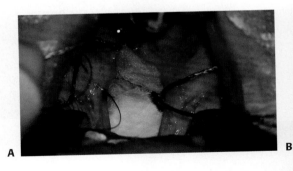
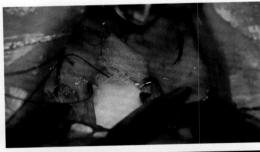
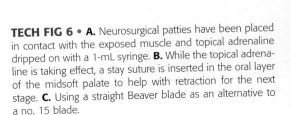
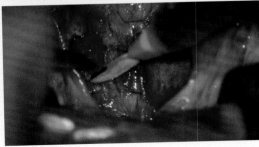

TECH FIG 6 • A. Neurosurgical patties have been placed in contact with the exposed muscle and topical adrenaline dripped on with a 1-mL syringe. **B.** While the topical adrenaline is taking effect, a stay suture is inserted in the oral layer of the midsoft palate to help with retraction for the next stage. **C.** Using a straight Beaver blade as an alternative to a no. 15 blade.

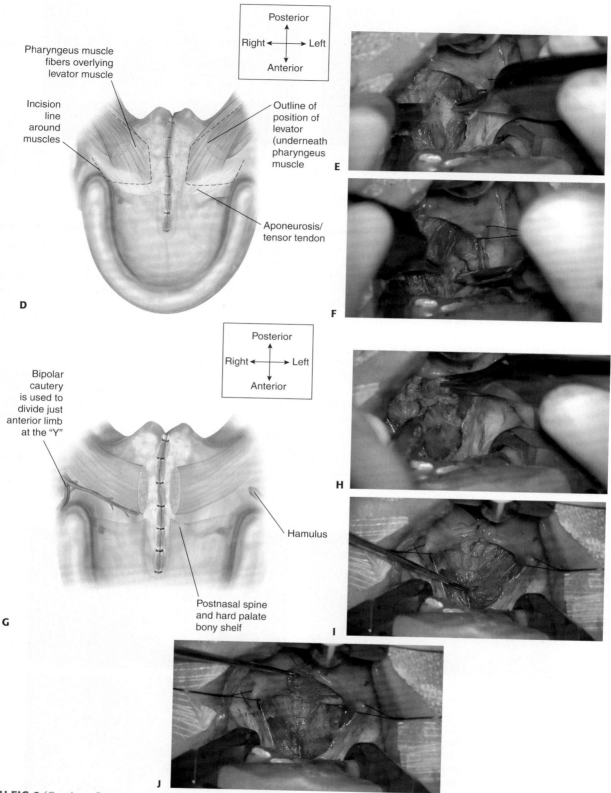

TECH FIG 6 (Continued) • **D.** Diagram showing the dissection of the soft palate muscles. (Oral layer not shown to allow clearer visualization.) **E.** Dissecting the medial extent of the soft palate muscles. The levator muscle is still not yet visible at this point in the dissection. **F.** Incision of the tensor aponeurosis off the back of the hard palate. Note how the forceps are used to tension the muscle toward the midline, which helps the dissection and reduces the chance of "buttonholing" the nasal layer. The sharp incision continues laterally to free the muscle from the hamulus. **G.** Key landmarks when freeing to muscle and of bipolar dissection. **H.** A dental flat plastic is slid between the levator (just visible as the slightly bluish muscle fibers under the brighter pink pharyngeus muscle fibers) and the nasal layer to complete the dissection. Before **(I)** and after **(J)** views of the muscles on the right side of the soft palate to show the extent of retropositioning after dissection is complete.

■ Closure

- The nasal layer closure can now be completed if necessary.
  - If the nasal layer has no holes, drainage holes can be incised laterally if required.
- The two sides of the muscle are now sutured across the midline (**TECH FIG 7A,B**).
  - We use a nonabsorbable monofilament suture such as 5-0 nylon to place reliable knots, minimize trauma to the muscle, and avoid inflammatory reaction from resorption.
  - There is also the potential benefit that the sutures act as a useful marker of the levator position if it becomes necessary to re-explore the palate in the future. A locked mattress suture (similar to a Kessler stitch) is used.
  - It is important to avoid tying the suture too tightly as this would strangulate the muscle with any postoperative swelling.

- It is also essential to cut the suture extremely short, right on the knot, so the knots can be laid flat as reef knots.
- The oral layer is closed with looped mattress sutures using a resorbable monofilament suture such as 4-0 Monocryl.
  - Modifying the mattress suture that sits just anterior to the muscle can close off the dead space between the oral and nasal flaps in the soft palate (**TECH FIG 7C**).
  - By picking up a bite of the fibrous/glandular tissue that was left behind on the nasal layer as the muscle was dissected, the mattress suture closes the two layers together (**TECH FIG 7D**).
- Finally, after closure is complete, the mouth is rinsed out, a nasal suction catheter is used to ensure there is no blood clot in the postnasal space, and if a throat pack was used, this is removed (**TECH FIG 7E**).

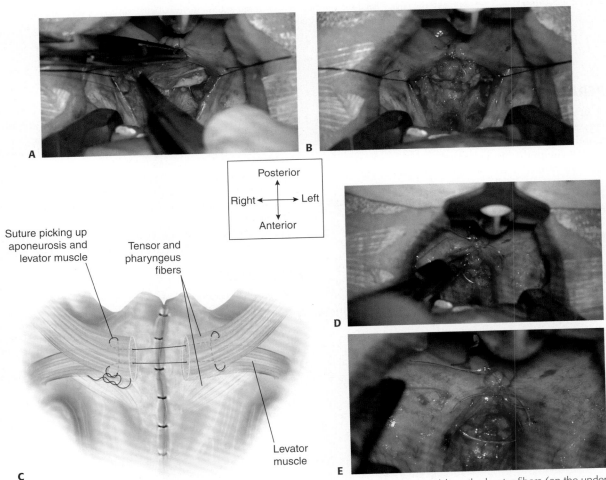

TECH FIG 7 • **A.** The mattress suture is placed in the muscle, aiming with each transverse bite to pick up the levator fibers (on the underside) as well as the aponeurosis tissue for a more reliable closure. **B.** The muscles on each side sitting at the posterior extent of the soft palate after suturing. **C.** Illustration (oral layer omitted) of the suture to appose the muscles on the two sides, just prior to tying. Locked mattress sutures pick up both keratin fibers (underneath) and tough tender aponeurosis tissue (anteriorly and on top) with each bite. **D.** The needle picks up a bite of the fibrous/glandular tissue that has been left attached to the nasal layer. **E.** The looped mattress suture, including the bite of the nasal layer, just prior to tying.

PEARLS AND PITFALLS

Timing of surgery	■ Careful optimization of the baby prior to surgery is important, progressive gain in length and weight as documented in a growth chart is a useful indicator—a thriving baby at the time of surgery is more important than a specific age.
Shared airway	■ As with all "shared airway" surgery, it is important for the anesthetist and surgeon to communicate well with each other—the WHO checklist and team brief are very useful for this.
Protecting the mouth and commissures	■ Steri-Strips are placed to protect the corners of the mouth from abrasion by instruments.
Operative microscope	■ The routine use of the operative microscope for palate repair gives excellent lighting and visualization of the operative field. It is also very helpful for giving trainees a better view and involvement, as well as reducing the strain on the surgeon's neck.
Muscle dissection	■ The key to dissecting the muscles (without putting holes in the nasal layer) is to place tension on the tissues by using a skin hook or forceps to draw the muscle bulk toward the midline and then to stroke the curve of the blade to get a neat division. The vascular plexus that is seen immediately superficial to the nasal layer is a useful marker.
Draping the patient	■ We use a clear plastic drape over the trunk, which allows the anesthetist to see the endotracheal tube and circuit without disturbing the surgical field. We avoid any adhesive drapes near the endotracheal tube because these have the potential to catch and dislodge the airway.
Postoperative elevation	■ Nursing the baby "head-up" in the recovery room and on the ward after surgery is very helpful for reducing postoperative swelling—cuddling the baby over the parent's shoulder tends to give ideal positioning.

POSTOPERATIVE CARE

■ Topping up the local anesthesia with a long-acting agent at the very end of the operation is useful for postoperative comfort and feeding.

■ Nurse the baby with the head elevated.

■ Babies can be offered feeds straight away once they are awake.

■ Monitor airway and oxygen saturation, especially during the first night after surgery.

OUTCOMES

■ The main outcome measures for cleft palate repair are fistula rate, structural speech problem rate, and impact on maxillary growth.[3]

■ Negative outcomes in any of these parameters can lead to the need for secondary surgery for their correction.

■ Sommerlad reported approximately 5% secondary surgery rates for VPI with a 10-year follow-up.[4]

  ■ He reported fistula rates that vary considerably by cleft type—35% in bilateral cleft lip and palate but an average of 12% in other cleft types.

COMPLICATIONS

■ Infection, significant bleeding, and transfusion are all rare after palate surgery.

■ Airway compromise is a potential risk, especially in babies with Pierre Robin sequence and in younger or smaller babies.

■ Fistula is often reported around the hard palate-soft palate junction, but there is wide variation between series and the extent and width of the cleft palate can be a major factor in the fistula rate.

■ Speech problems may occur for a variety of reasons, to include VPI and/or articulatory errors characteristic of cleft type.

REFERENCES

1. Kriens OB. An anatomical approach to veloplasty. *Plast Reconstr Surg.* 1969;43:29-41.
2. Khan K, Hardwicke J, Seselgyte R, et al. Use of the sphenoid flap in repair of the wide cleft palate. *Cleft Palate Craniofac J.* 2018;55:437-441.
3. Sitzman TJ, Allori AC, Thorburn G. Measuring outcomes in cleft lip and palate treatment. *Clin Plast Surg.* 2014;41:311-319.
4. Sommerlad BC. A technique for cleft palate repair. *Plastic Reconstr Surg.* 2003;112:1542-1548.

Two-Flap Palatoplasty

David K. Chong, Kathryn V. Isaac, and Kenneth E. Salyer

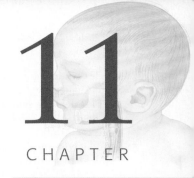

DEFINITION

- Cleft palate is the failure of fusion of the palatal shelves during embryological development.
- Cleft palate may occur in isolation or in combination with a cleft lip. It may occur as part of a syndrome or in the absence of associated anomalies.
- A cleft of the palate may lead to feeding difficulties, speech impairment, chronic Eustachian tube dysfunction, hearing loss, and altered facial growth.
- Varying surgical approaches for cleft palate repair are utilized depending on the type of cleft palate and beliefs regarding facial growth and speech repercussions.

ANATOMY

- Embryologically, the cleft may affect the primary or/and secondary palate.
- Anatomically, the cleft is defined according to the involvement of the hard and soft palate.
- The hard palate is the bony palate, and surgical anatomy involves
  - Palatine process of maxilla
  - Horizontal plate of palatine bone
  - Hook of hamulus and pterygoid plates of sphenoid bone
  - Vomer/septum
  - Greater palatine foramina
- Soft palate is the mobile part of the palate, and surgical anatomy involves
  - Levator veli palatini
  - Tensor veli palatini aponeurosis
  - Palatopharyngeus
  - Palatoglossus
- The Veau classification provides a clinically useful description of the cleft type according to the involvement of the alveolus, the hard palate, and the soft palate. It guides selection of the surgical treatment.
  - The two-flap palatoplasty is most commonly performed for clefts of the hard and soft palate. It is not commonly used for isolated clefts of the soft palate and is not used for submucous clefts.

PATHOGENESIS

- The etiology of cleft palate is multifactorial: environment, teratogen exposure (alcohol, anticonvulsants, steroids, diazepam), nutrition, maternal infections (rubella, toxoplasmosis), and genetics.

- Cleft palate repair restores anatomical closure between the oral and nasal cavities.
- An unrepaired cleft palate may result in impaired:
  - Breathing
  - Feeding
  - Speech
  - Hearing

NATURAL HISTORY

- Orofacial clefting is the most common craniofacial birth defect, occurring in 1:750 live births.
  - The incidence of cleft palate alone is 1:2000, with a female-to-male ratio of 2:1.
  - The incidence of cleft palate in combination with cleft lip is greater, estimated at 1:1000 with a reverse gender ratio.
- In the population of children with cleft lip and/or cleft palate (CL+/−P), approximately 50% will have CLP, 30% to 35% CP, and 15% to 20% CL.
- Approximately 40% of CP patients will have a syndrome, and 15% of CLP will have a syndrome.

PATIENT HISTORY AND PHYSICAL FINDINGS

- The diagnosis of a cleft palate is made by prenatal ultrasonography or by physical examination at birth and in early infancy. A detailed assessment is made of the child's breathing, feeding, growth, and development.
- Airway assessment must exclude presence of sleep apnea and micro-/retrognathia.
- Assessment of growth and weight is key to identify and monitor feeding difficulty, gastroesophageal reflux, and use of feeding aids (Haberman/Pigeon teat).
- Hearing and middle ear function must be assessed and treated early by an otolaryngologist.
- The plastic surgeon should define the cleft palate type according to the anatomic structures involved, the laterality, width of the palate, and presence/absence of a cleft lip.
- Also, the child should be assessed for associated anomalies suggestive of a syndrome: craniofacial dysmorphism, airway compromise, cardiac defects, ocular and auricular abnormalities, and musculoskeletal anomalies. A genetics referral is suggested if suspicious of syndromic cleft palate.[1]

DIFFERENTIAL DIAGNOSIS

- Syndromic cleft palate
  - van der Woude syndrome

- Stickler syndrome
- Robin sequence
- 22q11.2 deletion syndrome
- Treacher Collins syndrome
- Nager syndrome
- Ectrodactyly-ectodermal dysplasia
- Klippel-Feil syndrome

NONOPERATIVE MANAGEMENT

- It is very uncommon not to repair a cleft palate.
- If the child is unable to undergo surgical treatment secondary to airway concerns or medical fitness, a palatal obturator may be considered.

SURGICAL MANAGEMENT

- Cleft palate repair is ideally performed between 9 and 12 months of age,[2] with the infant weighing greater than 8 kg.
- Airway and middle ear disease assessment is performed and treated prior to or simultaneously with cleft palate repair.
- Risks of the procedure are hemorrhage/hematoma, airway compromise, wound dehiscence, infection, oronasal fistula, flap necrosis, velopharyngeal insufficiency, and reduced midfacial growth.
- The main objectives of the cleft palate repair are as follows:
  - To separate the oral and nasal cavities
  - To reposition to the velar musculature for restoration of the velopharyngeal sphincter, in particular the reconstruction of the levator muscular sling
  - To improve Eustachian tube function
  - To minimize detrimental effects on subsequent maxillary growth
- The main steps of the procedure are (a) marking and elevation of mucoperiosteal flaps off the hard palate; (b) isolation and lengthening of pedicles (greater palatine artery) for mobilization of the oral mucoperiosteal flaps; (c) dissection and separation of the nasal mucosa, velar musculature, and oral mucosa; (d) tension-free closure of nasal mucosal layer; (e) reconstruction of the velopharyngeal sphincter with repositioning of the levator sling; (f) recreation of the uvula; and (g) closure of the oral mucosal layer.

Preoperative Planning

- Active or passive dentofacial orthopedics is utilized for aligning the cleft maxillary arches by many teams today and is applied in the first few weeks of infancy. The orthopedic device is discontinued once the maxillary arches have been satisfactorily repositioned.
- With the patient anesthetized, the width of the cleft is measured at the junction of the soft palate and hard palate. The width of the cleft is important to predict difficulty of the cleft palate repair and anticipated amount of dissection required for closure. A cleft gap of:
  - Less than 11 mm closes with ease
  - 12 to 16 mm will require more extensive dissection to mobilize the greater palatine vessel and achieve nasal lining mobilization
  - Greater than 17 mm will require special maneuvers detailed below to achieve tension-free closure (greater palatine foramina osteotomy)

Positioning

- The patient is positioned supine with shoulder roll to allow neck extension. A south-facing oral RAE tube is carefully taped centrally with a mesentery. Corneas are protected with eye tapping.
- Access and visualization of the entire palate is very important and cannot be understated. It is especially important to ensure visualization from the uvuli to the anterior extent of the palate.
- It is essential for the surgeon to ensure that positioning is correct prior to scrubbing. This will facilitate the procedure.
- The surgeon should have a headlight or lighted instruments for optimizing visualization in the confined space and a skilled attentive assistant. It is also advantageous to have a bed that allows for Trendelenburg positioning. Some surgeons stand to perform palate surgery from below but having the baby's head supported with the surgeon seated operating upside down provides the best exposure and is the preferred position by many surgeons.

Approach

- The aim of cleft palate surgery is tension-free closure of the palate oral and nasal mucosal layers and restoration of the velopharyngeal muscular sphincter.
- Difficulties anticipated include the following:
  - Access
  - Lighting
  - Unforgiving tissue
  - Bleeding obscuring visualization
- Surgical approaches differ with regard to the amount of dissection performed to achieve tension-free closure and muscle repositioning.
- Importance lies in adequate exposure and dissection of tissues to allow comfort for the operating surgeon to achieve tension-free closure.
- Oral layer mobilization is largely dependent on careful mobilization of the greater palatine artery from its periosteal sleeve.
- Nasal layer mobilization is largely dependent on careful mobilization of the mucosa as a sheet from its dense bony attachments.

■ Two-Flap Palatoplasty for a Unilateral Complete Cleft Palate

Markings

- Carefully insert an intraoral gag and a throat pack (it is the surgeon's responsibility to insert and remove).
- Mark the incision lines:
  - Along the medial edges of the cleft from the uvuli to the anterior junction of the hard palate and alveolus
  - Laterally at the junction of the hard palate and maxillary alveolus, extending from the posterior maxillary tubercle to the anterior medial marking (**TECH FIG 1**)
- Inject local anesthetic with adrenaline into the hard palate and soft palate (average of 8 mL). The vasoconstrictive properties reduce blood loss and obstruction of the visual field. Local anesthetic also allows for hydrodissection of the mucoperiosteal flaps off of the hard palate and tissue expansion for ease of layer dissection in the soft palate.
- Wait 8 minutes or until injection sites stop bleeding.

Elevation of Oral Mucoperiosteal Flaps

- Perform incisions with needle tip cautery to reduce bleeding. Use a skin hook on the uvula or stay sutures for countertraction.
- Incisions, flap elevation, and pedicle dissection are done similarly on both the greater and lesser segments.
- Begin with lateral incisions: from the retromolar trigone along the junction of the alveolus and palate with diathermy down to bone and slightly angled medially to avoid injury of developing teeth.
- For the medial incisions, palpate the posteromedial edge of the hard palate before incising to ensure that the incision medially will be onto the bone (hard palate) as you can inadvertently cut into the nasal layer and do a "double cut" that reduces the available tissue for nasal layer closure. The incision medially is made with a scalpel.

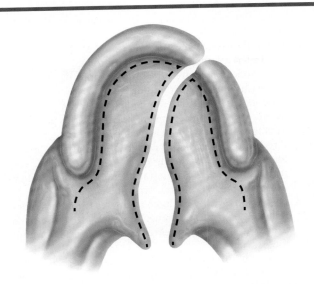

TECH FIG 1 • Markings of a two-flap palatoplasty for a unilateral complete cleft palate.

- Oral palatal mucosa is susceptible to tearing, so dissect continuously along the entire length of the lateral incision toward the cleft to elevate the mucoperiosteal flaps. Avoid "tunneling" as this can cause tearing of the hard palate mucosa due to dense periosteal attachments.
- Use a periosteal elevator to raise the mucoperiosteal flaps from lateral to medial (**TECH FIG 2A**).
- Then, use a skin hook at the leading anterior edge of the flap and dissect from anterior to posterior along the hard palate in sweeping motions toward the greater palatine foramina and posterior limit of the hard palate (**TECH FIG 2B**).

Isolation of Greater Palatine Vessels

- As you approach the greater palatine artery at the posterolateral edge of the hard palate, the vessel becomes visible on the undersurface of the flap.

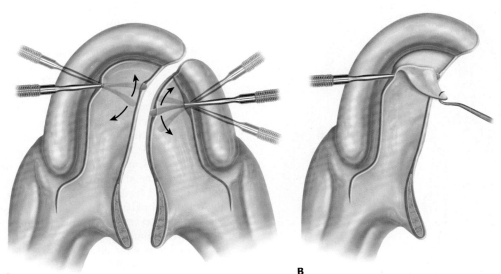

A   **B**

TECH FIG 2 • **A.** Dissection of the oral mucoperiosteal flaps. **B.** Elevation of the oral mucoperiosteal flap toward the pedicle, located posteriorly in the greater palatine foramina.

- The palatine artery has a circle of dense periosteal attachments around it.
  - Carefully dissect starting anterior and then working circumferentially around the foramina, staying on bone and taking care not to dissect into the artery or the leash of veins surrounding it.
  - To completely release the pedicle from its periosteal sleeve, careful and complete release of the periosteal attachments must be achieved by dissecting the flap directly off the posterior edge of the palatine bone.
  - Staying on bone during pedicle dissection is very important and rewarding as there are tethering ligaments that insert into the oral mucosa.
  - Dissection directly off bone facilitates the circumferential release of these ligaments, which otherwise make it exceedingly easy to tear the oral mucosa and injure the pedicle.
- Previous hydrodissection during local anesthetic injection will also aid in finding the bloodless plane between the oral layer mucosal glands and the muscular layer.
- Complete circumferential pedicle dissection is achieved once the periosteal sleeve is released behind the greater palatine foramina and velar muscle attachments to the posterior edge of the hard palate are visualized (**TECH FIG 3**).
- It is critical for the surgeon to approach the release of the periosteal sleeve patiently with gentle dissection and successive wider approach, which will allow the palatine artery to finally be freed without tearing the mucosa or creating excessive bleeding.
- Once pedicle dissection is achieved, use gentle traction with scissors to tease the vessel free out of the foramina. This will create enough freedom to close most palatal clefts.
- Very occasionally in the widest of clefts (>16 mm), osteotomy of the posterior wall of the foramina is required.
- Once sufficiently mobilized, retract the flaps out of the surgical field with stay sutures and secure to the intraoral gag/retractor.

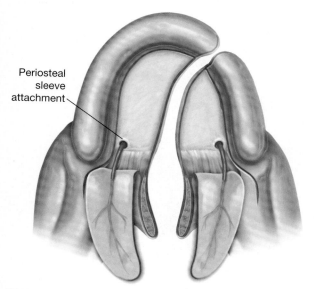

Periosteal sleeve attachment

TECH FIG 3 • Oral mucoperiosteal flap elevation is completed: pedicles are mobilized and velar musculature is visualized attached along the posterior hard palate.

- Under magnification, dissect in the plane between oral mucosal glands and the muscle layer posteriorly in the soft palate from the edge of the bony palate to the uvula.

Dissection of the Nasal Mucoperiosteum

- Mobilize the nasal mucoperiosteal layer with care, beginning on the lesser segment of the cleft. This requires the gradual and wide dissection of this continuous sheet of nasal mucosa, which is firmly attached to the hard palate along its medial and posterior edges, along the nasal surface of the bony palate and the medial surface of the medial pterygoid plate. The elevation of the nasal layer anteriorly on the greater segment will necessitate elevation off of the vomer.
  - The nasal mucosa is even more unforgiving than the oral mucosa, and once a tear occurs, it is very easy to propagate. Resist the temptation to tunnel before a whole edge has been liberated.
- Use a Mitchell's trimmer or similar blunt-edged instrument, starting at the cleft margin, and scrape the oral surface of the bone until the edge of the nasal mucosa starts to be defined and liberate the dense attachments to the medial hard palate. As the edge becomes apparent, elevate the nasal mucoperiosteum widely off the entire extent of the medial hard palate.
  - Judicious use of needlepoint diathermy on low setting can help to elevate firmly attached areas that are not easily released with the Mitchell's trimmer.
- Once the edge of the nasal mucoperiosteal flap is defined, slide the trimmer around the corner of the hard palate onto the nasal surface of the bone staying right on bone. If the edge is sufficiently liberated, then sweep anteriorly and posteriorly to liberate the entire sheet off of the nasal surface (**TECH FIG 4A**).
  - If a portion of the edge is still attached, resist further sweeping until releasing the portion that remains tethered to prevent a tear.
- This dissection is continued to the posterior nasal spine. At this juncture, there are always muscle attachments. Release these aberrant velar muscle attachments with needlepoint diathermy.
- Continue dissection along the nasal surface following the posterior edge of the bone cephalad and lateral toward the medial surface of the medial pterygoid plate (**TECH FIG 4B**).
- Release the nasal mucoperiosteum directly off the bony surface of the medial surface of the medial pterygoid plate with careful dissection of the fibrous attachments here. Be patient and careful during the release of this densely adherent portion of the nasal mucosa working posteriorly and cephalad along the pterygoid plate and palatine bone. Confirm complete release by directly visualizing the plane of the medial surface of the medial pterygoid plate. If further release is required, the origin of the tensor veli palatini (TVP) along the medial pterygoid plate may be severed to improve mobilization.
- The sheet of mucosa should now be freely mobile as one continuous sheet posteriorly and along the anterior medial hard palate. When extensive dissection is required for a wide cleft, there may be a noticeable reduction in the circumference of the oropharynx as the sheet mobilizes medially.

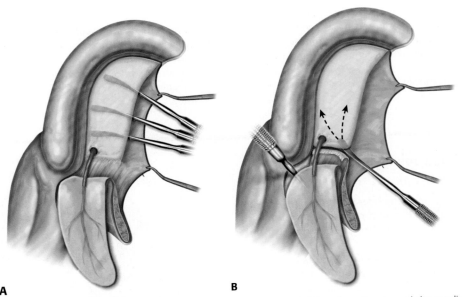

TECH FIG 4 • A. Elevation of nasal mucoperiosteal flaps. **B.** Nasal flap dissection toward the medial surface of the medial pterygoid plate.

- Attention is then turned to the greater segment.
  - The dissection of the nasal mucoperiosteal flap is identical posteriorly along the hard palate cleft margin.
  - Anteriorly, at the bony junction of the vomer and bony palate, the nasal mucoperiosteum is raised in continuity with the vomerine periosteum.
  - This vomerine flap is raised cephalad directly off bone and in continuity with the periosteum of the nasal surface of the hard palate.

Nasal Closure

- Nasal layer closure is then commenced once there is assurance that the repair is tension free by checking that both sides are sufficiently liberated.
- Meticulous closure with knots tied on the nasal side
- Small wedges are excised out at the base of the oral surface of the uvula to assist closure. Place eversion sutures during the closure of the uvuli to prevent notching or bifidity.

Dissection and Reconstruction of the Velar Musculature

- With the nasal layer completely closed, proceed with the muscle dissection and reconstruction of the velopharyngeal sphincter.
  - Three steps are critical for muscle repositioning:[3]
    - Identification and separation of levator veli palatini (LVP)
    - Velar musculature dissection and release from its attachments to the cleft margin and hard palate shelf
    - Velar musculature repositioning and repair
  - Deep to the muscles inserted into the back of the bony hard palate, the LVP inserts abnormally at the cleft margin in the anterior half of the velum.
- Using a scalpel, sharply dissect the velar muscle layer off of the nasal mucosa along the cleft margin. This is done with a paramedian incision lateral to the nasal mucosal closure line through muscle until the nasal mucosal surface is identified.

- It is easiest to separate the muscle layer once the nasal mucosa has been repaired to give a "trampoline" effect, providing tactile feedback and countertraction during this careful dissection.
- Also, it is important to note that the bulk and breadth of the muscle widen as you dissect laterally. This is analogous to the changing depth of a swimming pool, with a shallow end (paramedian) becoming deeper as one progressively dissects laterally.
- The velar musculature is raised off the nasal mucosa and separated from the tendinous fibers of the TVP. This separation is done laterally along the hard palate shelf at the junction of "salmon pink" velar muscle fibers and tendinous fibers of the TVP.
- The velar musculature is further dissected until it can be freely mobilized to lie parallel to the posterior hard palate margin and overlying the contralateral velar muscle bundle.
- You have completed the levator dissection when the "salmon pink"-colored longitudinal fibers of the levator are identified emerging from the skull base and the entire dissected muscle is free to be reoriented to a more functionally effective position in the posterior half of the soft palate.
- The dissection of the velar musculature is performed on both sides.
- Repair the muscles and reconstruct the levator muscular sling by suturing the muscles and securing with multiple sutures, knots facing the nasal surface.
- Ensure proper hemostasis is achieved.

Oral Closure

- Close the oral layer beginning with stay sutures placed anteriorly and progressing posteriorly toward the uvuli with horizontal mattress sutures.
  - There is no attempt of push-back of the flaps for lengthening with a V-Y closure.

T
E
C
H
N
I
Q
U
E
S

- During oral layer closure, place some full-thickness sutures through both the oral and nasal layers just posterior to the hard palate shelf (anterior to muscle repair) to help obliterate the dead space and position the muscle repair.
- Place interrupted simple sutures between each of the mattress sutures.

- Attempt to minimize raw bone exposure by closing palatal flaps to alveolus wherever possible.
- Recheck for adequate hemostasis, irrigate, and remove throat pack.
- If concerned for airway during postoperative period, consider nasopharyngeal tube insertion and a tongue stitch.

■ Two-Flap Palatoplasty—Bilateral Complete Cleft Palate

- In a bilateral cleft palate, the operative steps are similar to those outlined above except for the flap elevation and closure anteriorly along the junction of the primary and secondary palate.
- The oral and mucosal nasal incisions and dissections on the lesser segment are performed as outlined above.
- Bilateral vomerine flaps are raised from the premaxilla in continuity with the nasal mucoperiosteal flaps (**TECH FIG 5**).
- The anterior closure of the nasal and oral layers requires meticulous approximation and closure to eliminate the risk of an oronasal fistula at the junction of the primary and secondary palate.
- Careful and patient dissection is required to the dense attachments of mucoperiosteum to the posterior surface of the premaxilla to which the palatal flaps will be anchored.

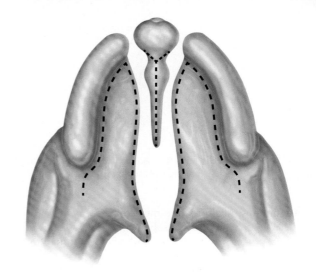

TECH FIG 5 • Markings of a two-flap palatoplasty for a bilateral complete cleft palate.

PEARLS AND PITFALLS

Headlight and positioning	■ Good lighting and access paramount importance
Loupe magnification	■ Especially helpful for dissection around palatine foramina and muscle when surgeon is less experienced
Hemostasis	■ Ensure meticulous hemostasis throughout case to optimize visualization. ■ Judicious use of needlepoint diathermy ■ Failure to do so may result in airway compromise, flap necrosis, and wound dehiscence.
Use needlepoint diathermy to make hard palate incisions.	■ Controls bleeding and persisting ooze
Work on broad front.	■ Avoid tunneling during dissection.
Patience and precision during dissection especially around palatine foramina	■ Bleeding obscures view, and careless dissection risks injury to pedicle and vascularity of the flap.
Handle tissues with care.	■ Nasal mucosa is especially susceptible to tears.
Inset palatal flaps with stay sutures to help control closure.	■ Helps to put the most difficult sutures anteriorly with stay sutures to judge closure and maintains good exposure
Do not attempt closure until all layers are sufficiently mobilized.	■ Prevents tearing ■ If sutures are prematurely placed, further attempts to mobilize tissue are more likely to result in tears. Prematurely suturing may also result in tears if tension is still present.
Oronasal fistula	■ Critical to achieve adequate tissue dissection, perfect approximation, and apposition of tissue layers with meticulous suture technique to prevent fistulae.

POSTOPERATIVE CARE

- Nasopharyngeal tube as required
- Remove tongue stitch in recovery if used.
- Analgesia to reduce blood pressure and distress (24 hours of intravenous opioids)
- Encourage feeding.
- Postoperative visit in 4 weeks

OUTCOMES

- Two-flap palatoplasty yields excellent speech outcomes with minimal surgical morbidity.
- In a 20-year long-term follow-up, the authors have recorded a 7% to 11% incidence of velopharyngeal insufficiency with no significant difference between cleft subtypes.[4]
- Speech results were normal to mildly impaired resonance (92%), no or inaudible nasal air emission (80%), and no compensatory articulation errors (98%).
- The fistula rate of a cleft palate repair with a unipedicled flap technique is 6.2% (95% CI, 4.3%–8.4%) according to a systematic review of international data.[5]
- The effect of palatoplasty on maxillary facial retrusion is controversial. Inherent maxillary growth deficiency, secondary scarring from palatal flap elevation, and timing of repair are all contributing factors to midfacial retrusion.[6] Deleterious growth has been shown to be greatest in patients treated by Veau push-back technique. Further long-term studies are required to compare the effect of palatal flap technique on maxillary growth restriction.

COMPLICATIONS

- Bleeding is a feared complication as it may lead to an emergency with airway obstruction and respiratory compromise. Additionally, hematoma may lead to compression of the pedicle or flap, with resultant flap necrosis, wound dehiscence, and oronasal fistulae. To prevent this complication, vigilant hemostasis is an absolute and adequate postoperative analgesia is necessary.
- Airway obstruction may occur in the absence of hemorrhage, and a tongue stitch or nasopharyngeal tube may assist in prevention of obstruction in infants at risk. Airway obstruction can also occur if a throat pack is utilized and the surgeon overlooks removal of the throat pack prior to extubation.
- Flap necrosis is rare and avoidable with careful dissection and release of the periosteal sleeve of the greater palatine pedicle.
- Infection and wound dehiscence leading to oronasal fistulae are detrimental. A small fistula secondary to delayed wound healing may heal with conservative measures. Failure of closure may necessitate reoperation with re-elevation and closure of oral and nasal flaps as well as possible augmentation using local flaps and/or biologic adjuncts.

REFERENCES

1. van Aalst JA, Kolappa KK, Sadove M. MOC-PS CME article: nonsyndromic cleft palate. *Plast Reconstr Surg.* 2008;121:1-14.
2. Rohrich RJ, Love EJ, Byrd HS, Johns DF. Optimal timing of cleft palate closure. *Plast Reconstr Surg.* 2000;106:413-422.
3. Kriens OB. An anatomical approach to veloplasty. *Plast Reconstr Surg.* 1969;43:29-41.
4. Salyer KE, Sng KW, Sperry EE. Two flap palatoplasty: 20-year experience and evolution of surgical technique. *Plast Reconstr Surg.* 2006;118:193-204.
5. Hardwicke JT, Landini G, Richard BM. Fistula incidence after primary cleft palate repair: a systematic review of the literature. *Plast Reconstr Surg.* 2014;134:618e-627e.
6. Lee YH, Liao YF. Hard palate repair technique and facial growth in patients with cleft lip and palate: a systematic review. *Br J Oral Maxillofac Surg.* 2013;51:851-857.

12

CHAPTER

Tongue-Lip Adhesion/Floor of Mouth Muscle Release for Pierre Robin Sequence

Chad A. Purnell and Arun K. Gosain

DEFINITION

- Pierre Robin sequence (PRS) is a clinical triad of glossoptosis, retrognathia, and airway obstruction.
- Cleft palate is present in approximately 50% of cases.
- PRS is associated with an identified syndrome in 30% to 60% of cases.[1]
- The most common syndromes associated with PRS are Stickler syndrome (11%–20%) and 22q11.2 deletion (velocardiofacial) syndrome (11%).[2]

ANATOMY

- The tongue in PRS is posteriorly displaced due to retrognathia. This results in an airway obstruction at the tongue base (**FIG 1**).
- Airway obstruction may also result from lesions lower than the tongue, such as laryngomalacia. Synchronous airway lesions are present in up to 28% of patients.[3]
- Cleft palate may be U- or V-shaped; a U-shaped palatal cleft is classically associated with PRS.

PATHOGENESIS

- Pathogenesis of PRS is incompletely understood and likely multifactorial.

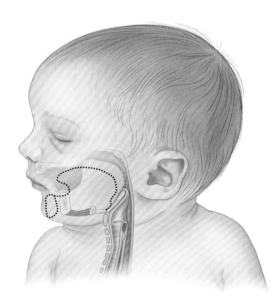

FIG 1 • Micrognathia results in a more posterior position of the mandible and tongue in PRS (*solid lines*) compared to a normal patient (*dotted lines*).

- Theorized mechanisms of PRS include mechanical obstruction to mandibular growth, delay in neuromuscular development of the tongue and oropharynx, connective tissue dysplasia, and teratogen exposure.[4,5]

NATURAL HISTORY

- PRS occurs on a spectrum that ranges from mild asymptomatic hypoplasia to critical airway obstruction requiring emergent endotracheal intubation at birth.
- In more severe phenotypes, PRS is often associated with feeding issues such as gastroesophageal reflux, failure to thrive, and abnormal oroesophageal motility.[6,7]
- Mortality has decreased dramatically with improved awareness and care. Mortality in 1946 was greater than 50% and has decreased to 16%, with all deaths occurring in syndromic patients.[8,9]

PATIENT HISTORY AND PHYSICAL FINDINGS

- A full birth history and physical examination should be performed. A key point of examination should be documenting the maxillomandibular discrepancy with the child upright and the mandible closed.
- A careful examination for syndromic features should include hearing and ocular exam to evaluate for Stickler syndrome.[10]
- Evaluation and treatment of any patient with PRS should be performed by a multidisciplinary team, which includes craniofacial surgery, otolaryngology, speech and feeding therapy, critical care/anesthesiology, and genetics.

IMAGING

- If the child is not intubated, a polysomnogram should be performed, including a portion with a nasopharyngeal airway in place in order to determine whether there is ongoing sleep apnea if upper airway obstruction is removed.
- Fiberoptic nasendoscopy is performed to evaluate whether the airway obstruction is isolated to the tongue base or whether there are additional sources of supraglottic airway obstruction, including laryngomalacia.
- Prior to any surgical intervention, bronchoscopy should be performed to evaluate for subglottic synchronous airway lesions.

NONOPERATIVE MANAGEMENT

- The majority of patients can be treated nonoperatively.
- Initial airway management is prone positioning to displace the mandible anteriorly.
- Supplemental oxygen may be added as well.

- A nasopharyngeal airway should be placed if desaturations continue. This airway has been utilized successfully as end-treatment at home by several centers.[11]
- If a nasopharyngeal airway does not resolve airway obstruction, emergent endotracheal intubation is indicated.
- Continuous positive airway pressure masks and palatal appliances have also been described for treatment.[12,13]

SURGICAL MANAGEMENT
Preoperative Planning

- Prior to any surgical treatment, bronchoscopy should be performed. In the presence of significant subglottic obstruction, tracheostomy is likely the only treatment option.
- Prior to performing a tongue-lip adhesion, a GILLS score should be calculated. One point is given for each of the following: gastroesophageal reflux, intubation preoperatively, late operation (greater than 2 weeks of age), low birth weight (less than 2500 g), and syndromic diagnosis. A score of 3 or more is predictive of failure of tongue-lip adhesion, and another option such as mandibular distraction osteogenesis or tracheostomy should be considered.[14,15]

Positioning

- The procedure is performed supine.
- Endotracheal intubation may be nasotracheal or orotracheal, with the tube taped to the side out of the operative field.

Approach

- Soft tissue procedures for PRS include tongue-lip adhesion, subperiosteal release of the floor of mouth, or both procedures performed concomitantly.[16,17]
- Subperiosteal release of the floor of mouth is an ideal addition to tongue-lip adhesion if the patient has a fixed, immobile tongue (ankyloglossia) and a tongue-based airway obstruction. This procedure is also performed in isolation for airway obstruction at some centers.
- Mandibular distraction osteogenesis is a skeletal technique to treat mandibular hypoplasia that may have more repeatable resolution of airway obstruction in a broader range of patients with PRS, with potentially higher complication rates.[18–20]

■ Subperiosteal Release of the Floor of the Mouth

Creation of Tongue and Lip Flaps

- 0.5% lidocaine with epinephrine is injected into all planned incisions for hemostasis.
- A transverse incision is made 1.5 cm in length in the lower lip (**TECH FIG 1A**).

- Incision is carried obliquely posterior into the muscle of the lip to create a superiorly based flap approximately 1.5 × 1 cm in area.
- A 1.5-cm transverse incision is made in the undersurface of the tongue approximately 2 mm inferior to the rugae (**TECH FIG 1B**).
- An inferiorly based 1.5- × 1-cm musculomucosal flap is elevated (**TECH FIG 1C**).

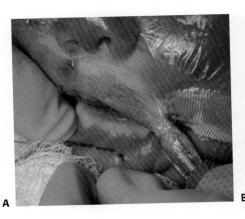

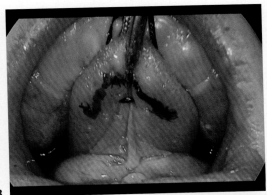

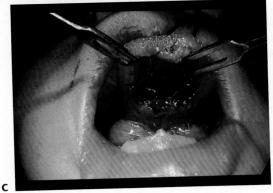

TECH FIG 1 • A. A 1.5- × 1-cm flap is marked in the mucosa of the inferior lip. **B.** A 1.5- × 1-cm inferiorly based flap is marked on the inferior tongue. **C.** See **TECH FIG 4**. Tongue musculomucosal flap after elevation.

TECHNIQUES

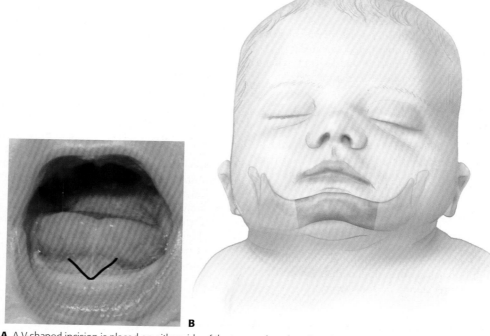

TECH FIG 2 • A. A V-shaped incision is placed on either side of the tongue frenulum for subperiosteal release of the tongue. **B.** Area of periosteal elevation of the lingual surface of the mandible.

Subperiosteal Release of the Floor of the Mouth

- A separate V-shaped incision is made around the base of the frenulum of the tongue (**TECH FIG 2A**).
- Dissection is carried anteriorly until the lingual surface of the mandible is reached. The periosteum of the mandible is incised.
- A periosteal elevator is used to completely elevate the periosteum of the lingual surface of the symphysis, parasymphyses, and bilateral mandible bodies (**TECH FIG 2B**).
- Incision is closed in a V-to-Y advancement fashion with 4-0 Vicryl in the muscle layer and 5-0 Monocryl for the mucosal layer.

Placement of Tongue Suspension Suture

- A loop of 4-0 silk suture is tied through one hole of a surgical button and left long as an emergency pullout suture.
  - The button is placed on a backer of adhesive foam to help prevent pressure sores (**TECH FIG 3A**).
- 2-0 polypropylene suture on a long, curved taper needle (2-0 Prolene on a CT-1 needle; Ethicon, Somerville, NJ) is used after straightening the needle slightly to allow the needle to capture the anterior tongue mass.
  - This suture is passed through the raw area created by the tongue flap, through the mass of the anterior tongue musculature, and out the posterior tongue mucosa at a point where the tongue starts to curve toward the oropharynx in a more vertical orientation.

- The needle is then passed through the button, then back through the tongue in a mattress fashion (**TECH FIG 3B**).
- The suspension suture is pulled forward to assess anterior movement of the tongue mass as the suture is brought under tension.
- If tongue movement is acceptable, the suture is brought through the incision in the lower labial sulcus, staying anterior to the mandible, to exit the skin in a submandibular crease.
  - The loose end of the suture can be threaded through a Keith needle and passed parallel to the first end to complete the mattress suture.
- Before removing the needles, both suture ends are passed through a foam-backed button, over which the suture will be tied. Foam should be firm and can be fashioned from the foam backing within an empty needle pack.
  - The button overlying the tongue mass does not require foam backing, whereas the submandibular button does require foam backing to avoid ulceration of the facial skin.

Closure and Tensioning of Tongue

- The posterior mucosa of the tongue is approximated to the inferior aspect of the labial sulcus incision using interrupted 5-0 Monocryl suture (Ethicon, Somerville, NJ).
  - Sutures are placed sequentially from one side of the incision to the other, taking care to place the knots such that they lie on the mucosal side of the closure (**TECH FIG 4A**).

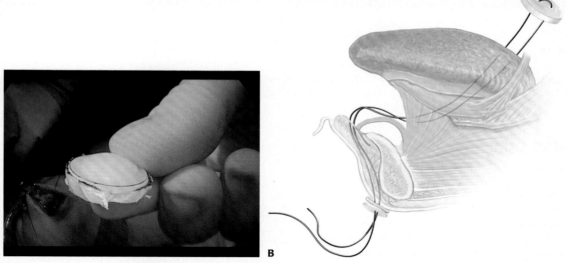

TECH FIG 3 • A. A backer of adhesive foam is placed on the back of the surgical buttons to prevent pressure sores from the buttons. **B.** Path of 2-0 polypropylene suspension suture through the tongue and surgical button and out the skin.

- The muscle of the tongue and the lip are approximated on either side and in the center of the limbs of the suspension suture using 4-0 Vicryl suture (Ethicon, Somerville, NJ). Three such sutures are usually sufficient.
- The anterior mucosa of the tongue is approximated to the superior aspect of the labial sulcus incision using interrupted 5-0 Monocryl suture. Sutures are placed sequentially from one side of the incision to the other, taking care to place the knots such that they lie on the mucosal side of the closure.
- Tension on the tongue suspension suture is determined by gently securing the first knot over the submandibular foam-backed button until the tongue

mass just begins to move forward. No further tension should be placed so as minimize pressure on the skin. Subsequent knots are placed to secure the suture (**TECH FIG 4B**).

  - The purpose of the suspension suture is simply to take pressure off of the mucosal and muscular layers of the closure for the first 7 to 10 days, and sequelae such as tongue edema or skin ulceration can be minimized by placing the least amount of tension on the suture required to move the tongue mass forward.
- The safety silk suture tied to the button in the mouth is taped to the cheek.
- A nasogastric tube is placed to facilitate feeding.

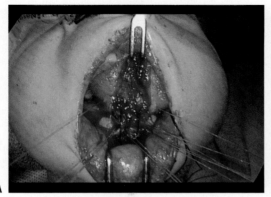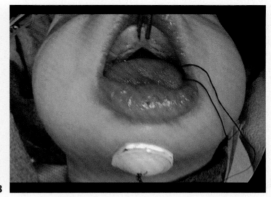

TECH FIG 4 • A. Posterior layer of mucosal flaps is closed with 5-0 Monocryl sutures. **B.** Suspension suture is tied over a button under the chin. Note the safety silk suture used to retrieve the intraoral button.

PEARLS AND PITFALLS

Preoperative screening	■ Nasendoscopy and bronchoscopy are essential prior to tongue-lip adhesion. The procedure should not be performed if there are any synchronous airway lesions.
Suspension suture	■ The suspension suture should be tensioned to pull the base of the tongue forward but should not be pulled maximally as to cause tissue necrosis and increased tongue edema.
Postoperative care	■ The adhesion should NOT be left in place until repair of cleft palate. This jeopardizes oromotor development and mobility of the tongue.

POSTOPERATIVE CARE

■ Extubation is carried out when deemed appropriate by anesthesiology or critical care. A nasopharyngeal airway is left in place for several days to manage the airway while surgical edema is present.

■ The suspension suture is left in place for 7 to 10 days.

■ The child is monitored carefully for resolution of airway obstruction. Postoperative polysomnography is performed.

■ If airway obstruction resolves, the patient is evaluated every 1 to 2 months. The tongue is monitored for active motion in response to touch, a sign of maturing tongue function.

■ If tongue motion has matured and MMD has decreased to 3 mm or less, the adhesion is taken down, usually by 6 to 7 months of age.

■ Early takedown of the tongue-lip adhesion is preferable so as to avoid oromotor delay in tongue function. Prior reports left the adhesion in place until the time of palate repair, often close to or later than 1 year of age. We believe that this can contribute to oromotor retardation. In addition, it is preferable to take down the tongue-lip adhesion well before the palate repair so as to assess adequacy of airway prior to further airway restriction that accompanies cleft palate repair.

OUTCOMES

■ Resolution of airway obstruction is variable in studies of tongue-lip adhesion, ranging from 43% to 89%.[15,21]

■ Complete resolution of feeding difficulties also is variable, but many authors report an approximately 60% rate of ability to oral feed without any tube-feeding supplementation. Variabilities may exist due to institution-based protocols for surgical feeding tube placement.[22,23]

■ Few studies comprehensively assess polysomnographic findings after tongue-lip adhesion. Sedaghat et al.[24] describe improvement in sleep study findings in 7/8 patients after adhesion, but only 3 patients had reduction to mild or no sleep apnea. Flores et al.[18] describe improvement in apnea-hypopnea index in 15 patients after adhesion, but improvement was significantly less compared to mandibular distraction patients.

■ Tongue-lip adhesion has minimal effects on long-term speech development.[25]

COMPLICATIONS

■ Dehiscence (greatly reduced in techniques that utilize a suspension suture)

■ Failure to completely resolve airway obstruction
  ■ In these cases, the airway should be reassessed for sites of synchronous airway lesions that may not have been appreciated, paying particular attention to supraglottic airway compromise and laryngomalacia.

■ If the only other site of airway compromise is some element of laryngomalacia, the multidisciplinary team should be consulted regarding potential role for mandibular distraction osteogenesis with or without supraglottoplasty.

■ If the patient is found to have laryngomalacia and is not felt to be a candidate for mandibular distraction osteogenesis with or without supraglottoplasty, or if synchronous subglottic airway compromise is identified (eg, tracheomalacia), then tracheostomy is recommended.

■ Requirement for prolonged nasogastric feeds or gastrostomy tube

REFERENCES

1. Izumi K, Konczal LL, Mitchell AL, Jones MC. Underlying genetic diagnosis of Pierre Robin sequence: retrospective chart review at two children's hospitals and a systematic literature review. *J Pediatr.* 2012;160(4):645.e2-650.e2.

2. van den Elzen AP, Semmekrot BA, Bongers EM, et al. Diagnosis and treatment of the Pierre Robin sequence: results of a retrospective clinical study and review of the literature. *Eur J Pediatr.* 2001;160(1):47-53.

3. Andrews BT, Fan KL, Roostaeian J, et al. Incidence of concomitant airway anomalies when using the University of California, Los Angeles, protocol for neonatal mandibular distraction. *Plast Reconstr Surg.* 2013;131(5):1116-1123.

4. Cohen M. Robin sequences and complexes: causal heterogeneity and pathogenetic/phenotypic variability. *Am J Med Genet.* 1999;84:311-315.

5. Chiriac A, Dawson A, Krapp M, et al. Pierre Robin syndrome: a case report. *Arch Gynecol Obstet.* 2008;277:95-98.

6. Daniel M, Bailey S, Walker K, et al. Airway, feeding and growth in infants with Robin sequence and sleep apnoea. *Int J Pediatr Otorhinolaryngol.* 2013;77(4):499-503.

7. Baudon JJ, Renault F, Goutet JM, et al. Motor dysfunction of the upper digestive tract in Pierre Robin sequence as assessed by sucking-swallowing electromyography and esophageal manometry. *J Pediatr.* 2002;140(6):719-723.

8. Douglas D. The treatment of micrognathia associated with obstruction by a plastic procedure. *Plast Reconstr Surg.* 1946;1:300.

9. Costa MA, Tu MM, Murage KP, et al. Robin sequence: mortality, causes of death, and clinical outcomes. *Plast Reconstr Surg.* 2014;134(4):738-745.

10. Antunes RB, Alonso N, Paula RG. Importance of early diagnosis of Stickler syndrome in newborns. *J Plast Reconstr Aesthet Surg.* 2012;65(8):1029-1034.

11. Abel F, Bajaj Y, Wyatt M, Wallis C. The successful use of the nasopharyngeal airway in Pierre Robin sequence: an 11-year experience. *Arch Dis Child.* 2012;97(4):331-334.

12. Leboulanger N, Picard A, Soupre V, et al. Physiologic and clinical benefits of noninvasive ventilation in infants with Pierre Robin sequence. *Pediatrics.* 2010;126(5):e1056-e1063.

13. Butow KW, Hoogendijk CF, Zwahlen RA. Pierre Robin sequence: appearances and 25 years of experience with an innovative treatment protocol. *J Pediatr Surg.* 2009;44(11):2112-2118.

14. Abramowicz S, Bacic JD, Mulliken JB, Rogers GF. Validation of the GILLS score for tongue-lip adhesion in Robin sequence patients. *J Craniofac Surg.* 2012;23(2):382-386.

15. Rogers GF, Murthy AS, LaBrie RA, Mulliken JB. The GILLS score: part I. Patient selection for tongue-lip adhesion in Robin sequence. *Plast Reconstr Surg.* 2011;128(1):243-251.

16. Argamaso RV. Glossopexy for upper airway obstruction in Robin sequence. *Cleft Palate Craniofac J.* 1992;29(3):232-238.

17. Caouette-Laberge L, Borsuk DE, Bortoluzzi PA. Subperiosteal release of the floor of the mouth to correct airway obstruction in pierre robin sequence: review of 31 cases. *Cleft Palate Craniofac J.* 2012;49(1):14-20.

18. Flores RL, Tholpady SS, Sati S, et al. The surgical correction of Pierre Robin sequence: mandibular distraction osteogenesis versus tongue-lip adhesion. *Plast Reconstr Surg.* 2014;133(6):1433-1439.

19. Master D, Hanson P, Gosain A. Complications of mandibular distraction osteogenesis. *J Craniofac Surg.* 2010;21:1565-1570.

20. Paes EC, Bittermann GK, Bittermann D, et al. Long-term results of mandibular distraction osteogenesis with a resorbable device in infants with Robin sequence: effects on developing molars and mandibular growth. *Plast Reconstr Surg.* 2016;137(2):375e-385e.

21. Li HY, Lo LJ, Chen KS, et al. Robin sequence: review of treatment modalities for airway obstruction in 110 cases. *Int J Pediatr Otorhinolaryngol.* 2002;65(1):45-51.

22. Kirschner R, Low D, Randall P, et al. Surgical airway management in Pierre Robin sequence: is there a role for tongue-lip adhesion? *Cleft Palate Craniofac J.* 2003;29:239.

23. Hoffman W. Outcome of tongue-lip plication in patients with severe Pierre Robin sequence. *J Craniofac Surg.* 2003;14(5):602-608.

24. Sedaghat AR, Anderson IC, McGinley BM, et al. Characterization of obstructive sleep apnea before and after tongue-lip adhesion in children with micrognathia. *Cleft Palate Craniofac J.* 2012;49(1):21-26.

25. LeBlanc SM, Golding-Kushner KJ. Effect of glossopexy on speech sound production in Robin sequence. *Cleft Palate Craniofac J.* 1992;29(3):239-245.

13

CHAPTER

Palatal Fistula

Gregory D. Pearson

DEFINITION

- A fistula is defined as an epithelialized tract between two cavities that are not meant to be communicating.
- A palatal fistula is an abnormal communication between the oral and nasal cavities.
- Palatal fistula can be intentional or unintentional.
  - Intentional fistulas are fistulas not repaired at the time of initial operation. Examples include:
    - The alveolar cleft with a Veau III or Veau IV (unless the surgeon elects to perform a gingivoperiosteoplasty)
    - A Veau IV with a "locked out" premaxilla
  - Unintentional fistula after palatoplasty[1-3]:
    - These fistulas are unwanted and not planned for during the initial operation.
    - Veau IV clefts are associated with the highest fistula rate.
    - No difference in risk for palatal fistula related to gender, age at time of repair, and race.
    - The difference in fistula rate between straight line repairs and Furlow-type repairs appears to be surgeon/institution dependent with no clear lower risk between the two types of repair.
- Palatal fistula repair can be an extremely challenging problem to solve and prevention is the best option.

ANATOMY

- The Pittsburgh fistula classification system classifies fistulas as I to VII, from a posterior to anterior location on the palate[4] (**FIG 1**).
  - Type I involves only the uvula (consisting of a bifid uvula).
  - Type II involves the soft palate.
  - Type III occurs at the junction of the hard/soft palate.
  - Type IV arises within the hard palate.

- Type V is located at the incisive foramen (reserved for Veau IV clefts).
- Type VI is a lingual alveolar communication on the alveolus.
- Type VII is located on the labial side of the alveolus.

PATHOGENESIS

- Occurrence rates of palatal fistula vary from 0% to 60% in reported literature.[1-3]
- Several factors have been associated with the prevention of palatal fistula:
  - Tension-free and watertight closure
    - Relaxing incisions advocated by von Langenbeck for tension-free closure.
    - Jackson et al. proposed "CHOP modification" of Furlow palatoplasty for soft palate repair.[2]
  - Complete two-layer closure of nasal and oral flaps
    - LaRossa promoted liberal use of vomer flaps for closure of the nasal floor.[5]
  - Infection prevention
    - The use of perioperative antibiotics is debated in the literature.

NATURAL HISTORY

- Palatal fistula will remain patent until the time of closure.
- A fistula can be symptomatic or asymptomatic

PATIENT HISTORY AND PHYSICAL FINDINGS

- Palatal fistula can occur after cleft palate repair, oncologic resection, trauma, or illicit drug use.
- Patients may report that the fistula is symptomatic.
  - Nasal escape of food or liquids
    - May be intermittent
    - Typically, viscous liquids like yogurt
  - Nasal escape of air
    - May be noted by patient as change in voice
- May be noted by speech pathologist as nasal turbulence or hypernasality
- Physical examination will demonstrate a hole or communication from the oral to nasal cavity.
  - Fistulas can range from small to large and vary in location on the palate.
  - Small fistulas can be difficult to see, but the patient can typically state/point to the location.
    - An examination under anesthesia with a lacrimal probe can be useful to determine the location, size, and orientation of a fistula.

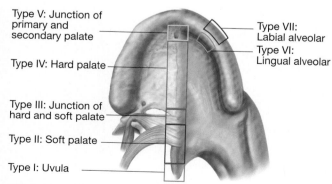

Type V: Junction of primary and secondary palate

Type IV: Hard palate

Type III: Junction of hard and soft palate

Type II: Soft palate

Type I: Uvula

Type VII: Labial alveolar

Type VI: Lingual alveolar

FIG 1 • Pittsburgh fistula classification system.

- A dental mirror can be useful in evaluating anterior fistulas.
- Deep crevasses or folds of mucoperiosteal tissue can simulate a fistula.
- Palatal expansion may open an occult fistula that was already present.

IMAGING

- Radiographic fistulograms (such as those performed for an enterocutaneous fistula evaluation) are not necessary.
- Physical examination should determine whether a fistula is present.
- Nasopharyngoscopy or video fluoroscopy should be employed to determine velopharyngeal gap size in patients with fistula and velopharyngeal dysfunction.

DIFFERENTIAL DIAGNOSIS

- Hypernasality from velopharyngeal dysfunction (VPD)
- Nasal escape of liquids/food secondary to poor oral motor planning/retrograde oronasal reflux

NONOPERATIVE MANAGEMENT

- Obturators/dental retainers can be fabricated by dentists or orthodontists to provide symptomatic relief (**FIG 2**).
  - Obtaining patient compliance for wearing the retainer can be difficult.
  - The dental brackets on the retainer may loosen and require retightening or fabrication of a new splint.
  - The patient must have enough teeth to properly support a retainer.

SURGICAL MANAGEMENT

- Surgical management and operative options are largely dictated by the location of the palatal fistula based upon the Pittsburgh classification system.
- When determining whether to repair a fistula, the surgeon should strongly consider and assess whether the fistula is symptomatic.
  - Nasal escape of fluids or foods, hypernasality, and preventing further surgical or orthodontic interventions (eg, bone grafting or orthognathic surgery) are all reasons for attempted fistula repair.
- Pittsburgh type I
  - Bifid uvula rate ranges from 1.34% to 19% of selected populations, but the true fistula rate is probably underestimated in the literature.
  - Because these fistulas tend to be asymptomatic as well as concerns about anesthesia on pediatric brain development, these fistulas are the least likely to be repaired as a primary objective for an operation.

- Pittsburgh type II
  - When determining the type of reconstruction choice for a soft palatal fistula repair, a surgeon should also make a determination related to a child's resonance (specifically if VPD is present) and the type of previous repair performed.
    - If the child has VPD, the fistula may be fixed but hypernasality will likely persist unless addressed with the repair.
  - If a child has normal resonance regardless of the type of primary palatoplasty performed, augmentation/reinforcement with acellular dermal matrix (ADM) can be used.[6]
  - For patients with a fistula after straight-line repair and concurrent VPD, addressing the VPD with either a palatal lengthening procedure or VPD surgery should be strongly considered.
    - A conversion to a Furlow double opposing Z-plasty typically allows repair of a type II fistula while addressing VPD in children with small velopharyngeal gaps on imaging.[7]
    - The CHOP modification with bilateral relaxing incisions can facilitate tension-free closure.
  - For larger velopharyngeal gaps and fistula or very large fistula (dehiscence), a superiorly based posterior pharyngeal flap may be necessary as conversion to Furlow may not lengthen the palatal sufficiently.
- Pittsburgh type III
  - Traditional teaching reports that the junction of the hard palate and soft palate remains the most common site of fistula, particularly when employing a Furlow palatoplasty.
  - As for type II fistula, the patient's resonance and type of previous repair should influence the operation considered for fistula repair.
- Pittsburgh type IV
  - There is significant overlap for techniques used to repair type III and IV palatal fistulas.
  - The mucoperiosteal flaps tend to scar, become stiffer, and have less mobility compared to flaps used in a primary palatoplasty, thus limiting their advancement or rotation potential.
- Pittsburgh type V
  - This is the second most common location of fistula as well as the most challenging to repair given the relative lack of palatal tissue in this area.
  - These fistulas are often the result of either poor inset of the lateral palatal mucoperiosteal flaps into the premaxillary segment or more commonly a premaxillary segment that is so anteriorly displaced out of the arch (a "locked out" premaxilla and intentional fistula) that closure at the time of initial palatoplasty is not possible.

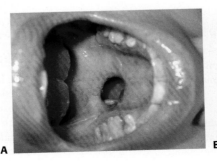
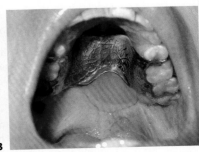

FIG 2 • Palatal fistula **(A)** covered with an obturator **(B)**.   A   B

- Pittsburgh type VI and VII fistulas pertain to the alveolar arch and labial sulcus and are addressed in the chapter on alveolar cleft repair.

Preoperative Planning

- The surgeon must discuss the possibility of palatal fistula recurrence after attempted closure with the patient and family.
- Assuring proper patient compliance with postoperative instructions prior to embarking upon repair is imperative.
- Depending on the type of repair technique used, a surgeon may consider having orthodontist fashion of a postsurgical retainer to protect repair while healing, particularly for type IV and V fistulas.
  - It is important to ensure the retainer does not put pressure on flaps or area of repair while still protecting the surgical site from tongue and food particulate.
- As previously stated, in rare instances, an examination under anesthesia with a lacrimal probe can be useful to determine the location, size, and orientation of a fistula.
- If a local flap is used, it must be protected from masticatory trauma during healing.

Positioning

- The patient should be orally intubated.
  - May use a regular endotracheal tube or oral RAE endotracheal tube depending upon surgeon and anesthesiologist's preferences.
  - The endotracheal tube may be positioned in the midline or laterally depending on the repair technique chosen.
- Typically, the patient should be placed in a horseshoe headrest with a shoulder roll and slight extension of the neck.
- A Dingman mouth prop or dental bite blocks (in which use depends on surgical technique to be employed) can be extremely useful for proper exposure of the intraoral cavity.

Approach

- Although multiple strategies can be performed for each site, the most common/useful approaches will be addressed according to the Pittsburgh classification system.
- Pittsburgh type I: Excision and reapproximation
- Pittsburgh type II:
  - Lateral relaxing incisions and rerepair
    - May consider augmentation with ADM
  - Conversion by Furlow palatoplasty
  - Posterior pharyngeal flap
- Pittsburgh type III:
  - Lateral relaxing incisions and rerepair
    - May consider augmentation with ADM
  - Posterior pharyngeal flap (if VPD present)
  - Buccal myomucosal flap
  - Facial artery musculomucosal (FAMM) flap
- Pittsburgh type IV:
  - Lateral relaxing incisions and rerepair with pushback technique
    - May consider augmentation with ADM
  - Elevation of mucoperiosteal flaps and pushback technique
  - Labial mucosal flap
    - If space in dental arch to pass through or if bite blocks employed
  - Buccal myomucosal flap
  - FAMM flap
  - Tongue flap
  - Free tissue transfer
- Pittsburgh type V:
  - Labial mucosal flap
  - FAMM flap
  - Tongue flap
  - Premaxillary turnover flap
    - Primarily used as nasal lining flap for fistula at anterior incisive foramen in Veau IV cleft
  - Free tissue transfer

T E C H N I Q U E S

■ Excision and Reapproximation

- Midline oral endotracheal tube placement; head placed in headrest with slight extension.
- Perform proper surgical time-out.
- Place Dingman mouth prop.
- Prep and drape the patient.

- Mark out medial epithelialized areas that must be excised.
- Inject with local anesthesia of choice. Author prefers ¼% Marcaine with 1:200 000 epinephrine.
- Excise medial portions of fistula.
- Repair with resorbable sutures. Author prefers 4-0 chromic sutures.

■ Lateral Relaxing Incisions and Rerepair
(TECH FIG 1)

Preparation for All Fistula Types

- Midline oral endotracheal tube placement; head placed in headrest with slight extension.
- Perform proper surgical time-out.
- Place Dingman mouth prop.
- Prep and drape the patient.
- Mark out lateral relaxing incisions (von Langenbeck style relaxing incision on the hard palate, soft palate, or both depending upon fistula type).

- Relaxing incisions typically need to be longer than initially thought due to relative immobility of soft tissues.
- Inject with local anesthesia of choice. Author prefers ¼% Marcaine with 1:200 000 epinephrine.

Pittsburgh Type II Fistula

- Incise lateral relaxing incisions on the soft palate.
- Incise medial fistula.
- Separate nasal mucosa from levator muscles with sharp dissecting scissors.
- Separate oral mucosa from levator muscles with sharp dissecting scissors.

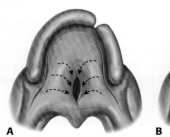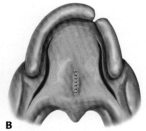

TECH FIG 1 • **A.** Lateral relaxing incisions. **B.** Rerepair.

- Make certain that levator muscles are not tethered to the hard palate, if so release sharply.
- Repair nasal mucosa with interrupted, buried (knot on nasal side) sutures. Author prefers 4-0 chromic.
- Repair levator musculature with re-establishment of levator sling. Author prefers 4-0 Monocryl.
- Repair oral mucosa with interrupted sutures. Author prefers 4-0 chromic.
- If augmenting closure with ADM, after muscle repair, place a thin piece of ADM over muscle with ample coverage beyond suture line. Author uses double-armed 4-0 Monocryl sutures suturing from underneath ADM through oral mucosa allowing knots to easily be placed and tied on oral mucosal side.
- Place tongue stitch and remove Dingman device.

Pittsburgh Type III Fistula

- Incise lateral relaxing incisions on the hard and soft palate.
- Incise medial fistula.
  - It is typically easier to recruit oral mucosa compared to nasal mucosa, so the initial markings should be slightly on the more lateral portions of the fistula to allow easier closure of the nasal mucosa.
- Use Joseph Periosteal Elevator to elevate mucoperiosteal flaps from the hard palate with care taken to preserve greater palatine vessels.
- Release soft palate lateral relaxing incision from hamulus and junction of the hard palate/end of alveolar ridge.
  - Dean scissors can be a useful instrument to release medial tissue off hamulus.
- Separate nasal mucosa from levator muscles (if present) and release nasal mucosa from nasal side of the hard palate.

- Separate oral mucosa from levator muscles with sharp dissecting scissors (if present).
- Make certain that levator muscles are not tethered to the hard palate, if so release sharply.
- Repair nasal mucosa with interrupted, buried (knot on nasal side) sutures.
- Repair levator musculature with re-establishment of levator sling (if previously released).
- Place liberal ADM prior to closure of oral mucosal flaps.
- Repair oral mucosa with interrupted sutures.
- Ensure hemostasis of lateral relaxing incisions.
- Place tongue stitch and remove Dingman.

Pittsburgh Type IV Fistula

- Incise lateral relaxing incisions on the hard and soft palate (if necessary depending on location of fistula in hard palate).
- Incise medial fistula.
  - It is typically easier to recruit oral mucosa compared to nasal mucosa, so the initial markings should be slightly on the more lateral portions of the fistula for easier closure of the nasal mucosa.
- Use Joseph Periosteal Elevator to elevate mucoperiosteal flaps from the hard palate with care taken to preserve the greater palatine vessels.
  - Determine whether fistula is too large for closure and if pushback technique will be required.
  - If pushback is required, continue lateral relaxing incisions more proximally, depending upon the location of fistula either incise from medial portion of fistula toward alveolus or fashion-like Veau-Wardill-Kilner–type palatoplasty.
- Separate/release nasal mucosa from nasal side of hard palate to allow medial mobilization.
  - A double hockey or Pigtail instrument or Woodson can be extremely helpful for this dissection.
- Repair nasal mucosa with interrupted, buried (knot on nasal side) sutures.
- Place liberal ADM prior to closure of oral mucosal flaps.
- Repair oral mucosa with interrupted sutures.
- Resuspend flaps to lateral relaxing incisions without placing undue tension on medial repair.
- Ensure hemostasis of lateral relaxing incisions.
- Place tongue stitch and remove the Dingman device.

■ Conversion by Furlow Palatoplasty

- Refer to Chapter on Furlow Palatoplasty (Chapter 8), for description of this technique.

- The CHOP modification should be encouraged if any concerns for tension on repair exist.

■ Posterior Pharyngeal Flap

- Please see chapter on Velopharyngeal Insufficiency (Chapter 14) for description of this technique.

- A palatal split technique (as described by Owsley[8]) should be considered over a fish-mouth technique as described by Argamaso.[9]

■ Labial Mucosal Flap

- Must be able to protect this flap from masticatory trauma by either having space to pass through dental arch or by having temporary bite blocks placed on the teeth.
- Midline oral endotracheal tube placement; head placed in headrest with slight extension.
- Perform proper surgical time-out.
- Placement of Dingman mouth prop.
- Prep and drape the patient.
- Mark out medial portions of the fistula.
  - Recruit tissue from oral side as previously described.
- Mark out flap on labial wet vermilion (this is a hinge- or finger-type flap).
  - The base of flap and point of rotation of flap can be unipedicle or bipedicle depending upon the location of fistula and Veau-type cleft.
  - Typically for Veau III clefts with recruitment of tissue from posterior segment.
  - Make certain to place incision line several millimeters above the attached gingiva so that closure of donor defect is made easier.
- Inject with local anesthesia of choice. Author prefers ¼% Marcaine with 1:200 000 epinephrine.

- Incise and repair medial portions of fistula as previously described.
- Incise buccal flap and elevate with sharp scissors.
  - Elevate this flap off the orbicularis muscle to maintain as much blood supply because this is a random pattern flap.
- Rotate flap into defect.
- Sew flap to raw oral mucosal edges (preferably through dental arch defect) (**TECH FIG 2**).
- Close donor defect with interrupted sutures.
- Place tongue stitch and remove Dingman device.

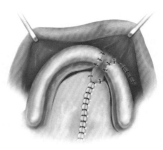

TECH FIG 2 • Design of a labial mucosal flap.

■ Buccal Myomucosal Flap

- Oral endotracheal tube placement; head placed in headrest with slight extension.
- Perform proper surgical time-out.
- Prep and drape the patient.
- Place Dingman mouth prop or dental mouth prop.
- Place several retraction sutures on the lip to aid in retraction/visualization.
- Identify Stensen duct.

- The flap is caudal to the duct.
- Mark out flap from area over ascending ramus transversely oriented to oral commissure (stay on wet vermilion) (**TECH FIG 3A,B**).
  - The base of flap is about 1.5 cm.
  - Narrow the flap distally.
- Inject with local anesthetic.
- Incise mucosa and sharply dissect from the distal end of flap toward base of flap (**TECH FIG 3C**).

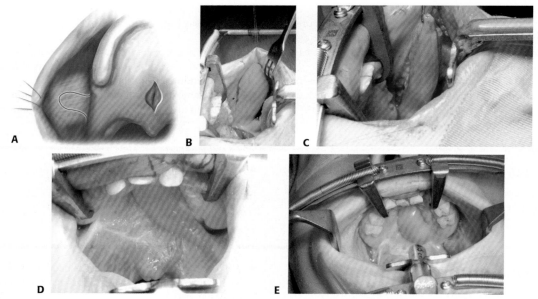

TECH FIG 3 • **A.** Design of a buccal myomucosal flap. **B.** Markings. **C.** Flap elevation. **D.** Flap inset into a palatal defect. **E.** Division of base of flap.

- A portion of the buccinator muscle is taken to improve the vascularity of the flap (as described by Mann,[3] this is an intramuscular dissection).
  - This flap can be elevated bilaterally if needed.
- Prepare fistula site so that some nasal mucosa can be rolled in (complete nasal mucosa closure is not critical).
  - Make certain to elevate raw edges of oral mucoperiosteal tissue to inset the flap.
- Rotate flap into defect and sew in place attaining excellent approximation of mucosal edges (**TECH FIG 3D**).

- Flap will need to be rotated posteriorly behind dental arch or through space in dental arch that can be protected from masticatory trauma (can use oral splints on teeth as well).
- Close donor site in a single layer.
- Place tongue stitch and remove Dingman/dental mouth prop.
- The base of this flap may be subsequently divided after 3 to 4 weeks (**TECH FIG 3E**).

■ Facial Artery Musculomucosal Flap[10]

- Oral endotracheal tube placement, place head in headrest with slight extension.
- Perform proper surgical time-out.
- Prep and drape the patient.
- Placement of Dingman mouth prop or dental mouth prop.
- Place several retraction sutures on the lip to aid in retraction/visualization.
- Identify Stensen duct.
  - Artery and flap should be anterior to the duct.
- Use handheld Doppler to identify the course of the facial artery.
- An obliquely designed flap is centered over the artery from retromolar trigone area to gingival buccal sulcus at alar base (should be anterior to Stensen duct).
  - Flap is 1.5 to 2 cm wide.
- Incise mucosa at distal end (either superiorly or inferiorly based) through mucosa and buccinators.
- Identify facial artery and ligate.

- Elevate flap deep to the artery taking a small cuff of buccinator muscle and orbicularis muscle (**TECH FIG 4A**).
  - Flap can be 8 to 9 cm in length.
  - This flap can be elevated bilaterally if needed.
- Prepare fistula site so that some nasal mucosa can be rolled in (complete nasal mucosa closure is not critical) (**TECH FIG 4B**).
  - Make certain to elevate raw edges of oral mucoperiosteal tissue to inset the flap.
- Rotate flap into defect and sew in place attaining excellent approximation of mucosal edges (**TECH FIG 4C**).
  - Flap will need to be rotated posteriorly behind dental arch or through space in dental arch that can be protected from masticatory trauma (can use oral splints on teeth as well).
- Close donor site in two layers (buccinators muscle and then mucosa) taking care to avoid the Stensen duct.
- Place tongue stitch and remove Dingman/dental mouth prop.

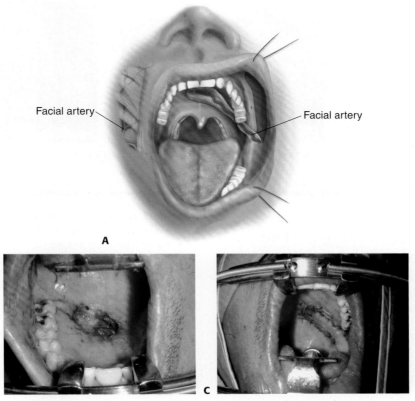

Facial artery   Facial artery

A

B   **C**

TECH FIG 4 • **A.** Design of a facial artery musculomucosal flap. **B.** Preparation of the fistula site. **C.** Flap inset.

■ Tongue Flap (Anteriorly Based)[9,11]

Raising and Insetting Flap

- Oral endotracheal tube placement to the right or left side; head placed in headrest with slight extension.
- Perform proper surgical time-out.
- Prep and drape the patient.
- Place bite block mouth prop.
- Inject palatal tissue with local anesthetic.
- Incise and elevate around palatal mucosa to become nasal floor.
  - Plan this incision so that you can have either complete nasal floor closure or at least significant nasal floor mucosa to place your tongue flap on.
- Close nasal floor if possible.
- Use the foil from a chromic stitch to make a template of the palatal defect.
- Place a traction suture through the tip of the tongue to improve exposure.
- Transpose the foil template onto the tongue with tip of flap at junction of anterior two-thirds and posterior one-third of the tongue.
- Mark out flap making certain to maintain at least a 2-cm pedicle base.
  - Can mark flap slightly larger than template for safety.
- Use a Colorado needle-tip Bovie to incise and elevate the flap from distal to proximal (**TECH FIG 5A**).
  - This dissection should include underlying longitudinal tongue musculature but can be thinned near the tip of the flap (down to 4 mm of muscle).

- This dissection is not a natural tissue plane and can bleed from the raw muscle edge.
- Inset tongue flap into edges of raw mucoperiosteal palatal flaps (**TECH FIG 5B,C**).
- The use of 4-0 double-armed Monocryl sutures with the knots on the palatal mucosa makes insetting of this flap much easier.
- This flap cannot be completely inset into the entire fistula as the pedicle width prevents complete inset (final inset is performed during division of flap).
- Closure of donor site of the tongue with horizontal mattress sutures to prevent bleeding.
- Extubate patient.
- Place light elastics on orthodontic brackets for gentle MMF and patient comfort.
- Wait for 3 weeks for revascularization.

Division of Flap

- A gentle rubber shod clamp can be used to test if neovascularization has occurred in OR prior to division.
  - If concerns for insufficient vascularity, postpone division.
- Plan division so that a portion of the pedicled base will fill remaining portion of the palatal fistula.
  - For incomplete nasal floor closure, some secondary healing from margins can occur.
- Divide flap and debulk the new portion to inset (typically about 10%–15% of flap).
- Complete inset of flap.
  - Double-armed sutures make inset significantly easier.
- Return unused pedicled tissue to the tongue by opening previous incision and closing with chromic sutures.

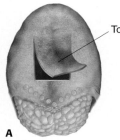
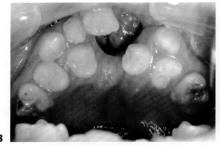
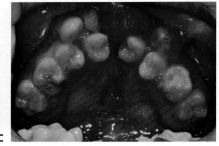

TECH FIG 5 • **A.** Design of a tongue flap. Fistula before **(B)** and after repair **(C)** with a tongue flap.

■ Premaxillary Turnover Flap (Fish-Mouth Technique into Hard Palatal Mucoperiosteal Flaps)[12]

- Midline oral endotracheal tube placement; head placed in headrest with slight extension.
- Perform proper surgical time-out.
- Place Dingman mouth prop.
- Prep and drape the patient.
- Mark junction of premaxillary gingiva and lingual side of incisors with lateral markings down the premaxilla along the cleft margin (**TECH FIG 6A,B**).

- Mark edge of mucoperiosteal flaps and lateral relaxing incisions along alveolar ridge (**TECH FIG 6C**).
- Inject with local anesthetic.
- Incise junction of the gingiva and lateral premaxilla and perform subperiosteal dissection of this flap.
  - The base of this flap narrows as you ascend toward the nasal cavity, so care must be taken in elevation (**TECH FIG 6D**).
- Use an angled blade to incise the edge of the mucoperiosteal flaps and make lateral relaxing incisions.
- Use a combination of periosteal elevators from lateral side and sharp scissor or knife dissection to re-elevate the mucoperiosteal flaps.

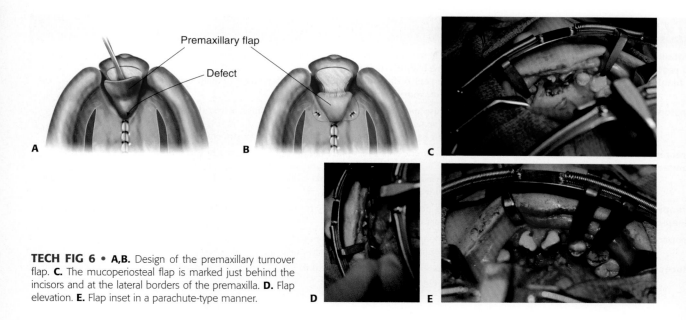

TECH FIG 6 • A,B. Design of the premaxillary turnover flap. **C.** The mucoperiosteal flap is marked just behind the incisors and at the lateral borders of the premaxilla. **D.** Flap elevation. **E.** Flap inset in a parachute-type manner.

- Care must be taken to preserve greater palatine vessels if dissection occurs that distally.
- Advance mucoperiosteal flaps if possible.
- Turn over premaxillary flap for inset.
  - The premaxillary gingiva will become the new nasal mucosa, and the periosteum of the premaxilla will be the oral side for this flap.
- Use parachuting sutures to tack the periosteal side of flap to raw surface of mucoperiosteal flaps.
  - The use of double-armed sutures coming through the premaxillary flap and out the palatal mucoperiosteal flap makes inset and parachuting much easier (see **TECH FIG 6A**).

- Do not attempt to tie these sutures until all have been placed for ease of placement.
  - Place sutures about 1 cm apart.
- After flap has been inset distally, close lateral aspect of flap to any raw areas of alveolus gingiva.
  - Work distally to proximally to close down posterior alveolar fistula.
  - Using a P2 needle and Castroviejo needle drivers facilitates this closure.
- May cover this flap with a thin piece of ADM if single layer closure is being performed.
- Place tongue stitch and remove Dingman device.

■ Free Tissue Transfer[13]

- Multiple donor sites have been described, including radial forearm free flap (**TECH FIG 7A**), anterolateral thigh free flap (**TECH FIG 7B**), and lateral arm flap.

- Thorough descriptions of and surgical techniques for the various free tissue flaps that have been described in the oncologic literature for palatal and maxillectomy defects are found in other chapters of this book.

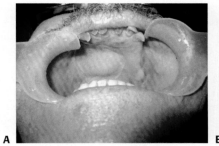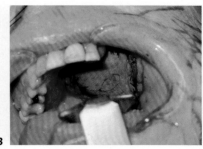

TECH FIG 7 • A. Radial forearm free flap for palatal fistula closure. **B.** Anterolateral thigh flap for palatal fistula closure.

PEARLS AND PITFALLS

Obtain a preoperative retainer to protect repair for type IV and V fistulas	▪ Have this item made 2 weeks before surgery and have patient wear it to check for compliance and become habituated to it. ▪ Meet with your orthodontist and patient with retainer to make certain it fits but does not compress on your repair.
Postoperative compliance	▪ Must discuss and ensure proper postoperative compliance with diet and activities in the preoperative setting. ▪ This author has had recurrence secondary to poor postoperative compliance.
Preoperative orthodontia for tongue flaps	▪ Have orthodontic colleagues place temporary orthodontic brackets on the permanent teeth. ▪ Saves time of placing some form of appliance while under anesthesia. ▪ Use light elastics instead of true MMF to decrease intraoral opening while attempting to provide more comfort to the patient.
Preoperative evaluation for sleep-disordered breathing	▪ If planning posterior pharyngeal flap for type II or III fistula, evaluate for obstructive sleep apnea with preoperative polysomnogram.
Proper exposure and visualization	▪ Make relaxing incision longer than expected. ▪ Dissect around greater palatine vessels under direct visualization.
Mucoperiosteal flap rigidity	▪ Remobilization of the mucoperiosteal flaps rarely provides as much mobility as desired as they are stiffer than primary repair.

POSTOPERATIVE CARE

▪ Patients should be observed overnight for pain control and to monitor for any airway issues.
▪ Patients should be started on a liquid diet for 24 to 48 hours after surgery (per surgeon's preference).
▪ Diet should then be advanced to a soft food diet for 3 to 4 weeks after surgery (per surgeon's preference).
▪ Some surgeons implement postoperative antibiotics, but the literature is divided about use.
▪ Peridex should be used (5 to 10 mL swish and spit) after every meal.
▪ Nasal precautions should be instituted.
  ▪ No nasal suctioning while in hospital.
  ▪ Avoid blowing of the nose.
  ▪ Sneeze with an open mouth if possible.
  ▪ No straws.
▪ If a postsurgical splint has been made, the retainer should be worn at all times and only taken out to clean.
▪ Follow-up within 1 week to assess healing.

OUTCOMES

▪ Recurrence rate is highly variable in the literature and dependent on technique/flap chosen and location of the fistula.[14]
▪ ADM shown to work in nine consecutive patients without recurrence for hard palatal fistula.[6]
▪ Buccal myomucosal flap has reported 7% to 18% failure rate for all uses.[3]
▪ FAMM flap has failure rates of 17% to 27%.[10]
  ▪ Secondary to venous congestion and flap tip necrosis
▪ Lateral relaxing incisions and pushback technique have 10% failure rate.[15]
  ▪ All failures are reported in bilateral cleft lip and palate.
▪ Tongue flap reported failure rates range from 8% to 15%.[9,16]
  ▪ Sohail et al. found no difference in complications or recurrence rates between FAMM flaps and tongue flaps for closure of large anterior palatal fistula.
  ▪ These authors found that the total operative time and fewer early postoperative complications with the FAMM flap.

▪ Free tissue transfer success rates are reported between 83% and 98%.[13]
  ▪ Most studies did not address any donor site morbidity though.

COMPLICATIONS

▪ Acute postoperative airway obstruction
  ▪ This situation can occur during emergence from anesthesia as tongue muscle tone can be slower to recover in patients compared with respiratory drive (effective glossoptosis).
  ▪ Can also occur when a tongue flap has been used.
  ▪ Prevention is key.
    • An oral airway device placed by the anesthesia team can disrupt/damage fistula repair.
    • Except in cases of tongue flap, I prefer to place a tongue stitch with 2-0 silk tied to a Raytec for resolution of acute postoperative glossoptosis.
▪ Bleeding
  ▪ Raw surfaces are frequently left after fistula repair (particularly when relaxing incisions have been used).
  ▪ Ensure hemostasis with normotensive anesthesia prior to extubation.
  ▪ Tell family/patient to expect some oozing from the mouth or nose for 24 hours.
  ▪ If nasal bleeding is severe, an endoscope can be used in the OR to evaluate the nasal repair.
▪ Recurrence[14]
  ▪ The most common complication after palatal fistula repair
  ▪ If a flap has been employed, usually from partial or full flap loss (see Outcomes section)
▪ Obstructive sleep apnea
  ▪ Can occur if a PPF has been employed in Pittsburgh type II or III fistula repairs
  ▪ May require modification, takedown of flap, or CPAP if persistent 6 months after surgery
▪ Halitosis
  ▪ Not a true complication but a frequent concern/question raised by family while wounds are healing

REFERENCES

1. Furlow LT Jr. Cleft palate repair by double opposing Z-plasty. *Plast Reconstr Surg.* 1986;78:724-736.
2. Jackson O, Low D, LaRossa D. The Children's Hospital of Philadelphia modification of the Furlow double-opposing Z-palatoplasty: 30-year experience and long-term speech outcomes. *Plast Reconstr Surg.* 2013;132:613-622.
3. Mann RJ, Fisher DM. Bilateral buccal flaps with double opposing Z-plasty for wider palatal clefts. *Plast Reconstr Surg.* 1997;100:1139-1143.
4. Smith DM, Vecchione L, Jiang S, et al. The Pittsburgh Fistula Classification System: a standardized scheme for the description of palatal fistulas. *Cleft Palate Craniofac J.* 2007;44:590-594.
5. LaRossa D. "The state of the art in cleft palate surgery." *Cleft Palate Craniofac J.* 2000;37(3):225-228.
6. Kirschner RE, Cabiling DS, Slemp AE, et al. Repair of oronasal fistulae with acellular dermal matrices. *Plast Reconstr Surg.* 2006;118:1431-1440.
7. Chen PK, Wu JT, Chen YR, Noordhoff MS. Correction of secondary velopharyngeal insufficiency in cleft palate patients with the Furlow palatoplasty. *Plast Reconstr Surg.* 1994;94:933-941.
8. Owsley JQ Jr, Blackfield HM, Owsley JQ Jr. The technique and complications of pharyngeal flap surgery: a continuing report. *Plast Reconstr Surg.* 1965;35:531-539.
9. Argamaso RV. The tongue flap: placement and fixation for closure of postpalatoplasty fistulae. *Cleft Palate Craniofac J.* 1990;27:402-410.
10. Pribaz J, Stephens W, Crespo L, Gifford G. A new intraoral flap: facial artery musculomucosal (FAMM) flap. *Plast Reconstr Surg.* 1992;90:421-429.
11. Pigott RW, Rieger FW, Moodie AF. Tongue flap repair of cleft palate fistulae. *Br J Plast Surg.* 1984;37:285-293.
12. Coe HE. The use of the premaxillary flap in the repair of bilateral cleft palate. *Plast Reconstr Surg.* 1953;123:194-197.
13. Schwabegger AH, Hubli E, Rieger M, et al. Role of free-tissue transfer in the treatment of recalcitrant palatal fistulae among patients with cleft palates. *Plast Reconstr Surg.* 2004;113:1131-1139.
14. Schultz RC. Management and timing of cleft palate fistula repair. *Plast Reconstr Surg.* 1986;78:739-745.
15. Pigott RW, Albery EH, Hathorn IS, et al. A comparison of three methods of repairing the hard palate. *Cleft Palate Craniofac J.* 2002;39:383-391.
16. Sohail M, Bashir MM, Khan FA, Ashraf N. Comparison of clinical outcome of facial artery myomucosal flap and tongue flap for closure of large anterior palatal fistulas. *J Craniofac Surg.* 2016;27:1465-1468.

CHAPTER 14

Velopharyngeal Insufficiency

Jennifer L. McGrath and Arun K. Gosain

DEFINITION

- Velopharyngeal insufficiency (VPI) refers to a structural inadequacy of the velopharyngeal apparatus, resulting in inadequate closure of the velopharyngeal port during speech.
- VPI may be congenital or acquired.
- It is characterized by nasal air emission and hypernasality of speech, articulation errors, decreased speech intelligibility, and nasal reflux of food and liquids.

ANATOMY

- The velopharyngeal sphincter is a complex, 3D arrangement of muscles that serves to separate the nasal cavity from the oral cavity during speech and swallowing.
- Muscles of the soft palate: levator veli palatini, tensor veli palatini, palatoglossus, palatopharyngeus, and musculus uvulae.
  - Paired levators are primarily responsible for velum closure by moving the velum posteriorly and superiorly.
  - Superior pharyngeal constrictor moves the posterior and lateral pharyngeal walls centrally.
- Innervation:
  - Predominantly CN IX and X: levator veli palatini and pharyngeal constrictors
  - CN V_3: Tensor veli palatini
- Three patterns of closure have been described:
  - Coronal: majority of closure from posterior movement of the velum
  - Sagittal: majority of closure from medial movement of the lateral pharyngeal walls to meet the velum
  - Circular: contributions of both movement of the velum posteriorly and movement of the lateral pharyngeal walls medially. Passavant ridge may contribute to closure.

PATHOGENESIS

- The cause of VPI may be structural, functional, or dynamic.
- Four main categories of VPI are frequently encountered. They include
- Postpalatoplasty: after primary cleft palate repair
  - Inappropriate levator veli palatini positioning
  - Palatal scarring preventing functional contraction of repaired levator sling
  - Length discrepancy preventing contact with the posterior pharynx
- Submucous cleft palate (SMCP)
  - May be classic (bifid uvula, palatal muscle diastasis) or occult
  - Often present later than cleft lip and palate

- Not always associated with VPI (see section Natural History below)
- Palatopharyngeal disproportion
  - No anatomic abnormality to reconstruct
  - Disproportion may result from a short palate and/or a deep nasopharynx.
  - May be seen after tonsillectomy and adenoidectomy
- Neurogenic
  - More common in adults than children
  - Etiology may be upper motor neuron, nuclear, or lower motor neuron or generalized hypotonia.
  - Examples: muscular dystrophy, neurofibromatosis, cerebral palsy, apraxia, dysarthria
  - This subset tends to do more poorly with surgery.

NATURAL HISTORY

- Transient VPI is common after primary palatoplasty.
  - Patients are referred to speech-language pathologist (SLP) as early as 2 weeks postoperatively.
  - Perceptual speech assessment (PSA) by a SLP is obtained when the patient is of a cooperative age, often age 3 or above.
  - The incidence of lasting VPI after primary palatoplasty is about 10% to 20%.[1,2]
- Submucous cleft palate (SMCP)
  - Not all patients with SMCP will develop VPI. Studies suggest roughly 5% to 10% of patients with SMCP will develop VPI warranting intervention.[3,4]
  - The incidence of VPI in the pediatric plastic surgery population is higher due to referral bias.
  - Children with SMCP should undergo PSA by a SLP. Intervention should be delayed until reliable PSA can be performed by a trained SLP, which is usually after age 3 years.
  - Some children with SMCP may improve with speech therapy. Surgery is indicated for SMCP only when VPI is present and cannot be corrected with speech therapy.
- VPI caused by palatopharyngeal disproportion tends to worsen as the tonsils and adenoids regress or are surgically removed.
- In general, if VPI is diagnosed on PSA by an SLP and is secondary to previous palatoplasty, submucous cleft palate, or palatopharyngeal disproportion, VPI will persist indefinitely.
- Speech outcomes are better when surgery is performed at a younger age, but there is not a specific age cutoff for surgical treatment. However, misarticulations are harder to correct as a child ages.

PATIENT HISTORY AND FINDINGS

- Patients are frequently identified by parents, teachers, and/or SLPs.
- Patients with a history of cleft palate are frequently followed by SLP as part of a multidisciplinary approach to cleft care.
- Patients and parents may report nasal regurgitation, liquids worse than solids.
- Hypernasal speech and nasal air emission are the classic findings. Nasal air emission is normally only observed in /m/ and /n/ sounds.
- Compensatory articulations occur when patients are unable to seal off the nasopharynx.

IMAGING AND OTHER DIAGNOSTIC STUDIES

- PSA by an SLP. Note that PSA is a *subjective* assessment of speech, one component of which is nasal air emission.
- Nasometry: *objective* test of nasal air emission, which can correlate subjective assessment of nasal air emission on PSA
- Imaging is indicated when VPI is documented on PSA.[2,4]
- Multiview videofluoroscopy
  - Quantify lateral wall motion on AP view
  - Quantify velopharyngeal gap on lateral view
  - Requires reference landmarks for quantification
- Nasendoscopy
  - Qualitatively assesses closure pattern
  - Helpful in identifying stigmata of SMCP in patients without overt clefting
  - Roughly quantifies closure ratio: fraction of the diameter of the velopharyngeal port that is closed off during attempted sphincter closure
  - Nasendoscopy does not provide reference landmarks, so it cannot quantify motion and gap as in videofluoroscopy. It does allow visualization of nasopharyngeal and oropharyngeal structures, such as the adenoids.

DIFFERENTIAL DIAGNOSIS

- Although the vast majority of patients will present with a history of previous palatoplasty or submucous cleft palate, it is important to recognize other mechanisms of velopharyngeal dysfunction that are less adequately treated with surgery.
- Velopharyngeal mislearning
  - Articulation errors with no anatomic disturbance; treat with speech therapy
- Velopharyngeal incompetence: neurologic or neuromuscular origin
  - Globalized hypotonia with no structural abnormalities
  - Poor muscular competence of the lip and tongue may predict poor surgical outcomes. However, many patients will benefit from traditional surgical approaches.

NONOPERATIVE MANAGEMENT

- Speech therapy: all patients should be evaluated and treated by an SLP prior to intervention to minimize articulation errors.
- Prosthetics
  - Speech bulb
  - Palatal lift
  - Disadvantages: compliance, fit, growth
  - Prosthetics may be a helpful training tool in conjunction with surgery to improve oromuscular coordination and articulation placement.

- If a true mechanical insufficiency exists, nonoperative management is not recommended if a patient can tolerate surgery.

SURGICAL MANAGEMENT

- The overall goal of surgical management is to recapitulate a velopharyngeal port that can be closed during speech.
- Surgical approach typically depends on deficiencies seen on videofluoroscopy and/or nasendoscopy. Common approaches include
  - Intravelar veloplasty
    - In cases of SMCP only, primary palatoplasty with intravelar veloplasty repositions the aberrant insertion of the levator veli palatine muscles to create a functional sling.
    - This approach does not increase palatal length and is often passed over for Furlow palatoplasty.
  - Furlow palatoplasty or double-opposing Z-plasty (DOZ)
    - Initially described by Leonard Furlow as a technique for primary repair of cleft palate, this technique has gained favor as an approach to the management of VPI due to its ability to lengthen the palate via Z-plasty while also opposing the levator veli palatini muscles to recreate an anatomic muscular sling.
    - The major benefits of this technique are as follows:
      - It does not mechanically alter the closure mechanism of the velopharyngeal port, leaving open the option of other surgical techniques for refractory cases.
      - It is not associated with airway obstruction as are other techniques.
  - Dynamic sphincter pharyngoplasty
    - Dynamic sphincter pharyngoplasty (DSP) uses myomucosal flaps transposed to the posterior pharynx to create a smaller, circular velopharyngeal port.
    - This procedure is typically selected for patients with a coronal or circular closure pattern. When lateral wall movement is poor, DSP narrows the velopharyngeal port and adds bulk to the posterior pharyngeal point of velum contact.
    - The senior author has advocated use of the DSP in conjunction with the DOZ in cases of large velopharyngeal gaps.[5]
  - Pharyngeal flap pharyngoplasty
    - Based on the palatopharyngeal adhesion described by Passavant in the 1800s, pharyngeal flaps have been described as a surgical treatment for VPI for over a century.
    - Superiorly based pharyngeal flaps are widely utilized as a preferred treatment for VPI.
    - We describe a high inset pharyngeal flap, which is used as a last resort procedure due to its association with airway obstruction.
  - Posterior pharyngeal wall augmentation
    - In cases of small gaps, implants and injectables have been used to augment the posterior wall of the pharynx to reduce the velopharyngeal gap.
    - Like many other applications of implants, implants in the posterior pharynx have been associated with failure due to migration, extrusion, and infection.
    - Silicone, Teflon, Gore-Tex, and polyethylene implants and calcium hydroxyapatite injections have been used. Despite successful reports, these techniques have not enjoyed widespread acceptance.

- Autologous fat grafting has gained popularity recently but is in need of standardized protocols and prospective studies to evaluate retention of the augmentation and its utility over time. Still, it is most likely only useful in small velopharyngeal gaps.[6-8]

Preoperative Planning

- Surgical procedures are usually selected based on the preoperative closure pattern and velopharyngeal closure gap.[9-11]
    - For sagittal closure, velum may be too short and/or not move well, but lateral wall movement is preserved; therefore:
        - For small gaps less than 9 mm, we recommend double-opposing Z-plasty (DOZ) to lengthen the palate.
        - For gaps larger than 9 mm, we recommend a superiorly based pharyngeal flap.
    - For coronal closure patterns in which lateral movement is poor, we recommend dynamic sphincter pharyngoplasty (DSP).
        - For gaps less than 9 mm, we recommend DSP alone.
        - For gaps greater than 9 mm, we recommend DSP in conjunction with DOZ.
    - For circular closure patterns, many approaches have been used. DOZ may be used in smaller gaps. Narrow pharyn-geal flaps or sphincter pharyngoplasty is recommended for larger gaps.[2]
- Pharyngeal flaps may have better outcomes in noncoronal closure patterns.[9]
- DSP may be most appropriate in coronal and circular closure patterns.[10]
- Combined DOZ and DSP can be used in very large velopharyngeal gaps.[2,5,12]
- Nasendoscopy can identify the point of maximal constriction and evaluate adenoid tissues for flap inset planning.

Positioning

- The patient is placed in the supine position on the operating table.
- A shoulder roll can be used to gently extend the neck.
- The head of the operating table can be extended to aid in visualization.
- The face and neck are prepped and draped such that the infraorbital face and submandibular region are adequately exposed.
    - Intraoral prep with chlorhexidine or Betadine swabs
    - Eyelids are taped closed to prevent corneal abrasions.
- A nasal RAE tube should be used for intubation.
- A Dingman retractor exposes the posterior pharynx and retracts the tongue inferiorly.

■ Furlow Palatoplasty or Double-Opposing Z-Plasty

Markings

- Z-plasty flaps are designed in two layers, oral and nasal, with one mucosal and one myomucosal flap in each layer.
    - Oral flaps: posteriorly based myomucosal flap and anteriorly based mucosa-only flap. By convention, the muscle-mucosa flap is on the patient's left side for the right-handed surgeon.
    - Nasal flaps: designed in opposite orientation to the oral flaps with a posteriorly based myomucosal flap (right side) and anteriorly based nasal mucosa flap
- The anterior limbs are designed near the junction of the hard and soft palate. Rather than the traditional 60-degree Z-plasty, we recommend a more obtuse angle, roughly 80 to 90 degrees.
    - Cheating the placement of the anterior limb to the more elastic soft palate tissue facilitates flap transposition (**TECH FIG 1**).

Dissection

- Oral flaps are incised and elevated. The surgeon should be conservative with the lateral extent of the mucosal incision as this dictates the inset location of the tip of the contralateral flap (**TECH FIG 2A,B**).
- It is critical to carefully identify the levator musculature within the myomucosal flaps to ensure recapitulation of the levator sling.
    - A muscle stimulator can aid in identification of functional muscle and facilitate complete release of muscle from scar in secondary palatoplasty. If a muscle stimulator is used, it is important to let the anesthesiologist know to avoid muscle relaxants or allow the relaxants to wear off prior to use of the muscle stimulator.
    - The muscle dissection often extends submucosally laterally to fully release the levator (**TECH FIG 2C**).
- Nasal flaps are transposed in the standard Z-plasty fashion, with the posteriorly based left-sided myomucosal flap rotated right and posterior and the mucosal flap left and anterior (**TECH FIG 2D**). The limbs of the nasal mucosa are closed with simple interrupted dissolvable sutures.
- Oral flaps are transposed in a similar manner. Transposition of the oral myomucosal flap completes reconstruction of a competent levator sling. The oral mucosal limbs are then closed (**TECH FIG 2E**).

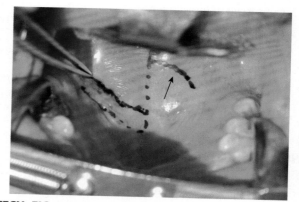

TECH FIG 1 • Markings for double-opposing Z-plasty. Z-plasty marked on the oral mucosa. The posteriorly based oromuscular flap is marked on the patient's left side for a right-handed surgeon (the end of the oromuscular incision is designated by the pointer). Note the curved arm of the anteriorly based Z-plasty (*arrow*) as well as its obtuse angle to the midline incision.

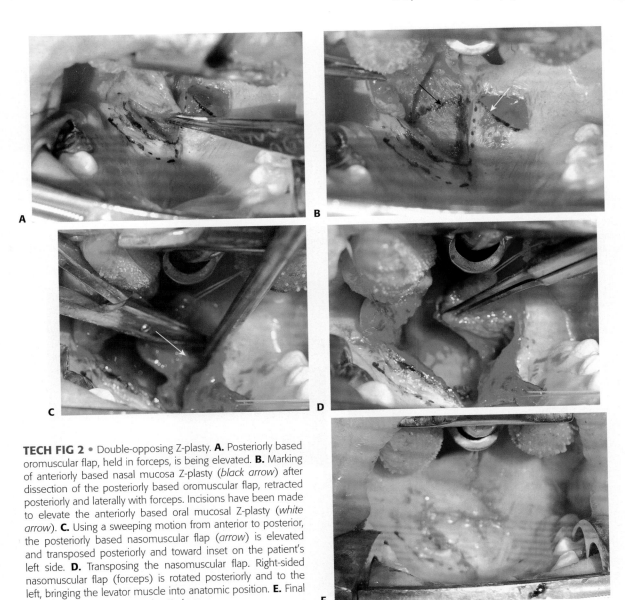

TECH FIG 2 • Double-opposing Z-plasty. **A.** Posteriorly based oromuscular flap, held in forceps, is being elevated. **B.** Marking of anteriorly based nasal mucosa Z-plasty (*black arrow*) after dissection of the posteriorly based oromuscular flap, retracted posteriorly and laterally with forceps. Incisions have been made to elevate the anteriorly based oral mucosal Z-plasty (*white arrow*). **C.** Using a sweeping motion from anterior to posterior, the posteriorly based nasomuscular flap (*arrow*) is elevated and transposed posteriorly and toward inset on the patient's left side. **D.** Transposing the nasomuscular flap. Right-sided nasomuscular flap (forceps) is rotated posteriorly and to the left, bringing the levator muscle into anatomic position. **E.** Final closure of the double-opposing Z-plasty.

▪ Dynamic Sphincter Pharyngoplasty

Markings

- The uvula can be reflected into the nasopharynx by suturing the tip to a red rubber catheter passed through the naris.
- The level of inset is based on the position of the adenoids (**TECH FIG 3A**).
  - Adenoids that extend inferiorly may hinder the ability to inset the flaps as adenoid tissue does not hold sutures well. Low-lying adenoid tissue should be identified preoperatively on nasendoscopy.
  - If the caudal extent of the adenoids is thought to compromise cephalic inset of the sphincter pharyngoplasty, then an inferior adenoidectomy should be considered prior to sphincter pharyngoplasty. In this case, we recommend delaying sphincter pharyngoplasty for at least 3 months following adenoidectomy.
- Superiorly based myomucosal palatopharyngeus flaps are designed on the posterior tonsillar pillars.

- The base of the flaps should be designed at the level of inset (**TECH FIG 3B**).
- A high inset should be anticipated, as the inset should be designed at the anticipated level of velopharyngeal contact during phonation.

Dissection

- Palatopharyngeus flaps are elevated to the height of the desired new nasopharyngeal port, typically the level of velum opposition from preoperative videofluoroscopy (**TECH FIG 4A**).
- Flaps are transposed to the posterior pharyngeal wall and inset in a transverse arrangement directly posterior to the desired nasopharyngeal port location. Flaps may be inset in a stacked or end-to-end manner (**TECH FIG 4B**).
- The size of the new sphincter should be roughly one fingerbreadth.
- Donor sites in the posterior tonsillar pillars are closed primarily with dissolvable sutures (**TECH FIG 4C**).

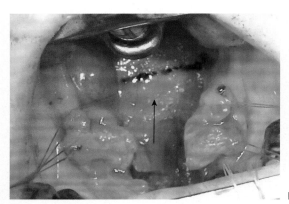
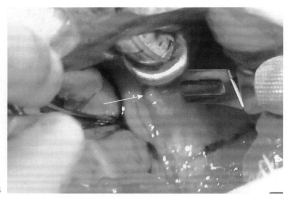

TECH FIG 3 • A. Horizontal marking at the level of inset of the sphincter pharyngoplasty. The position of the adenoids (*arrow*) may limit the superior extent of inset of the sphincter. **B.** Incision along the left posterior tonsillar pillar (*arrow*). Myomucosal flaps based on the palatopharyngeus are marked bilaterally.

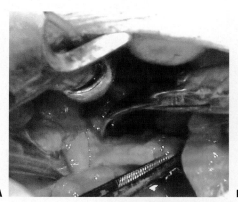
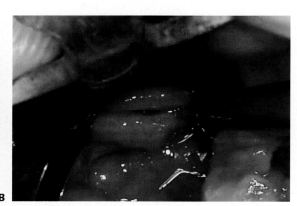

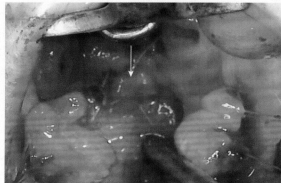

TECH FIG 4 • A. Elevating the left posterior tonsillar pillar, held in forceps, to the level of desired inset at the base of the adenoids. **B.** Setting the tension of the bilateral myomucosal flaps (tonsillar pillars). Flaps can be inset end to end or overlapping, depending on the desired tension. In this illustration, the tonsillar pillars are held in forceps in an overlapping configuration. **C.** Final inset of dynamic sphincter pharyngoplasty. Myomucosal flaps are inset (*arrow*) and donor sites are closed primarily (not shown).

■ Posterior Pharyngeal Flap

Markings

- Superiorly based myomucosal flap is marked on the central posterior pharyngeal wall. The base of the flap must be designed with awareness of the three-dimensional relationship of the flap to the velum. The width of the flap may vary depending on the velopharyngeal gap (**TECH FIG 5**).
- A transverse incision for flap inset is designed on the nasal side mucosa anterior to the uvula.

- A counterincision on the oral side creates a tunnel to pass and secure the flap. This transverse incision is located near the hard-soft palate junction. Incisions must be wide enough to accommodate flap width.

Dissection

- The pharyngeal flap is elevated deep to the pharyngobasilar fascia and superficial to the prevertebral fascia (**TECH FIG 6A**). This is crucial to safe use of this technique in cases of velocardiofacial syndrome (VCFS) in which the carotid arteries can be medially displaced.

- The carotid vessels lie deep to the prevertebral fascia and therefore will not be damaged irrespective of possible medial transposition, as long as the dissection remains superficial to the prevertebral fascia.
- A tunnel is created through the nasal and oral palate transverse incisions. This then allows the pharyngeal flap to be passed through using a clamp or forceps (**TECH FIG 6B–E**).
- Flap is inset into the oral mucosal incision. The tip of the flap is anchored to the periosteum at the posterior aspect of the hard palate to provide resistance to constriction and descent during healing.
- The donor site is closed with dissolvable sutures if possible. If too large to close primarily, it can be left raw to mucosalize. The posterior soft palate incision is also left to heal secondarily (**TECH FIG 6F**).
- Port size is checked by manual palpation using a finger. The new ports are typically stented in some manner. We choose 3-Fr endotracheal tubes trimmed short and passed through the nares into the ports.

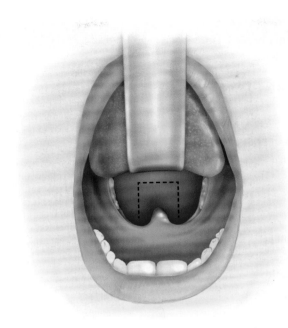

TECH FIG 5 • Marking of the superiorly based posterior pharyngeal flap. The location of the base of the flap can be determined by preoperative imaging.

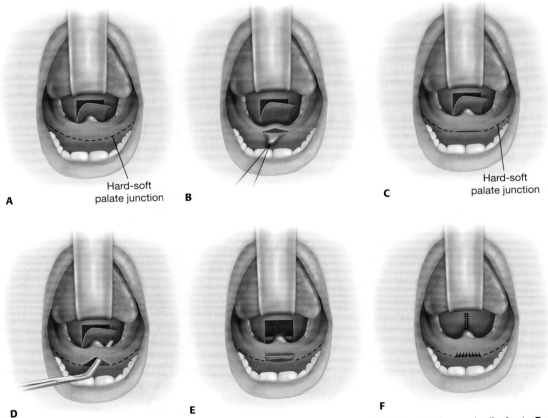

TECH FIG 6 • **A.** Flap elevation. The pharyngeal flap is elevated in a plane immediately superficial to the pharyngobasilar fascia. **B–E.** Flap inset into the velum. Incisions are made on the nasal **(B)** and oral **(C)** mucosa of the posterior soft palate to allow flap inset. A tunnel **(D)** is created between these incisions, and the flap is passed through and inset into the oral incision **(E)**. **F.** Final appearance after pharyngeal flap inset. The posterior pharynx donor site is closed primarily.

PEARLS AND PITFALLS

Tongue edema	▪ Release of the Dingman retractor every 90 minutes for 2 minutes reduces tongue edema and eliminates the need for a tongue stitch postoperatively.
Velocardiofacial syndrome (VCFS)	▪ VCFS disrupts the algorithm because outcomes are usually poorer. ▪ Assessment is the same, and selection of operation is not necessarily different. However, care must be taken during dissection to ensure surgical plane is deep to the pharyngobasilar fascia and superficial to the prevertebral fascia
DOUBLE-OPPOSING Z-PLASTY	
Flap design	▪ Design mucosal flaps more obtusely (80–90 degree) and arch to the desired end point. ▪ The oral myomucosal flap back cut should be posterior enough from the hard palate junction to lie within elastic soft palate tissue to facilitate closure. Placing the back cut too close to the hard palate will make it more difficult to achieve closure of the oral mucosa ▪ Limit the back cut of the anterior limbs of the mucosal flaps again to reduce difficulty closing. Muscular incision and dissection can extend beyond the mucosal incision.
Flap handling	▪ Careful flap handling, particularly of flap corners, is key to a satisfactory result.
DYNAMIC SPHINCTER PHARYNGOPLASTY	
Low adenoids	▪ Adenoid position should be assessed preoperatively. ▪ Attempts to inset the flaps into the adenoids will be unsuccessful and the adenoid tissue does not structurally hold sutures well. ▪ If adenoids are particularly inferior, consider preoperative inferior adenoidectomy. ▪ Inferior adenoidectomy should be at least 3 months prior to pharyngoplasty.
Flap inset	▪ Inset the flaps as high as possible, often immediately below the adenoids (2 mm inferior). ▪ Flaps should be inset at the point of maximum constriction, Passavant ridge, if developed.
Flap tension on inset	▪ Flaps can be inset overlapping or tip to tip. ▪ They should be placed on slight resting tension with residual elastic tone. ▪ Too tight at inset can cause airway obstruction. ▪ Too loose at inset can cause persistent VPI.
PHARYNGEAL FLAP PHARYNGOPLASTY	
Flap design	▪ Width of the flap should be tailored to the patient's needs.
Flap lining	▪ Line as much of the pharyngeal flap as possible. The raw surfaces will contract and the flap will narrow, creating a larger distance for the lateral pharyngeal walls to move for closure.
Flap descent	▪ Flaps tend to narrow and pull inferiorly over time. ▪ High inset allows more lining of the raw surface as well as a better anchor to the hard palate, resisting contraction and descent. ▪ High inset also shortens the exposed raw surface.

POSTOPERATIVE CARE

▪ Patients are observed in the hospital overnight for signs of airway obstruction.
  ▪ Some surgeons place a tongue stitch at the conclusion of the procedure to assist in clearing tongue-base obstruction in the postoperative period.
  ▪ Similarly, IV dexamethasone can be useful to reduce airway and tongue edema in immediate postoperative period.
▪ Although preoperative antibiotics are frequently given, postoperative prophylactic antibiotics are not routinely used, as there is no evidence to support their efficacy.
▪ Stenting of the reconstructed ports:
  ▪ Pharyngeal flap: Nasopharyngeal stents are left in place for 1 week postoperatively to prevent synechiae, while the raw surfaces of the pharyngeal flap are remucosalizing to maintain the newly constructed nasopharyngeal ports. We opt to use two small endotracheal tubes cut short that are passed through each naris into the pharynx. These are sutured to the caudal septum for stability. Tube size depends on the size of the ports, but a size 3 is often adequate.

  ▪ DSP: A larger caliber truncated endotracheal tube may be passed from the naris into the new port, but this is usually not necessary unless the reconstructed port is very tight. DSP is less prone to synechiae as there are fewer raw surfaces at the completion of the reconstruction.
▪ Oral rinses, especially after feeding, can help maintain oral hygiene. Older children may be prescribed chlorhexidine rinses if they are likely to be compliant with swishing and spitting. Alternatively, plain water rinses can aid in clearance of food and liquids from the oropharynx and flaps. We recommend that all patients drink clear liquids after eating to assist in clearance of food debris.
▪ Patients are placed on a soft diet for 6 weeks postoperatively. They are also instructed to drink from a cup only—no straws or suction.
▪ Patients return for follow-up 1 to 2 weeks postoperatively for an early incision check and at 6 weeks for a final assessment. At 6 weeks, all restrictions are lifted. If a fistula were to develop, this would most likely be visible at the 6-week appointment.

- Nasal resonance and articulation speech therapy are resumed after 6 weeks.
- PSAs are delayed until a minimum of 3 months postoperatively to allow for complete resolution of edema.

OUTCOMES

- Correction of VPI occurs in 80% or more of surgical patients, with slight variation across techniques. Head-to-head comparisons of techniques are difficult because most studies are based on treatment algorithms with groups differing in both preoperative VPI characteristics and surgical approach.
  - Randomized trials of DSP and pharyngeal flaps have shown no difference in residual VPI.[1,13]
  - DSP: 80% to 85% of patients demonstrated resolution of hypernasality.[14]
  - Pharyngeal flap: 85% to 95% improvement or resolution of VPI[1,11,15]
  - DOZ: 75% to 85% improvement or resolution of VPI[11,16,17]
    - DOZ may be slightly less effective in resolving VPI, but this is dependent on velopharyngeal gap size, supporting the use of an algorithmic approach to procedure selection.[18]

COMPLICATIONS

- Bleeding
  - Velocardiofacial syndrome: It is important to identify medial displacement of the carotids as this may alter surgical plan. Preoperative imaging with CTA or MRA is often obtained.
- Airway obstruction
  - Obstruction may occur acutely postoperatively or chronically.
    - Acutely, related to airway or tongue edema
    - Chronically, related to inadequate size of pharyngeal port
  - Pharyngeal flap has the highest incidence of obstruction.
    - Incidence of acute airway obstruction is as high as 38%,[19] but most resolve within the first few months postoperatively.
    - Chronic obstruction/obstructive sleep apnea incidence is roughly 10%. Pierre Robin sequence patients may be more susceptible.[20,21]
  - Sleep studies are useful in evaluating and quantifying obstruction.
  - Obstruction can be treated with CPAP or flap takedown in severe cases.
- Dehiscence or fistula: may be assessed at the 6-week visit, but we recommend waiting at least 6 months to intervene surgically.
- Scarring: particularly in the DOZ, scarring can limit functionality of the repair. We again emphasize dissection of functional muscle free from scar. Use of intraoperative muscle stimulation can serve as a guide to the distinction of functional muscle from scar.

REFERENCES

1. Ysunza A, Pamplona C, Ramirez E, et al. Velopharyngeal surgery: a prospective randomized study of pharyngeal flaps and sphincter pharyngoplasties. *Plast Reconstr Surg.* 2002;110(6):1401-1407.
2. Gart MS, Gosain AK. Surgical management of velopharyngeal insufficiency. *Clin Plast Surg.* 2014;41(2):253-270.
3. Weatherley-White RC, Sakura CY Jr, Brenner LD, et al. Submucous cleft palate. Its incidence, natural history, and indications for treatment. *Plast Reconstr Surg.* 1972;49(3):297-304.
4. Gosain AK, Conley SF, Marks S, Larson DL. Submucous cleft palate: diagnostic methods and outcomes of surgical treatment. *Plast Reconstr Surg.* 1996;97(7):1497-1509.
5. Gosain AK, Arneja JS. Management of the black hole in velopharyngeal incompetence: combined use of a Furlow palatoplasty and sphincter pharyngoplasty. *Plast Reconstr Surg.* 2007;119(5):1538-1545.
6. Bishop A, Hong P, Bezuhly M. Autologous fat grafting for the treatment of velopharyngeal insufficiency: state of the art. *J Plast Reconstr Aesthet Surg.* 2014;67(1):1-8.
7. Cantarella G, Mazzola RF, Mantovani M, et al. Fat injections for the treatment of velopharyngeal insufficiency. *J Craniofac Surg.* 2012;23(3):634-637.
8. Lau D, Oppenheimer AJ, Buchman SR, et al. Posterior pharyngeal fat grafting for velopharyngeal insufficiency. *Cleft Palate Craniofac J.* 2013;50(1):51-58.
9. Armour A, Fischbach S, Klaiman P, Fisher DM. Does velopharyngeal closure pattern affect the success of pharyngeal flap pharyngoplasty? *Plast Reconstr Surg.* 2005;115(1):45-52.
10. Abdel-Aziz M, El-Hoshy H, Ghandour H. Treatment of velopharyngeal insufficiency after cleft palate repair depending on the velopharyngeal closure pattern. *J Craniofac Surg.* 2011;22(3):813-817.
11. Yamaguchi K, Lonic D, Lee CH, et al. A treatment protocol for velopharyngeal insufficiency and the outcome. *Plast Reconstr Surg.* 2016;138(2):290e-299e.
12. Bohm LA, Padgitt N, Tibesar RJ, et al. Outcomes of combined Furlow palatoplasty and sphincter pharyngoplasty for velopharyngeal insufficiency. *Otolaryngol Head Neck Surg.* 2014;150(2):216-221.
13. Abyholm F, D'Antonio L, Davidson Ward SL, et al. Pharyngeal flap and sphincterplasty for velopharyngeal insufficiency have equal outcome at 1 year postoperatively: results of a randomized trial. *Cleft Palate Craniofac J.* 2005;42(5):501-511.
14. Riski JE, Ruff GL, Georgiade GS, et al. Evaluation of the sphincter pharyngoplasty. *Cleft Palate Craniofac J.* 1992;29(3):254-261.
15. Sullivan SR, Marrinan EM, Mulliken JB. Pharyngeal flap outcomes in nonsyndromic children with repaired cleft palate and velopharyngeal insufficiency. *Plast Reconstr Surg.* 2010;125(1):290-298.
16. Hudson DA, Grobbelaar AO, Fernandes DB, Lentin R. Treatment of velopharyngeal incompetence by the Furlow Z-plasty. *Ann Plast Surg.* 1995;34(1):23-26.
17. Chim H, Eshraghi Y, Iamphongsai S, Gosain AK. Double-opposing Z-palatoplasty for secondary surgical management of velopharyngeal incompetence in the absence of a primary furlow palatoplasty. *Cleft Palate Craniofac J.* 2015;52(5):517-524.
18. Chen PK, Wu JT, Chen YR, Noordhoff MS. Correction of secondary velopharyngeal insufficiency in cleft palate patients with the Furlow palatoplasty. *Plast Reconstr Surg.* 1994;94(7):933-941.
19. Lesavoy MA, Borud LJ, Thorson T, et al. Upper airway obstruction after pharyngeal flap surgery. *Ann Plast Surg.* 1996;36(1):26-30.
20. Wells MD, Vu TA, Luce EA. Incidence and sequelae of nocturnal respiratory obstruction following posterior pharyngeal flap operation. *Ann Plast Surg.* 1999;43(3):252-257.
21. Jackson P, Whitaker LA, Randall P. Airway hazards associated with pharyngeal flaps in patients who have the Pierre Robin syndrome. *Plast Reconstr Surg.* 1976;58(2):184-186.

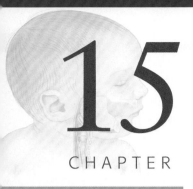

15
CHAPTER

Secondary Cleft Rhinoplasty

Ali Totonchi and Ji H. Son

DEFINITION

- Rhinoplasty remains one of the most challenging plastic surgery procedures for cleft patients. These patients present years after the initial cleft repair to correct residual nasal deformities.
- The nature of the procedure varies from patient to patient depending on the nasal deformities. Systematic reorientation of distorted nasal architecture and creation of a balanced platform for the lower lateral cartilages constitute some of the cardinal principles for correcting the cleft lip nose deformities.

ANATOMY

- Radix is the depth of the nasal root at the nasofrontal angle. This angle connects the brow and the dorsum through a soft concave curve. Although this angle can vary from 128 to 140 degrees, it is ideally 134 degrees in females and 130 degrees in males.
- Nasal dorsum is assessed using the curvilinear dorsal aesthetic lines traced from the supraorbital ridge to the tip-defining points. Ideally, the width of the dorsal aesthetic lines should match the width of either the tip-defining points or the interphiltral distance.
- Nasal deviation is evaluated by drawing a line from the mid-glabellar area to the menton, bisecting the nasal ridge, upper lip, and Cupid bow. Deviation of the nose from this line would most likely require septal surgery for correction.
- The upper lateral cartilage (ULC) overlaps the nasal bones, septum, and the lower lateral cartilages (LLCs). The internal valve is the angle formed by intersection of the nasal septum and the caudal margin of the ULC.
- LLCs comprise medial, middle, and lateral crura, which are connected to each other, the ULCs, and the septum by fibrous tissue and ligaments. Modification in any of these structures alters tip projection.
- The nasolabial angle is used to determine the degree of tip rotation. This angle is obtained by measuring the angle between a line coursing through the most anterior and posterior edges of the nostril and a line dropped perpendicular to the natural horizontal facial plane. This angle should be between 103 to 105 degrees in women and 95 to 100 degrees in men.
- The septum, turbinates, and nasal valves (internal and external) serve as the anatomic functional foundation for the nose, by contributing to respiration, filtration, humidification, temperature regulation, and protection.

PATIENT HISTORY AND PHYSICAL FINDINGS

- Although nasal deformities are partially corrected during cleft lip surgery, patients often present years after the initial cleft repair to correct residual nasal deformities.

- Efforts to correct nasal deformity in patients between the ages of 4 and 14 years may have a significant chance of supratip deformity and loss of tip definition, with widening and thickening of the skin.
- Many patients with bilateral and complete cleft lip deformities have other craniofacial abnormalities, particularly deformities of the maxilla. Correction of the skeletal deformity sets the stage for a more successful correction of the nasal deformity.
- Approximately 60% of patients with cleft lip nasal deformity have difficulty breathing through the nose. Correction of physiologic function of the nose should be addressed at the time of correction of the nasal deformity.
- Many of the patients may have asymmetry involving parts other than the nose and the lip. Therefore, it is important to assess the entire face and note asymmetry before analyzing the nose in detail (Table 1).[1]

Table 1 Detailed Nasal Analysis

Structure	Assessment
Skin	• Thickness • Quality of the tissue for reconstruction
Nasal bone	• Symmetry • Length • Distance from the midline • Depth of radix • Presence or absence of a dorsal hump
Midvault	• Upper lateral cartilage collapse • Vertical symmetry
Nasal tip	• Shape—bulbous, boxy, narrow, or parenthesis deformity? • Symmetry • Fullness • Projection • Infratip lobule size • Nasolabial angle • Direction of the columella
Alar base	• Comparison of thickness of the ala • Vertical position • Configuration of nasal sill
Nostrils	• Symmetry
Internal nose	• Stenosis of the internal and external valve • Presence or absence of a deviated septum • Size and shape of the turbinates • Synechiae • Septal perforation

Table 2 Features of Unilateral Cleft Lip Nasal Deformity

- The columella is shorter on the cleft side.
- The base of the columella is deviated to the noncleft side.
- The lateral crus of the lower lateral cartilage is longer on the cleft side.
- The nasal tip is displaced in both the frontal and the horizontal planes.
- The nasal tip is asymmetric.
- The ala is flattened, resulting in horizontal orientation of the nostril.
- The nostrils are asymmetric.
- The entire nostril is retropositioned because of the deficiency in the underlying frame.
- The base of the ala is displaced laterally and/or posteriorly and sometimes inferiorly.
- The nasal floor is caudal on the cleft side.
- A nasolabial fistula could be present.
- The septum and anterior nasal spine are shifted toward the noncleft vestibule.
- The nasal septum is deviated, resulting in a varying degree of nasal obstruction.
- The inferior turbinate on the cleft side is hypertrophic.
- The maxilla is hypoplastic on the cleft side.
- The premaxilla and the maxillary segments are displaced.

From Guyuron B. MOC-PS(SME) CME article: late cleft lip nasal deformity. *Plast Reconstr Surg.* 2008;121(4):1-11, with permission.

- It is crucial to recognize common features of unilateral cleft lip nasal deformity (Table 2) and bilateral cleft lip nasal deformity (Table 3).[1]

Table 3 Features of Bilateral Cleft Lip Nasal Deformity

- The columella is relatively short and the prolabium seems attached to the nasal tip.
- The nasal tip is flat and broad.
- The nasal alae are flat and sometimes drawn in an S-shaped fashion.
- The base of the ala is displaced laterally and sometimes inferiorly on both sides.
- Both nostrils are oriented horizontally.
- The lower lateral cartilages are severely deformed.
- The nasal floor is absent.
- The caudal cartilaginous septum and the nasal spine are displaced inferiorly relative to the level of the alar bases.
- The nasal tip and the nostril are commonly asymmetric.

From Guyuron B. MOC-PS(SME) CME article: late cleft lip nasal deformity. *Plast Reconstr Surg.* 2008;121(4):1-11, with permission.

IMAGING

- Imaging is not indicated for all of the patients undergoing secondary cleft rhinoplasty unless there is airway obstruction from sinus or cephalic septal pathology necessitating further imaging to aid in surgical planning.

SURGICAL MANAGEMENT

- One of the most important aspects of cleft lip rhinoplasty is the creation of symmetric nose.
- Patients commonly have maxillary deficiency and may need orthognathic surgery and maxillary bone grafting. Ideally, if maxillary surgery is contemplated, it should precede repair of the cleft lip rhinoplasty deformity.
  - Maxillary advancement is not advised before the age of 14 to 15 years for a female patient and 17 to 18 years for a male patient, unless serial cephalograms or hand radiographs demonstrate completion of bone growth before this age.
  - Otherwise, the patient may need another maxillary advancement if the maxilla is advanced and the mandible continues growing, which can alter the outcome of the initial cleft lip rhinoplasty.
- The operation may be performed through an endonasal or an open technique. Because of common asymmetry in the nasal frame, cleft lip–related nasal deformities are usually more successfully corrected through an open technique.
  - The advantages of an open technique are excellent exposure, good hemostasis, and flexibility in corrective procedures.
- The main objectives of the operation are to restore symmetry and harmony to the face as well as improve functional outcome.
- The nature of the operation varies tremendously from patient to patient.

Preoperative Planning

- Discuss risks, benefits, and expectations with parents and patients on the day of surgery. Specifically outline the risks including asymmetry, incomplete resolution or suboptimal correction of nasal deformities, and additional operations.
- It is paramount to do a detailed facial and midface analysis to address each component of the nasal deformity before the operation.

Positioning and Approach

- The patient is positioned supine.
- Depending on the choice of cartilage graft, either the ear or the chest wall is prepped in addition to the face.
- Previous incisions are used to minimize creating new scars when possible.

■ Open Cleft Lip Rhinoplasty

Incision and Dissection

- Incise the columella at the mid-columella, a stair-step incision helps to realign the columella at the end of the procedure (**TECH FIG 1A**). When possible, use an old scar in the nasal vestibule and avoid making a new incision.
  - Extend the incision behind the columella and upward, continue as an infracartilaginous incision on the non-cleft side.
  - On the cleft side, the incision is made to match the noncleft side, which may not coincide with an infra-cartilaginous incision.
- Dissect the columella. Find the loose areolar space between the medial crura and follow this upward in the lower lateral cartilage (LLC) to separate the LLCs from the fibrofatty tissue.

- The dissection extends to the pyriform rim laterally and nasal bone superiorly and should be symmetrical on both sides to allow for symmetric contracture after the operation (**TECH FIG 1B**).
- The course of the operation varies from patient to patient depending on the nasal deformities.
  - In our example, we present a patient with short medial crus, low dome, and excessive soft triangle soft tissue (**TECH FIG 1C**).

Shape Correction[1,2]

- After complete dissection and repositioning of the lower lateral cartilage on the cleft side, double hooks are placed to lift the alar domes symmetrically.
  - A 30-gauge needle is used to facilitate alignment of the medial crura when the columellar strut is placed (**TECH FIG 2A**).

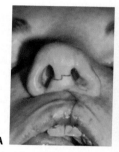 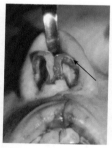 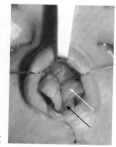

TECH FIG 1 • **A.** A columellar incision. **B.** In an open technique, the malformed lower lateral cartilage is exposed. The cleft lower lateral cartilage (*arrow*) has less projection relative to the noncleft side. **C.** Comparing the cleft side (*patient's left*) to the noncleft side (*patient's right*) with the skin retracted, the medial crus (*black arrow*) is shorter and the nasal dome (*white arrow*) is lower. From Guyuron B. MOC-PS(SME) CME article: late cleft lip nasal deformity. *Plast Reconstr Surg.* 2008:121(4):1-11, with permission.

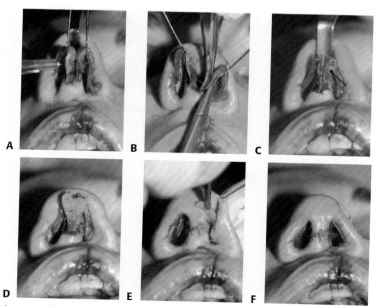

TECH FIG 2 • **A.** Medial crus is tattooed to facilitate alignment when columellar strut is placed. **B.** Columellar strut is placed. **C.** Columellar strut is secured using sutures. There is excessive soft triangle lining that will be trimmed (*arrow*). **D.** A shield graft is placed. **E.** Alar graft is placed for better shape and support. **F.** Internal and external splints are placed. From Guyuron B. MOC-PS(SME) CME article: late cleft lip nasal deformity. *Plast Reconstr Surg.* 2008:121(4):1-11, with permission.

- Tattoo marks can be made with methylene blue on either medial crus to mark the alignment.
- The columellar strut is fixed in position and 6-0 clear nylon sutures are placed in at least two or three sites guided by the previous tattoo marks (**TECH FIG 2B**).
- The final suture close to the domes will better align the medial crura. There is still excessive soft triangle lining that will be trimmed (**TECH FIG 2C**).
- A shield graft is placed in position to facilitate additional support and maintain central alignment of the nasal tripod (**TECH FIG 2D**).

- An alar rim graft is placed to support the ala in a better position, which will be further supported using external and internal stents (**TECH FIG 2E**).
- Upon completion of surgery, there is restoration of proper height and shape to the nostrils and the nasal tip; an external nasal silicone stent is positioned on the ipsilateral side to the cleft lip on the soft triangle (**TECH FIG 2F**).
- The columellar incision is closed using 6-0 fast-absorbing catgut.
- Turbinates are reduced to improve nasal airway passage, if needed.

■ Dorsal Correction

- Many patients require removal of a dorsal hump and reduction of the radix. Less frequently, there are patients with nasal deformities who may require augmentation of the radix and dorsum.
- Nasal bone deviation is corrected by nasal osteotomies when surgery is performed on skeletally mature patients. These techniques are discussed in the chapter on secondary rhinoplasty.
- If augmenting the radix and dorsum, diced cartilage graft can be utilized.
- Nasal bone asymmetry may require wedge osteotomy between the nasal bone and the midline structures for medial repositioning of the nasal wall.

■ Nasal Framework Correction

- The upper lateral cartilage (ULC) usually needs correction through separation, trimming, and repositioning.
  - Most cleft lip noses benefit from spreader grafts.
- If required due to septal deviation, septoplasty should include resection of the posterior portion of the quadrangle cartilage, vomer bone, and perpendicular plate of the ethmoid bone, leaving a strong and straight L-shaped frame to support the nose.

- This frame is straightened with or without scoring by application of bilateral spreader grafts anteriorly.
- The septum is then splinted using either a pair of Doyle stents or custom-fabricated stents.
- These stents are sutured in position using transseptal nonabsorbable sutures.
- The ULC is then fixed to the spreader grafts and the septum using 5-0 PDS suture (Ethicon Inc., Somerville, NJ).

■ Reshaping the Tip and Ala

- The dome on the affected side is posterior; the lateral crus extends laterally; and almost always, the medial crus is shorter than ideal, causing length deficiency in the columella.
  - A columellar strut is the most efficacious means of supporting the tip. Use of a columellar strut will:
    - Increase tip projection
    - Elongate the columella on the cleft side
    - Augment the subnasale, which is often deficient
    - Increase the nasolabial angle
    - Prevent the tip from shifting caudally
- Free up the lower lateral cartilage on the cleft side completely or bilaterally or advance in V-to-Y fashion to restore adequate projection on the cleft side.

- Reduce the thickness of the ala by removing some of the fibrofatty tissue, especially at the alar base and along the alar rim.
- Interdomal, transdomal, and lateral crural sutures may be required.
- A tip graft will only be used if the infratip lobule volume is inadequate, which is seldom the case.
- Placement of an alar rim graft and application of two stents externally and internally that are fixed with a through-and-through suture reduces the potential for recurrent alar thickening.

■ Nostril Correction

- Augmentation of the floor of the nostril and elevation of the nostril sill on the cleft side is achieved by placement of a cartilage graft.

- The alar bases are then narrowed as needed and repaired using 6-0 fast-absorbing catgut.

PEARLS AND PITFALLS

Physical findings	■ Careful selection of patients at a suitable age is required along with a cooperative patient and a caregiver. ■ Skeletal correction of the bony base must be performed before soft tissue correction.
Technique	■ Use old scars and avoid new scars if possible. ■ If length of the surgery lasts more than 1.5 hours, consider reinjecting vasoconstrictive agents to minimize bleeding intraoperatively and postoperatively. ■ Restoration of the distorted structures should be based on normal anatomy. ■ Careful tissue handling with meticulous alignment of landmarks is required. ■ Forcing the cartilage anteriorly to achieve symmetry is doomed to failure, as the cartilage will gradually shift the tip to the cleft side of the nose.

POSTOPERATIVE CARE

■ A nasal splint is applied for 7 to 8 days.
■ Patients are asked to refrain from heavy exercise for 2 to 3 weeks and use of eyeglasses for 4 to 5 weeks.

OUTCOMES

■ Cleft lip rhinoplasty addresses both functional and aesthetic nasal disturbance following initial cleft lip repair.
■ Patients are usually very satisfied following cleft lip rhinoplasty due to the resultant functional and aesthetic improvement.

COMPLICATIONS

■ The most common complication of secondary cleft lip rhinoplasty is asymmetry. Patients should be informed that they might need additional surgery. Most common sites of asymmetry are the alar base and nostril.[1-3]
■ Owing to the underlying condition, these patients have a higher chance of nasal obstruction preoperatively and sometimes postoperatively.[3]
■ Septal deviation may recur, or there may be residual septal deviation due to primary deformity. This may require additional procedures.

REFERENCES

1. Guyuron B. Late cleft lip nasal deformity. *Plast Reconstr Surg.* 2008;121:1-11.
2. Broadbent TR, Woolf RM. Cleft lip nasal deformity. *Ann Plast Surg.* 1984;12:216.
3. Rifley W, Thaller SR. The residual cleft lip nasal deformity: an anatomic approach. *Clin Plast Surg.* 1996;23:81.

Tessier 3 and 4 Clefts (Nasal-Cheek Region)

16

CHAPTER

Philip Kuo-Ting Chen and Vikram S. Pandit

DEFINITION

- The Tessier no. 3 facial cleft occurs at the junction of the frontonasal and maxillary process.
  - It involves the position of an ordinary cleft lip extending upward and passing through the alar base towards the medial canthal region.
  - The medial part of the eye is displaced laterally and inferiorly (**FIG 1A**).
- The Tessier no. 4 facial cleft is located lateral to the no. 3 facial cleft.
  - This cleft starts lateral to the philtral ridge and travels lateral to the alar base toward the medial canthal region.
  - The medial part of the eye is displaced laterally and inferiorly (**FIG 1B**).

ANATOMY

- The Tessier no. 3 and no. 4 facial clefts have similar soft tissue abnormalities resulting in shortened oculo-alar and oculo-oral distances.
- In the lip region, the cleft line is the same as ordinary cleft lip in no. 3 (**FIG 2A**) and is lateral to the philtral column in no. 4 (**FIG 2B**).
- Both clefts are accompanied by distortion or disruption of the orbicularis oris muscle. The cleft extends upward into the cheek with alar involvement in no. 3 and without alar involvement in no. 4.

- In both clefts, orbital dystopia is coupled with globe abnormalities and underlying skeletal deficiencies.
  - The medial canthus is displaced inferiorly, and the lacrimal canaliculus on the lower eyelid is usually disrupted.
  - Usually, it is possible to identify the punctum of the lower eyelid (**FIG 3**).
  - There is a coloboma of the lower eyelid (**FIG 4**).
- The involved muscles of facial expression are distorted in their orientation.
  - The alar base and the lateral part of the nasalis muscle are displaced upward, and the medial part of the cheek muscles is displaced downward.
- The underlying maxillary bone is depressed or separated according to the severity of the cleft.
- Patients may have independent pathology in their cheek region and lip (eg, an intact lip with the cleft only seen in the cheek region[1-4]) (**FIG 5**).

HISTORY AND PHYSICAL FINDINGS

- The history taking and physical examination are similar to other patients with craniofacial anomalies.
- The history should include the family history, medications during the first trimester, and prenatal diagnosis.
- Physical examination should include the extent and location of soft tissue cleft, eye condition, involvement of alveolus, palate, and also other associated systemic problems.[5]

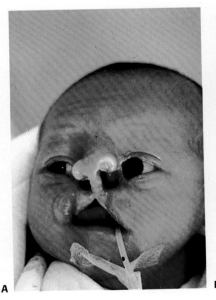
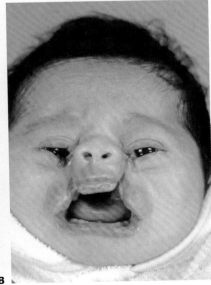

FIG 1 • A. Tessier no. 3 facial cleft. **B.** Tessier no. 4 facial cleft.

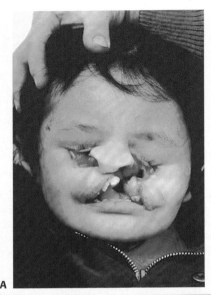

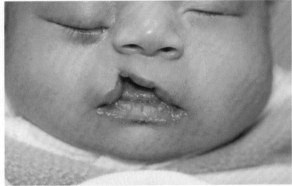

FIG 2 • **A.** The cleft lip of a Tessier no. 3 is similar to an ordinary cleft lip. **B.** The cleft lip of a Tessier no. 4 is lateral to the philtral column.

IMAGING

- Radiographic images are usually not necessary in the first visit.
- CT scanning is helpful to determine the extent of bony defect on orbital floor if the patient has severe orbital dystopia (**FIG 6**).

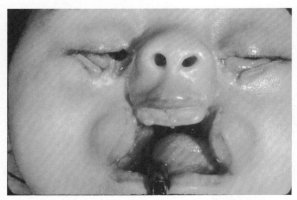

FIG 3 • The punctum can be identified lateral to the cleft.

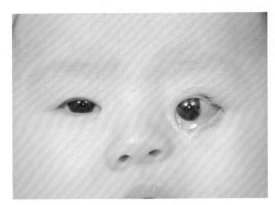

FIG 4 • Coloboma of left lower eyelid.

- Panoramic x-rays and CT scans are also helpful to evaluate the necessity of bone grafting in the alveolar or cheek region when the patient is older (**FIG 7**).
- In the author's center, cephalometric and panoramic radiographs and CT scans with 3D reconstruction are routinely recorded every 2 years from ages 5 to 17 years to monitor facial growth.

SURGICAL MANAGEMENT

- Surgical correction of the soft tissue problems is undertaken between 3 to 6 months of age. This correction should aim at the restoration of normal facial appearance and protection of the eye.
- Bony reconstruction of the alveolar clefts is similar to the timing of alveolar bone grafting in cleft patients, ie, in the mixed dentition period before the eruption of the teeth in the cleft region.
- The bony reconstruction for the skeletal defects on the face and orbit is generally not undertaken till the patient is at least 3 years of age and more commonly at the age of 5 years.
  - This allows the inner and outer tables of the calvarium to be split and therefore obtain a large amount of bone graft with minimal donor morbidity.
  - However, when there is severe bony deficiency on the orbital floor causing a significant dystopia of the globe, orbital floor reconstruction should be considered at an earlier age.

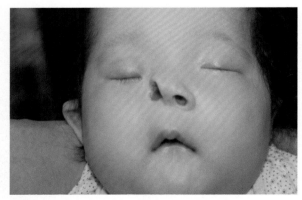

FIG 5 • Tessier no. 3 cleft with cleft on cheek region and intact lip.

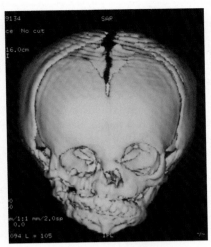

FIG 6 • 3D CT scan of a right Tessier no. 4 facial cleft.

■ The repair of the soft tissue deficit in the Tessier no. 3 and no. 4 craniofacial clefts is based on five basic components as outlined.[6]
  ■ A medial canthopexy with 2 mm overcorrection in an upward vertical position
    • The postoperative scar contracture will always pull the new medial canthus inferiorly.
  ■ Midface rotation advancement is performed with rotation of the medially based nasal flap, advancement of the laterally based cheek flap, and repositioning of the facial muscles.

• This helps to lengthen the shortened oculo-oral and oculo-alar distances while restoring normal facial expression.
• This is similar to the rotation-advancement repair in ordinary cleft lip.
• The lengthening achieved in the midface region should primarily be due to muscle repositioning rather than skin Z-plasties.
■ Placement of the surgical scars should be along the junction of the facial units, rather than placing multiple Z-plasties on the cheek, to avoid color mismatching due to skin differences in the nasal and cheek regions.
  • Placement of the scar lateral to the junction of the facial units will result in visible scars on the cheek region.[7-11]
■ Repair the cleft lip using the standard technique (ie, discard the redundant tissue lateral to the proposed philtrum to avoid an unnatural-looking lip).[12,13]
■ Downward and medially repositioning the involved alar base with 1 to 2 mm of overcorrection in vertical dimension
  • The postoperative scar contracture in cheek will always pull the alar base upward.

Positioning

■ The soft tissue repair is performed under general anesthesia.
■ The endotracheal tube is usually fixed to the center of the lower lip with tape.
■ The patient is placed in supine position with the face disinfected and draped.

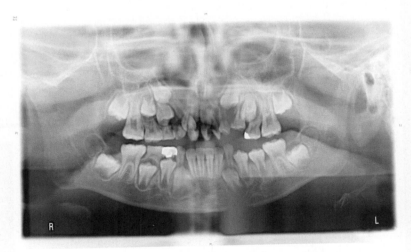

FIG 7 • Panoramic radiograph of a bilateral Tessier no. 4 facial cleft.

TECHNIQUES

■ Markings

- With the patient prepared under general anesthesia, the key elements of the cleft lip are marked, excluding the skin lateral to the philtral column on the cleft side.
- On unilateral facial clefts, the markings for the anatomical landmarks are relatively easy.
  - The positions of the displaced medial canthus, the alar base, and the peak of the Cupid's bow can be determined by comparison with equivalent landmarks on the noncleft side (**TECH FIG 1A**).
  - It should be emphasized that the position of the medial canthus and the alar base should be overcorrected, ie, 2 mm higher for medial canthus and 2 mm lower for alar base (**TECH FIG 1B,C**).

- It is much more difficult to determine these landmarks in the presence of bilateral facial clefts.
  - However, the position of the medial canthus can still be determined by the position of the lateral canthus, together with the width of the eyes.
  - The position of the alar base is determined by the position of the columella and the vertical height of the lateral lip, which is further determined by the vertical height of the prolabial segment.

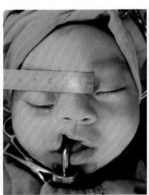 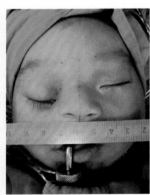 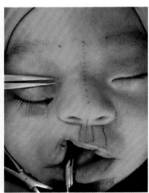

TECH FIG 1 • A. A case of bilateral asymmetric incomplete no. 4 facial clefts. The cleft lip on the left side is not at the typical location of an ordinary cleft lip. The left medial canthus is also slightly downward displaced. The reason that surgery is not performed on the cheek on the left side is because the deformity is so mild that it is not worthwhile to reposition the left medial canthus, with the resultant long paranasal scar. Hence, only the cleft lip is repaired in bilateral fashion, whereas unilateral repair is performed on the cheek. The ruler demonstrates the mirror-image position of the medial canthus on the cleft side. **B.** The ruler demonstrates the mirror-image position of the nasal floor and alar base on the cleft side. **C.** The new position of the medial canthus on the cleft side with 2 mm overcorrection.

■ Incisions

- Incision lines are marked along the margin of the nasal unit medially in a curvilinear fashion upward to the true medial canthus, then turning laterally, incorporating a triangular-shaped medially based flap on the upper eyelid.
- The incision then comes back medially to the proposed point of the new medial canthus.
- The lateral skin incision is made on the lateral cleft margin up to the medial canthus.
- The lip landmarks and incision lines are marked as regular unilateral or bilateral cleft lip repairs (**TECH FIG 2**).

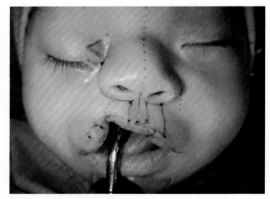

TECH FIG 2 • The incision lines: the prolabial width is similar to the design of an ordinary bilateral cleft lip. The tissue lateral to the proposed philtral column is discarded. A medially based triangular flap is designed on the upper eyelid.

■ Dissection and Facial Flap Elevation

- The redundant skin is excised and discarded to avoid an unnatural-looking repaired cleft lip.
- The extent of the muscle dissection is similar to that in an ordinary cleft lip repair (**TECH FIG 3A–C**).
- On the midface, the laterally based cheek flap is then elevated subperiosteally with a relaxing incision on the periosteum lateral to the infraorbital neurovascular bundle (**TECH FIG 3D,E**).
  - This allows the cheek flap to be advanced medially up to the lateral edge of the nasal flap and down to the philtral column.

- The muscle layer of the cheek is then separated from the skin for a few millimeters to facilitate the muscle approximation in later steps.
- The medially based nasal flap (in unilateral lesions) and the alar base are raised off the underlying nasal cartilages and the frontal process of the maxilla to allow downward rotation of the shortened oculoalar tissue. In patients with bilateral lesions, the nasal flap is based superiorly as there are incisions along both sides of the nose.
- The nasalis muscle is identified and dissected from the overlying skin in a sheet for about 5 mm for later muscle reorientation (**TECH FIG 3F**).

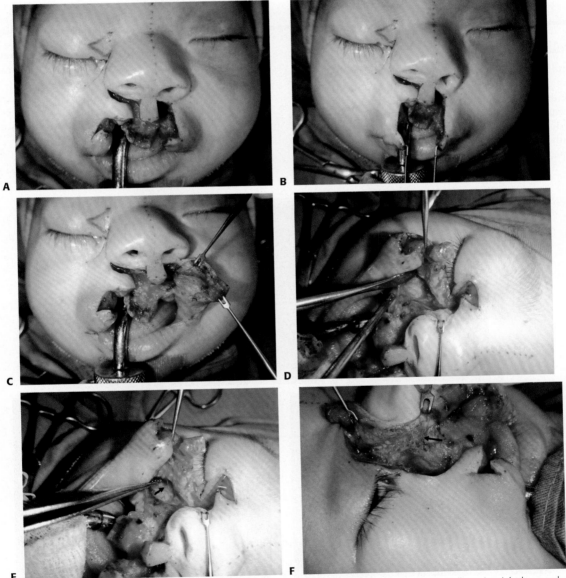

TECH FIG 3 • A. The incision of the lip part. The excessive tissue on the right lateral lip is preserved initially as it might be needed later for lengthening of the cheek region. **B.** The incision and dissection of the lip part is similar to a bilateral cleft lip repair. **C.** The extent of the muscle dissection on the lateral lip. **D.** Subperiosteal dissection of the cheek flap. **E.** A relaxing incision is made lateral to the infraorbital neurovascular bundle (*arrow*) to achieve adequate mobilization of the cheek tissue. **F.** The dissection of the nasalis muscle (*arrow*) in the nasal flap.

- In cases of complete no. 3 facial clefts, the nasal lining and the lining of the eyelid are repaired by local turn-over mucosal flaps between the nasal and cheek incisions (**TECH FIG 3G**).

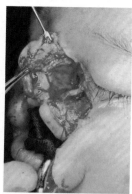

TECH FIG 3 (Continued) • **G.** Turnover flap along the cleft margin for reconstruction of the nasal lining.

■ Eyelid Correction

- Attention is then turned to the lower eyelid.
- After dissection and freeing of the displaced facial musculature, the subperiosteal mobilization of the later-ally based cheek flap is extended superiorly up to and including the inferior orbital rim (**TECH FIG 4A,B**).
- Usually, it is not very difficult to identify the remnant of the medial canthal tendon (**TECH FIG 4C**).

- The overlying lower eyelid tissue incorporating the tarsus and the attached conjunctiva are then transposed medially.
- If necessary, a lateral canthotomy may be required to facilitate the medial movement of the lower eyelid, correction of the coloboma, and reconstruction of the lower eyelid (**TECH FIG 4D**).

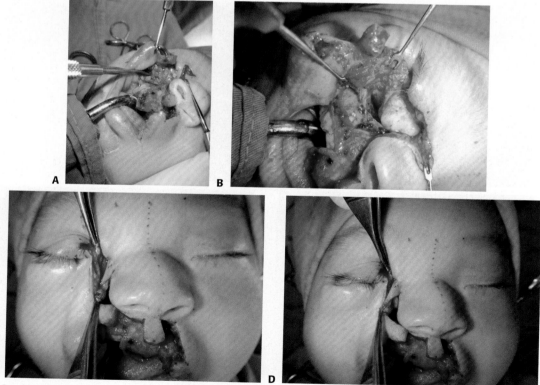

TECH FIG 4 • **A.** Dissection along the infraorbital rim. **B.** Dissection into the orbital floor. **C.** The remnant of the medial canthal tendon (upper forceps). **D.** The remnant of the medial canthal tendon and the lower eyelid are advanced medially and superiorly to the proposed position of the medial canthus.

Repositioning the Facial Musculature

- The lateral cheek flap is then advanced medially.
- A medial canthopexy is performed by transnasal wiring or directly suturing to the local periosteum using the medial edge of the tarsal plate and the remnant of the medial canthal tendon (**TECH FIG 5A**).
  - This will ensure adequate support for the lower eyelid.
- The orbicularis oculi muscle of the lower eyelid is identified and apposed to the superior limb of the newly created medial canthus (**TECH FIG 5B**).
  - It should be re-emphasized that this medial cantho-pexy always needs some overcorrection in cephalic direction for about 2 mm; otherwise, the position of the canthus will always be lower than its peer in the noncleft side after skin closure.
- The nasal complex of the medially or superiorly based nasal flap is then rotated downward matching the alar base on the noncleft side to achieve adequate oculoalar distance in unilateral lesions.
- For bilateral clefts, the positions of the alar bases are determined by the position of the columellar base (**TECH FIG 5C,D**).
- Repositioning of the remaining facial musculature, in particular the nasalis and the muscles of facial expression, is then performed.

- The sutures are placed more superiorly on the nasal muscles and more inferiorly on the cheek muscles to achieve a "rotation advancement" (**TECH FIG 5E**).
- With the redundant skin of the upper lip lateral to the philtral edge previously excised, a rotation-advancement repair of the cleft lip is performed in unilateral cases and bilateral cheiloplasty is performed for patients with bilateral lesions (**TECH FIG 5F**).
- The orbicularis oris is reconstituted and reapposed to the muscle bundle on the noncleft side.
- The medial edge of the cheek flap is then sutured to the lateral edge of the nasal flap with the suture line placed along the junction of the facial units.
- The medially based upper eyelid flap can be trimmed at this moment if the oculo-oral or oculonasal distance can be restored without difficulty, or can be placed as a small triangular flap on the lower eyelid under the medial canthus to further lengthen the oculo-oral or oculonasal distance, or to break down the straight line scar and to prevent possible postoperative scar contracture[14] (**TECH FIG 5G**).
- Repositioning the facial musculature and placing the suture line along the junction of facial units results in a more natural facial expression and therefore a better aesthetic result.

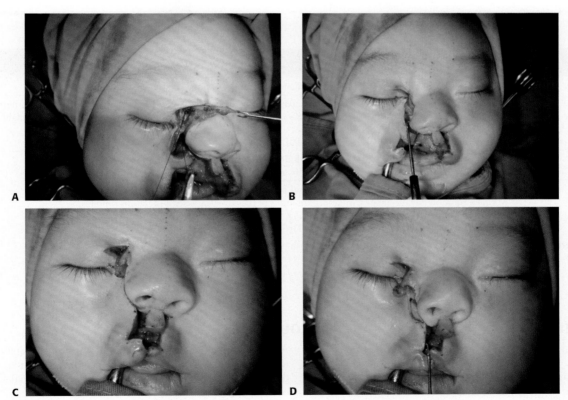

TECH FIG 5 • A. The medial canthal tendon is sutured to the periosteum of the new position of the medial canthus using 4-0 Prolene suture. **B.** The orbicularis oculi muscle of the lower eyelid is identified and apposed to the superior limb of the newly created medial canthus. **C.** The alar base position on the cleft side is determined by the base of columella. **D.** Excision of the excessive skin on the cheek flap helps for the lengthening of the oculonasal distance.

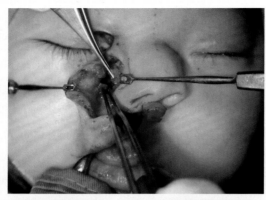

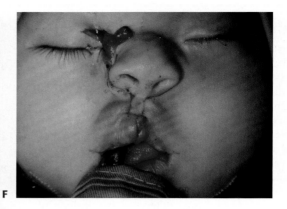

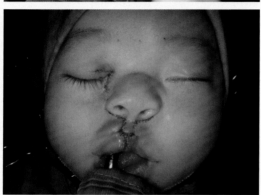

TECH FIG 5 (Continued) • **E.** Approximation of the muscle layer in cheek flap and nasal flap. The sutures are placed higher on the nasal flap and lower on the cheek flap to achieve the "rotation-advancement" movement. **F.** The lateral lips are approximated to the prolabium. The marking under the right nasal floor shows the skin needs to be excised for further downward movement of the nasal floor. The medially based upper eyelid flap is still preserved at this moment. **G.** The medially based upper eyelid flap is excised finally as the length of the oculonasal distance is adequate after reconstruction. The suture lines are placed along the junction of the facial units.

PEARLS AND PITFALLS

Markings	■ Precise marking of the anatomic position of the medial canthus and alar base
Incision	■ Make an incision along the cleft to raise the laterally based cheek flap and medially/superiorly based nasal flap. ■ The incision line of the lip is similar to ordinary cleft lip repair with special care not to preserve the redundant tissue lateral to the philtral column. ■ Design a medially based flap on the upper eyelid.
Dissection	■ Extensive subperiosteal dissection of the cheek tissue lateral to the infraorbital foramen ■ Extensive perichondrial dissection of the nasalis muscle
Reconstruction	■ Local turnover flaps for the lining of eyelid and nose ■ Midface rotation advancement with approximation of the cheek muscles and nasalis muscles ■ Medial canthopexy in an overcorrected position ■ Adjust the lower eyelid by the medial-based flap from the upper eyelid.
Aesthetic concerns	■ Placement of the suture lines along the junction of the facial subunits ■ Design for overcorrection of the oculonasal or oculo-oral distance (eg, move the proposed medial canthus upward and alar base downward)

POSTOPERATIVE CARE

■ The postoperative care is similar to that used for primary cleft lip repair.

■ The airway maintenance and chest care are as important as that in any patient who received general anesthesia.

■ The routine facial wound care in Chang Gung Craniofacial Center is to use normal saline wet dressing changed with the frequency of every 4 hours.

■ This wound care can be replaced by local antibiotic ointment if the wounds are clean without much discharge.

OUTCOMES

■ A retrospective review of the outcomes of surgical repair for rare facial clefts in Chang Gung Craniofacial Center was done in the early 2000s. The study reviewed the facial clefts over a period of 25 years.

■ Among the 41 different Tessier craniofacial clefts seen, most (17 patients) were Tessier no. 3 and no. 4 clefts. Patients could be roughly divided into two groups: a group of eight patients treated by the traditional Z-plasty principles and second group of nine patients treated with

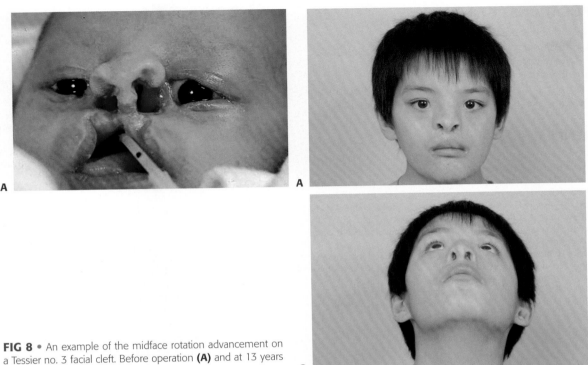

FIG 8 • An example of the midface rotation advancement on a Tessier no. 3 facial cleft. Before operation **(A)** and at 13 years old **(B and C)**.

the rotation-advancement technique described. Of these nine patients, five had Tessier no. 3 clefts and four had no. 4 clefts. Seven were primary cases, and the other two were secondary or tertiary revisions.

■ None of the patients in the Z-plasty group had a satisfactory result in terms of scar quality, color matching, or natural facial expression. The cases in the rotation-advancement group, while their medial canthus and alar base might not be well repositioned, still had much better results in their scar and facial expression[6] (**FIGS 8** and **9**).

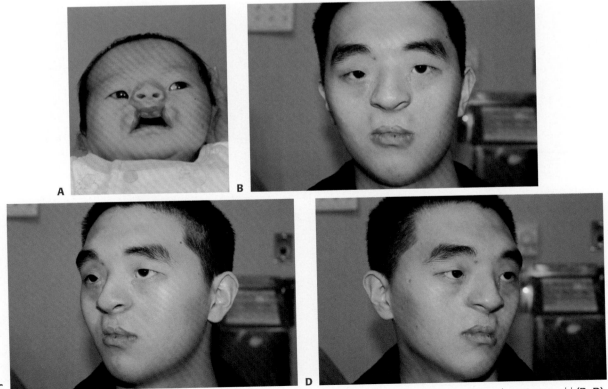

FIG 9 • An example of the midface rotation advancement on a Tessier no. 4 facial cleft. Before operation **(A)** and at 17 years old **(B–D)**.

COMPLICATIONS

- Postoperative bleeding
- Wound infection
- Wound dehiscence
- Hypertrophic scar formation
- Undercorrection with malposition of the medial canthus or alar base and persistent ectropion of lower eyelid.

REFERENCES

1. Tessier P. Anatomical classification of facial, craniofacial and latero-facial clefts. *J Maxillofac Surg.* 1976;4:69.
2. Kawamoto HK Jr. The kaleidoscopic world of rare craniofacial clefts: order out of chaos (Tessier classification). *Clin Plast Surg.* 1976;3:529-572.
3. van der Meulen JCH. Oblique facial clefts: pathology, etiology and reconstruction. *Plast Reconstr Surg.* 1985;76(2):212-224.
4. Ortiz Monasterio F, Fuente del Campo A, Dimopulos A. Nasal clefts. *Ann Plast Surg.* 1987;18(5):377-397.
5. Allam KA, Lim AA, Elsherbiny A, Kawamoto HK. The Tessier number 3 cleft: a report of 10 cases and review of literature. *J Plast Reconstr Aesthet Surg.* 2014;67:1055-1062.
6. Chen PK, Chang FC, Chan FC, et al. Repair of Tessier no. 3 and no. 4 craniofacial clefts with facial units and muscle repositioning by midface rotation advancement without Z-plasties. *Plast Reconstr Surg.* 2012;129:1337-1344.
7. Maeda T, Oyama A, Okamoto T, et al. Combination of Tessier no. 3 and 4: case report of a rare anomaly with 12 years' follow-up. *J Craniomaxillofac Surg.* 2014;42:1985-1989.
8. Alonso N, Freitas RS, Oliveira e Cruz GA, et al. Tessier no. 4 facial clefts: evolution of surgical treatment in a large series of patients. *Plast Reconstr Surg.* 2008;122(5):1505-1513.
9. Laure B, Picard A, Bonin-Goga B, et al. Tessier number 4 bilateral orbito-facial cleft: a 26-year follow-up. *J Craniomaxillofac Surg.* 2010;38:245-247.
10. Cizmeci O, Kuvat SV. Tessier no. 3 incomplete cleft reconstruction with alar transposition and irregular Z-plasty. *Plast Surg Int.* 2011;2011:Article ID 596569.
11. Versnel SL, van der Elzen MEP, Wolvius EB, et al. Long term results after 40 years experience with treatment of rare facial clefts. Part 1: oblique and paramedian clefts. *J Plast Reconstr Aesthet Surg.* 2011;64:1334-1343.
12. Noordhoff MS, Chen YR, Chen KT, et al. The surgical technique for the complete unilateral cleft lip-nasal deformity. *Operat Tech Plast Reconstr Surg.* 1995;2(3):167.
13. Chen PK, Noordhoff MS. Treatment of complete bilateral cleft lip-nasal deformity. *Semin Plast Surg.* 2005;19(4):329-341.
14. Longaker MT, Lipshutz GS, Kawamoto HK. Reconstruction of Tessier no. 4 clefts revisited. *Plast Reconstr Surg.* 1999;99(6):1501-1506.

Tessier 7—Macrostomia Repair

Patrick A. Gerety and Scott P. Bartlett

DEFINITION

- Macrostomia—enlarged oral aperture–related clefting of the oral commissure
- Tessier 7 cleft—lateral (transverse) facial cleft from the oral commissure to the zygomaticotemporal suture
- Cheilion—anatomic name for commissure point
- Commissuroplasty—recreation of oral commissure

ANATOMY[1]

- Oral commissure (FIG 1)
  - Position
    - Normal position: at a vertical line dropped from the medial limbus (some variability)
  - Shape
    - Normal shape: The upper and lower lip vermilion comes to sharp corner.
    - Macrostomic commissure: Oblique angle, gaping at rest, round with smile
- Tessier 7 cleft resulting in macrostomia
  - Variable in presentation—may be slightly wider oral commissure or severe cleft of skin, subcutaneous tissue, muscle, and bone
  - Trajectory—the cleft occurs along a line from the oral commissure to the zygomaticotemporal suture.

- Affected structures
  - Commissure—laterally positioned, anatomically abnormal (ie, made of cleft tissue [lighter in color than normal vermilion])
  - Orbicularis oris—interrupted and malinserted. The superior and inferior limbs contribute to the appearance of the lips on the macrostomic side (see FIG 1).

PATHOGENESIS

- Development of normal facial anatomy is dependent upon early first and second branchial arch embryology.
- The maxillary and mandibular prominences normally fuse in early embryologic development (weeks 4–6) forming the normal cheeks and lips.
- Stapedial artery is the blood supply before the external carotid system has developed.
- Stapedial disruption starves all tissue types—skin, fat, muscle, and bone.
- Macrostomia results as a presumed failure of this process.
- Interruption of embryologic development along the "oro-tragal" line can affect the oral commissure, muscles of mastication, muscles of facial expression, mandible, maxilla, and auricle.
- Isolated macrostomia is a disorder of the first branchial arch only.

NATURAL HISTORY[2]

- Incidence: rare, 1 in 225 000 live births
- Unilateral 80%, bilateral 20%
- As with cleft lip, the left side appears to be more commonly affected.
- May be associated with syndromes including the following:
  - Hemifacial microsomia
    - Including Goldenhar syndrome and variants of oculo-auriculovertebral spectrum
    - May account for as many as 25% of macrostomia patients
  - Treacher Collins syndrome
  - Auriculocondylar syndrome
- Tessier 7: the most common of the rare craniofacial clefts (5%–14%)

PATIENT HISTORY AND PHYSICAL FINDINGS

- Laterally displaced oral commissure
- Clefted/interrupted orbicularis oris
  - Oral incompetence may be encountered.
  - Gaping oral commissure in repose related to cleft orbicularis oris muscle

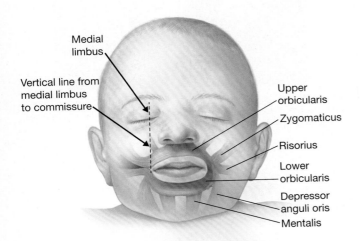

Medial limbus

Vertical line from medial limbus to commissure

Upper orbicularis

Zygomaticus

Risorius

Lower orbicularis

Depressor anguli oris

Mentalis

FIG 1 • Lateral facial cleft creates discontinuity of the orbicularis oris at the oral commissure. This in turn affects the location and insertion of the zygomaticus, risorius, and depressor anguli oris muscles.

- The cleft margin is demarcated. It does not contain normal lip elements (eg, white roll, dry vermilion), but it is mucosalized. The normal dark red vermilion can be seen to transition into a lighter colored cleft vermilion.
- Spectrum of the cleft[3]
  - Minor form—1 to 2 cm in length ending medial to the anterior border of the masseter muscle
  - Major form—cleft ends lateral to the medial border of the masseter. It may terminate at the tragus or at the tonsillar pillar with disruption of superficial and deep structures.
- The commissure is blunted/effaced, and when a baby with macrostomia cries, the commissural angle of an open mouth is more oblique than the normally formed commissure—this is thought to be related to disruption of the normally intact orbicularis ring.
- Associated anomalies
  - Preauricular tags
  - Microtia/ear anomaly
  - Mandibular hypoplasia
  - Condylar abnormality
  - Zygomatic arch abnormality
  - Hearing loss

IMAGING

- 3D craniofacial CT—if bony involvement is suspected, this may be obtained to evaluate anatomy.

SURGICAL MANAGEMENT

- Trilaminar repair—repair of oral mucosal, orbicularis muscle, and facial skin
- Repair consists of
  - Excision of abnormal cleft margin tissue (mucosa)
  - Repair/repositioning of orbicularis muscle
  - Recreation of the oral commissure
  - Rearrangement of the cutaneous scar to avoid deforming contracture
- Repair types (external cutaneous scar):
  - Straight line
  - Z-plasty
  - W-plasty

Preoperative Planning

- Standard facial photos should be obtained preoperatively including repose and animated (smiling) if possible.
- Appropriate expectations should be created with the parents in terms of realistic commissure appearance and the risk of scar hypertrophy/contracture.

- Evaluation for other anomalies and comorbidities with specialist consultation or multidisciplinary team as necessary
- 3D CT scan if cleft is thought to involve skeletal structures
- Timing—as with cleft lip surgery, macrostomia repair may be done early in life. It is also reasonable to delay until late infancy if there is minimal functional or feeding issue. Late treatment reported in the literature is a function of later age at presentation and is usually not due to planned delay in treatment.

Positioning (FIG 2)

- Nasal endotracheal tube allows unobstructed/distorted view of the mouth during surgery.
- Many groups use oral RAE intubation and midline taping that does not alter the lower lip (tape mesentery on chin).

Approach

- Determination of commissure position is most critical.
  - This can be mirrored from the contralateral lip in unilateral cases.
  - In bilateral cases, there are several considerations:
    - The cleft demarcation can be fairly obvious—normally demarcates with clefted tissue.
    - The normal position of the commissure lies below a vertical line that is dropped from the medial limbus. This can be marked.
    - Normative measures have been proposed for this use. However, these measures are highly variable and are not suitable for individual patient use.

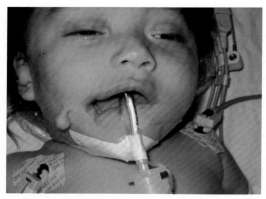

FIG 2 • Securing of the endotracheal tube in order to avoid lip and commissure distortion. Tegaderm is used to keep tape secure in a wet (Betadine) environment. (Note the commonly associated preauricular skin tags.)

■ Vermilion-Shifted Commissuroplasty With Optional Cutaneous Z-Plasty (Kaplan Technique)

- The senior author's (SPB) preferred technique for macrostomia repair was inspired by the work of Ernest Kaplan[4] and expanded upon by John Mulliken.[5]
- This repair uses mucosalized flaps to avoid scars directly within the commissure.

Markings

- Markings are performed using methylene blue ink and a pen point instrument.
- Important landmarks include the following:
    - Normal commissure (if present)
    - Peak of right and left Cupid's bow
    - Lower lip cutaneous midline
    - Vertical registration marks are also drawn above and below the normal and proposed commissures as reference (**TECH FIG 1**).
- In unilateral cases, the distance from the Cupid's bow peak to the normal commissure is reflected onto the cleft-side white roll of the upper lip.
    - The distance from the lower lip midline to the oral commissure is then reflected onto the white roll of the lower lip at the cleft commissure.
    - Because it is difficult to measure these distances around the curvature of the lip, it is often easier to create a vertical registration marking on the unaffected side and to then reflect that measurement to the affected side (see **TECH FIG 1**).

- In bilateral cases, the medial limbus is taken as the landmark for which to position the commissures upon repair.
    - Vertical registration lines are drawn down from the medial limbus.

Design (see **TECH FIG 2**)

- The commissure points are decided upon and tattooed with methylene blue at the upper and lower lip white roll.
- A vermilion flap is designed from either the upper or lower lip. The flap begins medial to the commissure (c') point on the chosen lip. It is rectangular in shape.
    - This flap will become the new mucosal commissure and importantly keep suture line outside of the commissure.
- The cutaneous margin of the cleft is marked—this tissue represents cleft/mucosal tissue that will be reflected initially into the mouth. Some tissue will be used for oral closure, and some will be discarded.
- On the lip (upper or lower) that will receive the vermilion flap, the incision at the cutaneous vermilion junction will also end medial to the commissure (c') point.
- The area of dissection is conservatively infiltrated with epinephrine-containing solution.

Dissection and Orbicularis Repair

- The markings are incised.
- The vermilion flap is incised and raised.
- The cleft mucosal tissue is freed and reflected intraorally with dissection to include the deep surface of the orbicularis muscles.

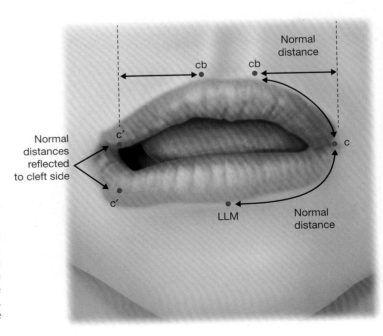

TECH FIG 1 • Landmarks for unilateral macrostomia repair: (c) normal commissure, (c') upper and lower lip cleft commissure, (cb) peak of Cupid's bow on each side of the upper lip, (LLM) lower lip midline. The distance from c to the ipsilateral cb and to *LLM* is measured. These measurements are then reflected to the macrostomic side. Vertical registration marks can allow for more accurate measurements and design.

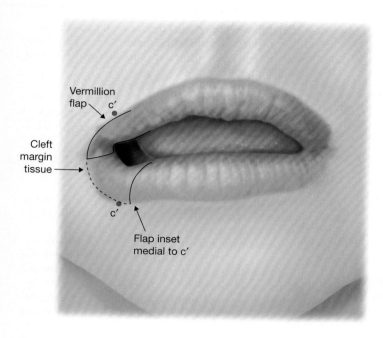

TECH FIG 2 • Repair design. A vermilion flap is designed that will bridge the new commissure in order to keep a scar line out of the repair. The cleft margin tissue shown with a *dotted line* is elevated and raised intraorally. The vermilion flap begins medial to the commissure point and will be inset medial to the commissure point on the recipient lip.

- The mal-positioned fibers of the orbicularis oris of the upper and lower lip are dissected free.
- The muscles are repaired in an overlapping fashion if enough muscle bulk exists for such a repair. Otherwise, they can be repaired end to end (**TECH FIG 3**).
- Repair is done with 3-0 or 4-0 Vicryl suture.

Commissuroplasty and Skin Closure

- The tattooed (c') points are united with a buried dermal suture.
- The vermilion flap is then inset with 4-0 chromic recreating the commissure.

- Excess mucosa intraorally may be trimmed, and intra-oral closure is completed with 4-0 chromic.
- Deep fascia is closed in the lateral skin wound.
- A small midincision Z-plasty is designed for transverse lengthening if needed.
- Skin closure is performed with buried deep dermal 5-0 Monocryl or with simple fast-absorbing gut sutures.
- Dermabond is used for the cutaneous incision with one Steri-Strip placed along the nasolabial fold.
- Franco et al. applied a similar concept, carrying the vermilion and orbicularis as a unit across the cleft to recreate the commissure (**TECH FIG 4**).[6]

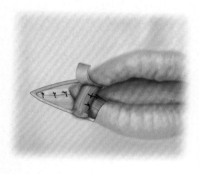

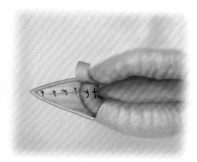

TECH FIG 3 • Orbicularis repair in macrostomia. **A.** Overlapping. **B.** end to end.

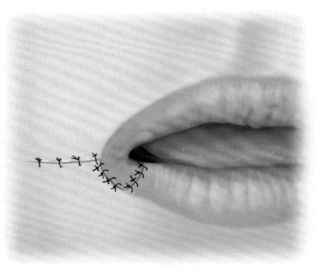
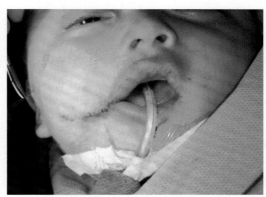

A   **B**

TECH FIG 4 • **A.** Vermilion flap inset after repair. **B.** Repaired macrostomia. The use of Z-plasty for cutaneous closure is an intraoperative decision.

■ Modifications of the Cutaneous Scar
(**TECH FIG 5**)

- Linear scar closure with no modification[7]
- Z-plasty closure along the nasolabial fold[4]

- W-plasty modification of the cutaneous scar for aggressive nonlinearization[8]

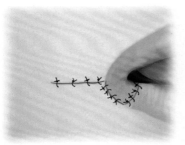
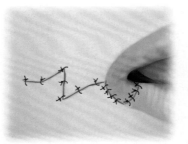
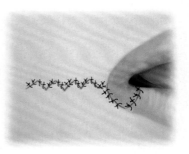

A   **B**   **C**

TECH FIG 5 • Cutaneous closure of macrostomia. **A.** Straight line. **B.** Z-plasty. **C.** W-plasty.

PEARLS AND PITFALLS

Endotracheal tube	■ If using an oral tube, the taping/securing must be closely guided by the surgeon. This ensures minimal commissure distortion and a secure tube throughout the case.
Local anesthesia	■ It is important to judiciously use epinephrine-containing local anesthetic. It helps keep the field relatively bloodless, but one must allow sufficient time for the effect to occur (ie, 5+ minutes). It is also important to not tumesce and thus distort the tissues.
Medial limbus	■ A critical landmark for commissure location in bilateral macrostomia cases.
Scar hypertrophy	■ Preoperative counseling, a proactive postoperative scar management program, and an established timeline for scar interventions are critical.
Lateralization and rounding	■ Many macrostomia repairs will result in lateral migration of the commissuroplasty and a nonanatomic commissure.

POSTOPERATIVE CARE

- For 3 to 4 weeks postoperatively, the scar is treated with massage and silicone gel.
- Hypertrophic scar may be treated with steroid injection at 3 to 6 months.
- Scar revision may be necessary 1 year or more postoperatively.

OUTCOMES

- Excellent, symmetric results can be achieved. Rogers and Mulliken (2007) reported on 13 patients[5]:
  - Age at surgery 11 months, follow-up 10.3 years
  - Commissure position averaged 1 mm difference
  - No lateral commissure migration

COMPLICATIONS

- Dehiscence
- Scar contracture with lateral commissure migration
- Scar hypertrophy

REFERENCES

1. Verheyden C. Anatomical considerations in the repair of macrostomia. *Ann Plast Surg.* 1988;20(4):374-380.
2. Woods R, Varma S, David D. Tessier no. 7 cleft: a new subclassification and management protocol. *Plast Reconstr Surg.* 2008;122(3):898-905.
3. Buonocore S, Broer P, Walker M. Macrostomia: a spectrum of deformity. *Ann Plast Surg.* 2014;72(3):363-368.
4. Kaplan EN. Commissuroplasty and myoplasty for macrostomia. *Ann Plast Surg.* 1981;7:136-144.
5. Rogers G, Mulliken J. Repair of transverse facial cleft in hemifacial microsomia: long-term anthropometric evaluation of commissural symmetry. *Plast Reconstr Surg.* 2007;120(3):728-737.
6. Franco D, Franco T, da Dilva Freitas R, et al. Commissuroplasty for macrostomia. *J Craniofac Surg.* 2007;18(3):691-694.
7. Kawai T, Kurita K, Echiverre N, et al. Modified technique in surgical correction of macrostomia. *Int J Oral Maxillofac Surg.* 1998;27(3):178-180.
8. Bauer BS, Wilkes G, Kernahan DA. Incorporation of the W-plasty in repair of macrostomia. *Plast Reconstr Surg.* 1982;70(6):752-757.

Tissue Expansion for Congenital Nevi

18

CHAPTER

Lee W. T. Alkureishi and Bruce S. Bauer

DEFINITION

- Congenital melanocytic nevi (CMN) are the most common congenital nevi.
- They are usually present at birth, but "tardive" CMN may arise within the first 2 years of life.
- CMN range from millimeter size to giant, covering the majority of the body.
- Implications include risk of melanoma, CNS involvement, and disfigurement.

PATHOGENESIS

- CMN result in a disturbance of neural crest cell migration between the 5th and 24th weeks of gestation, producing ectopic rests of immature melanocytes.[1]
- This is thought to be related to mutations in NRAS and, to a lesser extent, BRAF oncogenes.[2]
- Nevus cells can extend deep into the subcutaneous tissue, fascia, muscle, and/or periosteum (rare).
- Involvement of the leptomeninges or brain parenchyma is known as neurocutaneous melanosis (NCM).
- Histologic findings specific to CMN include cell clustering, a round shape, and location within eccrine ducts, in follicular epithelium or blood vessels, and in deeper tissues.

NATURAL HISTORY

Malignancy Risk

- Malignant melanoma may arise within the nevus or in extracutaneous locations, most commonly the CNS.
- Population heterogeneity, lack of standardized descriptors, and multiple treatment modalities lead to difficulty ascertaining the true melanoma risk in CMN.
- Earlier studies reported lifetime risk of up to 40%.
- More recent studies suggest much lower lifetime risk: less than 5% for all patients with large CMN and under 2% for smaller lesions.[3]
- Factors associated with increased melanoma risk include larger nevus size, truncal location, and multiple satellite lesions. The greatest risk may be extracutaneous.
- Risk of melanoma arising within a small CMN prior to puberty is extremely low.
- The same is not true for large (LCMN) and giant (GCMN) lesions; 50% of those developing malignancy do so within the first 3 years of life.[4]
- To date, there has not been a confirmed case of melanoma arising within a satellite lesion.
- Other tumors associated with CMN include lipomas, schwannomas, sarcomas, malignant cellular blue nevus, and undifferentiated spindle cell neoplasms.

- Reduction of the risk of melanoma is still viewed as a valid medical indication for excision.

NEUROCUTANEOUS MELANOSIS AND IMAGING

- The presence of nevus cells within the leptomeninges, brain, or spinal column is NCM.
- Symptoms can range from none to progressive, severe neurologic impairment, hydrocephalus, seizures, and death.
- Problems arise from either benign proliferation of nevus cells blocking cerebrospinal fluid flow or malignant degeneration.
- Exact incidence is unknown but thought to be around 5%.
  - Approximately 5% of these patients will be symptomatic, the vast majority developing symptoms before age 3.
- Prognosis of symptomatic NCM is poor, with over 90% dying within 3 years of diagnosis.
- The highest risk of NCM is thought to be in patients with LCMN of the posterior midline or greater than 20 satellite nevi. These patients should be strongly considered for MRI screening.[5]
- MRI demonstrates shortening of the T1 relaxation time and, less commonly, T2 relaxation time.
- For best sensitivity, MRI is recommended prior to 4 months of age due to the lack of myelinization in the newborn.
- In patients with symptomatic NCM, aggressive management of the cutaneous lesion needs to be decided on a case-by-case basis and is generally not recommended. This does not hold true for asymptomatic patients, in which the prognosis is more favorable.

DIFFERENTIAL DIAGNOSIS

- Blue nevus
- Mongolian spot
- Nevus of Ota/Ito
- Café au lait spot
- Nevus spilus
- Sebaceous nevus
- Spitz nevus

Classification

- Several classification schemes have been proposed, most of which use the projected adult size (PAS) of the nevus as the main feature.
- PAS is calculated by multiplying the largest diameter of the nevus in infancy by a factor that which varies by anatomical region (Table 1).
- Large CMN are considered as any nevus with a PAS of greater than 20 cm or greater than 2% of total body surface area.

Table 1 Projected Adult Size (PAS) of Congenital Nevi in Infancy (Data From Krengel et al., 2012)

Body Area	Projected Adult Size (PAS) Multiplication Factor
Head	1.7×
Neck, trunk, buttocks, arms	2.8×
Legs	3.3×

- The most inclusive classification system is that recently described by Krengel et al.[6] (Table 2).

Nevus Distribution

- CMN may arise anywhere on the body.
- Large and giant CMN often occur in recognizable patterns or distributions.
- Size and extent of involvement vary considerably between patients.
- Extensive nevi often involve multiple adjacent areas and/or cross the midline.
- Commonly encountered distributions include:
  - Scalp, forehead, root of nose, and upper eyelid
  - Face: cheek, nose, and lower eyelid
  - Trunk (posterior, anterior, or circumferential "bathing trunk" nevus)
  - Upper extremity (sleevelike distribution)
  - Lower extremity (as part of bathing trunk or isolated lower extremity)

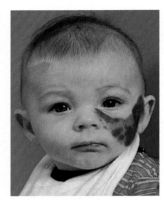

FIG 1 • Facial nevus, involving the unilateral cheek and abutting the lower eyelid.

- The surgical management of these patients is tailored to the location of nevus, extent of involvement, and presence of adjacent normal skin.
  - However, we describe common techniques and principles, many of which may be applicable for the management of nevi in any location.
- The example provided in this chapter focuses on a nevus involving the unilateral cheek and lower eyelid (**FIG 1**).

PATIENT HISTORY AND PHYSICAL FINDINGS

- Patients are often seen in infancy.
- Any changes in appearance of the lesion over time should be noted.

Table 2 Proposed New Classification of Congenital Melanocytic Nevi

CMN parameter	Terminology	Definition
CMN projected adult size	"Small CMN"	<1.5
	"Medium CMN"	1.5–10 cm
	"M1"	10–20 cm
	"M2"	>20–30 cm
	"Large CMN"	>30–40 cm
	"L1"	>40–60 cm
	"L2"	>60 cm
	"Giant CMN"	≥3 medium CMN *without a single, predominant CMN*
	"G1"	
	"G2"	
	"Multiple medium CMN"	
CMN localization[a]	"Face," "scalp"	No satellites
CMN of the head	"Neck," "shoulder," "upper back," "middle	50 satellites
CMN of the trunk	back," "lower back," "breast/chest," "abdomen,"	20–50 satellites
CMN of the extremities	"flank," "gluteal region," "genital region"	None, moderate, marked **c**olor heterogeneity
No. of satellite nevi[b]	"Upper arm," "forearm," "hand," "thigh," "lower	None, moderate, marked surface **r**ugosity
Additional morphologic characteristics	leg," "foot"	None, scattered, extensive dermal or subcutaneous **n**odules
	"S0"	None, notable, marked hypertrichosis ("**h**airiness")
	"S1"	
	"S2"	
	"S3"	
	"C0," "C1," "C2"	
	"R0," "R1," "R2"	
	"N0," "N1," "N2"	
	"H0," "H1," "H2"	

[a]One or more of these locations should be used to describe *preponderant* area of involvement.
[b]Refers to number of satellites within the first year of life; in case this number is not available, actual number should be mentioned.
CMN, Congenital melanocytic nevi.
Reprinted from Krengel S, Scope A, Dusza SW, et al. New recommendations for the categorization of cutaneous features of congenital melanocytic nevi. *J Am Acad Dermatol.* 2013;68(3):441-451, with permission from Elsevier.

- Nevus size and location and the presence of multiple satellite nevi should prompt screening for NCM.
- A family history of melanoma should be elicited.
- Potential psychological problems associated with this diagnosis should not be underestimated, especially in older children and adolescents.
  - Emotional, behavioral, or social problems are present in 30%.
- On initial examination, the extent of the nevus should be noted, including involvement of critical structures and any areas of adjacent normal skin for treatment planning.
- Serial examinations every 3 to 6 months are recommended.
- Darker pigmented areas or raised nodules may represent neural nevus rather than malignancy.
- Selective biopsy can be used to exclude malignancy for any suspicious areas but is rarely indicated if excision and reconstruction are already contemplated.

NONOPERATIVE MANAGEMENT

- Treatment of CMN is most often surgical, with excision and reconstruction. Other modalities include dermabrasion, curettage, and laser therapy. Some cases are best approached with observation alone.
- Some giant nevi are so extensive as to preclude excision, and regular follow-up by a pediatric dermatologist is recommended.
- Although many LCMN are amenable to surgical excision and reconstruction, the surgical experience needed for successful surgical management is not readily available in many areas of the world.

Dermabrasion and Curettage

- Dermabrasion and curettage are used to reduce, but not eliminate, the number of nevus cells within a lesion.
  - Dermabrasion is used to abrade away the surface cells within the epidermis and upper reticular dermis.
  - Curettage separates the cells at a natural cleavage plane between superficial and deep dermis.
- Both techniques are best performed within the first 15 days of life.
- Lightening of the nevus can be successful initially, but this is variable and the lesion may tend to redarken over time. Follow-up may also show marked hypertrichosis.[7]
- These techniques are theoretically less effective at reducing malignancy risk, due to persistence of nevus cells at deeper levels. Resultant scarring may also complicate surveillance of the lesion. Cases have been reported of melanoma arising within the field of previous dermabrasion.[8]

Laser

- Laser remains an attractive option, potentially reducing the level of pigmentation without scarring.
- Lasers used in the treatment of CMN include ruby, Q-switched, Er:YAG, and carbon dioxide, either alone or in combination with Nd:YAG or Q-switched ruby lasers.
- Serial treatments are required, and scarring can occur with aggressive treatment or improper settings.
- Hypo- and hyperpigmentation may also occur and may be transient or permanent.
- The disadvantages of laser treatment are similar to those of dermabrasion/curettage and include continued malignancy risk, scarring, difficulties with surveillance, and redarkening of the lesion over time.

- Despite their current limitations, nonoperative modalities do offer some benefits in certain situations.
  - For example, lightening a thin lesion on the eyelid
- Improvements in laser technology will likely continue to improve outcomes with this modality, expanding its usefulness in the future.

SURGICAL MANAGEMENT

- Surgical excision allows complete removal of nevus cells in the involved skin and subcutaneous tissue.
- Excision generally includes all tissue above the level of the deep fascia.
- Although skin grafts have been used for resurfacing, the mainstay of reconstruction is with tissue expansion.
  - Replacement of the excised tissue with similar thickness normal tissue (skin and subcutaneous fat) provides the most functional and aesthetic outcome.
- Early excision is recommended.
- Procedures can be safely carried out starting as early as 6 months of age.
- Those parents with concerns about multiple procedures under the age of 1 can delay initial surgery until after the first birthday (though in expander patients started at 6 months, the maximum additional surgeries under 1 year are only two).

FIRST STAGE: PLACEMENT OF TISSUE EXPANDER(S)

Preoperative Planning

- Treatment begins with the evaluation of the nevus extent and adjacent areas of unaffected skin amenable to placement of tissue expander(s).
- For lesions affecting the cheek and lower eyelid, a single expander placed in the lower cheek/neck is often appropriate.[9]
  - The size of expander chosen is dependent on the size of lesion, availability of adjacent unaffected tissue, and anticipated size of flap required.
  - For many infants, a 70- to 90-cc expander is the largest that can be placed.
  - With adequate expansion, the resultant flap can be designed to place incisions to lie less conspicuously at the junction of adjacent aesthetic subunits.
- For more extensive nevi involving the temporal forehead, scalp, or upper eyelid, an additional expander may be required in the forehead region.
- For nevus involving large portions of the nose, an expanded forehead flap based on the supraorbital or supratrochlear artery is the best option and must be done as the first expansion.
- The expanded forehead flap places the final scar along the brow rather than midforehead.
- For extensive forehead and nasal lesions, subsequent expansion and flaps can be safely done without risk to the prior nasal flap.
- Prior to surgery, the family undergoes extensive teaching regarding the procedures, postoperative care, technique of tissue expansion, and anticipated timing of the next stage.
- In the majority of cases requiring multiple rounds of expansion, each round is separated by at least 4 months.

Positioning

- The patient is placed supine on the operating table.
- A roll is placed under the upper back and shoulders, ensuring adequate neck extension.
  - This is especially important, as it is frequently necessary to dissect the pocket for the expander past the level of the mandible and into the neck.
- General anesthesia is administered via an oral RAE endotracheal tube.
  - Care is taken to ensure this is secured exactly in the midline, avoiding asymmetric distortion of the facial anatomy.
- If the nevus is hypertrichotic, a clipper is used to ensure the margins are clearly visible for incision planning.
- The face, scalp, neck, and shoulders are cleaned with surgical soap and saline, and drapes are applied.

Approach

- Considerations in planning the incision:

- The length of the incision should be adequate to facilitate dissection of the pocket and insertion of the expander, but no longer than necessary.
- The incision is generally placed within the nevus, at the inferior margin. By staying within the nevus, all healthy uninvolved skin is preserved.
  - In selected cases with a narrow inferior "finger" of nevus flanked by adjacent normal skin, it may be preferable to place the incision farther into the substance of the nevus. Although this will result in the nevus being partially expanded, it achieves maximal expansion of the normal skin.
- In patients with fine hairs along the border of the nevus, it may be preferable to place the incision just beyond the margin of the nevus, as those hairs may complicate cleaning the incision and increase the likelihood of secondary infection.
- The dimensions of the pocket for the expander are measured and marked on the skin.
  - The pocket measures 1 cm greater than the expander in both dimensions.

TECHNIQUES

- The incision line is infiltrated with lidocaine 1% and epinephrine 1:200 000.
- Incision is made with a 15c blade and deepened to the level of the subcutaneous fat.
  - Care is taken to stay perpendicular, avoiding unnecessary undermining of the nevus.
- With Iris scissors, the supra-SMAS plane is carefully developed under direct vision.
- Once the plane is established, the skin flap may be laid flat, and the majority of the remaining pocket can be dissected using the scissors without direct visualization.
  - The scissor blades can be seen on the surface of the skin, and the depth of the dissection can be accurately gauged by paying close attention to the tips.
  - This approach helps to minimize trauma to the thin skin flap.
- Particular care must be taken in the region just anterior to the mandibular angle, where the marginal mandibular nerve may be encountered. In addition, the facial artery and vein can potentially cause troublesome bleeding in this region. The depth of dissection is critical in this region, to avoid injury to the nerve below while maintaining a robust skin flap of sufficient thickness above. Of note is that the marginal mandibular nerve lies deep to the platysma, and if dissection remains superficial to the SMAS plane, the marginal mandibular nerve is spared.
- The dissection is carried over the mandible into the neck, to the extent of the pocket previously marked.
- The pocket is packed lightly with gauze for hemostasis, and attention is then turned to the expander.
- The location for the expander port is chosen and the length of tubing adjusted as needed.
  - A remote internal port is used in all cases.
  - The port should be placed over firm underlying structures to facilitate palpation.
  - The port should be placed through a limited tunnel to minimize risk of displacement or flipping.

- For lower face expanders, the temporal scalp is a typical location for the port.
- A narrow tunnel for the port is created using scissor dissection, a malleable retractor of similar width to the port, a urethral sound, or a combination of all.
  - The width of the tunnel should be limited to the diameter of the port, to prevent migration of the expander along the tunnel.
- A narrow gauge suction drain is placed into the expander pocket through a separate stab incision (19-G butterfly IV, reconfigured as a drain).
- The expander is filled with a volume of injectable saline dependent on size and location of the expander, filling enough to ensure a smooth contour.
- The port is generally inserted into the pocket first and guided into position with finger pressure or using a malleable retractor.
- The expander is rolled lengthwise, forming a thin tube with the edges rolled underneath, which is then easily inserted into the pocket.
  - Once the majority of the expander is within the pocket, it can be unfurled to lie flat.
  - Care should be taken to ensure that there are no folds present on the top surface of the expander, particularly in the face where the overlying skin flap can be very thin.
- The skin is closed in layers with interrupted 5-0 clear nylon for the dermal layer and a running 5-0 Prolene over this.
- The expander port is then accessed, and an additional small volume of saline may be injected.
  - The skin is observed and palpated during injection, to avoid overfilling.
  - In general, a total of approximately 15 cc is well tolerated at this stage.
- The site is cleaned and dressed with bacitracin, Xeroform gauze, gauze fluffs, and a loose SurgiNet dressing.
  - A tight dressing should be avoided over the expander, as this can easily compromise the skin flap.

PEARLS AND PITFALLS

Physical findings	▪ The appearance of CMN is widely variable, ranging from relatively inconspicuous flat, pale hairless nevi to dark or variably pigmented, highly rugous/nodular nevi with hypertrichosis.
Technique	▪ The use of Bovie electrocautery is limited, so as not to cause thermal injury in the dissection of thin, potentially tenuous skin flaps for the expander pocket. ▪ A 19-gauge "butterfly needle" makes for an excellent drain. The end of the tubing is perforated and placed into the pocket through a separate stab incision. Standard blood draw vacutainers can be used to provide suction. ▪ Avoiding folds and points on the superficial surface of the expander is key to minimizing the risk of skin breakdown and subsequent exposure of the expander.
Postoperative	▪ The key to successful expansion is to pay close attention to the skin's response to the fill. Aiming for a specified volume with each expansion will inevitably lead to problems. ▪ The first postplacement expander fill is typically 8–10 days postoperatively, and expansion then continues weekly. This can increase to q4-5 days in select cases if the overlying skin relaxes sufficiently.

POSTOPERATIVE CARE

- Patients can generally go home on the day of surgery, depending on parent comfort.
- Dressings are changed twice daily, keeping the incision and skin flap moisturized with Aquaphor or similar dressing.
- Drains are usually removed within 3 to 7 days, after which the dressing may be minimal.
  - Postoperative antibiotics are continued until the drains are removed.
- Expansion is begun at days 8 to 10.
  - The first expansion is performed under supervision in the clinic.
  - Subsequent expansions may be carried out at home or in the clinic depending on parents' preference.
- Parents are advised not to focus on a target volume for each fill but to assess the skin's response to the additional volume.
  - Skin turgor
  - Blanching indicates excessive fill, and some volume should be removed.
  - Expansion should not be painful; discomfort indicates excessive fill.
- Expansion is usually carried out weekly, unless the child has symptoms of upper respiratory infection or fever of unknown origin.
  - The frequency may be increased to q4-5 days in some cases.
- Total expansion time may range from 8 to 12 weeks.
  - Expansion may continue up until a few days before surgery (**FIG 2**).

SECOND STAGE: EXCISION OF NEVUS WITH EXPANDED FLAP RECONSTRUCTION

Preoperative Planning

- The planning of the second stage procedure begins prior to the first stage.
  - Position of the expander should take into account the anticipated flap design.
  - When advancing tissue from the neck to the cheek area, a transposition design is optimal.
  - This allows greater flap movement and helps align scars optimally along the junction between aesthetic subunits.
- The surgeon must decide whether to base the transposition flap laterally (most common) or medially.
  - The size and location of the lesion help to determine this.
  - Where early experience involved use of medially based flaps, the inferolaterally based flaps used today allow better reconstruction of the aesthetic unit with less risk of downward traction on the lower eyelid.
  - Smaller lateral based cheek lesions may be reconstructed with expanded inferomedially based flaps.
  - Even with expansion, the size of nevus that can be excised laterally without undue traction on the eyelid or oral commissure is limited.

Positioning

- Positioning, prepping, and draping are the same as for stage I.

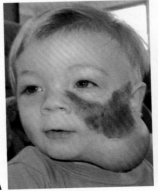 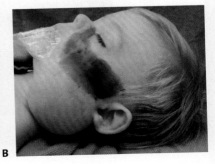

FIG 2 • **A.** Fully expanded lower cheek/neck tissue expander **(B)** ready for nevus excision and expanded flap reconstruction.

Approach

- The initial incision is planned to facilitate removal of the expander.
- The incision is marked around the inferior extent of the nevus, as before, but outside the nevus margin (**FIG 3**).
  - If the nevus margins are very light or indistinct, it is better to err on the side of preserving potentially uninvolved skin. Any areas that subsequently darken may be removed at the time of later scar revision or satellite removal.
  - In cases where the nevus margin is clear, a surgical margin of 1 to 2 mm is adequate.
  - Similarly, if only partial excision is planned/possible, then it is often better to keep as much of the scars within nevus tissue that will later be excised. In these cases, placing the incision within the nevus margin is advisable.

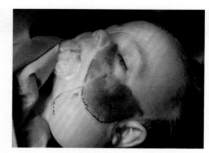

FIG 3 • Marking the incision for expander removal. The extent of the inferior extension of the incision is determined after expander removal.

- For laterally based flaps, the incision is often carried inferiorly in the line of the nasolabial fold, to facilitate flap transposition. However, the extent of this inferior incision is determined later, after expander removal.

■ Incision

- Incision is made with a 15c blade through the skin and deepened through the subcutaneous fat with electrocautery to the level of the expander capsule.
- The expander pocket is entered through the capsule.
  - The capsule is extremely important for the vascular supply of the flap. As such, it is important not to undercut the flap at this stage, as excessive removal of capsule can jeopardize the vascularity of the flap's extremes.
- The incision and deeper dissection are continued inferiorly for a short distance in the line of the nasolabial fold and marionette line, and once a large enough window has been created, the expander is removed.
  - The tubing connecting the expander to its port is cut, and the port is left in situ for now. Removal is often easier later in the procedure.
- The expander pocket is now fully accessible. The skin flap can be placed under moderate tension in the direction of the planned transposition, and limited release of the

capsule with electrocautery facilitates greater transposition without creating undue tension on the closure (**TECH FIG 1A**).
  - Care must be taken not to perform too much capsular release, as the importance of its vascular contribution cannot be overemphasized.
  - The extent of the dissection is a delicate balance between facilitating movement and preserving the viability of the flap.
- With the capsule is released, the skin becomes the limiting factor in achieving the desired transposition.
  - Options for skin release include extending the incision further down the nasolabial fold/melomental fold, backcutting into the flap, or both (**TECH FIG 1B**).
  - The type of extended incision or backcuts used is dependent on the extent and location of the nevus and the extent and location of uninvolved adjacent skin.
- Small triangles of uninvolved skin adjacent to the flap margins can often be used to fill in the defects created by backcuts.

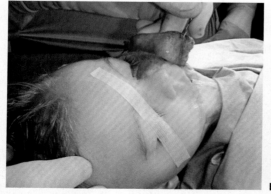
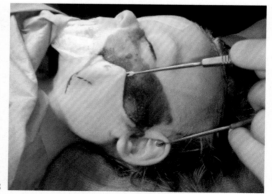

TECH FIG 1 • **A.** Limited release of the capsule with the skin flap on tension allows greater transposition of the flap without undue tension. However, the extent of release must be balanced with preserving as much vascular supply as possible. **B.** Options for skin release include extending the incision further down the nasolabial/melomental fold, backcutting into the flap, or both.

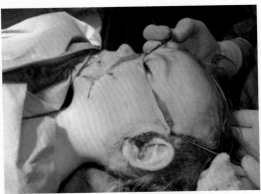

TECH FIG 1 (Continued) • **C.** The transposed flap, which covers the entire cheek at this stage.

- These small areas would otherwise be discarded, as they are covered by the transposed/advanced flap.
- Their interposition serves to allow a greater backcut, relieving tension and affording greater movement.
- Careful design of these small flaps can also break up the linear scar and/or place portions of the incision in the relaxed skin tension lines.
- The flap is again placed on moderate tension, and the extent of transposition is evaluated. At this point, the flap will often cover the entire cheek to the level of the lid crease, nose-cheek junction, and nasolabial fold (**TECH FIG 1C**).

- It can be helpful to temporarily tack the flap in place under moderate tension, allowing the areas of tension to be fully assessed.
- Further movement of the flap may be needed in the following situations:
  - Nevus involvement of the root of the nose or nasal sidewall
  - Nevus involvement of the upper lip
- In these cases, the inferior and medial-most extent of the flap can reliably reach these extremes. The additional backcuts into the flap should be designed to allow this.
- For all backcuts and incisions within the substance of the expanded flap, care should be taken to include sufficient capsule with the smaller or more tenuous of the created flaps. This helps to maximize vascular supply within the flap, particularly the venous drainage.
  - This may require beveling of the incisions in some cases, capturing more of the subcutaneous tissue and particularly the capsule.
- Upon flap transposition, a dog-ear of excess tissue will be apparent in the temporal region.
  - This is excised above the level of the lateral canthus, allowing secure flap fixation high enough to prevent the development of ectropion due to flap descent.
  - At this stage, the port for the expander is close to the level of dissection, and removal is relatively easy.

■ Excision

- Once the flap release is completed, the extent of nevus excision can be decided.
  - The defect created by excision should allow reconstruction without excessive tension on the flap.
  - In general, the superior extent of excision should be the lower eyelid-cheek junction. When the nevus also involves the lower eyelid, the very thin eyelid skin is best reconstructed with a full-thickness skin graft at a later stage.
  - The excision of nevus in this area should be delayed until the cheek flap is fully secured both medially and laterally.
  - If possible, the triangle of skin immediately lateral to the alar-cheek junction should be preserved if not involved by nevus.
    - This allows the scar in the nasolabial groove to terminate at the nose-cheek junction rather than the alar base.
- The nevus is excised at the level of the superficial musculoaponeurotic system (SMAS), and hemostasis is achieved with bipolar cautery (**TECH FIG 2**).

- This can be performed in stages, securing the flap to the deeper tissues at several points as the dissection progresses superiorly.
- This allows the most accurate determination of the flap's reach, ensuring that the distal portion of the flap is not placed under excessive tension due to overly aggressive nevus excision.

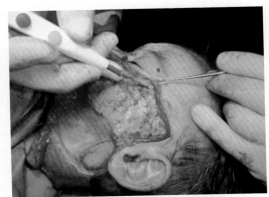

TECH FIG 2 • The nevus is excised at the level of the superficial musculoaponeurotic system (SMAS).

■ Suturing

- Deep sutures can be used to serve dual purposes.
  - Suturing the deeper tissue of the flap to the underlying periosteum with clear nylon can help prevent later downward migration of the flap.
  - Suturing the more superficial tissue of the flap to deeper tissues can help recreate anatomical grooves or folds (eg, at the alar base–cheek junction). At this site, through-and-through sutures into the nasal cavity are often used. Based on the requirements of the specific case, the flap can be anchored to the periosteum along the pyriform. On the flap side, the depth of the suture is dependent on how much of a groove is desired. Placing the suture higher (eg, grabbing part of the dermis) will create a deeper groove. The flap may also be anchored through and through into the nasal cavity at the level of the alar-cheek junction, using an absorbable suture.
- Key sites for deep suture fixation of the transposed flap:
  - Lateral orbital rim
  - Medial orbital rim
  - Nose-cheek junction
  - Alar base–cheek junction
- The remainder of the flap is inset with deep dermal sutures.
  - 5-0 clear nylon is used in areas with sufficient flap thickness.
  - 5-0 Monocryl (Ethicon, Inc., Somerville, NJ) is used in areas of thinner overlying tissue.
- It is of utmost importance to include the expander capsule along the entire border of the flap in the closure of the deep layer and in the placement of dermal sutures.
  - This ensures that the capsule is "unfolded," maximizing the venous return. Folds or wrinkles in the capsule

due to incomplete or incorrect inset can significantly affect the viability of the flap.
  - The flap may often appear congested until the capsule is fully unfolded.
- The final excision and inset along the nasolabial groove and melomental fold are not carried out until the above flap inset is near complete in order to avoid traction on the upper lip and commissure where final nevus excision will be required, leaving the lip intentionally "long" and the commissure pushed medially. This allows final excision to achieve symmetry.
  - With scar contraction, there is a tendency for the ipsilateral nostril to be pulled downward and the lip to be pulled upward.
  - The inset of the flap is designed to compensate for this, with the nostril slightly higher and the lip lower compared with the contralateral side (**TECH FIG 3**).

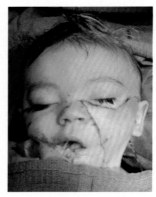

TECH FIG 3 • Flap inset is designed to compensate for subsequent scar contraction, with the ipsilateral nostril slightly higher and the lip lower than the contralateral side.

■ Closure

- A single butterfly drain is placed through a separate stab incision and secured as before.

- Skin closure is with running 6-0 chromic and 7-0 Vicryl (Ethicon, Inc., Somerville, NJ) sutures (**TECH FIG 4**).

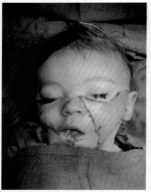 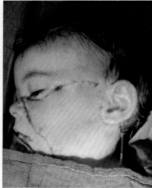 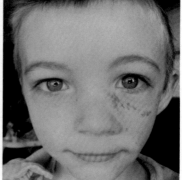

A   B   C

TECH FIG 4 • The completed reconstruction. **A,B.** On-table. **C.** Mature postoperative result, prior to excision of the small areas of residual nevus.

PEARLS AND PITFALLS

Technique	■ Transposition of the flap should be completed before completely excising the lesion, ensuring adequate flap coverage.
	■ The lower cheek/neck expanded flap can reach as far as the root of the nose or upper lip when needed.
	■ Deep suture fixation at several points is key to preventing downward migration of the flap and resultant ectropion.
	■ Through-and-through sutures at the alar base–cheek junction can help recreate the natural groove in this area.
	■ The thin skin of the lower eyelid cannot be satisfactorily reconstructed with a cheek flap and is best addressed with full-thickness skin graft at a subsequent procedure.
Postoperative	■ Postoperative care is essentially the same as for the first stage.

POSTOPERATIVE CARE

■ The face is cleaned and dressed with bacitracin, Vaseline gauze, gauze fluffs, and a loose SurgiNet dressing.
   ■ Ophthalmic bacitracin should be used around the eye.
■ Patients may go home on the day of surgery, depending on parent comfort.
■ Postoperative regimen is unchanged from the first stage.

OUTCOMES

■ In the authors' hands, expanded flap reconstruction with a laterally based lower face/neck flap provides the most pleasing results for this type of lesion.
   ■ The quality and thickness of the expanded flap match that of the uninvolved skin.
   ■ The contour of the lower cheek and neck is superior to that achieved with a medially based flap.
   ■ Deep suture fixation is effective in preventing later ectropion with vertical descent of the flap tissue.
■ For nevi involving the lower eyelid, a further stage is generally required.
   ■ This allows time for the flap to settle into its final position and any small adjustments to be made.
     • Medial or lateral canthopexy can be utilized to address any scar contraction or minor flap descent.
     • If further deep fixation is required at the lateral orbital rim, a permanent suture can be placed through a drill hole in the bone of the orbital rim.
   ■ The eyelid nevus is then excised and reconstructed with a full-thickness skin graft.
■ When excision of nevus involves expanded flap reconstruction of the forehead and scalp as well as neck, the reconstruction should be sequenced to address the scalp, forehead, and cheek; the cheek should be reconstructed last.
   ■ The cheek excision and reconstruction can commence once the forehead flap is inset in final position. Skin closure may be performed at the same time.

COMPLICATIONS

■ Infection during expansion can occur and is more common in the neck compared with other sites in the head and neck.
   ■ Infection can usually be managed with antibiotics, occasionally for the remainder of the expansion process.
   ■ Severe infection requiring removal of the expander is rare.[10]
■ Extrusion of the expander is rare.
   ■ Maintaining a flap of sufficient thickness minimizes this risk.
   ■ In older children where a 250-cc expander may be used, the most important part of expander placement is ensuring that the dissected pocket is large enough for the expander to be placed with minimal folds or irregular points.
■ The main complication of the second stage is vascular compromise of the expanded flap.
   ■ The increased vascularity afforded by expansion lowers this risk.
   ■ Flap compromise is always partial; total flap compromise does not occur.
   ■ Partial flap necrosis is generally limited to the distal aspect of the flap.
   ■ Sloughing is most often partial thickness and manageable with local wound care.
■ Infection is very rare following removal of the expander.
■ With placement of scars along the junctions of aesthetic subunits, the mature scar is very good in most cases. However, problems with hypertrophic or widened scars can occur and may require scar revision. This can often be combined with other planned procedures (eg, excision of satellite nevi).
■ When there is some extension of the nevus medial and inferior to the nasolabial fold, leaving that final excision until the scars have settled allows more precise final closure and may avoid the need for later scar revision.

REFERENCES

1. Cramer SF. The melanocytic differentiation pathway in congenital melanocytic nevi: theoretical considerations. *Pediatr Pathol.* 1988;8:253-265.
2. Roh MR, Eliades P, Gupta S, Tsao H. Genetics of melanocytic nevi. *Pigment Cell Melanoma Res.* 2015;28(6):661-672.
3. Krengel S, Hauschild A, Schaefer T. Melanoma risk in congenital melanocytic nevi: a systematic review. *Br J Dermatol.* 2006;155:1-8.
4. Marghoob AA, Schoenbach SP, Kopf AW, et al. Large congenital melanocytic nevi and the risk for the development of malignant melanoma. A prospective study. *Arch Dermatol.* 1996;132:170-175.
5. Marghoob AA, Dusza S, Oliviera S, Halpern AC. Number of satellite nevi as a correlate for neurocutaneous melanocytosis in patients with large congenital melanocytic nevi. *Arch Dermatol.* 2004;140:171-175.
6. Krengel S, Scope A, Dusza SW, et al. New recommendations for the categorization of cutaneous features of congenital melanocytic nevi. *J Am Acad Dermatol.* 2013;68(3):441-451.
7. Magalon G, Casanova D, Bardot J, Andrac-Meyer L. Early curettage of giant congenital naevi in children. *Br J Dermatol.* 1998;138:341-345.
8. Zutt M, Kretschmer L, Emmert S, et al. Multicentric malignant melanoma in a giant melanocytic congenital nevus 20 years after dermabrasion in adulthood. *Dermatol Surg.* 2003;29(1):99-101.
9. Bauer BS, Vicari FA. An approach to excision of congenital giant pigmented nevi in infancy and early childhood. *J Pediatr Surg.* 1988;23(6):509-514.
10. Adler N, Dorafshar AH, Bauer BS, et al. Tissue expander infections in pediatric patients: management and outcomes. *Plast Reconstr Surg.* 2009;124(2):484-489.

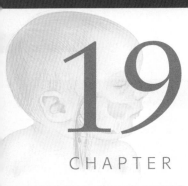

19
CHAPTER

Surgical Treatment of Congenital Midline Nasal Mass

Patrick A. Gerety and Scott P. Bartlett

DEFINITION

- Congenital midline nasal masses are a rare occurrence but require a thorough workup for an intracranial component, which then necessitates a transcranial resection.
- These masses typically represent one of three diagnoses: dermoid cyst, encephalocele, or glioma.
  - A nasal dermoid sinus cyst (NDSC) is lined by stratified squamous epithelium and contains dermal adnexal structures such as hair follicles and sebaceous glands. The cystic contents are sebum. If the mass has a punctum with drainage to the outside world, it is a dermoid sinus; otherwise, it is a dermoid cyst.
  - A nasal encephalocele is an extracranial protrusion of a cerebrospinal fluid (CSF)-containing dural mass. Twenty-five percent of all encephaloceles are in the nasofrontal region (sincipital). If brain matter is within the mass, this is referred to as meningoencephalocele.
  - A nasal glioma represents extracranial brain matter with no patent CSF connection.
- Intracranial extension—extension of midline nasal masses from extracranial nasal location to the anterior cranial fossa
- Transcranial approach—a combined extracranial and intracranial resection with reconstruction

ANATOMY

- Formation of a midline nasal mass results from disruption of early embryologic processes. The exact theory of embryology responsible for the formation of transcranial nasal masses remains debated.[1] Several operating theories lend rationale to the occurrence and anatomy of these masses. Some of these theories include the prenasal space theory, the nonseparation theory, and the ectodermal inclusion theory.
- Transcranial nasal congenital masses are believed to exist for two important reasons (**FIG 1**):
  - Failure of normal regression of a transcranial embryologic structure (dural diverticulum)
  - Embryologic contact of surface and neural ectoderm
- Per one theory, a dural diverticulum from the anterior cranial fossa normally exits the cranium via the nasofrontal junction (the fonticulus (naso) frontalis) and ends between the nasal bones and nasal soft tissues.
  - This diverticulum normally involutes and can be identified as the foramen cecum. This foramen has no contents typically but may contain a fibrous stalk.
  - If this process is disrupted, a persistent transcranial connection may be present at birth.
  - Importantly, the neural ectoderm of this diverticulum makes contact with the surface ectoderm of nasal skin.

Normally, this connection also regresses. If it does not, it may pull skin elements beneath the nasal skin resulting in an NDSC.
- The transcranial connection may occur at a number of anterior cranial fossa midline structures: cribriform plate, crista galli, foramen cecum, nasofrontal junction, or any combination of these.
- Anterior cranial encephaloceles can also occur via the nasofrontal, nasoethmoidal, or naso-orbital bony junctions.

PATHOGENESIS

- The etiologic basis of this occurrence is likely multifactorial with a genetic component. Family history and multiple siblings have been identified with these masses. Midline nasal masses are not related to any known syndromes or other known congenital anomalies.
- Conceptually and for disease categorization, these masses particularly the encephalocele are related to the embryologic failure of anterior neuropore (normally embryologic day 24) during early embryologic development.

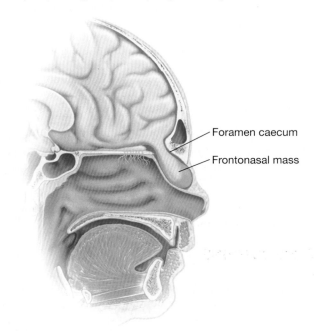

Foramen caecum

Frontonasal mass

FIG 1 • Embryologic origin of congenital frontonasal masses. Early embryologic connection between the nasal space and the intracranial space may lead to the presence of the congenital nasal mass. The existence of NDSC may be related to neural and surface ectoderm, which as the diverticulum regresses may draw skin contents into a subcutaneous position and in some case maintain a transcranial connection.

- A cranial defect must be present for either of the three main masses to be seen nasally and transmitted transcranially.
- Dermoid cysts likely result from trapping of skin structures subcutaneously as the dural diverticulum involutes normally.
- Encephalocele represents a neural tube defect. Terminology varies depending upon what the extracranial mass contains.
  - Meningocele—meninges only
  - Meningoencephalocele—meninges and brain matter
- Encephalocele and glioma represent neuroectodermal malformations.
- Dermoid cysts and sinuses represent a somatic (surface) ectodermal malformation.
- Intranasal gliomas and encephaloceles likely have a herniation point in the anterior cranial fossa that is more posterior (ie, posterior to the cribriform plate) as compared to masses that are seen on the nasal dorsum.

NATURAL HISTORY

- Congenital midline nasal masses are rare with an approximate incidence of 1 in 30 000 live births.
- These masses, particularly encephaloceles, occur in higher rates in Asia (Western incidence, 1 in 35 000; Asian incidence, 1 in 5000).
- NDSC—midline nasal cysts represent 3% to 12% of head and neck dermoid cysts.[2]
  - Intracranial extension of midline nasal dermoids has been found to be common among these masses on the order of 25% to 45% of cases.
- Encephalocele—approximately 80% are occipital and 20% frontonasal (sincipital).[3]
- Glioma
  - Approximately 15% have a transcranial connection; thus, nasal resection without intracranial exclusion can lead to CSF leak and meningitis.
  - 3:1 male predominance[4]
  - Sixty percent are extranasal, 30% are intranasal, and 10% are mixed.
- There is a reported association with other nonspecific congenital abnormalities (often quoted as approximately 40%). However, several series have not shown the same association. A transcranial midline nasal mass may occur in isolation.
- Risk of meningitis—with good soft tissue coverage and no sinus punctum, patients are likely at low risk of developing a meningeal infection even in the presence of intracranial CSF connection.

PATIENT HISTORY AND PHYSICAL FINDINGS

- Visible and palpable midline nasal mass (**FIG 2**)
- May occur from the columella to the radix but most commonly along the nasal dorsum
- Wide nasal bridge
- Hypertelorism—this may be true hypertelorism with total orbital widening or more commonly in this case interorbital hypertelorism with widening of only the medial orbital wall.
  - May be present in 70% of encephalocele patients
  - Normal interorbital distance increases from approximately 18 mm in infancy to 25 to 30 mm in adulthood.

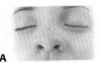

FIG 2 • Physical appearance of congenital midline nasal mass. **A.** Dermoid sinus with pathognomonic hairs from punctum. NDSC may also present as subcutaneous firm mass with no punctum. **B.** Nasal glioma with pathognomonic telangiectasia. This may be indistinguishable from a nasal dermoid without a dermal sinus. **C.** Nasal encephalocele with bluish hue, large size, hypertelorism, and positive fluid wave on exam.

- NDSC are firm, round masses.
  - NDSC may present with a punctum. The punctum may contain hair, which is a pathognomonic sign of the diagnosis.
  - If a punctum is present, patients are more likely to present with infection.
- Gliomas are firm, round masses.
  - Surface telangiectasia is present and this is pathognomonic.
  - May be extranasal, intranasal, or both
  - Does not transilluminate or change in size
  - Intranasal glioma may cause nasal airway obstruction or nasolacrimal dysfunction. Airway obstruction is particularly problematic in neonates/infants who are obligate nasal breathers.
- Encephalocele may occur through one of three sutures (junctions): nasofrontal, nasoethmoidal, and naso-orbital.
  - Often appear blue in color
  - Transillumination is pathognomonic because of CSF content.
  - Size change with crying may occur (Valsalva).
  - Size change may also be elicited by compression of the internal jugular veins (Furstenberg sign).
  - Patients may present with CSF leak or frank meningitis.
- The cranial exit point has been found to be fairly variable and may occur at the nasofrontal suture but also through other cranial bone junction points.
  - This can be difficult to differentiate on physical examination.

IMAGING

- Because of the occurrence of transcranial extension, there should be a low threshold for obtaining cross-sectional imaging of congenital midline nasal masses.
- In general, both a maxillofacial CT scan and brain MRI are obtained.
- CT scan provides a better examination of bony distortion and bony relationships.
- MRI is thought to be more sensitive and specific for transcranial soft tissue extension and for brain structural examination.[5]
- Typical imaging findings (**FIG 3**):
  - Interorbital distance—widened
  - Frontonasal cranial defect
  - Nasal bone—displaced and angulated
  - Bifid crista galli
- Tissue diagnosis via biopsy is contraindicated in these masses before a noninvasive, cross-sectional imaging workup has been performed.

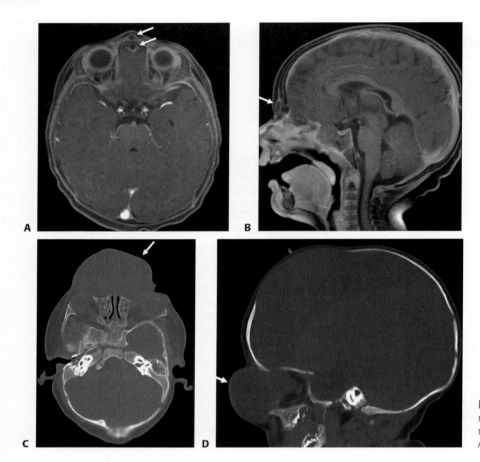

FIG 3 • A,B. MRIs reveal extra and intra components (*arrows*) in a 1-year-old girl with glabellar mass. **C,D.** Midline encephalocele is apparent in AP and lateral CT scans in a 4-month-old girl.

DIFFERENTIAL DIAGNOSIS

- The following are other diagnoses outside of NDSC, encephalocele, and glioma, which may occur on the nasal dorsum congenitally.[6]
  - Hemangioma/vascular malformation
  - Teratoma is pathologically distinct and contains all three layers, including endoderm, which is not present in NDSC.
  - Lipoma
  - Neurofibroma is often seen in concert with other neurofibromatosis cutaneous findings.

SURGICAL MANAGEMENT

Preoperative Planning

- Multidisciplinary collaboration
  - Plastic surgery
  - Neurosurgery
  - Ophthalmology—preoperative exam (interorbital, intercanthal, and interpupillary distances as well as eye movements), postoperative management of strabismus, and nasolacrimal management
- CT and MRI
- Hydrocephalus should be managed preoperatively by neurosurgery possibly with ventriculoperitoneal (VP) shunt before definitive correction (only pertains to encephalocele).
- Timing of surgery should be for at least late infancy (8 to 12 months) to allow better perioperative physiology and maturation of bone, which aids osteotomies and fixation.
- Transfusion and postoperative critical care are required.
- Computer-based 3D surgical planning may play a role in hypertelorism correction in the future.

Positioning

- Resection and reconstruction are done in a supine position.

Approach

- **FIG 4** is a decision-making algorithm for resection choice.
- Extracranial approach
  - Transnasal excision
  - Reduction of excess frontonasal skin
  - Open rhinoplasty—has been demonstrated when skin excess is minimal and there is no punctum. This can avoid dorsal nasal scar.
  - Intranasal—excision may be done through nares or open rhinoplasty approach if the mass is intranasal (more often with glioma).
- Intracranial
  - Frontal craniotomy
  - Limited craniotomy
  - Endoscopic minimally invasive approach
  - Immediate interorbital hypertelorism correction
- Dual approach
  - Extracranial
  - Intracranial
- Aims
  - Divide nasal and meningeal tissue and seal them apart.
  - Correct nasal soft tissue excess as needed.
  - Repair cranial base dural and bony defects.
  - Move medial orbits/medial canthi into normoteloric position if necessary.

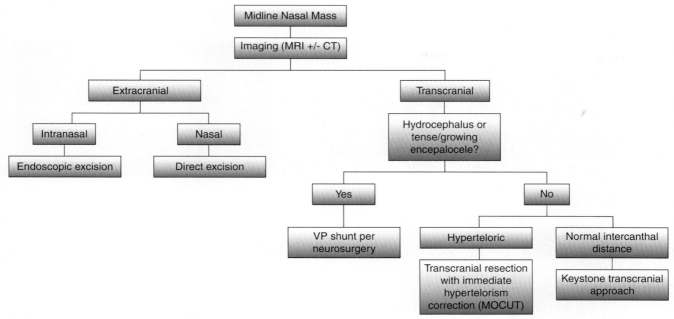

FIG 4 • Algorithm for choice of resection technique.

T
E
C
H
N
I
Q
U
E
S

■ Resection of Transcranial NDSC ("The Keystone Technique")

- Havlik et al. are responsible for describing and popularizing this technique.[7]

Nasal Approach/Frozen Biopsy

- In the case of dermoids with uncertain transcranial component, the mass is dissected down to its stalk. The stalk is biopsied for frozen section.[8]
- If it does not contain dermal contents, then the procedure is terminated with extracranial excision only.
- If dermal elements are present, an intracranial approach is followed (**TECH FIG 1**).

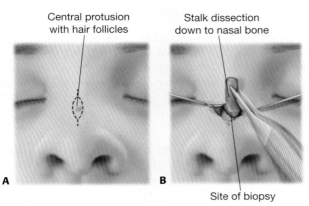

Central protusion with hair follicles

Stalk dissection down to nasal bone

A   **B**

Site of biopsy

TECH FIG 1 • External approach to midline nasal mass. This approach is combined with an intracranial approach when imaging, or intraoperative frozen biopsy confirms intracranial extension. **A.** Elliptical design for excising this nasal NDSC. **B.** The cyst and its stalk have been dissected down to the nasal bones, and a biopsy can be done at the deepest point.

Incisions, Dissection, and Craniotomy

- Bicoronal incision is designed at a symmetric point in the hairline just above the helical root. This is designed as a zigzag pattern to decrease visibility.
- Dorsonasal—a conservative elliptical skin excision is designed for nasal skin reduction and as access for dissection of the mass.
- An anterior scalp flap is raised in the areolar subgaleal plane (**TECH FIG 2A**).
- The pericranium should be carefully preserved.
- Upon approaching the orbits and nasofrontal junction, a plan for raising a subpericranial flap and subperiosteal dissection should be formulated.
- A large pericranial flap should be marked and raised to keep it in continuity with the scalp. This also allows full subperiosteal dissection of the orbits.
- The medial orbits and frontonasal defect edges are dissected subperiosteally with an elevator.
- A bifrontal craniotomy approximately 1cm above the supraorbital bandeau is performed by neurosurgery (**TECH FIG 2B**).
- The frontal lobes can be dissected and retracted to reveal the cranial base and the intracranial/dural extension of the mass (**TECH FIG 2C**).

Keystone Osteotomy and Dermal Sinus Excision

- To visualize the dermoid sinus tract, the frontonasal junction is osteotomized and removed (**TECH FIG 3**).
- This is done via vertical parasagittal osteotomies.
- This can be done to take only midline frontal bone or to include the nasal bones.
- Both approaches require reconstruction of the frontonasal junction or of the keystone area depending upon what is osteotomized.

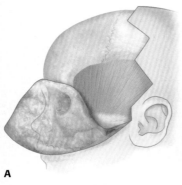

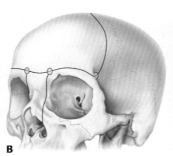

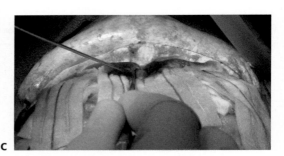

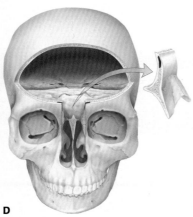

TECH FIG 2 • Transcranial approach to nasal dermoid. **A.** Design and reflection of coronal scalp flap. **B.** Design of frontal craniotomy and limited bandeau (so-called keystone approach—frontonasal osteotomy). **C.** Keystone osteotomy of frontonasal junction in order to access the transcranial component of the mass.

- The dermal sinus tract is resected from its dural connection following visualization.
- The NDSC, glioma, or redundant meningeal tissue is excised.
- At the site of the mass that is resected, a careful dural repair is performed by neurosurgery. Dural substitute is used as needed.

Bandeau/Frontal Bone Repair

- The keystone portion of the frontal bone is fixated back in place with resorbable hardware in infants and rigid hardware in older children.

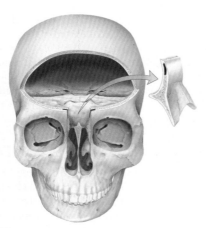

TECH FIG 3 • View of the transcranial component of the mass after frontal craniotomy.

- Fixation of the frontal bone should not compress or strangle the pericranial flap.
- Sizeable full-thickness cranial defects such as large bur holes can be filled with cranial bone shavings/particulate.
- A subcutaneous, closed suction drain is placed and the scalp is closed.

Cranial Base Repair and Seal

- If a bony defect is present in the cranial base, it should be treated with full or split calvarial bone graft (**TECH FIG 4A**). This bone is fashioned to the size and shape of the defect but not typically fixated.
- The pericranial flap harvested during scalp dissection (**TECH FIG 4B**) is then placed over the graft covering the cranial base.
- If possible, sutures are used to secure the flap. Fibrin glue is used to seal the edges of the flap (**TECH FIG 4C**).
- The pericranial flap acts to provide vascularized barrier both for the dural repair and the cranial base bone defect.

Completion

- The frontal sinus is not an issue in infants as the sinuses have not yet developed.
- In patients with delayed presentation and treatment, the frontal sinuses should be cranialized and the frontonasal duct should be obliterated with cautery and bone graft.
- The nasal skin redundancy is evaluated and additional skin is removed if necessary. The nasal skin is closed.

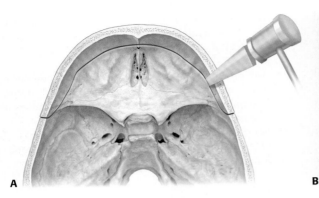

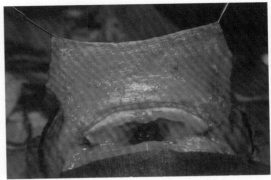

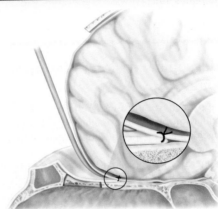

TECH FIG 4 • Seal of the anterior cranial base after transcranial resection. **A.** Bone graft (either full- or split-thickness calvarium) is placed in the cranial base defect. **B.** A pericranial flap is planned preoperatively for coronal scalp flap dissection. **C.** The pericranial flap is placed over the bone graft, and fibrin tissue sealant is used along with sutures to ensure a watertight seal.

■ Medial Orbit Composite Unit Translocation (MOCUT) Procedure

- This technique has been described and popularized by Boonvisut et al. for immediate hypertelorism repair in nasal encephalocele.[9]

Approach and Dissection

- The same coronal incision and bifrontal craniotomy as described for Resection of Transcranial NDSC above is utilized.
- The nose can be opened via either a vertical incision on the dorsum or through a conservatively designed vertical ellipse.
- Subperiosteal dissection is performed at the supraorbital bandeau into the orbits.
- Orbital dissection is limited to the medial aspects of each orbit between the supraorbital notches. Care is taken to keep the medial canthal tendon insertion intact.
- Careful subperiosteal dissection is used to ensure that the orbital and soft tissues are moved in concert in an uninterrupted fashion.
- The subperiosteal dissection is carried medially to the bone edges at the frontonasal defect.

Osteotomies, Resection, and Reconstruction

- Medial orbital wall is cut vertically from the craniotomy at the level of the supraorbital notch down to the inferior orbital rim (**TECH FIG 5A**).

- Via the nasal incision, a transverse osteotomy is performed from the piriform aperture to the inferior orbital rim to free the composite medial orbital unit.
- In the midline, bone will need to be removed from the medial orbital unit to establish the final interorbital distance.
  - This distance is planned preoperatively using a CT scan.
- Osteotomies are performed with a combination of conventional osteotomy, reciprocating saw, and ultrasonic scalpel.

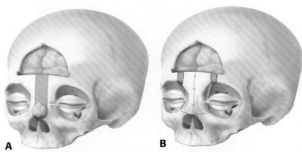

TECH FIG 5 • Encephalocele resection with transcranial approach and immediate hypertelorism correction. **A.** Bifrontal craniotomy is performed. Laterally vertical osteotomies are planned to descend from just medial to the infraorbital notch. A variable bony resection at the midline will be performed to allow medialization of the orbit and canthal units. The inferior horizontal osteotomy may be completed through the nasal incision. **B.** The medial orbit composite unit technique (MOCUT) can be seen here to immediately produce hypertelorism correction.

- Completion of the osteotomies mobilizes the orbital units allowing for improved exposure.
- The mass, typically an encephalocele with this approach, should be dissected free from its surroundings.
  - This is done via the nasal incision and the frontal craniotomy.
- Dural repair and cranial base/frontal sinus repair are as described above.
- The medial orbital units are joined at the midline with fixation (**TECH FIG 5B**).
  - This is typically done with a 30-gauge wire but may also be done using suture, permanent plates, or resorbable plates and screws.

- Transverse bony gaps at the supraorbital bandeau that have been created through orbital medialization should be treated with fixated interposition calvarial bone graft.
- Any disruption of the nasal cartilages to bone or of the nasofrontal junction should be repaired with suture.
- Redundant nasal skin should be conservatively resected. The nasal skin is closed.
- Some have argued for more complex nasal skin flaps. Our preference is for nasal skin revision at a second stage if necessary.

■ Endoscopic Excision of Intranasal Glioma

- The approach to intranasal gliomas also includes an external rhinoplasty approach and a lateral rhinotomy approach.[10] These specific approaches will not be discussed here.
  - In general, this approach has been used by those who practice endoscopic surgery and skull base approaches.
  - Many have argued that with evidence of transcranial extension, a traditional craniotomy should be performed to separate the nasal-intracranial connection. Others have demonstrated that intranasal glioma with intracranial extension can be successfully excised

endoscopically, thereby avoiding craniotomy.
- An angled endoscope is introduced intranasally to visualize the mass (**TECH FIG 6**).
- Electrocautery is used to incise the nasal mucosa along the mass.
- Retraction and blunt dissection define the mass.
- After defining the stalk, it is divided using electrocautery and the mass is removed.
- The base is examined for CSF leak. If necessary, it may be oversewn. Fibrin tissue sealant may also be used to ensure a seal.
- The nasal mucosa is closed with simple sutures.
- The affected nasal passage is packed. Nasal packing is removed in the early postoperative period.

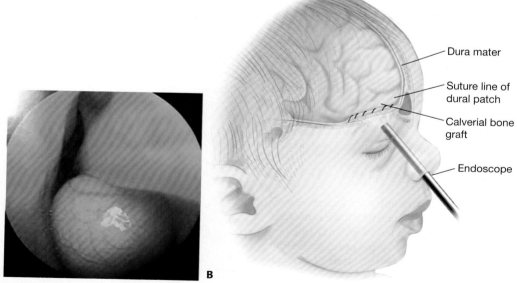

Dura mater

Suture line of dural patch

Calverial bone graft

Endoscope

TECH FIG 6 • Excision of intranasal mass. **A.** Endoscopic appearance of purely intranasal glioma. **B.** An endoscope may be used to visualize and aid excision of intranasal glioma. Endoscopic approaches to the cranial base are also well described.

PEARLS AND PITFALLS

Biopsy	■ Congenital nasal masses, particularly those occurring at or near the midline, should not be biopsied for diagnosis. Biopsy can lead to CSF leak and ascending/meningeal infection.
Radiologic evaluation	■ Congenital nasal masses should be evaluated radiographically. This often includes both a CT scan and MRI.
VP shunt	■ Decompression by neurosurgery in the setting of a large or growing encephalocele can allow surgery to be delayed until the patient is a better candidate for surgery.
Age at surgery	■ Timing of treatment, particularly with large lesions and encephaloceles, is a balance between the risk of infection/meningitis/family stress and the safety of surgery/quality of bone for reconstruction. We recommend waiting until late infancy if there are no other time-sensitive factors.
Intracranial seal	■ Transcranial approach requires careful reconstruction of the cranial base defect including bone grafting, pericranial flap, and fibrin glue seal.

POSTOPERATIVE CARE

- Pediatric ICU is mandatory with expected hospital stay of 5 to 7 days.
- Neurologic monitoring
- Routine labs for bleeding and infection
- Monitoring of nasal and drain output for CSF leak—the drain should be in place for at least 5 days.
- Close outpatient monitoring for the development of CSF leak, meningitis, and hydrocephalus
- Secondary nasal scar revision is often necessary.

OUTCOMES

- Complications
  - In these rare conditions, most case series are small.
  - Minor complications in any transcranial approach with nasal-intracranial communication should be expected to be moderate to high.
  - Catastrophic complications should be rare.
- Aesthetic outcome
  - Disruption of nasal growth and form is a high risk.
  - Revision of nasal scar/form and nasal reconstruction with rib graft should be expected.
  - Second hypertelorism correction may be necessary.

COMPLICATIONS

- CSF leak
- Meningitis
- Death
- Scar hypertrophy
- Residual hypertelorism

- Residual nasal deformity and skin excess
  - May require re-excision, local tissue rearrangement, onlay grafting of the nasal dorsum, and formal rhinoplasty at maturity

REFERENCES

1. Charrier J-B, Rouillon I, Roger G, et al. Craniofacial dermoids: an embryological theory unifying nasal dermoid sinus cysts. *Cleft Palate Craniofac J.* 2005;42:51-57.
2. Blake WE, Chow CW, Holmes AD, Meara JG. Nasal dermoid sinus cysts: a retrospective review and discussion of investigation and management. *Ann Plast Surg.* 2006;57:535-540.
3. Tirumandas M, Sharma A, Gbenimacho I, et al. Nasal encephaloceles: a review of etiology, pathophysiology, clinical presentations, diagnosis, treatment, and complications. *Child's Nerv Syst.* 2013;29(5): 739-744.
4. Rahbar R, Resto VA, Robson CD, et al. Nasal glioma and encephalocele: diagnosis and management. *Laryngoscope.* 2003;113:2069-2077.
5. Hedlund G. Congenital frontonasal masses: developmental anatomy, malformations, and MR imaging. *Pediatr Radiol.* 2006;36:647-662.
6. Bartlett SP, Lin KY, Grossman R, Katowitz J. The surgical management of orbitofacial dermoids in the pediatric patient. *Plast Reconstr Surg.* 1993;91:1208-1215.
7. Van Aalst JA, Luerssen TG, Whitehead WE, Havlik RJ. 'Keystone' approach for intracranial nasofrontal dermoid sinuses. *Plast Reconstr Surg.* 2005;116:13-19.
8. Sessions RB. Nasal dermal sinuses—new concepts and explanations. *The Laryngoscope.* 1982;92(8 Pt 2 Suppl 29):1-28.
9. Boonvisut S, Ladpli S, Sujatanond M, et al. A new technique for the repair and reconstruction of frontoethmoidal encephalomeningoceles by medial orbital composite-unit translocation. *Br J Plast Surg.* 2001;54:93-101.
10. Wu C-L, Tsao L-Y, Yang AD, Chen M-K. Endoscopic surgery for nasal glioma mimicking encephalocele in infancy. *Skull Base.* 2008;18:401-404.

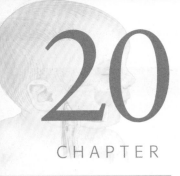

Section VI: Soft Tissue Masses

20
CHAPTER

Surgery of Neurofibromatosis in the Pediatric Patient

McKay McKinnon

DEFINITION

- Patients with cutaneous neurofibromatosis (NF), the most common of the myriad of phenotypic manifestations of the disease (and Von Recklinghausen's original case reports), can usually expect permanent relief of individual lesions by full-thickness excision. For those patients with so-called plexiform NF and/or malignant peripheral nerve sheath tumors (MPNST), the puzzlement of a permanent treatment (medical or surgical) has remained largely unsolved for most patients.
- For well over a century, the textbook recommendation for children with NF1 plexiform tumors has been to defer surgery until after puberty or until serious morbidity is evident. When surgery has been deemed necessary, it has most often been a superficial resection of the tumor, commonly referred to as "debulking." Subsequent recurrence of tumor has led to a default strategy of withholding surgery for pediatric patients, based upon fear of iatrogenic injury to normal structures, uncontrollable hemorrhage, and perceived inability to achieve permanent tumor removal.
- Over the past 30 years, the author has observed that radical resection of plexiform tumors in adults has resulted in permanent "nonrecurrence" of nearly all tumors, even those over 50 kg and some MPNST.[1] Despite a higher propensity for active tumor growth in children and adolescents, it seemed logical to extend the concept of radical surgical resection to pediatric patients.

ANATOMY

- Craniofacial
  - Most facial and frontotemporal scalp tumors derive from sensory branches of cranial nerve V. The ophthalmic division of the trigeminal nerve (**FIG 1A**) includes some sensory nerves that are within the musculofascial cone (annulus of Zinn) of the orbit. This area presents special risks of injury to the optic nerve and the extraocular muscles and should be avoided.
    - Orbital NF is often accompanied by a defect of the sphenoid greater wing, which may permit herniation of the temporal lobe into the orbit and subsequent orbital dystopia, pulsatile exophthalmos or enophthalmos, and pressure on the globe and optic nerve. Destruction of bone, ligaments, fascia, muscle, and skin may be present.
    - Tumor confined to the optic nerve (optic glioma) deserves neurosurgical management.
    - Motor nerves are not intrinsically involved with NF tumor.
  - NF tumors of the mandible, parotid, ear, and temporal scalp develop largely from the mandibular division of the trigeminal nerve, including the auriculotemporal nerve.
  - Tumors of the neck and posterior scalp derive from upper cervical sensory nerves (C1–C4), including the occipital nerves. Lower cervical nerves (C4–C8, sensory and motor) constitute most of the brachial plexus.
- Trunk and extremity
  - Plexiform NF can exist anywhere from the spinal cord to the sensory nerve terminus in the skin, bone, or viscera (**FIG 1B**).
  - Plexiform tumors most commonly appear between the deep fascia and the skin but may involve and destroy skin, muscles, bones, joints, and visceral organs. Careful dissection proximal to the tumor mass (toward their CNS origin) often reveals the specific sensory nerve origin. Large truncal lesions over time can develop paraspinal hypervascularity, which resembles an arteriovenous malformation. Scoliosis is common with posterior trunk lesions, and limb hyperplasia is common with extremity lesions.

PATHOGENESIS

- NF is an autosomal dominant condition, which can be attributed to a defect on chromosome 17, but mosaicism can also occur. The consequential lack of neurofibromin (a tumor inhibitor) permits growth of myelinated axonal tumors in any bodily location. Tumor types are cutaneous or plexiform. So-called plexiform tumors are solid tumors, which have an obligatory angiogenic influence, similar to other solid tumors. They express multiple angiogenic and neurogenic factors. Puberty, pregnancy, and childhood growth spurts can exacerbate their growth. Tumor vascularity increases proportionate to tumor growth. Transformation of benign NF tumors into MPNST can occur in plexiform tumors. This transformation may have a direct correlation to numerical tumor cell replication events.
- Tumor vessels in NF are pathologic arteries that reveal absent media and abnormally thin adventitia. Established tumors can exhibit vascular lakes and/or nests of abnormal vessels resembling a congenital vascular malformation.

NATURAL HISTORY

- Neurofibromas, once established as plexiform tumors, do not regress spontaneously. Their growth is unpredictable and nonregular, including possible onset throughout a patient's life of new lesions. Malignant transformation is more common in truncal/extremity lesions but is also unpredictable. Café au lait cutaneous spots do not necessarily signal

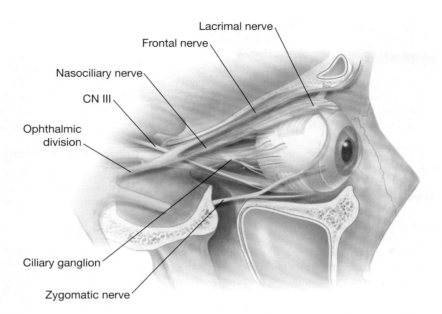

FIG 1 • Nerves of the orbit.

plexiform tumors, although they themselves represent microscopic tumor. If present at birth, plexiform tumors may have already inflicted defective tissue development of the newborn.

■ Eventual destruction by tumor of adjacent skin, bone, and other tissue should be expected without intervention. Hyperplasia and/or fragility of bone occurs in extremity lesions. Craniofacial tumors can also produce osteoclastic or osteoblastic pathology, likely as a consequence of tumor growth rate. Tumors involving the sphenoid and orbit can cause progressive orbital dystopia, blepharoptosis, and blindness. Paraspinal tumors inflict progressive scoliosis on the growing patient.

PATIENT HISTORY AND PHYSICAL FINDINGS

■ The myriad presentations of NF tumors should not deter accurate diagnosis, even in infancy, by the observant neurologist or experienced surgeon. If doubt of the diagnosis exists, a biopsy should be performed with exception at least of the optic nerve.

■ Physical findings are too numerous to justify an inclusive list, but palpable tumor, pain, and confirmatory imaging should precede surgical intervention in virtually all cases.

IMAGING

■ Pediatric patients with suspicion of plexiform NF tumor should have an MRI study, preferably with and without contrast. MRI of the CNS is appropriate as an early screening measure for all NF patients, even those without known tumors. T2- and STIR-weighted images usually give the clearest depiction of NF tumor.

■ MRI, especially with higher Tesla power, can frequently reveal the specific cranial or spinal nerve involved with tumor. This information (nerve mapping) should be sought out with the neuroradiologist.

■ High-resolution CT scans should only be ordered when and if the patient with skeletal destruction or high risk of skeletal pathology is being evaluated preoperatively.

DIFFERENTIAL DIAGNOSIS

■ NF tumors have been mistaken for vascular malformations, particularly by their hypervascular imaging on CT or MRI.

■ Hyperpigmentation of NF lesions has been confused by the inexperienced physician with congenital nevus. A biopsy can readily produce the correct diagnosis.

■ Most patients, even infants, with NF will present with at least three or more cutaneous lesions and/or café au lait lesions, axillary freckling, ocular Lisch nodules, or a subcutaneous plexiform mass.

■ Congenital ptosis can usually be differentiated from NF-derived ptosis by detection of an orbital mass, presence of enophthalmos or exophthalmos, and by MRI findings. Rapid increase of ptosis may be associated with orbital malignancy such as rhabdomyosarcoma, for which immediate incisional or excisional biopsy is required.

■ Diagnosis of MPNST or other orbital malignancies cannot be reliably made by symptoms, by imaging, or by clinical examination.

NONOPERATIVE MANAGEMENT

■ This default management decision is historically common but deserves renewed challenge because it is controversial. Observation of growing NF tumors is patently nontherapeutic yet may be justified if surgery is high risk, the patient has significant comorbidity, or the tumor has not reached a level of irreversible morbidity to vital structures. The surgeon and his or her medical colleagues should be prepared to intervene to prevent irreversible morbidity, even in young patients.

SURGICAL MANAGEMENT

■ An accurate diagnosis is the sine qua non of surgical management. With plexiform NF this should include determination of the tumor nerve origin(s), the degree of vascularity, bony deformity, proximity to other vital anatomy, and degree of skin destruction. In the craniofacial tumors, accurate diagnosis also should determine presence of brain herniation into the orbit (or elsewhere), orbital dystopia, ptosis vs pseudoptosis, ophthalmic pathology, and airway and carotid/jugular risks.

- Because all NF1 tumors are caused by pathologic sensory nerves, either of brain or spinal cord origin,[1] if a total interruption of the responsible sensory nerve(s) can be achieved (eg, a Sunderland V injury), permanent nonregrowth of tumor may also be achieved.[1] Thus, surgical strategy should aim to:
  - Radically resect the plexiform tumor and identify and amputate the responsible sensory nerve(s) proximal to the tumor
  - Dissect and preserve any motor nerves in the tumor proximity
  - Undertake tumor resection even in the pediatric patient because progressive tumor growth over time equates to more complex surgery, higher risk of morbidity to normal adjacent structures and function, and possibly more risk of malignant transformation of previously benign tumors
- All techniques are subservient to the principles of reconstructive surgery. A knowledge of and adherence to principles permit the surgeon to methodically approach virtually any surgical problem to arrive at an organized plan. The reconstructive surgeon's "creed" has been summarized by Millard: "Know the ideal beautiful normal. Diagnose what is present, what is diseased, displaced, or distorted, and what is in excess. Then, guided by the normal in your mind's eye, utilize what you have to make what you want—and when possible go for even better than what would have been!"
- No clinical condition presents to the surgeon a more variable array of pathology than neurofibromatosis. The NF

surgeon needs, therefore, to first make a strategy from application of principles. When the principles (such as making an accurate diagnosis, establishing priorities, making a plan and a backup plan, replacing lost tissue in kind, etc.) are applied, the surgical techniques will devolve naturally. The surgeon, much like his or her military counterpart, elucidates the goals and strategy of a military-type campaign before determining the specific technique(s) required.

Preoperative Planning

- Pertinent consultations with other specialists should be completed well prior to surgery, if feasible.
- Adequate warning to blood bank and ICU is made.

Positioning

- Most craniofacial procedures are done in the supine or lateral position with a standard OR table with a gel headrest.
- Trunk and extremity procedures are done in standard positions according to tumor site(s).

Approach

- Orbital tumors are approached via coronal, superior lid crease, and transconjunctival incisions as needed. Inferior orbital nerve (maxillary) tumors are accessed via a lower eyelid incision as in orbital floor exploration or via a nasojugal incision.
  - The surgeon should anticipate repeat procedures (ie, a subciliary incision is always a higher risk for ectropion).
- Posterior trunk tumors should be accessed via incisions that can resect not only the palpable tumor but also any feeding paraspinal sensory nerves (**FIG 2**).

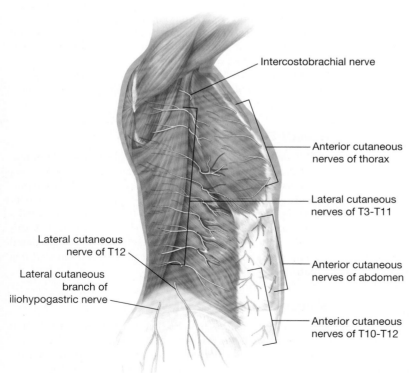

Intercostobrachial nerve

Anterior cutaneous nerves of thorax

Lateral cutaneous nerves of T3-T11

Lateral cutaneous nerve of T12

Lateral cutaneous branch of iliohypogastric nerve

Anterior cutaneous nerves of abdomen

Anterior cutaneous nerves of T10-T12

FIG 2 • Spinal sensory nerves of the trunk.

■ General Principles

■ The first priority of surgery in the child with NF is resection of tumor and reconstruction of bone. Large tumor resections can be aided by cautery devices such as LigaSure, but the surgeon should be facile in vascular surgical techniques.

■ Autogenous bone reconstruction is superior in virtually all cases to alloplastic reconstruction in NF, especially in the growing child.

■ Because resection of cranial nerve V tumors into the cavernous sinus is dangerous (and some tumor will necessarily remain there), reconstruction of the sphenoid defect should be undertaken with a combination of bone and plate/mesh to ensure permanence of brain-orbit separation (even in the enucleated patient). Bone should face the orbit to allow possible attachment of the levator muscle origin.

■ Early ptosis correction is important to avoid amblyopia, but definitive ptosis correction should be performed when the child can tolerate a nongeneral anesthetic for refinement of the correction by patient participation and tumor is not significantly present.

■ When approaching a large plexiform tumor, the surgeon should begin dissection in normal tissue and proceed to identify the plane at the tumor margin. Motor nerves that are within the tumor field should be identified by direct nerve stimulation.

■ Illustrative Cases

Case 1: Inferior Orbital Nerve Tumor

■ A 4-year-old girl demonstrated a rapid regrowth of a right inferior orbital nerve NF tumor 6 months following partial resection at an outside institution. The tumor was creating a vertical orbital dystopia (**TECH FIG 1A,B**).

■ A resection of the inferior orbital nerve tumor from the cheek to the posterior orbit was performed via the old nasojugal vertical scar (**TECH FIG 1C,D**).

■ Alternative approaches in an unoperated patient would be a transverse lower lid incision and a separate nasolabial fold incision, or even an intraoral incision, depending on extent of tumor.

■ Following resection, the marginotomy was repaired with a stainless steel wire in a corrected (inferior) reposition.

■ Over the subsequent 20 years, the patient presented multiple other tumors of alternate branches of the trigeminal nerve, but not of the inferior orbital (maxillary) nerve (**TECH FIG 1E,F**).

Case 2: Hypogastric Plexiform Tumor

■ A teenage girl presented a painful left hypogastric plexiform tumor recurrence 2 years after an attempted resection at an outside hospital (**TECH FIG 2A**).

■ MRI revealed the tumor extending from the skin to the deep abdominal fascia (**TECH FIG 2B**).

■ Resection via an extension of the old scar included dissection and resection of the pathologic hypogastric nerve lying deep to the external oblique muscle (**TECH FIG 2C–E**).

■ There had been no recurrence in 10 years of follow-up.

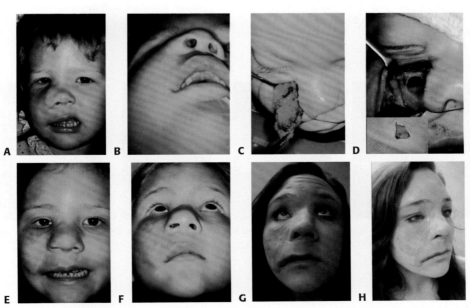

TECH FIG 1 • A,B. A 4-year-old girl with right inferior orbital nerve NF tumor 6 months after partial resection. **C,D.** A marginal osteotomy (a la Tessier) of the orbital rim allowed visualization and tumor resection in the posterior orbit to the cranial base. **E–H.** Postoperative photos.

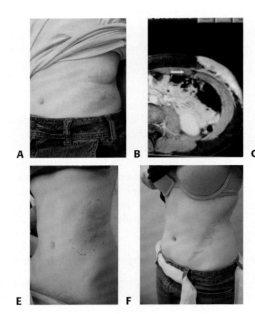
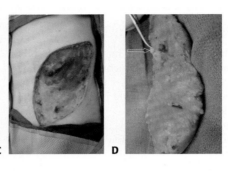

TECH FIG 2 • A. Teenaged girl with left hypogastric plexiform tumor recurrence 2 years after attempted resection. **B.** The tumor extended from the skin to the deep abdominal fascia, as shown on MRI. **C,D.** Dissection and resection of the pathologic hypogastric nerve lying deep to the external oblique muscle. **E,F.** The result 1 year after direct wound closure.

Case 3: Breast and Chest Wall Plexiform Neurofibromatosis

- A 15-year-old girl presented with right breast and lateral chest wall plexiform NF (**TECH FIG 3A**).
- At surgery, a simultaneous resection of a right intercostal tumor and a right breast reduction/tumor resection were performed (**TECH FIG 3B,C**).
- The intercostal nerve proximal to the tumor mass was located and amputated at the rib.
- No recurrence had been observed in over 8 years of follow-up (**TECH FIG 3D**).

Case 4: Left Orbital and Mental Nerve Neurofibromatosis 1

- A 12-year-old boy presented with left orbital and mental nerve plexiform NF1 (**TECH FIG 4A,B**), severe ptosis, and pulsatile exophthalmos.

- Through a coronal, left upper eyelid, and left nasolabial incisions (**TECH FIG 4C**), the tumor was radically resected.
- Via the coronal approach (without osteotomy), the temporal lobe dura was located inside the posterior orbit and dissected from the periorbitum (**TECH FIG 4D**) and then the brain/dura was repositioned into the cranial cavity and separated from the orbit by a cranial bone graft/titanium mesh reconstruction.
- The graft/implant was placed from the orbit into the cranial cavity and held in position by autoretention.
- In the same procedure, a cranial bone graft to the orbital floor and a moderate reduction of eyelid skin excess was performed.
- Vision was preserved (**TECH FIG 4E**). The patient will need future additional floor elevation and definitive ptosis correction.

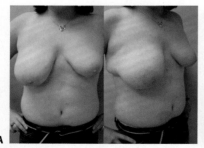
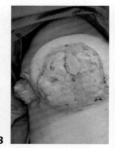
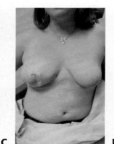
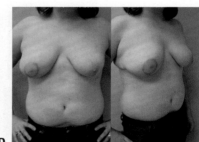

TECH FIG 3 • A. A 15-year-old girl with right breast and lateral chest wall plexiform NF. Simultaneous with resection of a right intercostal tumor **(B)**, a right breast reduction/tumor resection was performed **(C)**. **D.** Appearance at 8 years postoperatively.

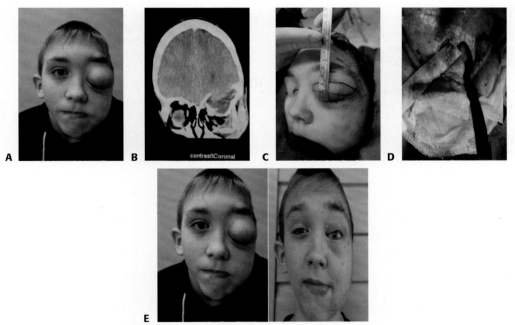

TECH FIG 4 • A. A 12-year-old boy with left orbital and mental nerve plexiform NF1, severe ptosis, and pulsatile exophthalmos. **B.** MRI demonstrated a plexiform tumor of the superior orbit and mental nerve, a large defect of the sphenoid greater wing, and prolapse of the temporal lobe into the orbit. **C.** Markings for coronal, left upper eyelid, and left nasolabial incisions. **D.** Dissection of the temporal lobe dura inside the posterior orbit from the periorbitum via the coronal approach. **E.** Postoperative appearance.

PEARLS AND PITFALLS

Diagnosis	■ The most common pitfall in NF surgery is inaccurate diagnosis. ■ When recommending a tissue biopsy for definitive diagnosis, avoid biopsy within a highly vascular region of NF tumor or adjacent to the optic nerve. ■ Tumor heterogeneity on MRI may indicate a benign tumor adjacent to a malignant tumor.
Surgical strategy	■ The NF surgeon should avoid underestimation of tumor extent and potential hemorrhage, underdissection with nerve stimulation of motor nerves along the path of the tumor, and underestimation of a surgical strategy that anticipates tumor recurrence in young patients. ■ Lifetime surveillance by the surgeon should be assumed because the medical specialists are ill prepared to have a surgical perspective of NF. ■ The occasional NF surgeon will inevitably experience high morbidity and low patient satisfaction.
Technique	■ The surgical term "debulking" in NF1 represents a common pitfall of partial, superficial resection. Rapid recurrence of tumor normally ensues. Debulking of intraorbital tumors may, however, be justified to save vision. ■ It should be clear to the NF surgeon that vision is also at risk due to possible glaucoma, hemorrhage, tumor/brain pressure on the optic nerve, glioma of the optic nerve, severe orbital dystopia, severe ptosis (amblyopia), and palpebral incompetence.
Other specialists	■ Orthopedic surgeons, neurosurgeons, and ophthalmologists frequently treat pediatric patients with NF. ■ If limb hypertrophy or spinal scoliosis is present in conjunction with a tumor that is resectable, the plastic NF surgeon should champion primary tumor resection prior to orthopedic attempts to reduce epiphyseal growth, reconstruct joints, to correct scoliosis, or even to amputate parts. This should be intuitive as correct general surgical principle, not a pearl of wisdom. Likewise, strabismus and/or ptosis surgery should not precede tumor resection and orbital bone reconstruction.

POSTOPERATIVE CARE

- The NF surgeon should use drains freely due to the vascularity and vessel pathology of NF tumors, following extensive resections, which predispose to seroma formation.
- Suction drainage may be hazardous near the dura and may exacerbate hemorrhage near fragile-walled, residual tumor vessels.

- Since many NF surgeries overlap into other surgical specialties, the plastic NF surgeon should include those specialists in the postoperative care but remain the captain of care and assume ultimate responsibility.

REFERENCE

1. McKinnon M. Why patients with neurofibroma don't need allotransplantation. *Plast Reconstr Surg.* 2012;130:12.

Vascular Anomalies

Arin K. Greene and Jeremy Goss

DEFINITION

- Vascular anomalies are a group of lesions that can affect any part of the vasculature.
- Lesions are divided into tumors (with dividing endothelium) and malformations (structural anomalies with minimal endothelial turnover).[1]
- Eight types of vascular anomalies (four tumors and four malformations) constitute approximately 95% of lesions.

ANATOMY

- Vascular anomalies most commonly involve the integument (although they can affect any anatomical structure).
- The most common morbidity is lowered self-esteem because of a deformity.
- Lesions involving the head and neck are more likely to be problematic.

NATURAL HISTORY

- The somatic mutations responsible for most vascular anomalies recently have been identified.
- Some vascular tumors improve over time (infantile hemangioma, rapidly involuting congenital hemangioma, kaposiform hemangioendothelioma).[2]
- Vascular malformations slowly worsen, particularly during adolescence.
- Following treatment of vascular malformations, recurrence is common and patients often require repeated procedures.

PATIENT HISTORY AND PHYSICAL FINDINGS

- Ninety percent of vascular anomalies can be diagnosed by history and physical examination.
- Before considering management, the type of vascular anomaly must be identified because lesions have different natural histories and treatments.[3]
- The most common vascular anomalies encountered in clinical practice are (in order of frequency) pyogenic granuloma, infantile hemangioma, and capillary malformation.
- A handheld Doppler can determine whether the lesion has fast flow, which aids the diagnosis.
- Lesions with fast flow include infantile hemangioma, congenital hemangioma, kaposiform hemangioendothelioma, and arteriovenous malformation. Slow-flow anomalies are capillary malformation, lymphatic malformation, and venous malformation.

IMAGING

- Less than 10% of patients require imaging to diagnose their vascular anomaly.
- If the diagnosis is unclear by history and physical examination, ultrasound is the first-line imaging study because it is easy to perform and does not require sedation in children.
- If the diagnosis remains uncertain after ultrasonography, then MRI with contrast is obtained.
- Imaging is not required prior to resection of hemangiomas, pyogenic granulomas, or capillary malformations.
- Before operative intervention for a venous malformation, lymphatic malformation, or arteriovenous malformation, MRI typically is obtained to determine the extent of disease.

DIFFERENTIAL DIAGNOSIS

- Fibrosarcoma
- Neurofibroma
- Pilomatrixoma
- Teratoma

NONOPERATIVE MANAGEMENT

- Nonoperative intervention is the mainstay of treatment for vascular anomalies; lesions are benign and often can be observed.
- Less than 10% of infantile hemangiomas require treatment. Problematic lesions during the proliferative phase can be managed with topical timolol, corticosteroid injection, prednisone, propranolol, or rarely, resection.
- Kaposiform hemangioendothelioma is treated with vincristine or sirolimus.
- First-line intervention for problematic vascular malformations typically is nonsurgical: capillary malformation (pulsed-dye laser), venous malformation (sclerotherapy), lymphatic malformation (sclerotherapy), arteriovenous malformation (embolization).[4-7]

SURGICAL MANAGEMENT

- Operative treatment of vascular anomalies generally is performed for symptomatic patients who are not candidates or have failed nonoperative interventions.
- Residual infantile or congenital hemangiomas causing a deformity can only be improved with resection (or pulsed-dye laser for telangiectasias).
- The primary treatment of pyogenic granuloma is full-thickness skin excision or cautery (curettage, laser, and cryotherapy have a recurrence rate as high as 50%).

- Capillary malformation can cause overgrowth of tissues beneath the stain, which can be improved by resection.
- Operative intervention for venous malformation is reserved for small lesions that may be removed for cure or for a residual deformity following sclerotherapy.
- Macrocystic lymphatic malformation may have redundant skin following sclerotherapy that can be resected. Microcystic lesions are not amenable to sclerotherapy, and thus, excision often is first-line treatment.
- Arteriovenous malformations generally are removed if they remain symptomatic following embolization.

Preoperative Planning

- A critical principle is that vascular anomalies are benign and thus do not require radical resection; the scar and reconstruction should not cause a worse deformity than the appearance of the lesion.
- Vascular anomalies typically are diffuse and involve multiple tissue planes; consequently, most resections are subtotal.
- The goal of operative management is to improve the patient's symptoms by removing enough of the lesion to reduce pain, bleeding, and/or ulceration and/or improve appearance.
- Symptomatic infantile hemangiomas are best excised between 3 and 4 years of age after they have completed involution.
- If possible, resection should be postponed until the child is at least 6 months of age to reduce the anesthetic risk.
- Consideration should be given to improving deformities before 4 years of age to minimize impact on self-esteem.

- Venous, lymphatic, and arteriovenous malformations usually are removed after they have been treated with sclerotherapy or embolization; these interventions reduce the size of the lesion, decrease bleeding, create fibrosis, and facilitate the operation.

Positioning

- The table is turned 90 degrees during resection of head/neck lesions.
- To limit blood loss, the head of the bed is elevated for facial vascular anomalies.

Approach

- Intraoperative antibiotics are not administered except when resecting large lymphatic malformations because they are prone to infection.
- After marking the extent of the resection, bupivacaine with epinephrine is infused throughout the operative site to reduce blood loss and pain.
- Markings are tattooed for lesions located on the vermillion or mucosa.
- To reduce blood loss, cold epinephrine-soaked sponges can be applied to the operative field; clips may be applied to the skin edges to decrease bleeding.
- After making the incision, hemostasis should be obtained prior to proceeding with further excision to avoid significant blood loss.
- Margins are not required; the least amount of tissue as possible should be removed to achieve the operative aims.
- A pressure dressing usually is applied to minimize the risk of postoperative hemorrhage.

TECHNIQUES

■ Lenticular Excision and Linear Closure

- Most vascular anomalies act as a tissue expander, and thus, adequate skin is available to close the wound (**TECH FIG 1**).
- The majority of resections are subtotal, and thus, missing integument is rare.
- Skin grafts or local/regional flaps rarely are necessary to reconstruct an area following extirpation.

- Incisions are designed to be as inconspicuous as possible (eg, relaxed skin tension lines, hairline, etc.).
- Vascular anomalies often cause local ischemia because of insufficient oxygen delivery; consequently, interrupted rather than continues sutures are preferred for closure.
- After resecting a facial lesion in children who are less able to tolerate suture removal, 7-0 chromic followed by cyanoacrylate glue and tape can be used.

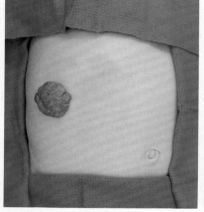 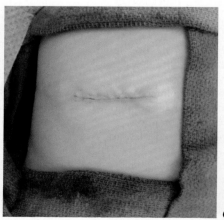 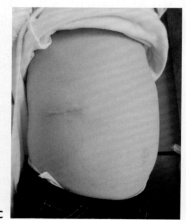

TECH FIG 1 • A 3-year-old with an involuted infantile hemangioma managed with lenticular excision and linear closure. **A.** Preoperative appearance. **B.** Following resection. **C.** Early postoperative view.

◼ Circular Excision and Purse-String Closure

- This technique is useful for round lesions to limit the length of the scar, which would be 2 to 3 times the diameter of the lesion if it was excised lenticularly (**TECH FIG 2**).[8,9]
- Circular excision is most commonly performed for infantile hemangiomas after they have involuted, but can be used for any round skin lesion.
- Almost all procedures are conducted on the face where it is important to limit the length of the scar; round lesions involving the trunk or extremity usually undergo lenticular excision because the linear scar is concealed and appears favorable in a relaxed skin tension line.

- A contraindication to circular excision is the scalp because there is minimal tissue laxity, a circular scar can cause visible alopecia, and it is not critical to limit the length of a scar in the scalp because it is camouflaged by hair.
- When closing the circular excision, it is important to undermine the skin edges to reduce tension; I usually prefer a Vicryl purse-string suture. After the purse-string closure, I approximate the epidermis/dermis with interrupted chromic or nylon suture (depending on the age of the patient) followed by cyanoacrylate glue and tape.
- Disadvantages of this technique are that there is an increased risk of wound dehiscence compared to linear closure and a second stage may be required to convert the circular skin into a line.

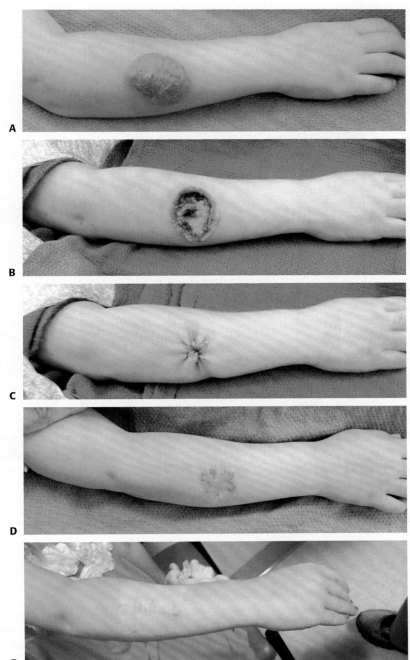

TECH FIG 2 • A 3-year-old with an involuted infantile hemangioma of the arm. The lesion was managed with circular excision and purse-string closure to limit the length of the scar in a visible location on the dorsum of the extremity. If the lesion was removed as an ellipse, the scar would be at least twice the diameter of the lesion. **A.** Preoperative view. **B.** Following circular resection. **C.** Purse-string closure. **D.** Appearance prior to second stage conversion of the round scar and residual telangiectasias into a line. **E.** Linear scar 6 weeks postoperatively approximates the diameter of the hemangioma that was removed.

- Approximately 50% of patients are satisfied with the round scar and do not wish to have a second procedure (the circular scar can look like an acne or chickenpox scar).
- If the circular scar is converted to a line during a second stage, its length will approximate the diameter of the original lesion.
- I wait 6 to 12 months after the circular excision before considering a second stage to convert it into a line.

Transverse Mucosal Resection and Linear Closure

- Vascular anomalies involving the lip often cause overgrowth and a deformity.
- Unlike malignant labial lesions, subtotal resection of benign vascular anomalies can be performed to improve the patient's appearance.
- This technique avoids the placement of a scar on the cutaneous lip (**TECH FIG 3**).

- An elliptical excision is designed along the keratinized and nonkeratinized vermillion; the markings are tattooed prior to injection of local anesthetic.
- Diseased vermillion, mucosa, submucosa, and a portion of orbicularis muscle are removed.
- The incision is closed with interrupted Vicryl and chromic suture.
- The patient is maintained on a full-liquid diet for 2 weeks.
- If the lesion regrows, it can be debulked again using the same incision.

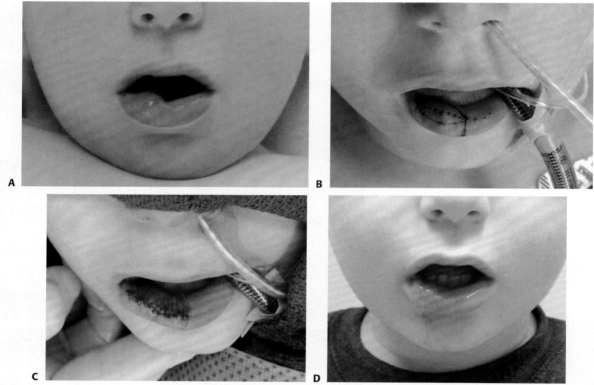

TECH FIG 3 • Transverse mucosal resection of an involuted infantile hemangioma of the lip. **A.** Appearance of the lesion at 3 years of age. **B.** Markings for excision. **C.** Suture line following resection. **D.** Postoperative appearance.

Suction-Assisted Lipectomy

- Several types of vascular anomalies are amenable to suction-assisted removal when they are located primarily in the subcutaneous plane: infantile hemangioma, capillary malformation, lymphatic malformation, and other lesions that have a significant adipose component (**TECH FIG 4**).[10]

- This technique allows the removal of diseased tissue without long incisions, raising skin flaps, and "open" excision, which has increased morbidity and recovery compared to liposuction.
- Stab incisions are placed in nonconspicuous areas and tumescent solution is infused (1 mL of epinephrine 1:1000, 1000 mL normal saline, 50 cc 1% lidocaine) not to exceed 35 mg/kg of lidocaine.

TECHNIQUES

- Cannulas of 3 mm typically are used for the face, 4 mm for the upper extremity, and 5 mm for the trunk or lower extremity.
- The aspirate is one-half to equal the amount of tumescent that was infused.

- I usually do not use a tourniquet for extremity lesions.
- A pressure dressing is applied, and the incisions are closed loosely to allow drainage.

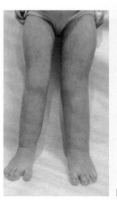 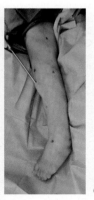 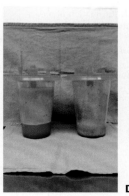 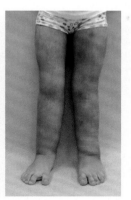

TECH FIG 4 • A 10-year-old female with a capillary malformation and overgrowth of her left lower extremity managed with suction-assisted lipectomy. **A.** Preoperative appearance. **B.** Intraoperative view. **C.** Lipoaspirate. **D.** Reduced circumference of her leg postoperatively.

PEARLS AND PITFALLS

Diagnosis	■ Vascular anomalies are commonly misdiagnosed. ■ Ensure accurate diagnosis prior to operative intervention to prevent erroneous treatment.
Nonoperative management	■ First-line treatment of vascular anomalies often is not operative intervention.
Operative indications	■ Resection of vascular anomalies is indicated for small lesions or those that have failed or are not candidates for other treatments.
Hemostasis	■ Despite being vascular, significant intraoperative hemorrhage rarely occurs. ■ Blood loss can be reduced using epinephrine, elevation, cold saline gauze, cutaneous clips, and careful hemostasis with cautery.
Operative technique	■ Complete excision is not required. ■ Subtotal resection to improve symptoms typically is the goal of operative intervention. ■ Most lesions outside of the face are excised using lenticular excision and linear closure. ■ Round lesions on the face often are best removed using circular excision and purse-string closure.

POSTOPERATIVE CARE

- Individuals who have had significant resections of the head/neck spend 24 to 48 hours in the hospital and are given Decadron to reduce swelling.
- Generally, patients may shower 2 days postoperatively and the occlusive dressing and underlying Steri-Strips are allowed to "fall off."
- Children are managed with dissolvable sutures whenever possible.
- Individuals are examined 2 to 3 weeks postoperatively and 6 to 12 months later if a second stage is being considered.
- Incisions are reinforced with Steri-Strips and are protected from the sun for 1 year.

OUTCOMES

- Patients and their families are counseled that the area involving the vascular anomaly cannot be made to look exactly like the anatomy without the lesion.

- The best outcomes typically are obtained by improving the area of deformity with the simplest approach rather than radical resection and reconstruction.
- The most favorable results are by surgeons who have experience managing vascular anomalies.

COMPLICATIONS

- Operative management of vascular anomalies has a higher risk of perioperative hemorrhage compared to resection of other types of lesions.
- Because the tissues usually are ischemic, suture line dehiscence is more likely than removal of nonvascular lesions; interrupted sutures that are not removed too early can reduce this risk.
- Intraoperative blood loss can predispose the patient to iatrogenic injury of important structures.
- Circular excision and purse-string closure is more likely to have dehiscence than lenticular resection and linear closure.

REFERENCES

1. Wassef M, Blei F, Adams D, et al.; ISSVA Board and Scientific Committee. Vascular anomalies classification: recommendations from the International Society for the Study of Vascular Anomalies. *Pediatrics.* 2015;136:e203-e214.
2. Greene AK. Management of hemangiomas and other vascular tumors. *Clin Plast Surg.* 2011;38:45-63.
3. Hassanein A, Mulliken JB, Fishman SJ, Greene AK. Evaluation of terminology for vascular anomalies in current literature. *Plast Reconstr Surg.* 2011;127:347-351.
4. Greene AK, Perlyn C, Alomari AI. Management of lymphatic malformations. *Clin Plast Surg.* 2011;38:75-82.
5. Greene AK, Alomari AI. Management of venous malformations. *Clin Plast Surg.* 2011;38:83-93.
6. Greene AK, Orbach DB. Management of arteriovenous malformations. *Clin Plast Surg.* 2011;38:95-106.
7. Maguiness SM, Liang MG. Management of capillary malformations. *Clin Plast Surg.* 2011;38:65-73.
8. Hassanein A, Couto J, Greene AK. Circular excision and purse-string closure for pediatric facial skin lesions. *J Craniofac Surg.* 2015;26: 1611-1612.
9. Mulliken JB, Rogers GF, Marler JJ. Circular excision of hemangioma and purse-string closure: the smallest possible scar. *Plast Reconstr Surg.* 2002;109:1544-1554.
10. Couto JA, Maclellan RA, Greene AK. Management of vascular anomalies and related conditions using suction-assisted tissue removal. *Plast Reconstr Surg.* 2015;136:511e-514e.

Functional Burn Reconstruction

22
CHAPTER

David A. Billmire and Kim A. Bjorklund

DEFINITION

- The hallmark of burn injury in children is burn scar and burn scar contracture.
- The tendency toward hypertrophic scarring in children is a major challenge.
- Hypertrophic scars tend to develop in wounds that require greater than 3 weeks to close.
- These scars are raised, red, tight, hard, and often itchy.
- Hypertrophic scarring after burns is common and creates a wide range of cosmetic and functional problems.[1]
- Contractures (inability to perform full range of motion) result from factors such as limb positioning, duration of immobilization, and muscle, soft tissue, and bony pathology.[2]
- Scars result in restriction in movement, particularly when they cross a joint, and increase the likelihood of contracture development.
- A similar burn injury in an adult that requires only initial resurfacing of the wound may require repeated releases and other procedures during subsequent growth and development of a child.
- Growth can be affected with restriction, distortion, and, in some cases, elongation.
- Heterotopic ossification (HO) resulting from ectopic bone formation in the soft tissue around joints can significantly affect extremity motion and function.
- Functional issues are frequently coupled with aesthetic concerns regarding loss of structures, obliteration, and distortion of normal anatomy.

ANATOMY

- Major problems tend to occur across joints and sites of active movement.
- The shoulder, elbow, and hand are most commonly affected by contractures.[2]

PATHOGENESIS

- In normal acute wound healing, myofibroblasts provide collagen and fibronectin deposition and aid in wound contraction over approximately 7 to 10 days.[3]
- However, the presence of myofibroblasts following a burn injury can result in excessive extracellular matrix deposition leading to a pathologic contracture and hypertrophic scarring.[3]
- Although in adults scars typically mature within 12 months, in children, the scarring diathesis may take years to resolve.

NATURAL HISTORY

- The natural history of a burn wound is to heal with re-epithelialization in superficial partial-thickness burns within 10 to 14 days.
- Deep partial-thickness or full-thickness burns heal by combination of contracture and re-epithelialization and are unlikely to heal within 14 days.
- Accordingly, burn wounds that are unlikely to re-epithelialize by 2 weeks should be treated with early operative intervention for excision and split-thickness skin grafting (STSG).
- Sheet grafts should be used in critical areas such as the face and hands.
- Less cosmetically sensitive areas can be covered by mesh graft techniques.
- We have found early sheet grafting of burn wounds (where adequate donor sites allow) to dramatically reduce the need and extent of subsequent reconstruction.
- Wound coverage is followed by an aggressive rehabilitation program with appropriate splinting and positioning in the immediate postoperative period, followed by ongoing physiotherapy, splinting, and the use of pressure garments.

PATIENT HISTORY AND PHYSICAL FINDINGS

- Examination should focus special attention on critical areas, beginning with the airway (neck) and eyes.
- A history of previous airway problems such as inhalation injury and need for tracheostomy should be noted.
- The presence of dry eye symptoms can be subtle in children, and coverage of the globe needs to be ascertained.
- Major joints and hands should be examined closely for restriction of growth and movement.
- Range of motion and functional limitations from scar contractures or HO should be carefully documented.
- In females, the breast buds and/or breasts should be examined to evaluate need for release or reconstruction.
- A systematic anatomic approach to catalogue affected structures is important. Complete or partial loss of limbs, digits, eyes, ears, nose, breast buds/breasts, genitalia, skull, and hair-bearing scalp should be noted.
- Previous donor sites and uninjured skin should be evaluated for future reconstructive efforts.
- Putting all of this together allows one to plan and sequence the reconstructive effort.

IMAGING AND DIAGNOSTIC TESTS

- X-rays should be obtained for significant hand burns.
- Most major joints usually do not require imaging unless the burn wound extended into the joint.
- Joints with functional limitations may benefit from x-rays to look for HO.
- Facial burns (especially those requiring face masks in a growing child) may benefit from monitoring with serial cephalograms to track facial growth and change.

NONOPERATIVE MANAGEMENT

- Nonoperative management begins in the acute phase of the burn injury.
- Many of the secondary problems in pediatric burn injuries can be avoided or lessened by the initial wound management.
- The use of sheet grafting in sensitive areas such as the head and neck and hands can dramatically reduce the need for subsequent reconstruction.

- A rehabilitation program using splinting, stretching exercises, and pressure garments can be effective in modifying the maturing burn wound and scar.

SURGICAL MANAGEMENT

- Secondary burn reconstruction ideally begins when the burn wound matures.
- Burn maturation is a lengthy process that is unpredictable and may take years in children.
- Immature burn scars are hyperemic, red, and raised and should become softer, pale, and flatter as they mature.
- While the scar is maturing, nonoperative methods previously described above should be employed.
- Certain problem areas require early intervention with the knowledge that they may need to be treated multiple times.

TECHNIQUES

■ Contracture Release

- Contractures that may interfere with growth in a child should be addressed surgically.

■ Airway, Eyes, and Lips

- The airway (neck contracture), eyes (ectropion/lagophthalmos), and contractures of the lips result in significant functional deficits including exposure keratitis, blindness, and oral dysfunction that limits eating and mouth care.[4]
- These critical areas should be treated first and early in secondary burn reconstruction (**TECH FIG 1**).

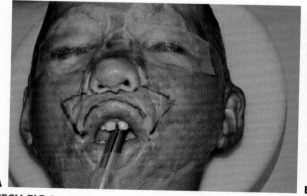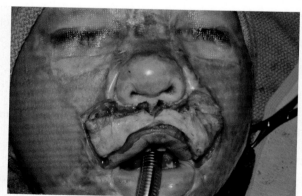

TECH FIG 1 • A. Planned release dart into adjacent unit. **B.** Appearance following release prior to excision of scar.

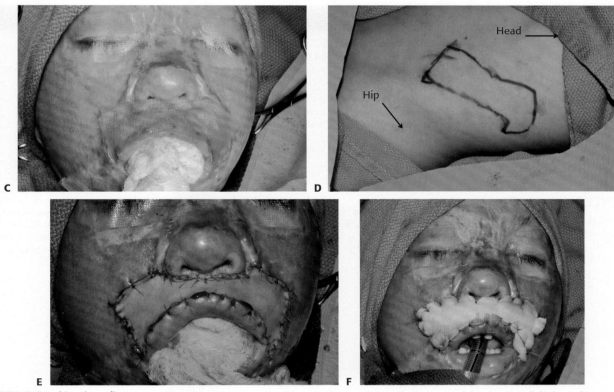

TECH FIG 1 (Continued) • **C.** Creating a template pattern for skin graft; the mouth is packed to expand the site. **D.** Full-thickness harvest site based upon template. **E.** Graft sewn in place. **F.** Stented with bolster tie over dressing.

■ Burn scar contractures

- In approaching burn scar contractures, one should start centrally and work peripherally.
- The neck, axilla, and elbow should be addressed first to allow access to the hand and provide a safe airway (**TECH FIG 2**).

- Depending on donor-site availability, numerous releases can be performed with a variety of techniques from thick-split grafts to free flaps.
- The most common reconstructive techniques include split- or full-thickness skin grafts and local flaps.

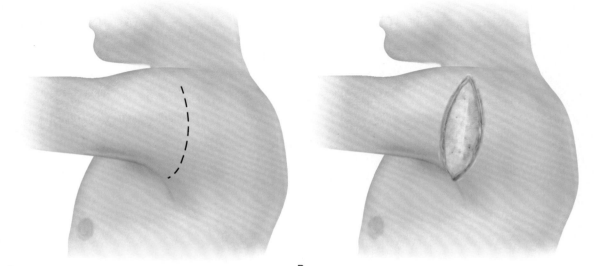

TECH FIG 2 • **A.** Planned incision for tight axillary region release. **B.** Appearance of axilla following release and skin grafting.

TECHNIQUES

PEARLS AND PITFALLS

Contractures	■ Burns unlikely to re-epithelialize by 2 weeks should be treated with early excision and split-thickness skin grafting to reduce the likelihood of hypertrophic scarring and contractures. ■ Early initiation of splinting, stretching, and pressure garments can help prevent contractures and improve functional motion, especially in burn injuries across joints.
Reconstructive planning	■ A systematic approach that examines all affected areas and potential donor sites should always be employed when undertaking burn reconstruction. ■ Critical areas (neck, eyes, lips, and hands) are a priority and should be treated early in secondary burn reconstruction.

REFERENCES

1. Bombaro KM, et al. What is the prevalence of hypertrophic scarring following burns? *Burns*. 2003;29(4):299-302.
2. Schneider JC, et al. Contractures in burn injury: defining the problem. *J Burn Care Res*. 2006;27(4):508-514.
3. Van De Water L, Varney S, Tomasek JJ. Mechanoregulation of the myofibroblast in wound contraction, scarring, and fibrosis: opportunities for new therapeutic intervention. *Adv Wound Care*. 2013;2(4):122-141.
4. Egeland B, et al. Management of difficult pediatric facial burns: reconstruction of burn-related lower eyelid ectropion and perioral contractures. *J Craniofac Surg*. 2008;19(4):960-969.

Harvesting a Skin Graft

David A. Billmire and Kim A. Bjorklund

DEFINITION

- Skin grafts are an integral part of burn reconstruction.
- Various graft options include full thickness, split thickness, allografts, cultured (engineered) skin, dermal substitutes Integra, and Alloderm.
- Full-thickness grafts consist of the entire dermal layer with the overlying epidermis.
- Split-thickness grafts include a portion of the dermis and the overlying epidermis.
- Allografts or skin substitutes are used for temporary coverage and may be biologic or synthetic.
  - Human cadaver allograft, porcine xenograft, and amniotic membrane are biologic temporary skin substitutes.[1]
  - Biobrane double-layer dressing (silicone with nylon-containing collagen) and TransCyte double-layer dressing (silicone with nylon-containing neonatal fibroblasts) are examples of synthetic skin substitutes.[1]
- Cultured skin such as cultured epithelial autograft (CEA) is typically grown from the patient's own cultured keratinocytes and may be coupled with an engineered dermal substrate.
- Dermal substitutes provide an engineered dermis (Integra) or allograft dermis (Alloderm) in preparation for eventual grafting with split-thickness grafts.

Advantages

- Virtually all reconstructive grafting needs can be met by either autogenous full-thickness or split-thickness grafts.
- Allografts may be used temporarily to stabilize burn wounds and create an acceptable bed.[2]
- Dermal substrates may allow the use of thinner split-thickness grafts in donor-limited patients.

NATURAL HISTORY

Split-Thickness Skin Grafts

- Scarring of the donor site is dependent on the site and depth of harvest, patient age, and genetic makeup.
- Once healed, the graft may exhibit dyschromia, increased scar contracture, and decreased durability.

Full-Thickness Skin Grafts

- Typically closed primarily, but in large grafts may require closure with a split-thickness graft
- Less color change and scar contracture and greater elasticity and durability

Prognosis

- Highly dependent on the quality of the wound bed and influenced by factors including vascularity, bacterial contamination, fluid collection under the graft, and shearing

ANATOMY

- Skin grafts can be harvested from virtually any part of the body.
- Physical, functional, and aesthetic characteristics of the recipient site may dictate the preferable donor site location.
- Glabrous or hairless skin can typically be harvested from areas including the sole of the foot, hypothenar eminence, retroauricular, inner upper arm, and potentially the lateral flank areas, depending on the patient.
- Full-thickness grafts can be harvested in areas with redundant skin such as the abdomen, groin, upper arms, and supraclavicular regions.

SURGICAL MANAGEMENT

Preoperative Planning

- Wound bed preparation is critical and must be debrided to healthy well-vascularized tissue. If uncertain of the readiness of the wound bed, it may be prudent to temporize with a skin substitute following debridement.
- Donor-site choice should be matched to the recipient site for characteristics such as color, hair bearing, thickness, and texture.
- Type of graft (split or full) is chosen based upon donor availability and recipient needs.

■ Split-Thickness Graft Harvest

- Tumescence of donor site is frequently performed to facilitate harvest, as well as reduce pain and blood loss. A Pitkin solution (1 L of Normosol with 2 mg of epinephrine [1/500 000]) and ropivacaine 0.5% (maximum dose 3 mg/kg or 10 mL spread out over the entire volume of solution needed) or other tumescent solution of choice may be used (**TECH FIG 1A,B**).
- Split grafts are typically harvested using a dermatome, which is electric, drum, or air powered (**TECH FIG 1C**).
  - For average depth split-thickness grafts, the appropriate depth of the dermatome is 12 to 15 thousands of an inch (**TECH FIG 1D–F**).
- For thick split-thickness grafts, the depth is set to 20 thousands of an inch, whereas for thinner grafts, it is set around 10 thousands of an inch.
- Manual harvesting knives such as the Humby, Watson, or Braithwaite may be used as an alternative to a dermatome. These typically require experience to ensure grafts are harvested at a uniform thickness.
- The graft may be meshed depending upon recipient site goals and availability of donor sites for harvest.
- Meshing will increase the graft surface area and allow for egress of fluid but is not cosmetically desirable.
- Grafts are typically meshed 1:1.5; however, the ratio may be increased to cover a recipient greater area.

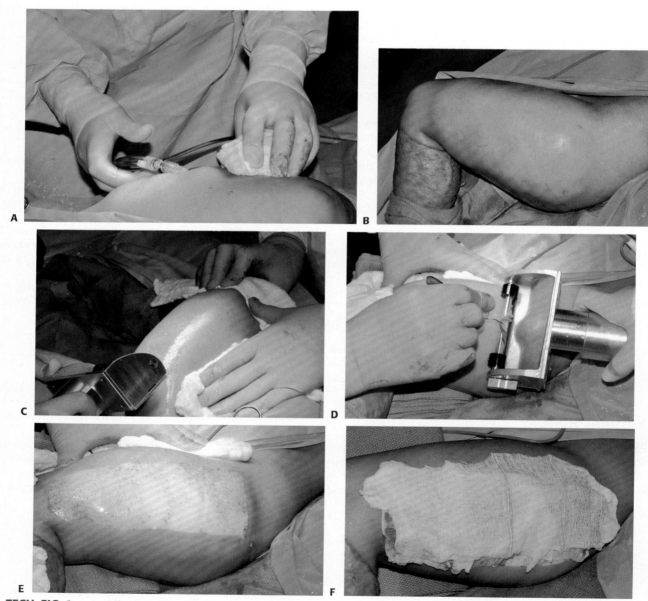

TECH FIG 1 • A. Infiltrating Pitkin solution. **B.** Postinjection. **C.** Harvesting with powered dermatome. **D.** Stopping to check thickness. **E.** Harvested site. **F.** Dilute lidocaine with epinephrine soak.

Fixation

- Absorbable sutures, tissue glue, and staples may be used to tack the graft in place.

- The recipient bed should be healthy, well-vascularized tissue with no evidence of infection. The site should be dry to avoid a hematoma.
- Donor site can be covered with bulky dressing (**TECH FIG 2**).

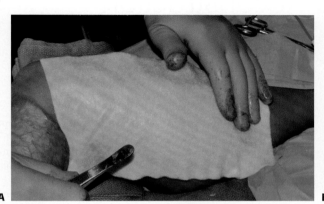 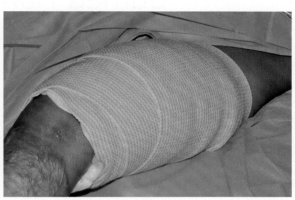

TECH FIG 2 • **A.** Applying Kaltostat alginate dressing. **B.** Bulky occlusive dressing.

■ Full-Thickness Graft Harvest

- A template or specific measurements of the recipient site defect should be used to avoid harvesting unnecessary graft.
- The full-thickness graft is typically harvested in an elliptical fashion to allow for primary closure without dog ears.
- Depth of harvest should include the epidermis and complete dermis.
- Subcutaneous tissue should be removed completely prior to insetting the graft.

- The donor site should be closed primarily in layers.
- Sutures are typically used to secure the graft to the recipient site.

Graft Dressing

- Nonadherent gauze, antibiotic ointment (Bacitracin), bulky dressing, tie over bolster, Reston Foam, and splint should be applied with either a split- or full-thickness graft.

PEARLS AND PITFALLS

Dermatomes	■ Always stop and check dermatome thickness prior to beginning split-thickness harvest.
Tumescent solution	■ Use of tumescent solution facilitates harvest by stabilizing and smoothing the surface, and reducing pain and bleeding.
Boluses	■ Reston foam boluses sewn with absorbable sutures allow excellent fixation, protection, and mobility and may aid in splinting the site.

POSTOPERATIVE CARE

- The graft should remain immobilized until an initial dressing change at 5 to 7 days for split-thickness grafts and 7 to 10 days for full-thickness grafts.
- Erythema, drainage, or foul odor at the graft site should prompt a concern for graft infection and necessitate an earlier graft takedown.

REFERENCES

1. Calota DR, et al. Surgical management of extensive burns treatment using allografts. *J Med Life.* 2012;5(4):486.
2. Shores JT, Gabriel A, Gupta S. Skin substitutes and alternatives: a review. *Adv Skin Wound Care.* 2007;20(9):493-508.

Burned Hand Reconstruction

David A. Billmire and Kim A. Bjorklund

DEFINITION

- More than 80% of all severe burns involve the hand.[1]
- These injuries may be devastating with long-term functional consequences and significant morbidity.
- Burns of the pediatric hand are common and are most frequently thermal type injuries (scald, contact, or flame burns).[2]
- Injuries tend to occur accidently as children explore their environment with their hands.
- However, a glove or stocking appearance to a burn, or an injury not consistent with the history, should prompt concerns for abuse.
- Hand function may be affected through tissue loss, burn scar contractures, impaired growth, and abnormal sensation.

ANATOMY

- Pediatric skin is thinner and has not yet developed the thickened palmar epidermis of an adult.[3]
- Dorsal skin is thin and pliable and provides less protection for underlying extensor tendons and bone.

PATHOGENESIS

- Thin dorsal skin places underlying structures at particular risk for exposure and stiffness.
- Extensor tendons are particularly at risk at the PIP joints where the central slip may attenuate or rupture with exposure, resulting in a boutonniere deformity.
- Burned hands tend to assume a position of wrist flexion, MCP hyperextension, PIP flexion, thumb adduction, and interphalangeal hyperextension.[4]
- Early elevation, splinting, and escharotomies when indicated affect postburn edema and help prevent the development of burn contractures.
- Altered sensation and motor and nerve function may occur secondary to the burn.

NATURAL HISTORY

- Untreated or inadequately treated hand burns frequently result in contractures and long-term functional impairment.
- Early involvement of a multidisciplinary team with aggressive elevation, splinting, hand therapy, and early excision and grafting for deep burns is essential.
- Hand burns that are unlikely to heal within 2 weeks of injury should undergo tangential excision and skin grafting.[5]
- Palmar burns are more likely than dorsal burns to heal spontaneously from glabrous skin appendages and may be less likely to require grafting.
- Approximately 78% of pediatric palm burns heal without the need for grafting; however, flexion contractures of the fingers

and/or shortening of the thenar-hypothenar distance may occur when burns take greater than 2 to 3 weeks to heal.[6,7]
- Secondary burn deformities may occur as a child grows because burn scars do not grow at the same rate as the rest of the child's hand and may impede overall bone and soft tissue growth.[3]
- Secondary burn deformities include intrinsic minus deformities ("claw hand"); palmar cupping deformity; web space deformities; hypertrophic scars and/or scar bands; finger deformities including boutonniere, swan neck and mallet deformities; and deformities of the nail.[8]

PATIENT HISTORY AND PHYSICAL FINDINGS

- Evaluation of the location, size, depth, and previous treatment of the burn
- Mechanism of injury (thermal, contact, chemical, electrical)
- Previous splinting and hand therapy
- Nature of the contracture (extension, flexion)
- Skin and soft tissue adequacy and contracture
- Tendon function—flexor and extensor
- Assessment of sensation and vascular status of the hand and digits
- Joint contractures—passive and active range of motion
- Bony deformities and inadequate growth
- Assessment of the entire upper extremity
  - Wrist or elbow contractures may need to be addressed to adequately position the hand in space.

IMAGING AND DIAGNOSTIC TESTS

- Plain radiographs of the hands and digits should be assessed for bony deformities, joint contractures, or destruction.

SURGICAL MANAGEMENT

- Surgical intervention is warranted for functionally significant contractures not improving with stretching and splinting.[3]
- Multiple surgeries may be required as a child grows for recurrent contractures.
- Thumb reconstruction
  - The thumb contributes up to 50% of function of the hand, and secondary reconstruction is critical in restoration of hand function.
  - When thumb loss remains distal to the interphalangeal joint, function is reasonably well preserved.[9]
  - Web space deepening in these cases can help maximize function with techniques such as the 4 or 5 flap Z-plasty and release with full-thickness skin graft (FTSG) as described above.
  - As the thumb loss extends proximal to the interphalangeal joint, function becomes increasingly more impaired.

- Procedures to lengthen the thumb in these cases include pollicization of the index finger, osteoplastic reconstruction, distraction lengthening, and toe-to-thumb transfer.
- Soft tissue is frequently limited and groin flaps or free tissue transfers are often necessary as a first stage to provide a sufficient soft tissue envelope for the transplanted toe.[9]

Preoperative Planning

- An operative plan should be developed based upon the structures affected: skin, tendon, joint, and bony structures should be addressed based upon their involvement in the contracture.
- Advanced joint destruction may warrant arthroplasty or arthrodesis.

- Hand mobility, strength, and sensation are important to overall function and should be carefully assessed in conjunction with an experienced hand therapist.
- It is important to consider how the burn has previously been treated and if previous surgery has been performed, as it may change the operative approach.

Positioning

- The patient is positioned supine on the operating table. A hand board is attached to the table and centered on the patient's axilla. The affected extremity is then extended with the hand positioned either dorsal or volar on the table.
- A malleable lead hand may be used to secure the hand and fingers.
- A nonsterile tourniquet may be used on the upper arm.

■ Z-Plasty (Standard, 4- or 5-Flap, Multiple Z-Plasties in Series) for Thumb Reconstruction

- Z-plasties are used to break up a tight linear scar when there is unscarred soft tissue that can be transposed and is particularly useful for the web spaces of the hand (**TECH FIG 1A**).[9]
- In circumstances where flaps to be transposed are significantly scarred, consider an alternative procedure such as release and grafting.

- 4-Flap or 5-flap "jumping man" Z-plasties are typically used for web space contracture release and are designed with the transverse limb parallel to the web space and all limbs being equal in length.
- With the 4-flap Z-plasty, 90-degree flaps are drawn at the end of each central limb and bisected to give 45-degree flaps.
- Multiple Z-plasties in series should be used to break up a long vertical scar band (**TECH FIG 1B,C**).
- Incisions are made down through subcutaneous tissue and flaps are elevated as thick as possible, allowing for preservation of blood supply (**TECH FIG 2A**).

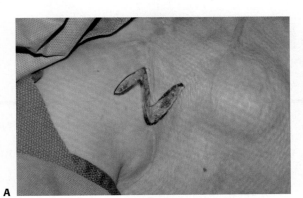

A

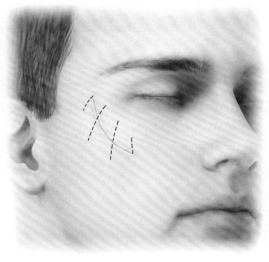

B

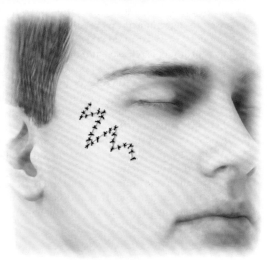

C

TECH FIG 1 • A. Scar band across axilla. **B.** Z-plasty in series. **C.** Final appearance of Z-plasty in series following closure.

- Flaps should be dissected until they transpose easily without any tension (**TECH FIG 2B,C**).
- In the 1st web space, care should be taken in the dissection to avoid injury to the index radial neurovascular bundle, which lies beneath the flap.

- The tourniquet should be released and flaps checked for viability. Hemostasis should be achieved with pressure and cautery.
- Flaps should be transposed into position and secured with 4-0 or 5-0 suture (**TECH FIG 2D**).

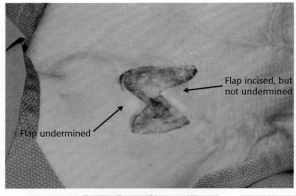
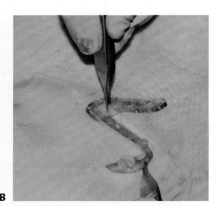

Flap incised, but not undermined

Flap undermined

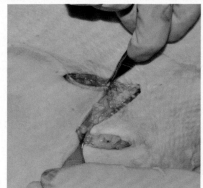
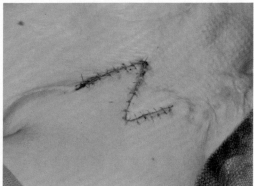

TECH FIG 2 • **A.** Flaps elevated. **B,C.** Transposition of flaps. **D.** Closure.

■ Contracture Release With Full-Thickness Skin Grafting

- Indicated for flexion contractures of the digits, contractures of the dorsal or volar of the hand, and web space contractures or syndactylies

Incision and Release

- Scar contracture is assessed for area of maximal tightness and transverse incision marked at this location (**TECH FIG 3A,B**).
- Incision must extend into unscarred tissue on either side of the contracture band to provide complete release (**TECH FIG 3C**).
- Release is performed by pushing into the scar contracture with the blade while counter tension is applied to the digit by stretching it into extension. The tight thick scar will give way in the release using pushing movement with a fresh blade, whereas the underlying neurovascular bundle will be unharmed, under the appropriate pushing tension.

- Continue to use pushing technique against scar until complete release is achieved.
- Identify underlying flexor tendons and neurovascular bundles and avoid injury.
- Slow passive stretch on a digit can help further stretch soft tissue.
- Following soft tissue release, the contracture is reassessed to determine if any release of checkrein, collateral ligaments, or volar plate is required.
- The tourniquet is released and digits assessed for capillary refill and color. If the digit appears pale with slow capillary refill, it may not tolerate the extent of the contracture release due to the stretch on the neurovascular bundles. In this case, the digit should be extended only to the point where it retains normal color and capillary refill.
- Meticulous hemostasis of the defect site is achieved.
- If there is significant memory of the digit following contracture release, a K-wire can be placed across the joint to maintain its position in extension (**TECH FIG 3D**).
- Color and capillary refill should be checked again after K-wire placement to ensure the digit can tolerate the extended position.

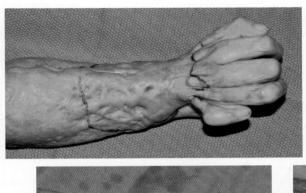
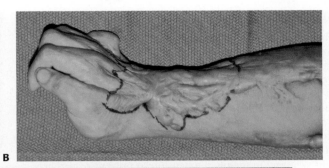
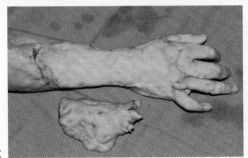
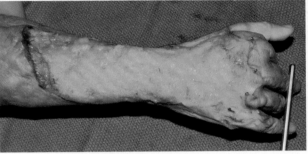

TECH FIG 3 • **A,B.** Dorsal hand burn. **C.** Following release. **D.** Following release and pinning of MCPs.

Graft Placement

- The defect from the soft tissue release outlined using a template from suture packet or Esmarch bandage.
- The template is transposed to desired site of full-thickness skin graft (FTSG) harvest (upper arm if available) and outlined in ellipse.
- FTSG is harvested and defatted. Donor site is closed in layers.

- FTSG is secured at the defect site with 5-0 chromic or plain gut suture.
- A thick split-thickness graft may also be used (**TECH FIG 4A**).
- Saline irrigation with a syringe and catheter tip beneath the graft to flush any clots is performed.
- A compression dressing with wet cotton and gauze is applied to the graft site, followed by a splint to maximally protect position of release and graft (**TECH FIG 4B**).

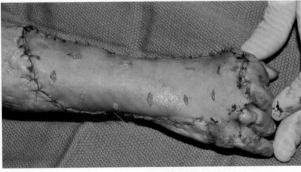
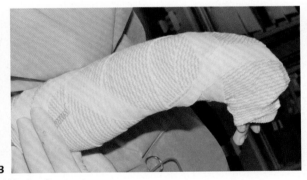

TECH FIG 4 • **A.** Resurfaced with thick split graft. **B.** Dressed with dorsal block splint.

PEARLS AND PITFALLS

Neurovascular limitations	■ It is critical to recognize signs of digital neurovascular compromise intraoperatively and ensure the digit is returned to a position where the neurovascular structures are under less tension, in particular with the PIP joint release when the neurovascular structure may be under tension with full stretching of the joint after release.
Incomplete contracture release	■ Soft tissue contractures must be completely released and joint and ligamentous structures examined in sequence if the contracture remains.
Immobilization of the graft site	■ An inadequate compression dressing or failure of extremity immobilization may result in suboptimal skin graft take.
Therapy	■ Postoperative splinting is critical to preventing recurrence of contractures.

TECHNIQUES

POSTOPERATIVE CARE

- To avoid any mobility at the graft site, a cast is applied (long arm in young child).
- Healing and graft take is assessed at 7 to 10 days, and daily dressings are performed if healing is incomplete.
- If a K-wire is present, it is removed at 4 to 6 weeks. The patient should remain in a cast to protect the K-wire for the duration.
- Activities may be resumed once grafts are completely healed and K-wires removed.
- Night splinting in maximal extension to prevent recurrence of the deformity should continue for 3 to 6 months.

COMPLICATIONS

- Infection
- Wound healing problems
- Limited mobility from recurrent contractures
- Hypertrophic or keloid scarring
- Pain

REFERENCES

1. Pruitt BA Jr, Dowling JA, Moncrief JA. Escharotomy in early burn care. *Arch Surg.* 1968;96:502-507.
2. Choi M, Armstrong MB, Panthaki ZJ. Pediatric hand burns: thermal, electrical, chemical. *J Craniofac Surg.* 2009;20(4):1045-1048.
3. Birchenough SA, Gampper TJ, Morgan RF. Special considerations in the management of pediatric upper extremity and hand burns. *J Craniofac Surg.* 2008;19(4):933-941.
4. Hentz VR. Burns of the hand: thermal, chemical, and electrical. *Emerg Med Clin North Am.* 1985;3:391-403.
5. Pham TN, et al. Results of early excision and full-thickness grafting of deep palm burns in children. *J Burn Care Rehabil.* 2001;22(1):54-57.
6. Sheridan RL, et al. Acute hand burns in children: management and long-term outcome based on a 10-year experience with 698 injured hands. *Ann Surg.* 1999;229(4):558.
7. Barret JP, Desai MH, Herndon DN. The isolated burned palm in children: epidemiology and long-term sequelae. *Plast Reconstr Surg.* 2000;105(3):949-952.
8. Achauer BM. Reconstruction of the burned hand. *Eur J Plast Surg.* 1995;18(4):166-170.
9. Gulgonen A, Ozer K. The correction of postburn contractures of the second through fourth web spaces. *J Hand Surg Am.* 2007;32(4):556-564.

Reconstruction of Burned Eyelids

David A. Billmire and Kim A. Bjorklund

DEFINITION

- The majority of ocular sequelae following facial burns occur as a result of secondary eyelid deformities.[1]
- Burn scar contracture can lead to cicatricial ectropion and lagophthalmos, which may in turn produce exposure keratopathy and in severe cases result in corneal scarring.

ANATOMY

- The eyelids are complex structures providing protection and lubrication for the surface of the globe.
- They contain an anterior and posterior lamella, which are separated by the orbital septum.
- In children, the levator muscle is rarely involved.
- Eyelid skin is naturally thin and may result in a deeper burn than a similar heat exposure elsewhere in the body.
- Contractures most often affect the lower lids.
- Reduction of motion and coverage may be the result of direct scar contracture to the lid itself (intrinsic) or burn scar contracture in sites remote to the lids such as the cheeks, mouth, neck, and forehead.

PATHOGENESIS

- Burn scar contracture affects the motion and excursion of the lids and consequently the coverage of the cornea.
- With deeper burns, lagophthalmos of the lids develops and places the eye at risk.
- Bell phenomenon reflex helps prevent corneal epithelial defects and may be problematic if absent such as in heavily sedated or paralyzed patients.[1]

NATURAL HISTORY AND PHYSICAL FINDINGS

- Patients frequently present with an inability to fully close their eyes and may complain of irritation and discomfort.
- The eyes should be carefully examined to determine the etiology of the dysfunction, noting if the anterior or posterior lamellae are affected and whether there are additional extrinsic burn scars contributing to the contracture.
- These symptoms tend to be better tolerated in children than adults.
- The depth and extent of the eyelid burns should be noted, as well as presence of eyebrows and eyelashes.[1]
- The eyelids tend to demonstrate stiffness and fail to completely cover the eyes, which may be most noticeable when the patient is asleep. Parents should be queried about the status of the lids when the child sleeps. It is also easily noticed when the child is under anesthesia.
- The conjunctiva of the lower lids may be everted and pulled down onto the cheeks.
- The upper lids may demonstrate "clotheslining" where a band of scar runs from the lateral canthus to medial canthus and functions as a fixed point holding the lid up and preventing closure.
- Reconstructive planning should include examination of both upper and lower eyelids, extent of surrounding scar, including cheek and forehead, and donor sites for potential FTSG.

NONOPERATIVE MANAGEMENT

- In mild to moderate cases, eye drops and lubricants and taping can be used temporarily until definitive release is performed.
- In the acute burn phase, corneal exposure may be managed by a temporary tarsorrhaphy, which is replaced as soon as the patient is stable with a formal eyelid release-resurfacing.
- The eyelids are delicate structures and tarsorrhaphies routinely pull out and fail and should not be relied upon for an extended period of time.

SURGICAL MANAGEMENT

- Operative intervention to protect the cornea and counteract lid retraction should be considered a priority in burn reconstruction.
- The timing of surgery is dictated by evidence of lagophthalmos with signs and symptoms of corneal exposure.[1]
- If both lids will require release, it is best to stage them by addressing the more involved lid first for appropriate overcorrection.
- Lower lid
  - Both extrinsic and intrinsic sites of the contracture should be released, but even in a minimally involved lower lid attention should first be directed to the lid itself.
  - As with all burn scar contractures, it should be overcorrected.
  - Although an extrinsic contracture with an unaffected lower lid may be released, often the lower lid will still not achieve a normal position. In these cases, the lower lid will need to be released and overcorrected, even though there is no scar.
- Upper lid
  - The surgical approach is similar to the lower lid.
  - Again the levator muscle is rarely involved and when involved actually results in ptosis. This could be the result of dehiscence or destruction.
  - The lid should be resurfaced and released prior to addressing the ptosis.
  - Depending on the state of the levator, it can be repaired or a suspension technique utilized.

Preoperative Planning

- Review photographs and carefully examine the patient to determine etiology of the problem.
- Choose an appropriate donor site, preferably glabrous and thin. Acceptable sites are an unburned opposite lid, retroauricular or preauricular, supraclavicular, or the inner upper arm for full-thickness skin grafts.

Positioning

- Supine, with shoulders elevated by a shoulder roll.
- Ensure the donor site is accessible.

■ Lower Lid Reconstruction

- The approach is the similar to a blepharoplasty approach for both the upper and lower lids.
- Local anesthetic with epinephrine should be injected.
- In the lower lid, a subciliary incision is performed with a 15 blade and dissected down to the orbicularis oculi muscle.
- The incision should be continued from canthus to canthus, extending beyond the medial and lateral canthi to ensure a complete release.[1]

- Hooks or a Frost suture is used to apply steady traction to the lid margin pulling superiorly as you release the scar.
- The release should continue until the lid margin easily approximates the globe.
- Orbicularis muscle may require dissection if scarred, but typically, the orbital septum is not involved and should not be violated.
- A lateral canthotomy and cantholysis with subsequent canthoplasty may need to be performed.

■ Upper Lid Reconstruction

- Approach is similar to a blepharoplasty with an incision along the likely tarsal crease, approximately 1 cm along the lash line (**TECH FIG 1A**).
- The incision should be extended more medially and laterally than in a standard blepharoplasty (**TECH FIG 1B**).
- Apply gentle traction and continue to divide the scar until the lid comes down.
- As with the lower lid, the release should be overcorrected.
- Do not violate the orbital septum.
- The conjunctival surface should easily redrape over the globe.
- A pattern of the defect is made and transferred to the donor site (**TECH FIG 1C**).

- Harvest a full-thickness graft and defat as necessary.
- In extensive burn cases, a split-thickness graft may be necessary.
- Sew the graft in place with an absorbable suture, such as 6-0 chromic.
- A bolster should be applied such as a thin Reston foam tailored stent over a nonadherent gauze (Adaptic) impregnated with an ophthalmic ointment. The bolster should be sewn in place again with an absorbable suture and left for 7 to 10 days (**TECH FIG 1D**).
- A tarsorrhaphy is unnecessary with this technique as the bolster holds the eyelid in position and allows the child to have some vision in the affected eye.
- Using this method, release and reconstruction of both eyes may be performed at the same time.

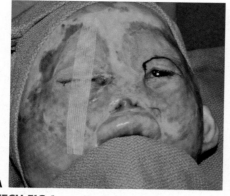 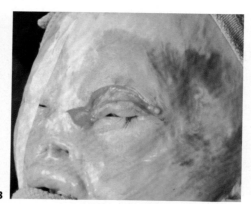

TECH FIG 1 • **A.** Planned incision. **B.** Lid released with medial and lateral extensions.

TECHNIQUES

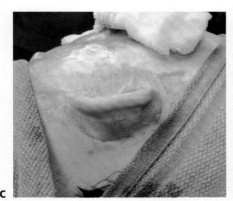

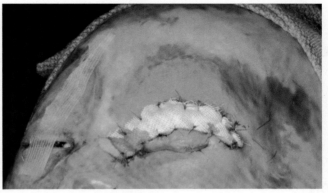

TECH FIG 1 (Continued) • **C.** Post auricular donor site. **D.** Graft placed and stented.

PEARLS AND PITFALLS

Early intervention	▪ Burn scar contracture of the eyelids may result in exposure keratopathy and corneal scarring; thus early intervention is critical.
Tarsorrhaphy	▪ Tarsorrhaphy techniques should only be relied upon temporarily until appropriate scar release and reconstruction can be performed.
Contracture	▪ Careful examination of the eyelids should determine if intrinsic or extrinsic contracture is present.
Surgical approach	▪ Surgical approach is similar to a blepharoplasty for upper and lower lids, and the orbital septum should remain intact. ▪ Full-thickness skin grafts from a thin glabrous donor site are ideal for reconstruction.

REFERENCE

1. Malhotra R, Sheikh I, Dheansa B. The management of eyelid burns. *Surv Ophthalmol.* 2009;54(3):356-371.

26
CHAPTER

Burn Neck Contracture Release

David A. Billmire and Kim A. Bjorklund

DEFINITION

- Burn scar contractures of the neck are relatively common and should be a priority in surgical reconstruction when indicated.
- Burn contractures of the neck may result in deformities that impair functions such as eating and speaking.
- If severe, the contracture can compromise the airway, make intubation difficult, and distort growth of the facial skeleton.[1]

ANATOMY

- Anterior neck contractures have been classified based upon the location of the band and the degree of flexion and extension away from the anatomical position of the neck and jaw.[2]
- The width of the contracting segments and availability of supple surrounding skin is also considered in the classification of the deformity.[2]
- The key anatomical considerations are the burn scar crossing the mobile cervical-mental angle or the manubrium.
- Burn scarring above the cervical-mental angle will primarily affect the chin, lower lip, and mandible.
- When the burn crosses the angle, the mandible and head are pulled into flexion.

PATHOGENESIS

- Neck burn scar contractures in the pediatric patient can be severe secondary to the propensity to hypertrophic scarring, which may develop rapidly in the initial weeks following the injury.
- Significant neck burn scarring creates a persistent downward force on the lower lip, chin, and eyelids resulting in ectropion and AP growth restriction of the mandible.[3]
- Contractures may be severely disfiguring and functionally impair neck motion, making eating and communication problematic.
- The airway may become compromised and intubation difficult.
- In extreme cases, scarring pulls the chin down to the chest wall, elongating the mandible and severely affecting the airway.

NATURAL HISTORY

- The natural history and progression is dependent on the depth of the burn wound, the inherent tendency toward scarring, the age of the child, and the initial treatment and management.

- Neck burn scar can exert considerable pressure on the growing mandible and adversely affect growth.
- Depending on the vector of pull, the AP growth of the mandible can be negatively affected and require later genioplasty or even a BSSO with advancement.[1]
- In the most severe cases where the mandible is drawn down to the chest, mandibular lengthening and eventual setback may be required.

PATIENT HISTORY AND PHYSICAL FINDINGS

- A detailed assessment of the patient's functional limitations is documented.
- Previous treatment of the neck burn injury should be noted as well as compliance with stretching and splinting.
- Note the specific anatomic location of the neck burn contracture, width of scar bands, and whether supple non-burned soft tissue is present.
- Deformities such as lower lip and eyelid ectropion affected by the neck contracture should be noted.
- Occlusion is assessed—loss of chin projection and class II occlusion may develop over time.
- Range of motion and ability to extend the head and neck should be measured.
- The patient should be assessed for potential intubation difficulty.
- Availability of potential donor sites for surgical planning should be assessed.

IMAGING

- Imaging is rarely required unless growth disturbances are suspected.
- A standard lateral cephalogram is useful to follow the patient.

NONOPERATIVE MANAGEMENT

- In the scar maturation phase of the burn wound, splinting and stretching are recommended to reduce the contracture.

SURGICAL MANAGEMENT

- Depending on the severity and extent, contracture releases may be accomplished by a variety of techniques including split-thickness or full-thickness skin grafting, local flaps, tissue expansion, and local flaps or a free flap.
- Operative intervention is warranted for functional deformities that are not amenable to stretching and splinting.

- The majority of neck contractures can be managed with a thick split-thickness skin graft and may also be staged by initial release with a skin graft to assure a safe airway and at a later date resurfaced with tissue expansion or flap.
- In a growing child, releases may need to be repeated.
- Recurrence is also significantly affected by the use of long-term postoperative splinting:
  - In a study of 143 neck release procedures with Z-plasties or STSG, the postoperative use of a neck hyperextension brace for over 1 year following skin grafting decreased the recurrence rate by 40% to 50%.[4]

Preoperative Planning

- Consultation preoperatively with anesthesia is critical for any potential for a compromised airway and difficult intubation.
- Although fiberoptic intubation has facilitated the process, in severe cases, it is appropriate that the surgeon be at the bedside to do an emergent release if the anesthesiologist is unable to establish a safe airway.

Positioning

- The patient is positioned supine on the operating table.
- A transverse shoulder roll is placed to allow maximum extension of the neck.

■ Incision and Release

- Local anesthesia with epinephrine may be injected to help with hemostasis and developing a dissection plane.
- The neck is typically incised along the cervicomental angle and extends from mid axis to mid axis or further if necessary to obtain complete release (**TECH FIG 1A,B**).
- The incision is carried down to a scar-free plane, which usually includes division of the platysma with the lateral extension into the unburned skin on either end.

- The wound is then spread using digital traction or retractors to achieve release of the scar.
- This is aided by extending the neck as much as possible and using continuous slow traction to release the contracture as much as possible.
- It is important to overcorrect the contracture release as there will be subsequent secondary contracture with healing.
- Care should be taken to avoid injury to neurovascular structures deep to platysma.

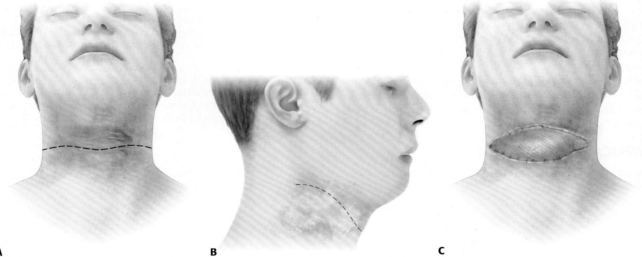

A　　　　　　**B**　　　　　　**C**

TECH FIG 1 • Incision for neck flexion contracture release, anterior view **(A)** and lateral view **(B)**. **C.** Appearance of neck following release and grafting.

■ Reconstruction

- When the wound is spread to its fullest extent, meticulous hemostasis is achieved.
- A thick split-thickness graft (14 to 16 thousands of an inch) sheet graft is harvested, pie crusted, and sewn into place (**TECH FIG 1C**).
- The graft is then stabilized with a tailored Reston foam stent sewn over a nonadherent gauze (Adaptic) coated with Bacitracin ointment.

- Alternatives to Reston foam include a bolster dressing.
- In difficult recurrent cases, it may be necessary to consider the use of a flap as opposed to a graft. Options include trapezius fascial or myocutaneous flaps,[5] supraclavicular flaps,[6,7] or a free flap of choice.
- Integra dermal substitute has also been described as a reconstructive option.[8]

T E C H N I Q U E S

PEARLS AND PITFALLS

Contractures	■ Burn contractures of the neck require early treatment to prevent compromise of the airway and impairment of functions such as eating, speaking, and growth of the facial skeleton. ■ Anatomically, it is critical to note burn scars crossing the cervical-mental angle, which result in a flexion deformity as the mandible is drawn to the chest.
Airway	■ Preoperative anesthesia assessment is critical for potential compromised airway and difficult intubation.
Surgical technique	■ Ensure complete contracture release in plane deep to platysma with incision along the cervical-mental angle.
Postoperative splinting	■ Postoperative management with neck splinting to prevent recurrence of the contracture until the scar is fully mature is essential.

POSTOPERATIVE CARE

- The foam bolster is left in place for 10 to 14 days.
- Following removal, a neck brace is crafted to hold the neck in an extended position.
- It will be worn ideally 24 hours a day until the scar matures and may be beneficial for up to a year.
- For small releases one can also consider a soft collar.

OUTCOMES

- Despite a successful release, it may have to be repeated due to subsequent contracture secondary to growth in children.
- Factors include the age of the patient, the degree of scar response and the adherence to the postoperative regimen.[9]
- Failure due to significant hypertrophic scarring may require the use of a flap; however, even flaps can fail as surrounding scar may create tension and result in vascular compromise to the flap.
- Once a stable neck release is obtained, it is often possible to replace the grafted area at a later date by using tissue expansion to expand the unburned skin on the lateral neck and supraclavicular area if available.

COMPLICATIONS

- The major complications are graft loss and recurrence of the contracture.

REFERENCES

1. Katsaros J, et al. Facial dysmorphology in the neglected paediatric head and neck burn. *Br J Plast Surg*. 1990;43(2):232-235.
2. Onah II. A classification system for postburn mentosternal contractures. *Arch Surg*. 2005;140(7):671-675.
3. Upadhyaya DN, et al. Our experience in reconstructing the burn neck contracture with free flaps: are free flaps an optimum approach? *Indian J Burns*. 2013;21(1):42.
4. Waymack JP. Release of burn scar contractures of the neck in paediatric patients. *Burns*. 1986;12(6):422-426.
5. Zheng XY, et al. Extended lower trapezius myocutaneous flap in burn scar reconstruction of the face and neck of children. *Pediatr Surg Int*. 2011;27(12):1295-1300.
6. Margulis A, et al. The expanded supraclavicular flap, prefabricated with thoracoacromial vessels, for reconstruction of postburn anterior cervical contractures. *Plast Reconstr Surg*. 2007;119(7):2072-2077.
7. Pallua N, Demir E. Postburn head and neck reconstruction in children with the fasciocutaneous supraclavicular artery island flap. *Ann Plast Surg*. 2008;60(3):276-282.
8. Lorenz C, et al. Early wound closure and early reconstruction. Experience with a dermal substitute in a child with 60 per cent surface area burn. *Burns*. 1997;23(6):505-508.
9. Germann G, Cedidi C, Hartmann B. Post-burn reconstruction during growth and development. *Pediatr Surg Int*. 1997;12(5-6):321-326.

Adolescent Burned Breast Reconstruction

David A. Billmire and Kim A. Bjorklund

DEFINITION

- Burned breast contractures and loss are a common occurrence in females who sustain major burns injuries prior to adolescence.
- Knowledge of the importance of preserving the breast bud in preadolescent females has lessened the need for complete reconstruction.[1,4]
- In the acute burn phase, debridement should be kept to a minimum in the area of the nipple areolar area.[2]

PATHOGENESIS

- With the onset of puberty, the breast bud will begin to grow and expand the overlying skin acting much like a tissue expander.[4]
- Any overlying scar can cause restriction and/or distortion of the maturing breast mound.
- Additionally, full-thickness tissue loss from the burn injury surrounding the breast bud will cause additional loss in the eventual volume of the breast.
- Complete loss of the breast bud itself will result in a smaller or absent breast.
- Burn wounds may also result in the loss of the nipple areolar complex, despite the development of an acceptable breast mound.

NATURAL HISTORY

- Full-thickness and deep second-degree burn injuries to the female chest warrant special care in the acute burn wound and careful management in the subsequent time period prior to development of the breast.[3-5]
- Care should be taken with axillary releases, especially when considering the use of Z-plasties. An inappropriately designed Z-plasty can unknowingly transpose the breast bud into the axilla.
- As the breast develops, the amount of constriction and distortion will become apparent.
- It is advisable to delay release/reconstruction until the breast has reached its full size.
- Rarely, the release may be warranted prior to growth completion and will most likely need to be repeated.

PATIENT HISTORY AND PHYSICAL FINDINGS

- Long-term follow-up for young females with significant chest burns is critical to identify any problems during adolescence.[4]
- Once the breast has begun developing, the patient should be evaluated about every 6 months to assess potential problems.
- The soft tissue envelope of the breast, breast tissue, and nipple areolar complex should be assessed, noting location and degree of scar contracture.
- Age and stage of breast development should be determined at each visit.

- Restriction can be complicated by inherent underlying congenital deformations such as constricted breast, tubular breast deformity, or Poland syndrome. These should be considered in addition to the burn injury deformity.

SURGICAL MANAGEMENT

Preoperative planning

- All areas of constriction and distortion should be noted.
- Breasts are treated with almost entire release and grafting and/or resurfacing.[4,5]
- Typical areas of release are the inframammary, intermammary, and the periareolar sites.
- Reconstruction is typically performed with split-thickness sheet grafts, although dermal templates such as Integra have been described.[6]

Positioning

- The patient is placed supine on the operating table with a shoulder roll and the arms abducted at 60 degrees.
- Graft donor site should be exposed, typically the thighs or legs. The back is also a good choice but requires turning the patient.

Approach

- Both inframammary and intermammary releases are frequently performed at the same time.
- The inframammary release should be at the level of the inframammary fold (which is frequently obliterated by burn scar) and will curve up at the midline, joining the incision from the opposite side (**FIG 1**).

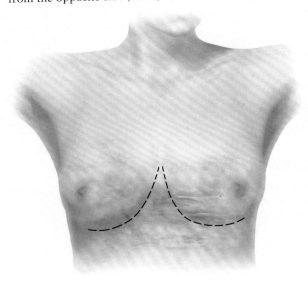

FIG 1 • Incision design for breast release along inframammary fold.

- The incision is made as indicated.
- The underlying breast mound is pulled superiorly to open the release and define the inframammary fold.
- At the midline, the breasts are retracted laterally to separate the breasts into two distinct mounds and define the cleavage (**TECH FIG 1**).
- A periareolar release may be performed following the curve of the areolar, although it may be delayed to a second operation if necessary.

- Sheet grafts (approximately 15/1000ths thick) are harvested with a dermatome from the chosen donor site.
- Grafts are sewn in place and tacking sutures are placed along the inframammary crease. The graft may be piecrusted to allow escape of underlying fluid.
- The grafts are dressed with nonadherent gauze and antibiotic ointment. Moist fluffed gauze is molded along the inframammary fold followed by a tailored Reston foam bolus, which can be sewn or stapled into place.

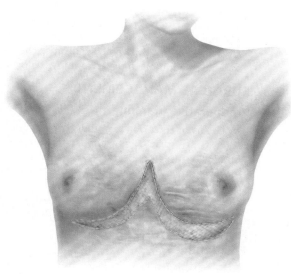
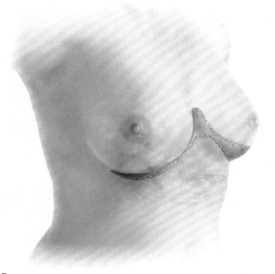

A **B**

TECH FIG 1 • Appearance of breasts following release and grafting—inframammary and intermammary definition apparent, anterior view **(A)** and lateral view **(B)**.

PEARLS AND PITFALLS

Burned breast deformity	■ In the burned breast with inherent congenital deformities (such as constricted or tuberous breast), release and correct the burn deformity first and approach the congenital deformity secondarily. ■ Address the nipple areolar deformity at a later date once scars have matured and edema has settled. ■ Volume loss can be treated with fat grafting at a later date.
Loss of the breast	■ Complete loss of the breast can be approached by any of the techniques used in breast cancer reconstruction ranging from tissue expansion,[7] pedicled flaps such as latissimus dorsi[8] or TRAM flaps, to free tissue transfer. ■ The reconstruction should consider the state of the breast site, the quality of the tissue, and available donor sites. ■ Nipple areolar reconstruction likewise can be addressed by the standard techniques used for breast cancer patients. ■ Contralateral breast procedures to address asymmetry may be required if only one breast is affected.

POSTOPERATIVE CARE

- Bed rest is not required, and early ambulation should be encouraged.
- The dressings are left on for 10 to 14 days.

- After the initial dressings are removed, the patient is dressed in a light padded gauze dressing and a longline or surgical bra until the grafts are stable.
- The patient is then switched to silicone inserts molded for the inframammary fold to apply pressure the maturing graft.

REFERENCES

1. Neale HW, Smith GL, Gregory RO, Macmillan BG. Breast reconstruction in the burned adolescent female (an 11-year, 157 patient experience). *Plast Reconstr Surg.* 1982;70(6):718-724.
2. Armour AD, Billmire DA. Pediatric thermal injury: acute care and reconstruction update. *Plast Reconstr Surg.* 2009;124(1):117e-127e.
3. McCauley RL, et al. Longitudinal assessment of breast development in adolescent female patients with burns involving the nipple-areolar complex. *Plast Reconstr Surg.* 1989;83(4):676-680.
4. Foley P, et al. Breast burns are not benign: long-term outcomes of burns to the breast in pre-pubertal girls. *Burns.* 2008;34(3):412-417.
5. MacLennan SE, Wells MD, Neale HW. Reconstruction of the burned breast. *Clin Plast Surg.* 2000;27(1):113-119.
6. Palao R, Gomez P, Huguet P. Burned breast reconstructive surgery with Integra dermal regeneration template. *Br J Plast Surg.* 2003;56(3):252-259.
7. Versaci AD, Balkovich ME, Goldstein SA. Breast reconstruction by tissue expansion for congenital and burn deformities. *Ann Plast Surg.* 1986;16(1):20-31.
8. Bishop JB, Fisher J, Bostwick J III. The burned female breast. *Ann Plast Surg.* 1980;4(1):25.

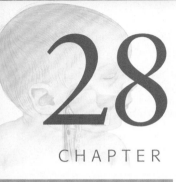

28

CHAPTER

Pressure Injuries (Sacral and Pelvic Region, Columella—From CPAP)

David A. Billmire and Kim A. Bjorklund

DEFINITION

- A pressure injury is a localized injury of skin and underlying tissue secondary to prolonged pressure, frequently in combination with shear forces.
- Severity ranges from nonblanchable erythema to full-thickness tissue loss.
- Common locations are over bony prominences such as the sacrum, coccyx, ischium, and heels.
- In the pediatric population, children with special needs and those who are critically ill are at particularly high risk for pressure injuries.[1]

PATHOGENESIS

- Pressure injury formation is a complex process that involves numerous factors.[2]
  - Extrinsic contributing factors include pressure, friction, and shear.
  - Intrinsic factors include local tissue ischemia, decreased autonomic control, infection, loss of sensation, decreased mental status, fecal or urinary incontinence, anemia, and hypoproteinemia.[3,4]
- As muscle is more sensitive to pressure than is skin, areas with a significant amount of muscle may be susceptible to an inverted cone pattern of injury, in which most of the necrosis is deep to the skin.[5]
- Particular risk factors in the pediatric population have been identified[1,6]:
  - Paraplegia, sensory impairment
  - Cognitive impairment
  - Kyphoscoliosis or kyphosis
  - Chronic fecal or urinary soiling
  - Trauma
  - Immobility
  - Poor nutrition

NATURAL HISTORY[7]

- Nonblanchable erythema may be observed within 30 minutes of unrelieved pressure and typically disappears within 1 hour after pressure is eliminated.
- Ischemia develops after pressure is present for 2 to 6 hours.
- Necrosis may occur if pressure is not relieved within 6 hours.
- Ulceration tends to occur over bony prominences within 2 weeks after development of necrosis.

PATIENT HISTORY AND PHYSICAL FINDINGS

- Determine factors contributing to the pressure injury (extrinsic and intrinsic) and whether they can be eliminated postoperatively.

- Note any chronic medical conditions contributing to the pressure injury, such as myelodysplasia, cerebral palsy, paraplegia, and scoliosis.
- Note any temporary conditions contributing to the pressure injury (prolonged immobility, repetitive trauma) that require resolution.
- Ambulatory status
- Previous pressure injuries
- Compliance and motivation with treatment
- Assess risk factors using Braden Scale, including mobility, activity, sensation, moisture, friction/shear, and nutrition.
- Assess sensation and lower extremity motor function, including spasticity.
- Palpate for any fluctuance or bony prominences.
- Note any signs of infection such as warmth, erythema, tenderness, purulent drainage, and systemic signs of infection.
- Assess ongoing factors that may be contributing to wound breakdown, such as items causing pressure, spasticity, and fecal or urinary incontinence.
- Staging of pressure injuries based on the updated guidelines of National Pressure Ulcer Advisory Panel[8]:
  - Stage 1: Nonblanchable erythema of intact skin
  - Stage 2: Partial-thickness skin loss with exposed dermis
  - Stage 3: Full-thickness skin loss
  - Stage 4: Full-thickness skin and tissue loss
  - Unstageable pressure injury: Obscured full-thickness skin and tissue loss
  - Deep tissue pressure injury: Persistent nonblanchable deep red, maroon, or purple discoloration

IMAGING AND DIAGNOSTIC STUDIES

- Nutritional assessment (including albumin, prealbumin, electrolytes)
- Wound cultures if concern for infection
- WBC and ESR if concern for infection/osteomyelitis
- MRI or CT scan may help in identification of osteomyelitis and communicating sinus tracts.
- Bone biopsy and culture if concern for osteomyelitis prior to treatment with antibiotics

NONOPERATIVE MANAGEMENT

- Generally indicated for stage 1 and 2 pressure injuries
- Correct nutritional deficiencies and medical comorbidities.
- Control spasticity.
- Treat infection with local wound care and culture-directed antibiotics.
- Cleaning, debridement (mechanical, autolytic, enzymatic, sharp), and local wound care of pressure injuries

- Local wound care should be adjusted based on the nature of the wound (exudative, granulating, fibrinous).
- Pressure relief through frequent repositioning and protective padding; support surfaces that minimize pressure and reduce shear.
- Prevent contamination from urinary and fecal soiling.
- Routine inspection by caregivers for early pressure changes and timely referrals during growth spurts for assessment of orthotics, prosthetics, or wheelchairs are critical.

SURGICAL MANAGEMENT

- Surgery is indicated for large stage 3 or 4 pressure injuries that require debridement and reconstruction.
  - Goals include preventing osteomyelitis and protein loss through the wound; improving function, hygiene, and quality of life; and reducing rehabilitation and wound care costs.[8]
- Ischial pressure injuries: Common reconstruction options include gluteal muscle rotation flaps, posterior thigh V-Y advancement flap (hamstring muscles may be included if nonambulatory), or gracilis musculocutaneous flap.

- Sacral pressure injuries: Common reconstruction includes bilateral V-to-Y gluteus advancement, gluteus maximus myocutaneous flap, and superior gluteal artery perforator flap.[8]
- Coccygeal pressure injuries can be treated with coccygectomy.
- Trochanteric pressure injuries are typically reconstructed with tensor fascia lata flap.

Preoperative Planning

- Identify and address causes of the pressure injury.
- Control comorbidities.
- Optimize nutritional status, including serum albumin and hemoglobin.
- Consider diverting colostomy and catheterization to minimize urinary and fecal soiling.
- Careful consideration of future pressure sores in planning of operative technique

Positioning

- The patient is positioned prone on the operating table with pressure points well padded.
- General anesthesia is administered.

■ Debridement

- Completely excise injured area, bursa, scar, and all necrotic tissue.
- Debride all nonviable bone and calcifications.
- Bony debridement should continue until healthy bleeding bone is apparent.
- Biopsy of underlying bone should be sent for culture and pathology.

- Reconstruct by filling dead space with well-vascularized muscle or fascial flaps inset without tension.
- Pressure injury recurrence or formation in new locations should be carefully considered in reconstructive planning.
- Drains should be placed under the flap.

■ V-Y Advancement Flap for Ischial Pressure Injuries

- V-Y biceps femoris musculocutaneous advancement flap design for ischial pressure injury (**TECH FIG 1A**).
- Reconstructed ischial pressure injury with V-Y biceps femoris flap (**TECH FIG 1B**).

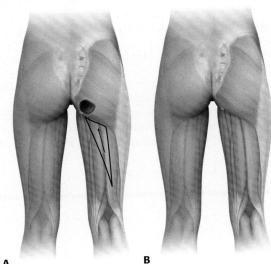

A **B**

TECH FIG 1 • A. V-Y biceps femoris musculocutaneous advancement flap design for ischial pressure injury. **B.** Reconstructed ischial pressure injury with V-Y biceps femoris flap.

■ Gluteus Maximus Myocutaneous Flap

- Unstageable right ischial pressure injury prior to debridement (**TECH FIG 2A**)
- Following debridement, a gluteal rotation flap design is outlined (**TECH FIG 2B**).
- The defect from the pressure injury is triangulated with the apex toward the flap pedicle.

- Rotation flap is outlined approximately 5 times the length of the defect base.
- Gluteal skin and muscle are incised, and the flap is elevated until it can be mobilized into the defect (**TECH FIG 2C**).
- A small back cut can be performed at the end of the rotation flap.
- Flap should be closed in layers over suction drains (**TECH FIG 2D**).

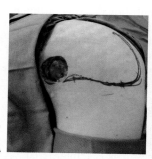 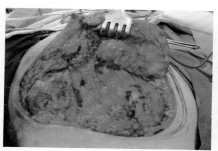 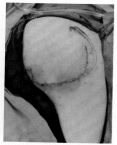

TECH FIG 2 • A. Ischial defect following debridement with gluteal rotation flap design outlined. **B.** Gluteal skin and muscle are incised and the flap elevated until it can be mobilized into the defect. **C.** Flap should be closed in layers over suction drains.

■ Bilateral V-to-Y Advancement of Gluteal Muscles

- Following debridement of sacral pressure injury, bilateral V-Y gluteal flaps are marked extending from the edges of the debrided pressure injury at the sacrum medially and including the entire gluteal region (**TECH FIG 3A**).
- Skin incisions are performed, and the gluteus maximus muscle is identified.
- It is detached from sacral attachments medially and iliac crest attachments superiorly.
- Superior and inferior gluteal vessels must be preserved.
- The lateral and inferior aspects of the myocutaneous flap are incised and elevated at the edges to allow for advancement.
- Gluteus myocutaneous flaps are then advanced to the midline.
- Closure is performed in a V-to-Y fashion (**TECH FIG 3B**).
- Suction drains are placed under each flap.
- Large absorbable sutures such as 2-0 Vicryl or PDS should be used for deep tissue approximation.
- Deep dermal and subcuticular layers should then be closed.

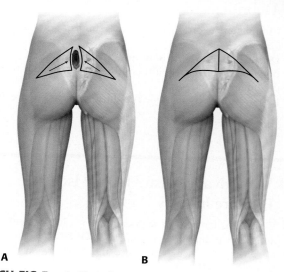

TECH FIG 3 • A. Bilateral V-Y gluteal myocutaneous flaps extend from the edges of the sacral pressure injury at the sacrum medially and include the entire gluteal region. **B.** Closure is performed in a V-to-Y fashion.

PEARLS AND PITFALLS

General	■ Ensure the underlying etiology of the pressure injury is corrected prior to surgical reconstruction. ■ Comorbidities, nutritional deficiencies, fecal/urinary contamination, infection/osteomyelitis, and postoperative pressure relief plan must be addressed prior to reconstruction. ■ Plan flap reconstruction accounting for possible recurrence of the pressure injury and new pressure injury.
Debridement	■ Adequate debridement for the pressure injury is critical to a successful outcome. ■ Complete excision of the bursa as well as any nonviable tissue is essential. ■ Failure to adequately debride bone or bursa may lead to failure of the reconstruction. ■ Consider staging the reconstruction if there are uncertainties regarding infection or tissue/bone viability.
Ischial, sacral, trochanteric pressure injuries	■ Ambulatory status of the patient must be determined if considering use of gluteal or hamstring muscles in flap reconstruction. ■ Gluteal rotation, posterior thigh, and TFL flaps must be designed with adequate dimensions to fill the defect. ■ Ensure the vascular pedicle is preserved in design and dissection of flap. ■ Ensure the flap is not inset under tension. ■ Do not excise dog ears or extra tissue. ■ Always close flaps over a drain.

POSTOPERATIVE CARE

■ Patients should be non–weight bearing on the operative site for up to 6 weeks postoperatively.

■ Prone or lateral decubitus positioning should be maintained to avoid pressure on the site.

■ Pressure relief adjuncts such as low air loss beds should be used to prevent development of additional pressure injuries.

■ Nutrition status should be closely monitored in the postoperative period to promote good wound healing.

■ After wounds are healed, sitting protocols should be used to gradually increase the amount of time spent sitting.

■ Pressure relief should be performed every 15 minutes when in the seated position.[9]

OUTCOMES

■ Pressure injuries represent a major burden of illness, affecting the quality of life of patients and their families.[10]

■ For patients at high risk for pressure injuries, it is critical that pressure relief measures—such as specialized support surfaces, frequent repositioning, and efforts to minimize shear, moisture, and spasticity—are adhered to.

■ Optimizing nutrition and limiting medical comorbidities are also essential in avoiding a high likelihood of recurrence.

■ High-risk patients should be followed regularly by a physiatrist for evaluation and care.

■ Education on prevention and treatment of pressure injuries is critical to successful outcomes.

COMPLICATIONS

■ Hematoma
■ Seroma—important to maintain suction drain beneath reconstruction until minimal output

■ Wound dehiscence—if small, may heal with local wound care and offloading pressure

■ Wound infection

■ Recurrence is high if patients who are noncompliant or do not have medical management optimized preoperatively are at high risk of postoperative recurrence.

REFERENCES

1. Okamoto GA, Lamers JV, Shurtleff DB. Skin breakdown in patients with myelomeningocele. *Arch Phys Med Rehabil.* 1983;64(1):20-23.
2. Crenshaw RP, Vistnes LM. A decade of pressure sore research: 1977-1987. *J Rehabil Res Dev.* 1989;26:63.
3. Enis J, Sarmiento A. The pathophysiology and management of pressure sores. *Orthop Rev.* 1973;2:26.
4. Maklebust J. Pressure ulcers: etiology and prevention. *Nurs Clin North Am.* 1987;22:359.
5. Bouten CV, Oomens CW, Baaijens FP, Bader DL. The etiology of pressure ulcers: skin deep or muscle bound? *Arch Phys Med Rehabil.* 2003;84:616.
6. Pallija G, Mondozzi M, Webb AA. Skin care of the pediatric patient. *J Pediatr Nurs.* 1999;14(2):80-87.
7. Edberg EL, Cerny K, Stauffer ES. Prevention and treatment of pressure sores. *Phys Ther.* 1973;53:246.
8. National Pressure Ulcer Advisory Panel (NPUAP). NPUAP Pressure injury stages. NPUAP website. http://www.npuap.org/resources/educational-and-clinical-resources/npuap-pressure-injury-stages/. Published April 13, 2016; accessed October 18, 2017.
9. Kierney PC, Engrav LH, Isik FF, et al. Results of 268 pressure sores in 158 patients managed jointly by plastic surgery and rehabilitation medicine. *Plast Reconstr Surg.* 1998;102:765.
10. Franks PJ, Morfatt CJ. Focus on wound management: quality of life issue in chronic wound management. *Br J Community Nurs.* 1999;4(6):283-284.

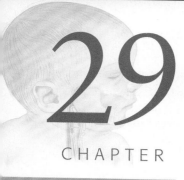

29
CHAPTER

Pressure Injuries

Lawrence J. Gottlieb and Maureen Beederman

DEFINITION

- A pressure injury is a soft tissue injury due to the complex interplay of tissue deformation, stress, strain and ischemia from unrelieved pressure, shear, and friction typically overlying bony prominence.[1]
- The standard for classifying pressure injuries is based on the four grades originally described by Shea in 1975.[2]
- Grades I and II have potentially reversible acute inflammatory reactions involving all soft tissue layers; grade III has full-thickness tissue loss, extending to fascia; and grade IV extends through the deep fascia to bone.
- Skin loss in grades I and II is thought to be more likely due to shear, friction, and maceration rather than pressure per se.
- Over time, refinements have been made to this classification with the most recent being a six-stage classification by The National Pressure Ulcer Advisory Panel during their 2016 Staging Consensus Conference.[3]

ANATOMY

- Pressure injuries typically occur over bony prominences and are dependent on patient positioning.
  - Supine: greatest pressure overlying heels, sacrum, occiput, and scapula
  - Sitting: greatest pressure at ischial tuberosities, elbows
  - Lateral decubitus: greatest pressure over greater trochanters (often accompanied by hip flexion contractures), fibular head, and malleoli
- Pressure injuries also occur due to inadvertent pressure from external objects pressing on the skin (ie, IV connectors, side rail of bed pressing on the skin or small object in shoe of the patient with neuropathy) or securing devices too tight (ie, nasal tubes, CPAP devices).
- Extrusion of internal objects (ie, hardware or internal prosthetic or tubing) is generally caused by the same pathophysiology of classic pressure injuries over bony prominences.

PATHOGENESIS

- Unrelieved pressure
  - External pressure greater than capillary pressure leads to decreased blood flow and tissue ischemia, eventually causing tissue necrosis.
  - Pounds-per-square-inch pressure highest in thin patients over bony prominences. Obese patients are able to distribute pressure better.[4]
- Reperfusion injury
  - Tissue loss after restoration of blood flow and generation of oxygen free radicals after relief of pressure

- Deformation injury of cells
  - Local cell damage and death
- Tissue breakdown may also occur due to
  - Friction
  - Shearing forces
  - Moisture/maceration
- Tissue breakdown is more likely with circulatory disturbances.
- The presence of infection and edema can influence the wound environment and ultimately the extent of necrosis.

NATURAL HISTORY

- Pressure injuries are "inside-out" injuries caused by soft tissue damage from unrelieved pressure on the skin, typically overlying bony prominences.
- Tissues most sensitive to pressure die first.
  - Nerve and muscle are the most sensitive to ischemia from pressure, which is why there is no muscle or major nerves between the skin and bony prominences in any area of the body.
  - Subcutaneous fat dies first in the typical pressure injury occurring over bony prominences.
  - Skin is one of the most resistant tissues to pressure. The earliest changes seen in the skin (ie, swelling and erythema of stage 1 pressure injuries) generally reflect injury to the tissues beneath.
  - Skin breakdown without underlying tissue loss (stage II) is generally due to shearing, friction, and maceration and not pressure per se.
  - The tissue type most resistant to pressure is fascia, which has very low metabolic demands.
- "Iceberg effect": by the time that there is any evidence of pressure injury in the skin, there is significant tissue destruction beneath; the skin findings are only the "tip of the iceberg."
- Although pressure injuries are typical in debilitated, immobile, and/or insensate patients, they are not inevitable and indeed should be preventable in most situations.
- Prevention is directly related to educating and motivating patients and or caregivers in
  - Recognizing risks in various situations
  - Pressure-relief training
    - Relieving pressure every 15 minutes when seated or for 5 minutes every 2 hours when in decubitus position will generally prevent pressure injuries.
  - Providing resources (eg, cushions for seats)
  - Compliance
- Change in caregivers and/or intermittent psychological disturbance (such as depression) correlate with pressure injury development and recurrence.

- Evaluation and coordination with a rehabilitative team preoperatively leads to the least incidence of recidivism.[5,6]

PATIENT HISTORY AND PHYSICAL FINDINGS

- Patients at risk
  - Patients with diminished mobility
    - Paralyzed patients
      - Spinal cord injury, disease, or dysfunction
      - Patients under anesthesia or deep sedation during surgery or undergoing procedure or treatment requiring prolonged immobilization (eg, ECMO)
    - Patients requiring others to move them
      - Patients with quadriplegia
      - Patients who are debilitated due to cerebral dysfunction (stroke, intoxication, infection)
  - Debilitated patients in acute care and long-term care facilities
  - Patients with diminished sensation
    - Spinal cord injury, disease, or dysfunction
    - Peripheral neuropathy
- Assess for muscle spasticity, which increases the risk of shearing forces and friction and postoperative healing issues if not controlled.
- Assess for joint contractures, which make avoiding pressure on bony prominences very difficult for health care providers.
- Assess for tunneling and pseudobursa formation.
- Assess for involvement of joint spaces and other adjacent structures.
- Assess for bone exposure.
- Assess for infection: soft tissue and bone.
- Assess for urinary tract infections, in patients with spinal cord dysfunction.
- Assess patient and caregiver knowledge, home resources, likelihood of being compliant, and potential social/psychological issues, all of which can affect incidence of recurrence.

IMAGING

- X-rays are helpful for assessment of osteoporosis, fractures, and heterotopic ossification.
- Radionuclide bone scans are helpful in assessing activity of heterotopic ossification.
- MRI is the best diagnostic imaging to evaluate for acute osteomyelitis; however, bone biopsy remains gold standard for the diagnosis of osteomyelitis.
- CT scan or MRI and sinograms are helpful to evaluate for sinus tracts, fluid collections, and tunneling in the pelvis or possible involvement of rectum.

NONOPERATIVE MANAGEMENT

- Nonoperative management of pressure injuries is appropriate in patients who
  - Are prohibitive surgical risk due to comorbidities
  - Demonstrate that they would not be compliant with postoperative regimens
  - Need to be prepared for possible operative management in the future
- Optimize nutrition (sufficient protein, vitamins/minerals).
- Monitor prealbumin levels.
- Check vitamin D levels.
- Promote optimization of general medical care.
- Evaluate cardiovascular, pulmonary, and genitourinary systems.
- Promote smoking, alcohol, and drug cessation.
- Promote treatment of depression.

- Optimize wound conditions.
  - Quantitative bacteriologic assessment of wound with wound tissue biopsy
  - Pathologic assessment of long-standing (more than 5 years) wounds with wound tissue biopsy
  - Offloading/frequent turning for pressure relief
    - Air mattresses/cushioning
- Provide patient and caregiver education.
- Prevent spasticity.
  - Medical management: baclofen, dantrolene, diazepam, botulinum toxin
  - Surgical management: rhizotomy, baclofen pump, peripheral nerve blocks
- Infection control
  - Assess colonization vs infection of wound using quantitative cultures.
    - If quantitative culture shows greater than 10^5 organisms per gram, use a topical antimicrobial (eg, silver sulfadiazine, mafenide acetate, dilute hypochlorite solution).
    - If unable to control bacteria with topical, it may need surgical debridement.
  - Systemic antibiotics used for treatment of cellulitis, osteomyelitis, or joint space infections as well as for any distant infection of genitourinary or respiratory tracts
    - If repeat quantitative culture shows greater than 10^5 organisms per gram, consider additional debridement and/or change in topical antibiotic treatment prior to definitive closure.

SURGICAL MANAGEMENT

- All patients are candidates for surgical debridement, but not all patients are candidates for surgical closure.
  - Candidates for closure should demonstrate (along with their caregivers) an understanding, commitment, and motivation to prevent future injuries.
  - In addition, they must demonstrate compliance with nonoperative management (including nutrition, pressure relief, and wound care) and have the necessary resources available prior to definitive surgical closure.
  - Evidence of improvement of wounds with nonoperative management is a good indicator that patient/family are motivated, have the appropriate resources, and will likely abide by postoperative protocols.
- Surgical options for pediatric patients and adult patients are similar.
  - Consider whether child (or adult) has the potential to become ambulatory in the future when deciding best reconstructive option.
- Optimize nutrition, minimize muscle spasms, and obtain bacteriologic balance in the wound prior to definitive surgical closure.
- Ensure that adequate debridement is performed prior to definitive closure.

Preoperative Planning

- Preoperative evaluation and coordinating with the multidisciplinary rehabilitative team that will care for patient postoperatively has been shown to minimize recurrence.[5,6]
- Assess location, size, and depth of wound.
  - Is there a pseudobursa that needs resection?
  - Is there a bony prominence that needs to be flattened?

■ Is their evidence of osteomyelitis?
  • Does it need to be resected?
■ Is there heterotopic ossification?
  • Does it need to be resected?
■ Review previous surgical interventions and incisions.
■ Consider ambulatory status of the patient.
■ Plan closure with skin graft or flap depending on location of wound and goal.
  ■ If the wound is amenable to closure with a graft, is it the best technique to use or would a flap give a better result?[7]
  ■ If a flap is chosen; determine whether it should be a muscle, musculocutaneous, fasciocutaneous, cutaneous, or perforator flap.
■ Plan obliteration of anticipated dead space.
■ Plan flaps with the understanding that recurrence of pressure injuries is frequent and the ability to reuse a flap is frequently helpful.

Positioning

■ Need to ensure that all bony prominences and pressure points are protected and padded to avoid creating new pressure injuries during surgery.
■ Posterior wounds are generally best positioned prone but may be put in lateral decubitus position if needed.
  ■ Airway needs to be secured well.
  ■ The hips should be flexed for insetting of thigh-based flaps.
■ Ischial injuries may be addressed in lithotomy position.

Approach

■ Adequate debridement includes removal of the pseudobursa and all necrotic, devitalized, and infected tissue as well as removal of all scars if possible.
■ Preliminary bedside debridement can be helpful to obtain tissue cultures and decrease the wound burden of nonviable tissue.
  ■ Long-standing (greater than 5 years) wounds should be biopsied to rule out Marjolin ulcer.
■ Bedside debridement is rarely adequate because of inability to remove all dead tissue without too much bleeding or pain in patients with sensation.
■ The use of methylene blue dye during operative debridement will assist in removing pseudobursa and ensuring all surface tissue is removed, especially in irregular wounds with tracts and tunneling.
■ Bony prominences should be flattened.
■ All nonbleeding infected bone should be removed.
■ Pre- and postdebridement tissue cultures should be obtained of soft tissue and bone.
■ Many patients require more than one operative debridement to optimize the wound or allow for optimization of a systemic condition prior to definitive surgical closure.
■ Once a wound is adequately debrided, determine if the next goal is to close the wound or to reconstruct the part.

■ Closure should be preceded by adequate debridement.
■ The techniques below describe typical debridement techniques and examples of closure or reconstructive options utilizing standard principles and concepts.

■ Surgical Debridement

■ Paint the wound (and/or inject sinuses) with methylene blue dye to stain the pseudobursa, granulation tissue, and other surface tissue to ensure complete removal (**TECH FIG 1A,B**).
  ■ This is particularly important in irregular wounds with tracts and tunneling.
■ An incision should be made through normal skin circumferentially around the wound (**TECH FIG 1C**).

■ Incision should be carried down through normal subcutaneous tissue, beneath all blue-stained as well as indurated tissue and scar converging on any bony prominences if present.
  ■ Wounds that have bony prominences such as ischial and trochanteric pressure injuries should have these prominences flattened, typically with an osteotome.
■ Pre- and postdebridement samples of soft tissue and bone should be sent for quantitative bacteriologic assessment.
■ Postdebridement bone biopsy samples should be sent for pathologic assessment to rule out osteomyelitis.
■ The entire debrided wound should be sent for pathologic assessment, especially in long-standing chronic ulcers (**TECH FIG 1D**).

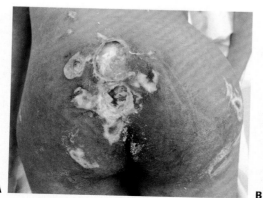
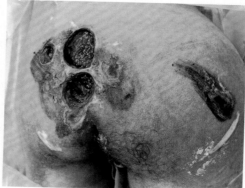

TECH FIG 1 • Debridement. **A.** Sacral and trochanteric pressure injuries after bedside debridement. **B.** After application of methylene blue to help guide debridement.

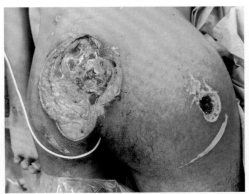
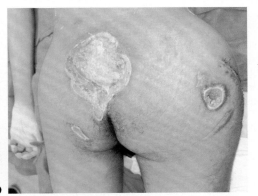

TECH FIG 1 (Continued) • **C.** Immediately after excisional debridement of sacral and trochanteric pressure injuries. **D.** Five weeks later after nutritional repletion.

■ Sacral Pressure Sore Closure

- Sharp surgical redebridement into normal tissue as described above.
- Determine location of perforator vessels with handheld Doppler.
- Large left-sided inferiorly based rotation perforator flap is designed (**TECH FIG 2A**).

- Incisions are made and the flap is elevated above the muscle to large medial perforator (**TECH FIG 2B,C**).
- Skin overlying the left gluteal muscle rotated clockwise to close most of the wound and contralateral skin overlying the right inferior gluteal muscle rotated to close the rest without tension (**TECH FIG 2D**).

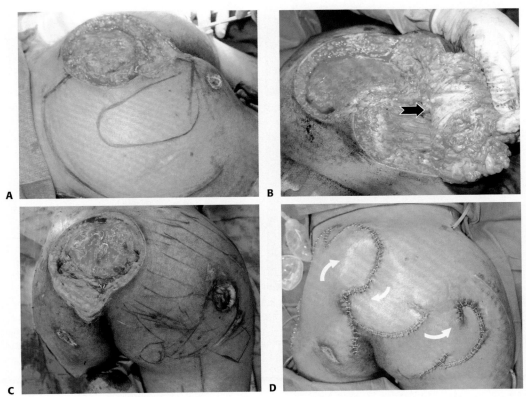

TECH FIG 2 • Sacral and trochanteric pressure injuries. **A.** Design of the left superior gluteal perforator fasciocutaneous rotation flap. **B.** Flap elevated. *Arrow* points to perforator. **C.** Design of the right inferior gluteal myocutaneous flap. **D.** Sacral and right trochanteric pressure injuries closed. *Arrows* demonstrate direction of skin rotation.

■ Ischial Pressure Sore Closure

- Sharp surgical debridement into normal tissue as described above.
- Previously used left posterior thigh flap, based on the descending branch of the inferior gluteal artery, was re-elevated and transposed, and along with a gluteal perforator rotation flap, the left ischial pressure sore was able to be closed.
- Right ischial pressure sore closed with a crescent VY inferior gluteal myocutaneous flap with distal muscle extension to be "tucked" underneath to fill dead space (**TECH FIG 3**).

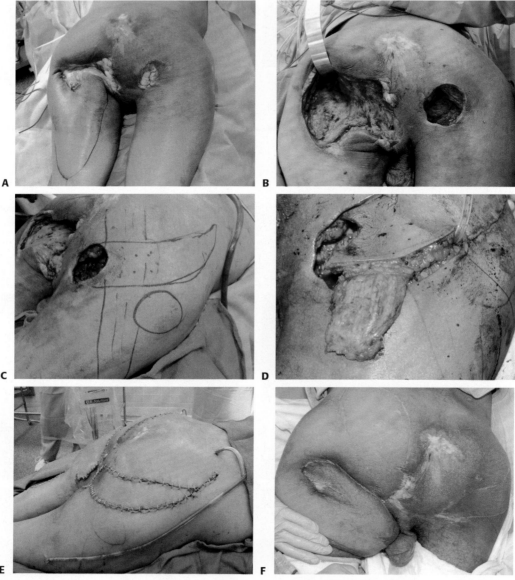

TECH FIG 3 • Bilateral ischial pressure injuries. **A.** Left side recurrent, note design of previous posterior thigh flap. **B.** After debridement. **C.** Design of right ischial closure with inferior gluteal myocutaneous flap with the skin designed to be moved as a V-Y and muscle extension to be folded under to fill dead space. **D.** Inferior gluteal muscle before it is folded under to fill dead space. **E.** V-Y closure of cutaneous portion of flap. **F.** Six-month follow-up of left ischial closure by transposing previous posterior thigh flap and right with inferior gluteal myocutaneous flap.

■ Medial Inframalleolar Perforator Flap

- After determining location of perforator vessels and direction of venous flow, the flap can be designed with the anticipated pivot point centered over perforator vessels.
- Incision is made and carried down through the subcutaneous tissue.
- The flap is elevated toward the perforator.
  - Transposition of flap is less than 90 degrees, so the perforator vessels do not need to be skeletonized.
- The flap is transposed and inset.
- Donor site is closed with a split-thickness skin graft (**TECH FIG 4**).

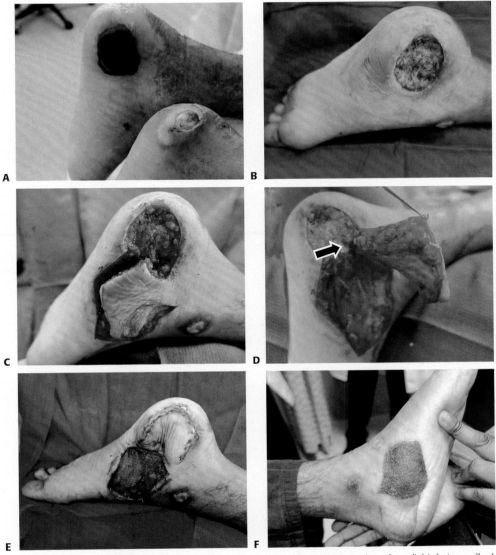

TECH FIG 4 • Pressure injury of left medial heel. **A.** Initial eschar. **B.** After debridement. **C.** Design of medial inferior malleolar perforator flap. **D.** Elevation of flap (*arrow* points to perforator). **E.** Flap transposed and donor site closed with a skin graft. **F.** Stable closure demonstrated 6 months later.

■ Skin graft

■ Flaps are not required for all wounds.

■ A well-vascularized wound bed may be closed with skin grafts or allowed to close by secondary intention (**TECH FIG 5**).

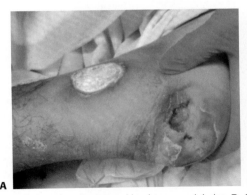

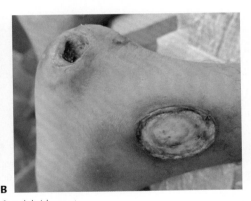

TECH FIG 5 • **A.** Right lateral malleolus and heel pressure injuries. **B.** After debridement

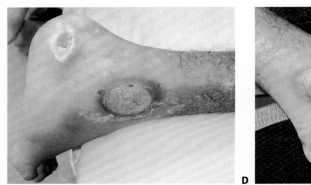
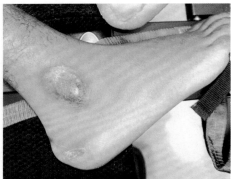

TECH FIG 5 (Continued) • **C.** Five weeks after wound care and nutritional repletion wound closed with a skin graft. **D.** Six months stable coverage of malleolus. Heel closed by secondary intention.

■ Propeller flap

- After debridement as described above make an incision to verify location of the perforator.
- Elevate the flap and skeletonize the perforator.
- Turned 180 degrees and flap inset (**TECH FIG 6**).

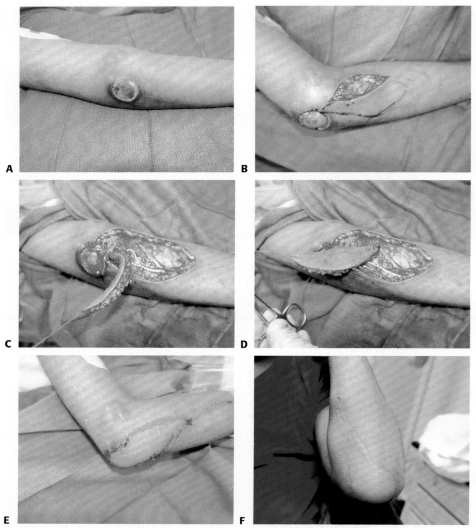

TECH FIG 6 • **A.** Left elbow pressure sore. **B.** After debridement and incision to verify location of perforator. **C.** Propeller flap elevated. **D.** Propeller flap turned 180 degrees. **E.** Flap inset. **F.** Stable closure demonstrated 6 months later.

PEARLS AND PITFALLS

Debridement	■ All patients are candidates for surgical debridement, but not all patients are candidates for surgical closure.
	■ Wide local debridement prior to definitive surgical closure is necessary for successful pressure ulcer coverage.
Methylene blue	■ Paint wound and inject sinuses to help facilitate adequate debridement.
Infection	■ Obtain bacteriologic balance prior to definitive closure.
	■ Assess soft tissue and bone by tissue biopsy cultures.
Flaps	■ Flaps should be well vascularized, inset without tension, and able to obliterate dead space.
	■ Do not burn bridges with closure options; consider flaps that can be reused if recurrence occurs.
Skin grafts	■ Skin grafts tolerate pressure but do not tolerate shear forces well.

POSTOPERATIVE CARE

- Use perioperative antibiotics only, unless postdebridement cultures are positive.
- Closed suction drains should be used to help obliterate dead space, improve tissue apposition, and minimize fluid collections.
- Patients should be nursed on a specialized mattress, air fluidized bed, or in prone position for 3 to 6 weeks postoperative.
- Gradually progress advancement of activity.
- Control/prevent spasticity.
- Continue optimization of nutritional support.

OUTCOMES

- Despite optimization, recurrence rate is high for many patients.
- Minimize recurrence by working with multidisciplinary rehabilitative team preoperatively and postoperatively.[4,5]

COMPLICATIONS

- Acute wound breakdown is generally related to poor surgical planning, with either ischemic flap edges or excess tension on suture lines or a complication such as hematoma.
  - Hematomas are thought to be more common in patients with spinal cord injury due to loss of sympathetic vascular tone and inability to vasoconstrict blood vessels.

- Subacute recurrence (wound breakdown) is generally related to failure to obliterate dead space with fluid collection, which may subsequently get infected.
- Delayed recurrence is generally related to inadequate compliance with pressure preventing protocol.

REFERENCES

1. Olesen CG, de Zee M, Rasmussen J. Missing links in pressure ulcer research—an interdisciplinary overview. *J Appl Physiol.* 2010;108:1458-1464.
2. Shea JD. Pressure sores: classification and management. *Clin Orthop Relat Res.* 1975;(112):89-100.
3. http://www.npuap.org/resources/educational-and-clinical-resources/npuap-pressure-injury-stages/
4. Lindon O, Greenway RM, Piazza JM. Pressure distribution on the surface of the human body. I. Evaluation in lying and sitting positions using a "Bed of Springs and Nails". *Arch Phys Med Rehabil.* 1965;46:378-396.
5. Singh DJ, Bartlett SP, Low DW, Kirschner RE. Surgical reconstruction of pediatric pressure sores: long-term outcome. *Plast Reconstr Surg.* 2002;109(1):265-269.
6. Kierney PC, Engrav LH, Isik FF, et al. Results of 268 pressure sores in 158 patients managed jointly by plastic surgery and rehabilitation medicine. *Plast Reconstr Surg.* 1998;102:765.
7. Gottlieb LJ, Krieger LM. Editorial: From the reconstructive ladder to the reconstructive elevator. *Plast Reconstr Surg.* 1994;93(7):1503-1504.

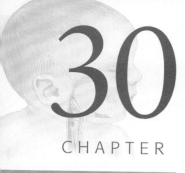

30

CHAPTER

Vascular Lesions

Benjamin C. Garden and Jerome M. Garden

DEFINITION

- Vascular lesions can be classified into two main categories: proliferative and malformations.[1]
- Vascular proliferative lesions are characterized by a proliferation of blood vessels.
  - Infantile hemangiomas are the most common form of vascular proliferative lesions.
  - Other vascular proliferative lesions include kaposiform hemangioendotheliomas, tufted angiomas, and pyogenic granulomas.
- Vascular malformations are characterized by vessels with abnormal structure and normal endothelial cell turnover. Types of malformations include capillary, venous, lymphatic, arterial, and arteriovenous malformations (AVMs).
  - Capillary malformations include nevus simplex (salmon patch) and nevus flammeus (port-wine stain, PWS).
  - Venous malformations (VM) are a fairly common slow-flow type of vascular malformation present at birth. Various names used to describe these lesions include venous angioma and cavernous angioma.
  - Lymphatic malformations (LM) are composed of interconnected lymphatic channels.[2]
    - Older terminologies used include cavernous lymphangioma, lymphangioma circumscriptum, and cystic hygroma.
    - LM can be further differentiated into macrocystic and microcystic depending on the size of the involved channels.
  - AVMs are rare vascular malformations consisting of both arterial and venous components with AV shunting.[2]

ANATOMY

- Vascular lesions may occur on any cutaneous surface but are most commonly found on the head and neck.
- Hemangiomas have been noted to have a nonrandom distribution, with the majority of lesions occurring on the central face at sites of development fusion.[3]
- Capillary malformations are often, but not always, unilateral.

PATHOGENESIS

- Hemangiomas are thought to occur due to a first-trimester developmental error regarding angiogenesis or a result of embolized placental cells. There is a suggested autosomal dominance inheritance.[4]

- Although their exact cause is unknown, PWSs evolve due to a progressive ectasia of the superficial vascular plexus. This progression is likely due to an abnormal neural regulation of blood flow. PWSs have significantly less nerve density and a higher vessel to nerve ratio.[4]

NATURAL HISTORY

- Infantile hemangiomas become evident in the first weeks of life and exhibit a proliferative phase, with continued growth, until around 8 to 12 months. This is followed by a plateau phase, followed by a period of spontaneous regression as the lesion involutes.
  - Initial involution is usually noted with a color change from the original bright red to dull red or gray.
    - It is estimated that completed involution occurs at a rate of 10% per year, such that 30% have involuted by 3 years of age, 50% by 5 years of age, and greater than 90% by 9 to 10 years of age.[3]
    - These lesions occasionally have residual changes, including telangiectasias, atrophy, scarring, or fibro-fatty material.
  - Ulcerations occur in 5% to 13% of infantile hemangiomas.
    - Most frequent locations include the lip, perineum, and intertriginous areas.
    - Ulcerations are painful, increase the risk of infection, and can cause scarring and textural changes.[3]
- Vascular malformations tend to be present at birth and persist for a lifetime.
  - PWS may darken progressively over many years, and occasional lesions develop secondary vascular blebs on their surface. They may also become hypertrophic later in life.
  - VMs are present at birth but may not become obvious until later in life. Occasionally, a patient first notices the lesion after trauma to the overlying area. In those cases, the trauma may cause the underlying vessels to temporally enlarge allowing the patient to notice it for the first time.

PATIENT HISTORY AND PHYSICAL FINDINGS

- The preoperative evaluation for patients with vascular lesions includes a detailed history and exam to determine the type of lesions and to assess the risks of the patient having any associated complications or syndromes.
- Infantile hemangiomas may occur as superficial, deep, or mixed lesions.
  - Superficial lesions tend to appear as bright red nodules or plaques (**FIG 1A**).

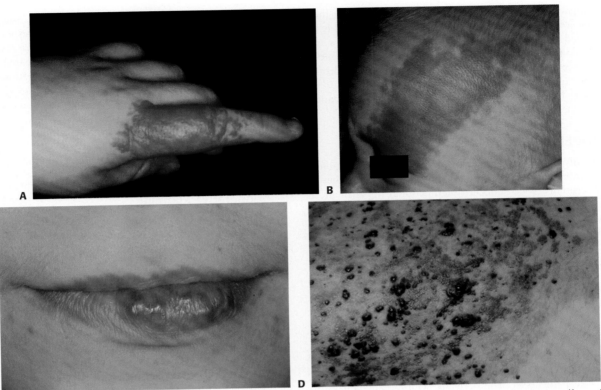

FIG 1 • A. Superficial infantile hemangioma. **B.** Port-wine stain. **C.** Venous malformation. **D.** Mixed microcystic lymphatic and venous malformation.

- Deep hemangiomas are subcutaneous nodules, and usually present with an overlying blue hue, venous network, or telangiectatic vessels.
- Hemangiomas in certain locations may suggest a higher probability of complications or associated findings.[3]
  - With periorbital hemangiomas, an ophthalmologic examination is generally recommended in many cases.
  - Larger lesions of the beard area require evaluation for potential airway obstructions.
  - Hemangiomas on the tip of the nose, the lip, and the parotid areas can have very slow involution periods.
- PWSs are normally easy to recognize with their well-defined red macular stains (**FIG 1B**). They do not proliferate, but will grow proportional to the child's growth. Patients with PWS should be assessed for any associated syndromes that would necessitate additional referrals.
  - The most common syndrome is Sturge-Weber syndrome (SWS), which most commonly occurs with a PWS occurring in the distribution of the ophthalmic branch of the trigeminal nerve (V1).
  - PWS can be associated with many other syndromes including Klippel-Trenaunay, Parkes-Weber, Proteus, Cobb, Rubinstein-Taybi, and Beckwith-Wiedemann syndrome.
- VMs usually present as blue to purple nodules in the skin (**FIG 1C**). They may have prominent surrounding veins and calcified phleboliths within the lesion. These lesions may expand with dependent drainage of venous blood; this may be elicited by placing the patient in the Trendelenburg position or by performing the Valsalva maneuver.[2]
  - Most VM are asymptomatic, although they may occasionally become painful in association with their gradual enlargement and pressure on surrounding structures.

- They may be found in association with syndromes, including Maffucci and blue rubber bleb nevus syndrome.
- Macrocystic LMs, sometimes referred to as cystic hygromas, present as large, translucent masses under normal-appearing skin. Microcystic LM usually present as erythematous to flesh-colored papules, which may be somewhat translucent, and have traditionally been compared to the appearance of frog spawn (**FIG 1D**).
- AVMs may be clinically pulsatile and warm and have a thrill. They present as a vascular stain at birth, with increasing erythema and size with age. They can spontaneously bleed.

IMAGING

- One should strongly consider doing a liver MRI in those patients having five or more hemangiomas due to the increased potential of having visceral lesions.[3]
- Large segmental facial hemangiomas should prompt imaging to assess possible PHACES syndrome:
  - *Posterior fossa malformations*
  - *Hemangiomas*
  - *Arterial anomalies*
  - *Coarctation of the aorta*
  - *Eye abnormalities*
  - *Sternal or supraumbilical raphe*
- Perineal hemangiomas should prompt evaluation for PELVIS syndrome:
  - *Perineal hemangiomas*
  - *External genital malformations*
  - *Lipomyelomeningocele*
  - *Vesicorenal abnormalities*
  - *Imperforate anus*
  - *Skin tags*

- In patients with a PWS, imaging may be necessary if there is concern for a related syndrome, such as SWS. MRI is the preferred screening modality of SWS. Patients with a vascular malformation located in the midline lumbar location may have an underlying AVM, as seen in Cobb syndrome, which would be imaged by an MRI.
- VM can be confirmed or the depth of involvement can be ascertained with MRI with and without contrast.

NONOPERATIVE MANAGEMENT

- Generally, appropriate treatment for infantile hemangiomas is nonintervention.[5] However, in those lesions where there is high visibility, social concern or functional impairment, as well as complications such as ulceration, infection or bleeding, therapy may be warranted.[4,6]
  - Topical timolol can be useful in the treatment of superficial hemangiomas.
  - Treatment using oral propranolol may be indicated for functional impairment, significant ulceration, or lesions with potential for significant disfigurement.
  - Topical wound care is also necessary for ulcerated lesions.

SURGICAL MANAGEMENT

- Lasers are designed to deliver energy precisely into the target chromophore with minimal damage to surrounding tissue.
  - To keep the laser from causing widespread damage to other tissues, the laser exposure should occur faster than the amount of time it takes for the heat to extend significantly beyond the target.
  - Safe and effective heating occurs using a pulse duration equal to or less than the target's thermal relaxation time (TRT). TRT is the amount of time for the tissue to lose half the heat gained from the laser.
    - For PWS, the target venules have a TRT of tens of milliseconds.[4]
- Surgical intervention with lasers for hemangiomas should be used cautiously but can be very helpful, especially for lesions in areas of high visibility or areas of high risk for ulcerations, such as the anogenital area.
  - Laser treatment of ulcerated hemangiomas can lead to decrease in pain and more rapid healing. However, care must be taken because aggressive laser treatment can occasionally induce ulcerations.
  - Lasers can also be used for the treatment of involuted lesions with residual telangiectasis or residual dermal vascular involvement.[7]
  - Lasers can be used successfully in conjunction with propranolol.[8]
  - Excisional surgery of hemangiomas can lead to a more unsatisfactory result than an untreated lesion, and therefore, the risks and merits of surgical intervention should be discussed with the family and surgical removal performed on a case-by-case basis.
- PWS should be treated with laser surgery as early as possible with the natural evolution of these lesions to become more hypertrophic over time. Additionally, children younger than 1 year seem to have the most effective lightening and require fewer treatments than older patients.[4]
  - One should note that laser surgery can be helpful in treating PWS, but some PWSs can partially recur over an extended period of time with aging.

- PWS lesions on the periorbital region, midforehead, lateral cheeks, chest and proximal arms respond best to treatment, whereas the other areas are more resistent.[6]
- The superficial components of VMs may be treated with laser therapy. However, more extensive malformations may be treated via sclerotherapy prior to eventual surgical excision.[2]
- Carbon dioxide lasers used in a nonfractional mode can be used to treat the superficial blebs of lymphatic lesions, vaporizing the tissue nonselectively and sealing the lymphatic channels.
- Embolization and surgical resection are the mainstay of treatment of AVMs.

Preoperative Planning

- A pretreatment consultation is advisable to discuss potential lesional response, number of treatments, expected and potential adverse effects, and aftercare.
- Visual examination of lesion and of patient skin type assists in planning of laser treatment. Optimal coherence tomography, three-dimensional photography, and reflectance spectrophotometry are newer technologies that are being evaluated to assist in objective quantification of preprocedure and postprocedure lesional depth, volume, and color.[9]
- Patients should be advised to practice strict sun protection for at least 4 to 8 weeks prior to treatment. Treatment of a patient with a tan can result in permanent hypopigmentation.
- Patients with darker skin are at risk for hypopigmentation and hyperpigmentation.
- An assessment of the child's ability to tolerate treatment should be made prior to choosing an anesthesia option. Options include topical, intralesional, and general anesthesia.
  - Although topical anesthetics such as topical liposomal lidocaine and a eutectic mixture of local anesthetics (EMLA cream, 2.5% lidocaine/2.5% prilocaine) have been used, topical anesthetics may cause significant blanching of the vascular lesions, making them more difficult to be effectively treated with the laser, as there is less hemoglobin to act as a target chromophore.
    - Special care should be used with prilocaine in infants as it is associated with an increased risk of methemoglobinemia.
  - Most infants less than 1 year of age are restrained and treated without general anesthesia.
  - General anesthesia is appropriate in older children. However, general anesthesia also may be associated with blanching of the lesion. Care should be taken to limit the use of the general anesthetic to as low a dose as safely possible to reduce blanching.[6,9]
- Photographs should always be taken before the initial treatment. Photographs before subsequent treatment sessions to the same area are at the discretion of the clinician.
- Flammability is a risk when using lasers. Water or clear non–alcohol-based viscous lubricants can be used to diminish singeing terminal hairs.

Positioning

- The patient should be placed in a position that allows the clinician to manipulate the laser handpiece without difficulty.
- Infants and young children, who will be undergoing the treatment without general anesthesia, are recommended to be held and restrained with a bear hug by a parent or assistant. Placing an infant in a papoose may be of help in addition to immobilization by an assistant.

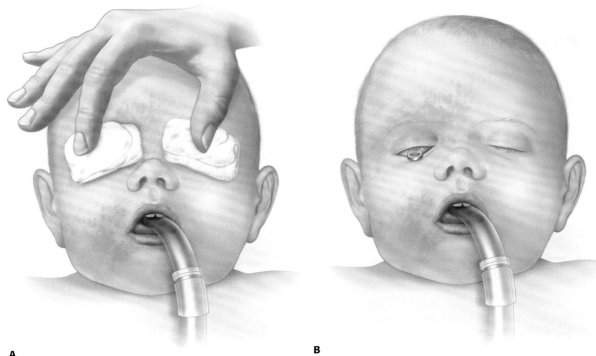

A   **B**

FIG 2 • A. Overlapping white gauze held with a firm hand should be used to cover the periorbital area in young children in whom the protective eye glasses would be too large. **B.** Globe eye shields should be used when lasering close to the orbit. Note the postoperative purpura from the pulsed dye laser.

- Everyone present must use appropriate eye protection during laser treatment.
  - Most glasses and goggles may be too large for small children.
  - Overlapping white gauze held with a firm hand should be used to cover the periorbital area, as these will reflect laser light (**FIG 2A**). The gauze should be moistened with water if used with general anesthesia. Pressure should be placed on the orbital rim and not on the eye itself.
  - Globe eye shields must be used if lasering close to the eye (**FIG 2B**).

Approach

- The most commonly used laser for superficial or ulcerated hemangiomas is the pulsed dye laser (PDL). Suggested settings are dependent on the various chosen parameters and may include wavelengths of 585 to 595 nm, fluences of 4 to 8.5 J/cm^2, pulse durations between 0.45 to 3 ms, spot sizes of 5 to 10 mm, and a concomitant cooling device.
  - Deeper parts of the lesion can respond to long-pulsed Nd-YAG or alexandrite lasers, although there is a higher risk of scarring and pigmentary complications.

- The PDL is the most commonly used laser for PWS treatment. General settings to be used could include 585 to 595 nm for wavelength, 5.5 to 11 J/cm^2 for fluence, 0.45 to 3 ms for pulse duration, and 7 to 12 mm for spot size. Lasering is most safely performed in combination with epidermal cooling (Table 1).
  - A larger spot size allows the laser beam to penetrate deeper into the lesion. However, lower fluences are used for larger spot sizes to maintain a high safety profile.
  - Changing the pulse duration may allow targeting of different sized vessels. Treatment often begins at 1.5 ms, and this can be adjusted down to 0.45 ms and up to 3 ms. Lower fluences are required for shorter pulse durations.
- PWS have a nonuniform response to laser surgery, likely due to variously sized blood vessels, different flow rates, and different depths of involvement.
- One should not use a cookbook approach to the settings used. Each lesion is unique. It is strongly recommended that test sites be placed with each patient. Or, if there are overriding reasons not to place test sites, initially use only very low-energy parameters for the first treatment, especially in infants. If one is in such a situation that limits the placement of test sites, one may treat a larger area at a low-energy setting and place discreet test sites with slightly higher settings during the first treatment session.

Table 1 General Settings Used With Pulsed-Dye Laser

Vascular lesion	Wavelength (nm)	Fluence (J/cm²)	Pulse Duration (ms)	Spot Size (mm)
Hemangioma	585–595	4–8.5	0.45–3	5–10
Port-wine stain	585–595	5.5–11	0.45–3	7–12

■ For older patients who prefer a treatment without purpura, one can use an intense pulsed light (IPL) device (**FIG 3**). These systems are less safe around the eyes and with higher skin types. Each IPL system is manufactured differently and is applied in a unique approach appropriate to the particular system. It is recommended to be very familiar with the device that is to be used and always place test sites.

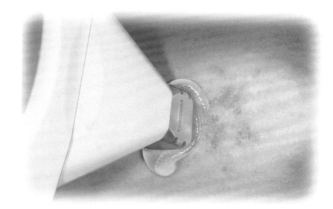

FIG 3 • Use of an intense pulsed light (IPL) device on a partially treated port-wine stain.

■ Test Sites

■ One should perform test sites prior to treatment of the entire lesion. In larger lesions, especially over multiple anatomical regions, test pulses should be performed over the various regions and clinical lesional variations. Patients are evaluated dependent on their age anywhere from 4 to 8 weeks after test site placement to assess response of the test sites.

■ Laser Treatment of Vascular Lesion

■ Once the clinician has determined appropriate settings from the test pulses, one can treat the entire lesion. If the test site outcomes were not decisive, one should not hesitate to place additional test sites with even the same and other parameters until one feels comfortable proceeding. One often treats different anatomical regions with different parameters. Even the same anatomical region may be treated with different parameters dependent on symmetry of lesional involvement.

■ In those patients having ill-defined borders and especially for those patients receiving general anesthesia that induces fading of the lesions, prior to treatment, it may be helpful to outline the borders of the lesion. Place the outline marker slightly beyond the margin of the lesion because the marker material itself may absorb laser energy resulting in undesired damage to the skin.

■ The laser handpiece should be pressed gently, perpendicularly, against the skin (**TECH FIG 1**). Avoid aiming tangentially at the skin, as this may alter the fluence and the cooling device effectiveness.

■ To regulate the amount of laser energy impacting the skin, thus reducing the chance of undesired adverse effects, only single passes are generally placed with pulsed dye laser and intense pulsed light (IPL) systems. Pulse overlap should also be avoided or at least limited to less than 10% overlap.

■ Throughout the treatment, the clinician should always be monitoring the tissue for the desired tissue changes such as tissue darkening or edema. When there is any deviation, stop the procedure and check the laser and parameters or reassess the lesional area being treated. In those patients who are not anesthetized and are old enough to give reliable feedback, a change in pain level is also an indicator that parameters should be reconsidered. Ask the patient to inform the clinician if there is any change in baseline procedural discomfort.

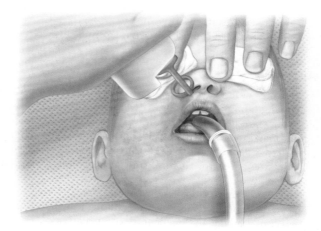

TECH FIG 1 • The laser handpiece should be pressed gently, perpendicularly, against the skin. Note the physician is protecting the patient's eye with white gauze.

PEARLS AND PITFALLS

Eye protection	■ For children, cover the periorbital area using overlapping white gauze held firmly. ■ Pressure should be placed on the orbital rim and not on the eye itself. ■ If there is use of inhalation anesthesia, the gauze should be thoroughly wetted with water or saline. Tape or similar nonflammable material may be placed on the closed eyelid to ensure it remains closed. ■ With any lasering near or into the orbital rim, a full global eye shield should be placed.
Clinical endpoint	■ Always pay attention to tissue response to each pulse. ■ Any deviation from previous responses or blistering or vesiculation is a cause of serious concern, mandating stopping the procedure and reassessing the laser and parameters.
Therapeutic outcome	■ Ideally, total lesional resolution is desired. With port-wine stain vascular malformations, this is achieved only in a small minority of cases after a series of many treatment sessions. ■ If after an initial trial no further lesional regression is accomplished, it is probable that one has achieved the maximum lesional reduction possible with the current therapeutic approach. Either another approach should be tested or therapy should be suspended, and the family should be informed of the ineffectiveness of further therapy using the current approach.
Skin color	■ The higher the skin type the greater is the absorption of laser energy by melanin in the epidermal layer and the increased chance of cutaneous damage resulting in permanent hypopigmenation. ■ This concern is greatly enhanced if the patient has additional coloring from the sun. Since even a modest amount of darkening from the sun is associated with a significant increased risk, do not treat patients who have any appreciable color from the sun. Wait for it to fade.

POSTOPERATIVE CARE

■ After treatment, all patients experience local swelling and discomfort. The discomfort is transient with the intensity dramatically reducing over the first 30 to 60 minutes. Ice packs, cooling gels, and nonsteroidal anti-inflammatory medications may minimize discomfort.

■ Patients should practice proper sun protection for weeks after the treatment to minimize risk of pigmentary changes.

■ Emollients should be applied routinely until clearing of the immediate postlaser changes.

■ Topical antibiotics should be initiated if crusting or scabbing occurs, as these can raise risks of secondary bacterial infection.

■ Postadjuvant antiangiogenesis therapy is currently being evaluated. Treatment with topical imiquimod 5% and topical rapamycin in between laser treatments has been shown to prevent reformation and reperfusion of blood vessels in small trials.[10,11]

OUTCOMES

■ Approximately 20% of PWS can be lightened completely or almost completely with the PDL. About 70% will lighten by more than 50% and about 10% to 20% of lesions will only respond minimally.[12]

■ For best results, vascular lesions will require multiple treatments. Very rarely does a lesion clear after a few sessions. Typically, lesions would be treated for at least 8 to 10 treatments at a minimum of 4- to 12-week intervals.

■ More resistant or hypertrophic PWSs may not respond to PDL and may be better suited for treatment with longer wavelength lasers. Proven lasers include the long-pulse alexandrite (755 nm), long-pulse 1064 nm Nd-YAG, and dual 595 nm/1064 nm lasers. These lasers are only recommended for skilled laser surgeons, as there is a very small therapeutic window, and the risk of scarring is higher.[4,6,9]

COMPLICATIONS

■ Skin darkening usually will develop immediately with PDL treatment and may persist for 10 to 14 days.

■ Transient erythema and swelling typically persists for 4 to 8 days with the PDL and less with the IPL.

■ Blistering and crusting can also develop, more commonly with higher fluences or with overlapping pulses.

■ Transient or permanent hyper- and hypopigmentation can occur, especially in darker-skinned patients and if one treats patients with a tan.

  ■ Pigmentary risks can be reduced in darker skin types with using appropriate epidermal cooling, longer pulse durations and lower fluences. Treatment efficacy is also likely to be reduced when using longer pulse durations and lower fluences.

■ Alopecia can occur if using lasers in areas that have pigmented hairs. Care, especially over the eyebrows, is necessary to prevent permanent hair loss.

■ The risk of scarring after PDL treatment of PWS is very low (less than 1%). These risks can be minimized by using test sites.

REFERENCES

1. Mulliken JB, Glowacki J. Hemangiomas and vascular malformations in infants and children: a classification based on endothelial characteristics. *Plast Reconstr Surg.* 1982;69:412-422.
2. Hoff SR, Rastatter JC, Richter GT. Head and neck vascular lesions. *Otolaryngol Clin North Am.* 2015;48(1):29-45.
3. Bruckner AL, Frieden IJ. Hemangiomas of infancy. *J Am Acad Dermatol.* 2003;48:477-493
4. Stier MF, Glick SA, Hirsch RJ. Laser treatment of pediatric vascular lesions: port wine stains and hemangiomas. *J Am Acad Dermatol.* 2008;58(2):261-285.
5. Batta K, Goodyear HM, Moss C, et al. Randomized controlled study of early pulsed dye laser treatment of uncomplicated childhood hemangiomas. *Lancet.* 2002;360:521-527.
6. Craig LM, Alster TS. Vascular skin lesions in children: a review of laser surgical and medical treatments. *Dermatol Surg.* 2013;39(8):1137-1146.

7. Garden JM, Bakus AD, Paller AS. Treatment of cutaneous hemangiomas by the flashlamp-pumped pulsed dye laser: prospective analysis. *J Pediatr.* 1992;120(4 Pt 1):555-560.

8. Reddy KK, Blei F, Brauer JA, et al. Retrospective study of the treatment of infantile hemangiomas using a combination of propranolol and pulsed dye laser. *Dermatol Surg.* 2013;39(6):923-933.

9. Brightman LA, Geronemus RG, Reddy KK. Laser treatment of port-wine stains. *Clin Cosmet Investig Dermatol.* 2015;12;8:27-33.

10. Tremaine AM, Armstrong J, Huang YC, et al. Enhanced port-wine stain lightening achieved with combined treatment of selective photothermolysis and imiquimod. *J Am Acad Dermatol.* 2012;66(4):634-641.

11. Griffin TD Jr, Foshee JP, Finney R, Saedi N. Port wine stain treated with a combination of pulsed dye laser and topical rapamycin ointment. *Lasers Surg Med.* 2016;48(2):193-196.

12. Woo WK, Handley JM. Does fluence matter in the treatment of port-wine stains. *Clin Exp Dermatol.* 2003;28:556-557.

Laser Burn Scar Revision

C. Scott Hultman and Yuen-Jong Liu

DEFINITION

- Mortality from burn injury has markedly decreased in the second half of the 20th century as wound sepsis, wound coverage, kidney failure, and shock have been largely overcome.
- Burn injury is the result of high-energy transfer to a significant surface area of the skin or soft tissues and can be categorized by the form of energy:
  - Contact with high temperature solids (contact), liquids (scald), or gases (flame)
  - Contact with low temperatures (frostbite)
  - Exposure to chemicals (acids, alkalines, or other caustic reagents)
  - Electricity
  - Friction or abrasion
- Burn wounds frequently heal in the form of hypertrophic scars, which hamper functional and aesthetic outcomes.
- Symptoms include pruritus, burning pain, and hyperesthesia, which may be treated with antihistamines, narcotic analgesics, and non-narcotic analgesics.
- Functional deficits may vary from tightness or tethering of the surrounding skin to contractures that limit range of motion.
- Hypertrophic burn scars may be erythematous due to hypervascularity.
- Treatments include occupational therapy, physical therapy, compression garments, moisturizing agents, sunblock, and scar massage.[1,2]
- Evidence for the efficacy of laser therapy in the treatment of hypertrophic burn scars is now well documented in individual cohort studies,[3] review articles,[4] and a rigorous meta-analysis of 28 well-designed clinical trials.[5]
- The exact biologic mechanism for improvement has yet to be elucidated, but pulsed dye laser (PDL) improves the inflammatory component of hypertrophic burn scars, which have excess pathologic vascularity, whereas fractional carbon dioxide (CO_2) laser improves remodeling of dermal collagen, which is disorganized and abnormal in hypertrophic burn scars.
- Best practices involve six to eight laser sessions, performed every 4 to 6 weeks, using a combination of these two lasers, plus on occasion the Alexandrite laser, to ablate hair follicles in cases of chronic folliculitis of the burn scar.
- Substantial, rapid improvement in hypertrophic burn scars is now observed through objective measures, such as the Vancouver Scar Score (height, erythema, pliability), as well as subjective reports, such as the UNC 4P Scar Score (pruritus, paresthesias, pliability, and pain).[6]
- A major benefit to both the patient and the payer is that multiple, minimally invasive laser sessions may decrease or prevent the need for more complex and more invasive surgical procedures, decreasing patient risk, reducing overall cost, and potentially achieving outcomes not previously possible.

ANATOMY

- Burn scars may affect any part of the body.
- Hypertrophic scars across joints may cause contracture.
- Contractures on the face may interfere with competence of the eyelids or the mouth.
- Burn scars are especially disfiguring on the face due to its high aesthetic importance.
- Neuropathic pain may be observed in burned areas, grafted regions, and even donor sites.

PATHOGENESIS

- The incidence of hypertrophic scarring after burn injury ranges from 5% to 40%, depending on anatomic location, depth of burn, method of closure, and genomic response to healing.
- Hypertrophic scarring and contractures can develop in burn scars that heal by secondary intention or re-epithelialization, in split-thickness skin grafts over excised burns, along the seams of full-thickness grafts, and in donor sites that had delayed healing, due to infection of excessive depth of harvest.
- Hypertrophic scars may be associated with an imbalance of collagen types 1 and 3, as well as TGF beta 1 and TGF beta 3.
- Hypertrophic scarring can be viewed as an abnormal physiologic response after wound closure, in which collagen deposition and angiogenesis continue beyond their desired end points.

NATURAL HISTORY

- Neuropathic symptoms, such as pruritus, searing pain, hyperesthesias, and paresthesias, are a source of frustration for the patient, can limit quality of life, and may prevent return to school, work, and social functions.

- Hypertrophic scarring may cause disability ranging from minor discomfort to joint contracture.
- Hyper- or hypopigmentation, erythema, and abnormal texture may cause the burn scars to be aesthetically unacceptable.

PATIENT HISTORY AND PHYSICAL FINDINGS

- Complete patient history should be elicited, focusing on the type of energy delivered: scald, electrical, flame, contact, chemical, cold, friction, abrasion, or other.
- Previous treatments and their effects should be noted, including skin grafting, laser treatments, topical scar treatments, moisturizing agents, sunblock, systemic medications, occupational therapy, physical therapy, compression garments, and massage.
- The patient should have had no significant improvement in symptoms for at least 3 months on maximal medical therapy.
- Relative contraindications to laser therapy include connective tissue disorders, utilization of systemic steroids or immunosuppressive medications, and chemotherapy or radiation therapy. Patients with moderate to severe lymphedema should also be treated with caution, as healing from ablative lasers may be delayed.
- Complete physical exam should be performed, focusing on the burned area, noting whether it is a native burn scar or burn scar after skin grafting.
- The burned areas should be well healed without open wounds or evidence of cellulitis.
- Total body surface area of the burn injury should be noted, as extremely large areas should be staged, in terms of laser treatment.
- Functional deficits should be recorded, such as loss of range of motion or loss of sensation.
- Aesthetic concerns should also be considered, especially in burns of the face and the hands.
- The patient's Fitzpatrick skin type should be documented, and this will advise the initial energy settings for the laser.
- Photographs are useful for insurance submission and to track progression of the scar between laser treatments.

IMAGING

- Imaging is not required. However, medical photography is often needed for preauthorization from insurance companies.
- For patients enrolled in a clinical trial, other imaging modalities might be helpful to measure extent of hypertrophic scarring and quantify changes:
  - Ultrasound to measure thickness of scar
  - Chroma meter to measure light-dark axis and degree of redness from erythema
  - Cutometer to measure elasticity of scar

SURGICAL MANAGEMENT

- The patient is routinely consented for a series of laser treatments, involving selective photothermolysis with the PDL, ablative resurfacing using the fractional using CO_2 laser, and either Alexandrite or diode lasers to rupture hair follicles.

- A series of 6 to 8 sessions is submitted for insurance coverage at a time, though a patient may reach maximal benefit before 6 to 8 sessions or may continue to experience symptomatic improvement beyond eight sessions.
- We strongly recommend maintaining a burn scar registry, which includes preoperative, operative, and postoperative data, which can be used for practice-based learning, retrospective and prospective cohort analysis, insurance preauthorization and payment, and medical-legal documentation.
- We recommend working with a board-certified anesthesiologist who has completed additional specialization in pediatric anesthesia or has significant clinical experience with children and has expertise in ambulatory and office-based anesthesia.
  - Multimodal anesthesia has been shown to significantly decrease patient pain, need for intravenous opioids during recovery, and time to discharge from the postanesthesia care unit.[7]
- Patients must be treated in an accredited surgery facility, which can include a hospital-based ambulatory surgery center and an office-based surgery facility.
  - Control of airway is paramount, even with mild sedation; burn patients may have compromised airways from previous tracheostomy scars and/or prolonged intubation and mechanical ventilation.
- To maximize throughput with our practice, patients do not return until their next laser session, which is typically 6 to 8 weeks later.
  - The next session serves as both the postoperative visit from the previous treatment and the preoperative visit for that day's session.
  - At that time, we ask the patient for feedback about their symptoms and tailor the treatment for that day based on these observations, which can include changing the energy levels as well as type of laser used.

Positioning and Preparation

- Our burn patients usually receive a Propofol drip and boluses of fentanyl, ketamine, and midazolam as appropriate.
- The burn scar should be clean but sterile preparation is not necessary.
- Sterile drapes are not necessary.
- All operating room personnel must wear tinted eyewear for PDL or clear eyewear for CO_2 laser to protect against laser backscatter.
- The patient's eyes should be closed and covered with a saline-moistened towel.
- Fire prevention is of paramount concern for all laser cases, and patient safety protocols for reducing the potential for an oxygen-enriched environment must be followed.
  - This includes lower the inspired oxygen concentration to the lowest needed FIO_2, using room air only when discharging the laser in the head and neck region, avoiding towels or drapes that can serve as a reservoir for oxygen, and alerting all OR personnel when discharge of the laser commences.
- The lasers must be calibrated and tested on the back table, before treating the patient, to confirm that the appropriate amount of energy will be delivered.

◼ Pulsed Dye Laser

Anesthesia

- For small areas below the clavicles, as well as test areas, in adult patients only, no anesthesia is necessary, except for the cooling of the cryogen jet, which is administered milliseconds before the laser is discharged.
- All children, adults with large surface areas, and patients with hypertrophic scars on the face and neck require some type of anesthesia, which can range from oral anxiolytics and narcotics to TIVA (total intravenous anesthesia); general anesthesia with inhalation agents is rarely used, but patients will often benefit from a LMA (laryngeal mask airway) to control the tongue and epiglottis.
- Of note, most topical anesthetics constrict the capillary targets in the dermis, so we almost never utilize these agents, to ensure that the target receives and absorbs adequate energy for selective photothermolysis.

Laser Application

- We use a Candela V-Beam, 595-nm wavelength, PDL.
- The laser is set to 1-cm diameter circular spot size, cryogen mix of 30/20, and 1.5-ms pulse duration or pulse width (**TECH FIG 1A**).
- The energy or fluence setting is titrated to mild bruising without blistering. 6.5 J/cm^2 is a reasonable level for a patient's first session for Fitzpatrick class 1 and 2 patients. For patients with Fitzpatrick grade 3 and 4

pigmentation, acceptable starting energy settings are 4.5 to 5.0 J/cm^2. Patients with Fitzpatrick class 5 and 6 skin types must be counseled that they are at high risk for mild blistering and hypopigmentation and should be treated with minimal fluence, such as 3.5 J/cm^2.

- The energy setting for subsequent sessions is increased if the patient experiences minimal skin changes in the days following the procedure. Conversely, the energy setting is decreased if the patient experiences severe bruising, blistering, or epidermolysis in the days following the procedure.
- As the operator fires the laser sequentially over the burn scar, there should be mild overlap between successive bursts (**TECH FIG 1B**).
- Each laser burst can be expected to sting as if struck by a drawn rubber band.
- End points for titrating the fluence, in the OR, include slight ecchymosis of the skin. Immediate blistering or purpura indicates that too much energy has been applied and that reduction in fluence is required.

Wound Care

- We use topical antimicrobial ointment for several days, until bruising begins to resolve.
- Oral antibiotics and antiviral agents are almost never given, except in cases of recurrent cellulitis or frequent outbreaks of herpetic infection in the treated areas.

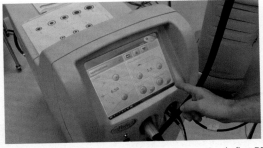 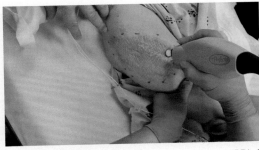

TECH FIG 1 • A. We typically use these settings for a patient's first PDL treatment session on our Candela V-Beam, 595 nm, PDL. The laser is set to 6.50-J/cm^2 fluence, 1-cm diameter spot size, cryogen mix of 30/20, and 1.5 ms pulse duration. **B.** The PDL handpiece is held so that the distance guide (*purple ring*) is flat at skin level. The treatment area of hyperemic autografted burn scar is encircled with marked *dots*. There should be mild overlap between successive bursts.

◼ Fractional CO_2 Laser

Anesthesia

- Fractional CO_2 laser ablation is extremely painful.
- For small areas below the clavicle, in adults who have minimal baseline neuropathic pain, topical anesthetics including lidocaine and bupivacaine mixtures can be applied for 20 to 30 minutes, to create enough anesthesia that the laser can be tolerated, when using 15 to 30 mJ/micropulse.
- However, most burn patients already have neuropathic symptoms from their hypertrophic scars, so most require at least intravenous sedation and analgesia, but total intravenous anesthesia is usually employed.

Laser Application

- We use a Lumenis UltraPulse fractional CO_2 laser at wavelength of 10 600 nm.
- The laser is set to 30 to 60 mJ/micropulse, 1- × 1-cm^2 square spot size, 250 to 300 Hz for the micropulses, 0.3- to 0.5-second delay between sequential firing, and 5% to 3% density in terms of tissue surface area (**TECH FIG 2**).
- Higher energies of 60 to 90 mJ/micropulse can be delivered safely, provided that density is dropped to 1%. We rarely use energy of this magnitude, expect in very thick hypertrophic scars that require a greater depth of penetration, to yield fine, punctate, capillary bleeding. The efficacy of using such high energies has not been

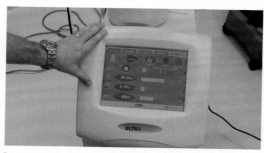
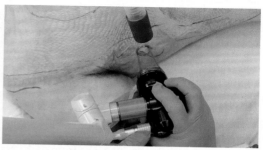

TECH FIG 2 • A. On our Lumenis UltraPulse fractional CO_2 laser, initial settings consist of 30 to 60 mJ/micropulse, 1- × 1-cm² square spot size, 0.5-second delay between sequential spots, 300-Hz firing rate, and 5% density. **B.** The CO_2 laser handpiece is held so that the distance guide (translucent grey ring) is flat at skin level. The treatment area of indurated autografted burn scar is outlined by skin marker. There should be minimal or no overlap between successive bursts. An assistant suctions vaporized tissue smoke with the tip of the evacuator (purple end of plastic tubing) held a few centimeters from the laser spot to remove vaporized tissue smoke.

rigorously studied, and we cannot recommend using energy of this magnitude routinely.

- While some surgeons use very high energies to treat keloids, we prefer to manage burn scar keloids by direct excision and fractionated, immediate postoperative radiation. In children, patients with keloids of the neck (where the thyroid and parathyroid glands could be in the field of irradiation), and patients with a history of XRT, we instead close the wound through complex repair, tissue rearrangement, or skin graft and then proceed with laser therapy to reduce the incidence of recurrence.
- The laser should be tested on a wooden tongue depressor, to confirm orderly and consistent ablation, evidenced by a regular pattern of burn marks on the tongue depressor.
- As the operator fires the laser sequentially over the burn scar, there should be minimal or no overlap between successive bursts (**TECH FIG 2B**).
- An assistant should suction away vaporized tissue smoke, as this may be dense and irritating. Furthermore, the

plume may contain viral particles that could theoretically infect members of the OR team. For that reason, the surgeon must wear a tight-fitting, filtered mask.

- The energy setting is titrated to pinpoint bleeding, indicative of penetration into the reticular dermis.
- Char is left in place.

Wound Care

- The treated areas are immediately dressed with a topical antibiotic ointment and cooled with ice packs.
- We routinely apply topical corticosteroids, dosed to patient weight, through vigorous massage into the fresh channels.
- Patients with a history of significant postoperative itching or pain are also treated with topical antihistamines and lidocaine, respectively.
- These pharmacologic agents are kept in contact with the treated areas with semiocclusive dressings, which are then gently and snugly wrapped with circumferential gauze, which is removed in 1 to 2 days.

PEARLS AND PITFALLS

Anesthesia	■ All patients require a personalized plan, which can range from topical agents to general anesthesia, depending on patient age, location of burn scar, type of laser used, and energy applied. Almost all patients can be discharged on the day of surgery, except for those infrequent patients who may require monitoring of airway or who experience postoperative nausea and vomiting. It is critical to use only the amount of anesthesia necessary to produce the desired level of comfort.
End points	■ PDL: slight bruising or reactive erythema. ■ CO_2: fine punctate bleeding with reactive erythema. ■ Diode and alexandrite: rupture of hair follicle with flash of light and audible crackle.
Complications	■ Blistering can occur with PDL, especially in patients with higher Fitzpatrick scores; this is very superficial and is treated with topical ointment until wound re-epithelializes. ■ Hypopigmentation is quite common. ■ Postinflammatory hyperpigmentation can occur with UV radiation exposure and should be treated with topical corticosteroids. ■ Allergy to topical antibiotics can occur after prolonged use of these agents and typically resolves with cessation of use. ■ Cellulitis is rare but does respond quickly to oral antibiotics, which include coverage of MRSA. ■ Wound breakdown and infarction is extremely uncommon and may be due to a combination of technical issues with too much energy delivered and superimposed infection.
Cessation of therapy	■ Most patients achieve maximum benefit after 4–6 sessions, but continued improvement can occur well beyond this series of treatments. We typically stop treatments when both the patient and provider agree that signs and symptoms have reached maximum improvement.

POSTOPERATIVE CARE

- The patient should be advised to expect reactive erythema, bruising, and occasional superficial blistering within 3 to 5 days.
- The patient should apply bacitracin ointment daily to the treated area.
- Patients must avoid sunlight to prevent UV radiation exposure.
- Postprocedure pain should be adequately covered by over-the-counter analgesics such as acetaminophen and NSAIDs.
- We do not routinely prescribe narcotic analgesics after PDL.
- The CO_2 laser is painful, and we routinely prescribe a small amount of narcotic analgesics for postprocedure pain.
- Dressings can be taken down by the family 1 to 3 days after treatment.
- Occupational and physical therapy can be started at that time.
- Compression garments can be worn when the scab formation occurs, typically 5 days after treatment.
- Children often go back to school, and adults return to work, within 1 to 2 days.

OUTCOMES

- Some degree of symptomatic improvement can be expected in all patients, though returns tend to diminish with each successive treatment (Clayton, Levi). We objectively measure improvement with the Vancouver Scar Score, in which the provider rates thickness, redness, color, texture, and pliability. Patients provide subjective feedback through the use of the UNC 4P scale, in which patients rate pain, paresthesias, pliability, and pruritus. Interestingly, patients often report continued subjective improvement, after the provider notes plateau in objective clinical findings.
- Patients who reach maximum improvement are re-evaluated in 2 to 3 months and then at yearly intervals thereafter. Children will often experience recurrence of symptoms during and after puberty and may benefit from an additional series of sessions, sometime many years later.
- One unexpected finding is that many burn patients with chronic neuropathic pain, whose hypertrophic scars have been treated with lasers, present with focal anatomic causes of their pain, such as nerve compression or neuroma formation. Laser therapies treat the generalized inflammatory and hypertrophic response, often unmasking surgically treatable causes of chronic neuropathic pain. Diagnosis of an anatomic cause can be made by clinical exam, with elicitation of a Tinel sign, as well as nerve block, which can be assisted with ultrasound guidance. If an anatomic cause is identified, then patients may undergo a combination of nerve decompression and transposition, neuroma resection with subfascial or intramuscular implantation, or fat grafting. In our experience, laser treatment of hypertrophic burn scars improves chronic neuropathic pain in 80% to 90% of patients, as defined by reduction of symptoms and de-escalation of pharmacologic regimen. In the remaining patients, 80% to 90% have an anatomic cause of neuropathic pain that is amenable to surgical intervention. One guiding observation is that over the past 10 years of treating hypertrophic burn scars with laser therapies, the more we look for discrete anatomic causes of neuropathic pain, the more likely we are to find abnormalities that respond to a combination of nerve decompression and neuroma resection. Fat grafting has also proven to be a highly successful form of treatment in refractory cases.

COMPLICATIONS

- Adverse events are minor and include hyperpigmentation, hypopigmentation, mild blistering, pain, rash, fever, and infection (Clayton).
- In our 10-year experience, involving 800 sessions per year, we have observed one case of herpetic whitlow, one case of wound breakdown with delayed healing, and two cases of postoperative pulmonary insufficiency, requiring intubation (one patient with aspiration at end of case, the other patient with myasthenia gravis).

REFERENCES

1. Friedstat JS, Hultman CS. Hypertrophic burn scar management: what does the evidence show? A systematic review of randomized controlled trials. *Ann Plast Surg.* 2014;72(6):S198-S201.
2. Tredget EE, Levi B, Donelan MB. Biology and principles of scar management and burn reconstruction. *Surg Clin North Am.* 2014;94(4):793-815.
3. Hultman CS, Edkins RE, Wu C, et al. Prospective, before-after cohort study to assess the efficacy of laser therapy on hypertrophic burn scars. *Ann Plast Surg.* 2013;70(5):521-526.
4. Hultman CS, Edkins RE, Lee CN, et al. Shine on: review of laser- and light-based therapies for the treatment of burn scars. *Dermatol Res Pract.* 2012;2012:243651.
5. Jin R, Huang X, Li H, et al. Laser therapy for prevention and treatment of pathologic excessive scars. *Plast Reconstr Surg.* 2013;132(6):1747-1758.
6. Hultman CS, Friedstat JS, Edkins RE, et al. Laser resurfacing and remodeling of hypertrophic burn scars: the results of a large, prospective, before-after cohort study, with long-term follow-up. *Ann Surg.* 2014;260(3):519-529.
7. Edkins RE, Hultman CS, Collins P, et al. Improving comfort and throughput for patients undergoing fractionated laser ablation of symptomatic burn scars. *Ann Plast Surg.* 2015;74(3):293-299.
8. Clayton JL, Edkins R, Cairns BA, Hultman CS. Incidence and management of adverse events after the use of laser therapies for the treatment of hypertrophic burn scars. *Ann Plast Surg.* 2013;70(5):500-505.
9. Levi B, Ibrahim A, Mathews K, et al. The use of CO_2 fractional photothermolysis for the treatment of burn scars. *J Burn Care Res.* 2016;37(2):106-114.

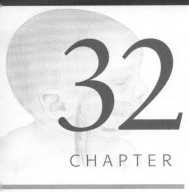

32 CHAPTER

Fat Grafting for Nerve Entrapment Within Burn Scars

C. Scott Hultman and Yuen-Jong Liu

DEFINITION

- Mortality from burn injury has markedly decreased in the second half of the 20th century as wound sepsis, wound coverage, kidney failure, and shock have been largely remedied.
- Patients who have undergone tangential excision of burn injuries, escharotomies, and autografting often develop symptomatic scars.
- Superficial sensory nerves may become entrapped in burn scars and cause debilitating paresthesias, such as burning pain, tingling, or hyperesthesia.
- Although nerve decompression and neurolysis are the primary treatments for entrapment, fat grafting is a low-risk adjunct procedure that can mitigate neuropathic symptoms by capitalizing on anti-inflammatory effects and physical cushioning by autologous fat.[1-7]
- The principles of fat grafting for burn scars may also be applied to scars from other etiologies, such as chemical exposure, frostbite, abrasion, electrical injury, or a combination of injurious energy transfer to the skin and superficial soft tissues.

ANATOMY

- Nerve entrapment may occur at any location of the body where there are sequelae of burn injury.
- Superficial sensory nerves are affected, frequently in the extremities, such as the superficial radial nerve, the medial antebrachial cutaneous nerve, the saphenous nerve, the sural nerve, and lateral dorsal cutaneous nerve.

PATHOGENESIS

- Hypertrophic scarring and contractures develop in burn scars or in split-thickness skin grafts over excised burn scars.
- The fibrotic tissues constrict around superficial sensory nerves and cause a combination of pain, hyperesthesia, and paresthesia.
- Sensory receptors in the damaged skin may also received aberrant innervation from sensory nerves, as the integument heals.

NATURAL HISTORY

- The neuropathic symptoms are a source of frustration for the patient, often preventing return to school and work.
- They require narcotic and non-narcotic analgesics and may become tolerant.
- Adjunct analgesics include gabapentin and pregabalin, which have adverse effects of varying severity.

PATIENT HISTORY AND PHYSICAL FINDINGS

- Complete patient history should be elicited, focusing on the type of energy delivered: scald, electrical, flame, contact, chemical, cold, friction, or abrasion.
- Previous treatments and their effects should be noted, including skin grafting, laser treatments, topical scar treatments, and medications.
- Complete physical exam should be performed, focusing on the burned area, noting whether it is a native burn scar or burn scar after skin grafting.
- Total body surface area of the burn injury should be observed, as this often dictates algorithms for treatment, that include medical therapy (compression, silicone), laser photothermolysis and ablation, nerve decompression, and fat grafting.
- Functional deficits should be noted, such as loss of range of motion or loss of sensation.
- Gentle percussion around the symptomatic area can elicit Tinel sign corresponding to the location of nerve tethering or entrapment.
- The Tinel sign can be followed to assess the effectiveness of treatment.

DIFFERENTIAL DIAGNOSIS

- Nerve compression amenable to decompression and possible transposition
- Discrete neuroma formation that may benefit from exploration, resection, and implantation of nerve below fascia or into muscle or even bone
- Persistent hyperemia of hypertrophic burn scar, which may respond to laser resurfacing

IMAGING

- Imaging is not required, although ultrasound may be helpful in guiding diagnostic nerve blocks, to confirm diagnosis of entrapped nerve vs neuroma, and to provide temporary relief.

SURGICAL MANAGEMENT

- Fat grafting is a modality that can offer significant relief of neuropathic symptoms, after patients have been considered for or treated with laser resurfacing, nerve decompression, or neuroma resection.
- Fat grafting involves surgically controlled incisional release of the integument from the underlying subcutaneous tissues and fascia.

- The grafted fat contains adipocytes and possibly stem cells, which are thought to have anti-inflammatory effects on the entrapped nerves and scar tissue.
- The grafted volume provides mechanical padding that decreases nerve sensitivity by effectively burying afferent end fibers, deeper and away from direct contact.
- Other reasonable surgical options include scar subcision and open neurolysis.
- LipiVage is the preferred system for small volume grafting, and Puregraft is preferred for large volume, structural fat grafting.

Preoperative Planning

- Overall, fat grafting is indicated for patients with any of the following criteria:
  - Require significant pharmacologic therapy for neuropathic pain
  - Have previously undergone laser therapies for hypertrophic burn scars
  - Have multiple areas of dysesthesias not necessarily corresponding to the anatomic distribution a sensory nerve
  - Have already undergone major peripheral nerve decompression, neurolysis, and neuroma resection
- The senior author prefers to use fat grafting as "rescue" therapy for patients with chronic, neuropathic burn scar pain, who have undergone other modalities with documented success in the literature, such as laser resurfacing and peripheral nerve decompression.
- Patients with large burn scar surface areas, who are on medications for neuropathic pain, should first undergo laser treatments with pulsed dye laser to reduce hyperemia, fractional CO_2 laser resurfacing to improve pliability of burn scar, and laser-assisted drug delivery (usually kenalog) to reduce inflammatory component.
- Patients with a discrete Tinel sign, suggestive of neuroma or entrapment, as well as those with motor dysfunction,

should first undergo surgical exploration, nerve decompression, and possibly neuroma resection.
- Patients who have multiple Tinel sign, who have undergone other modalities such as laser resurfacing, and who have previously had peripheral nerve surgery, can be considered optimal candidates for fat grafting.
- Another indication for fat grafting is the patient who is on an aggressive pharmacologic regimen for chronic neuropathic pain and who wants or needs to de-escalate medications, which often lose efficacy and cause side effects of decreased level of alertness, poor sleep hygiene, and peripheral swelling.
- The role for early fat grafting, within the first 6 to 12 months after wound closure, is unknown and would benefit from prospective clinical studies.
- The role for fat grafting in prepubertal children is also not known and requires prospective clinical trials.

Positioning

- Supine, to access fat from anterior abdominal wall and lateral trunk
- Shoulders abducted at 85 degrees for upper extremity surgery, with pressure points padded
- Lower extremities prepped such that ankles, knees, and hips can be mobile

Approach

- Fat grafting is often performed in multiple sessions, as there is a limit to how much fat can be grafted into and below a burn scar, especially when there is a paucity of subcutaneous tissue present.
- The authors plan harvest and use 0.5 to 1.0 cc of fat for every cm^2 of surface area grafted.
- Regular liposuction or power-assisted liposuction may be used to harvest the fat.

■ Port Creation and Cannula Use

- The port sites of the donor and recipient sites are first injected with a wheel of local anesthetic, typically 1% lidocaine with epinephrine, to minimize bleeding at locations.
- Donor sites ports typically include the inferior umbilicus, the flanks near the anterosuperior iliac crest, or previous surgical scars on the abdomen.
- The donor sites are tumesced with approximately 200 mL, targeting above and below the superficial fascial system using a solution of 1 L lactated Ringer's containing 1 mL of 1:100 000 epinephrine and 50 mL of 1% lidocaine.
- Tumescent is allowed to diffuse for 10 minutes.
- Port sites, of 1 to 2 mm, are made with stab incisions, proximal to the symptomatic burn scar. At least two port sites are made, to allow for a radial, fanning, cross-hatched matrix, with overlapping tunneling and at different levels in the burn scar.

- A subcision cannula is tunneled anterograde, from proximal to distal, to decrease risk of avulsing nerve branches (**TECH FIG 1**).
- Rigotomy is performed with advancement of the cannula. Usually, a blunt-tipped or semi–blunt-tipped cannula can be advanced through the scar, but occasionally, a sharp pickle-fork cannula is needed to perform discrete rigotomies.
- Fat is injected on withdrawal of the cannula, in aliquots of 0.1 to 0.2 cc, up to 0.5 mL with the bevel up and another 0.5 mL with the bevel down, over a distance of 2 to 6 cm.
- Additional passes of the subcision cannula are repeated in a fanning fashion through each fat grafting port, centering on the focus of nerve entrapment. Care is taken to stay superficial, directly under the burn scar, to avoid disruption of the deeper afferent neural plexus.

TECHNIQUES

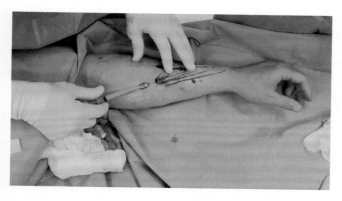

TECH FIG 1 • A subcision cannula is tunneled anterograde, from proximal to distal, to decrease risk of avulsing nerve branches.

■ LipiVage

- The tubing set attached to the LipiVage Harvester is connected to an aspirator and the vacuum level is set to approximately 60% of its capacity, ensuring a gentle vacuum (**TECH FIG 2**).
- The transfer adapter is removed, and the recommended aspiration cannula is attached. The senior author prefers to use a serrated, 1 to 2 mm cannula with multiple side ports, which is helpful for extracting fat during repeat harvests.
- Fat is harvested for approximately one minute, and then fluids are drained for a few seconds, from the trap mechanism with the LipiVage system.
- The nearly bloodless lipoaspirate is then washed with normal saline, within the closed system, before processing on the back table. Fat is then transferred into 3 cc injection syringes using the transfer adapter supplied. Harvesting steps are repeated for additional fat if needed.
- The filter is simply rinsed for a few seconds, and the plunger tip is used to wipe the inner walls of the filter clean in between harvests.
- Fat cells collect in the filter chamber suspended within the harvester body.
- Fat cells are gently pulled toward the inner walls of the filter and collect along the length of the front of the blue plunger tip, while fluids wash through.
- Once inside, the fat is gently cleaned by the accompanying tumescent fluid.

- Fluid and oils pass through the fat and the filter walls and are then carried to the waste receptacle via the tubing set.
- Due to the low vacuum levels, there is very little oil present to begin with because fewer fat cells are damaged during harvesting.
- After fluids are drained, the concentrated and cleaned fat is immediately ready for injection.
- The unique LipiVage plunger tip design gently wipes the fat from the inner filter walls and transfers the fat as the plunger is pushed forward gradually.
- The processed fat grafts are allowed to settle on the back table for at least 10 minutes, with the 3 cc syringes upside down, so that any additional tumescent fluid and oil can separate and be discarded, prior to fat grafting.

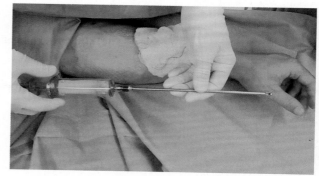

TECH FIG 2 • Attaching tubing set to the LipiVage Harvester.

■ Puregraft

- Fat is aspirated into a syringe.
- The lipoaspirate is injected into a Puregraft drain bag (**TECH FIG 3**).
- The lipoaspirate is washed lactated Ringer's solution.
- The filtered fat is aspirated from Puregraft drain bag into small syringes for grafting.

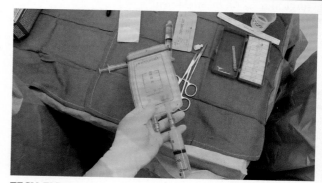

TECH FIG 3 • The lipoaspirate is injected into a Puregraft drain bag.

PEARLS AND PITFALLS

Port sites: harvest	▪ Usually, all of the lipoaspirate needed for fat grafting can be obtained through an infraumbilical incision. ▪ If multiple rounds of fat grafting are anticipated, we usually harvest fat from the right and left lower quadrants first, followed by the central infraumbilical fat second, and possibly the flank on repeat harvests. This is done to yield a desirable, symmetric abdominal wall contour. ▪ We always avoid harvesting fat from the right and left upper abdominal wall quadrants, to avoid injury to the liver or spleen, in case an aberrant pass is deflected deeper from the costal margin and into the peritoneal cavity. ▪ Recipient sites are closed with 4.0 plain gut and a Steri-Strip.
Port sites: recipient	▪ Port sites are almost always placed proximal to area of concern, so that the rigotomy can be done from proximal to distal, parallel to the topical distribution of the cutaneous nerves. ▪ Several port sites enable a cross-hatched matrix, which increases the amount of fat that can be transferred and should survive. ▪ Recipient sites are closed with 4.0 plain gut and a Steri-Strip.
Fat harvest	▪ We recommend against energy-assisted liposuction, such as laser or ultrasound, as this may decrease the viability of the grafted fat. ▪ The LipiVage system is used most of the time, as this allows for efficient harvest of the small volumes required for fat grafting. Structural fat grafting, which requires larger volumes to replace deficient tissue, is better served by the Puregraft system.
Engraftment	▪ For burn scars in the extremities, no tourniquet is used. ▪ After the cannula is advanced from proximal to distal, effecting a rigotomy, fat is injected in 0.1 to 0.2 cc aliquots, from distal to proximal. ▪ Pre-tunneling is not performed in order to decrease the risk of hematoma. ▪ We use 3 mL syringes for injecting fat during grafting, as the small size gives adequate control over delivering 0.2 mL aliquots without having to change syringes often. ▪ Our formula for volume of final processed and purified fat needed for grafting is 0.5 to 1.0 cc of fat for every cm^2 of surface area treated. Of note, we typically harvest lipoaspirate 2–3 times the volume needed for fat grafting ultimately needed, discarding tumescent fluid and oil as these elements separate.

POSTOPERATIVE CARE

▪ Acute postoperative pain from donor sites and at fat grafting sites lasts no more than 2 weeks. Typically, the patient experiences more pain in the donor site than the recipient site.

▪ Patients are kept on their neuropathic pain regimen but do require additional narcotics, especially for the donor-site pain.

▪ One dose of IV antibiotics is given at induction of anesthesia, and 5 days of oral antibiotics are given in the immediate postoperative period.

▪ The donor site is wrapped with gentle compression for 4 weeks to minimize the risk of seroma and hematoma. For abdominal donor sites, an abdominal binder is recommended at all times except when showering.

▪ The patient is advised against strenuous physical activity and heavy lifting (greater than ten pounds) for 4 weeks.

▪ The recipient site is dressed in clean, dry, gauze to absorb any drainage from the injection ports, and the initial postoperative may be removed on the 2nd day and reapplied as needed.

▪ The recipient site is treated with moderate compression during early engraftment, to prevent significant edema or hematoma. We believe that similar to the principle of needing a bolster to immobilize a skin graft, during the imbibition and inosculation phases, this compression helps with engraftment of the fat, in recipient sites, which may have less than optimal vascularity. The patient is advised to avoid direct pressure on the recipient site for 4 weeks, to prevent fat liquefaction or fat necrosis.

OUTCOMES

▪ Fat grafting reduces neuropathic pain, in approximately 90% of patients, permitting reduction in medication regimens.

▪ Fat grafting reduces scar symptoms such as pruritus, hyperesthesia, paresthesia, and tethering to deep structures.

▪ Fat grafting can improve tendon gliding in the hand and foot.

▪ Fat grafting improves scar pliability, texture, and color.

COMPLICATIONS

▪ Complications at the donor site are essentially complications from liposuction, which are rare, but include seroma, hematoma, and infection at the donor site.

▪ Complications at the recipient site have not been reported but may include infection and graft loss. Infections are exceedingly rare. In the author's practice, postoperative cellulitis occurs less than 2% of the time and can successfully be treated with oral antibiotics, continued compression, and extremity elevation.

▪ A small subset of patients report no improvement in neuropathic symptoms after fat grafting, but the overwhelming majority of patients report relief, measured by reduction of pain and/or reduction in need for medications. In fact, relief from neuropathic symptoms can be dramatic, suggesting that rigotomy may be the primary mechanism of early improvement. Maintenance of relief argues toward the mechanical cushioning effects of the fat graft, or possibly the ability of the adipocyte stem cells to stabilize fibrotic recipient sites or even regenerate normal afferent innervation.

REFERENCES

1. Byrne M, O'Donnell M, Fitzgerald L, Shelley OP. Early experience with fat grafting as an adjunct for secondary burn reconstruction in the hand: technique, hand function assessment and aesthetic outcomes. *Burns.* 2016;42(2):356-365.
2. Condé-Green A, Marano AA, Lee ES, et al. Fat grafting and adipose-derived regenerative cells in burn wound healing and scarring: a systematic review of the literature. *Plast Reconstr Surg.* 2016;137(1):302-312.
3. Fredman R, Edkins RE, Hultman CS. Fat grafting for neuropathic pain after severe burns. *Ann Plast Surg.* 2016;76(suppl 4):S298-S303.
4. Fredman R, Katz AJ, Hultman CS. Fat grafting for burn, traumatic, and surgical scars. *Clin Plast Surg.* 2017;44(4):781-791.
5. Huang SH, Wu SH, Chang KP, et al. Autologous fat grafting alleviates burn-induced neuropathic pain in rats. *Plast Reconstr Surg.* 2014;133(6):1396-1405.
6. Klinger M, Caviggioli F, Klinger FM, et al. Autologous fat graft in scar treatment. *J Craniofac Surg.* 2013;24(5):1610-1615.
7. Piccolo NS, Piccolo MS, Piccolo MT. Fat grafting for treatment of burns, burn scars, and other difficult wounds. *J Craniofac Surg.* 2015;42(2):263-283.

Section VIII: Ear Reconstruction

Auricular Reconstruction for Microtia and Post-traumatic Deformities

33

CHAPTER

Charles H. Thorne

DEFINITION

- Microtia literally means small ear but is used to refer to a spectrum of auricular anomalies (**FIG 1**) that are almost always associated with aural atresia (absence of the external auditory canal).
- From a practical point of view, any congenital deformity of the auricle that requires insertion of a complete or near-complete cartilage or synthetic framework is an example of microtia.
- As discussed below, the principles for reconstruction of other auricular deformities such as post-traumatic deformities are similar.

ANATOMY

- As depicted in **FIG 1**, the anomalies that constitute microtia vary from almost complete anotia to cases that demonstrate an almost normal lower 2/3 of the auricle. Microtia has been classified in various ways, but the most useful is the classification of Nagata: lobular microtia, small concha microtia, and large concha microtia. Complete anotia is almost never seen.
- Patients with microtia almost always have absence of the external auditory canal (aural atresia) with complete bony separation of the auricular remnant and the middle ear structures (**FIG 2**).
- The middle ear is underdeveloped and also presents variable abnormalities. If an apparent external auditory canal is present, it is almost always blind or stenotic. Patients with microtia, therefore, almost always have total conductive hearing loss on the affected side.
- Microtia is more common on the right side; 90% of cases are unilateral, and those patients usually have normal hearing in the contralateral ear.

- In the 10% with bilateral involvement of microtia and aural atresia, the patients are functionally deaf and require bone conductive hearing aids on an urgent basis in order to develop speech.
- There are several anatomic differences between microtia and post-traumatic deformities:
  - The skin quality in post-traumatic cases may present problems because of scarring around the remnant.
  - Post-traumatic auricular remnants almost always contain a canal and a tragus, making reconstruction of near-normal auricle more likely.
  - Post-traumatic remnants may be distorted by scar but are almost always in the correct position, as opposed to microtic remnants that are often malpositioned.

PATHOGENESIS

- The auricle and the middle ear develop together from the first and second branchial arches, explaining the concomitant anomalies of those two structures.
  - The inner ear is almost always normal in microtia patients because it arises separately in embryonic development and is not a branchial arch derivative.
- Microtia is the second most common congenital deformity affecting the head and neck (after cleft lip and palate) and is more common in patients of Southeast Asian descent.

PATIENT HISTORY AND PHYSICAL FINDINGS

- Microtia and aural atresia fall within the larger spectrum of craniofacial microsomia or first and second branchial arch syndrome. Craniofacial microsomia can present with either unilateral (ie, hemifacial microsomia) or bilateral involvement.

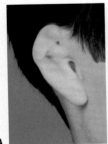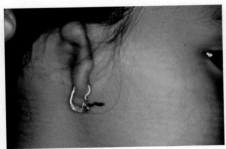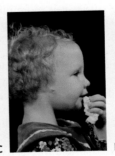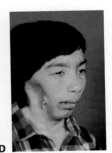

A **B** **C** **D**

FIG 1 • Variable presentation of microtia. The term microtia refers to a wide variety of presentations. **A.** Small conchal-type microtia. **B.** Lobular-type microtia. **C.** Almost complete anotia. **D.** Atypical microtia with hemifacial microsomia.

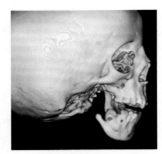

FIG 2 • Aural atresia. Microtia is almost always accompanied by aural atresia. Note the absence of an external auditory canal and, in this case, an extremely hypoplastic mandibular ramus.

- Most patients with microtia have symmetrical or nearly symmetrical faces, but radiographs usually show some asymmetry of the ipsilateral mandibular condyle indicating that microtia is part of the craniofacial microsomia spectrum.
  - A minority have more obvious underdevelopment of the tissues of the face including mandible, soft tissue, facial nerve, and auricle.

SURGICAL MANAGEMENT

- The autogenous method of auricular reconstruction is the technique with which this author is most familiar.[1-3] If the reader is interested in a technique using synthetic frameworks, the publications of John Reinisch are recommended.[4]
- The ideal age to perform reconstruction of a missing auricle is age 10 years.
  - At this age, the contralateral ear has reached adult size, and the rib cartilages are large enough to create an adult size ear framework. In a patient who is small for his/her age, delaying surgery until the patient is approximately the size of an average 10-year-old is recommended.
- Prior to age 10, the focus of patient management is on the hearing.
  - As mentioned, a patient with unilateral microtia has a total conductive hearing loss on the affected side but normal hearing in the unaffected ear. These patients can hear normally in quiet environments, but the lack of binaural input causes difficulty with localizing sound and in discriminating sounds in noisy environments. For example, a unilateral patient will have difficulty playing football when his/her name is yelled. The patient may have trouble immediately determining the direction of the sound and may look in the incorrect direction initially. In addition, in a room with multiple voices, it is more difficult for a microtia patient to screen out the background noise to focus on a conversation. These patients benefit from a bone conduction hearing aid (**FIG 3**).
  - Patients with bilateral microtia, on the other hand, absolutely require conduction aids because they are functionally deaf and will not develop normal speech without appropriate aids.
- Hearing can be restored either surgically or by use of a bone-anchored hearing aid (BAHA).
  - Reconstruction of the external auditory canal and ossicles can be surgically performed in approximately half the cases of aural atresia. In the other 50% of cases, the anatomy is too deranged for surgical repair.

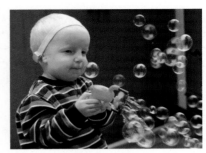

FIG 3 • BAHA soft band. Infants with unilateral microtia benefit from the BAHA soft band, which will provide binaural hearing. Patients with bilateral aural atresia must have a bone conduction aid in order to hear and to develop normal speech.

  - BAHAs are so effective, however, and less prone to complications when compared to canalplasty, that they are more commonly employed than surgical reconstruction of the canal (**FIG 4**).

Preoperative Planning

- When planning the auricular reconstruction, a tracing of the contralateral ear is made (**FIG 5**) that can be sterilized for intraoperative use. From that tracing, the surgeon then makes a drawing of the framework that would be required to produce that size auricle.
  - Because the skin has a certain thickness (approximately 2 mm), the framework must be at least 4 mm shorter than the desired auricle (or shorter depending on how deep in the native lobule the framework will be placed).
  - In addition, each of the convexities of the auricle must be much thinner and the concavities wider than the desired thickness on the ultimate auricle because the skin will make any raised portion of the framework (such as the helical rim) much thicker.
  - Once the drawing of the framework has been made, separate drawings of each component can be made.
- At the time of surgery, only two markings must be made on the affected side prior to the induction of anesthesia:
  - The lowest point on the unaffected side must be transferred to the affected side so the craniocaudal position of the ear is accurate. If this is not performed, then the lobules (and earrings) will not be in symmetrical positions.
  - The angle that the ear makes with the vertical: Most auricles are approximately 15 degrees off vertical and slightly less angulated than the line created by the dorsum of the nose. There is some variability, however, and the correct angle should be marked.

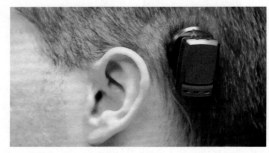

FIG 4 • A bone-anchored hearing aid is secured by a magnet that is attached to a titanium implant in the skull.

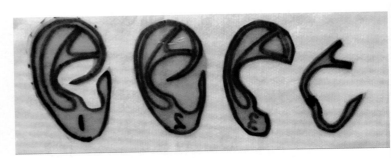

FIG 5 • Templates. Tracings are made from the contralateral ear and sterilized for intraoperative use.

- The remaining measurements and drawings can be made after the patient is under anesthesia.
  - Because some patients with microtia have more severe forms of facial asymmetry and may have airway issues, it is important to discuss airway management with the anesthesiologist. These patients may require more sophisticated intubation techniques or even, in the case of Treacher Collins patients, tracheostomy.

■ Stage One

Markings and Anesthesia

- Once the patient has been intubated and prepping and draping has occurred, the plastic templates that were made preoperatively are used to draw the precise location, size, and orientation of the new auricle.
- A decision is made about the skin incision, which most commonly involves either rotation of the vertically malpositioned lobule or an incision that will allow dissection of the pocket and placement of the framework without rotation of the lobule.
- If an appropriate lobule is present and rotation will result in its being in the correct position at the caudal aspect of the new auricle, rotation is performed.
  - If on the other hand, there is an inadequate lobule or one that is located such that rotation into the correct position is impossible, then an incision without lobule rotation is performed.
  - Local anesthesia with epinephrine is injected and attention is directed to the chest.

Graft Harvest

- An incision is made over the caudal aspect of the ipsilateral rib cage, and the muscles are divided to expose the rib cartilages.
- Using the sterile, plastic templates, decisions are made about which cartilages to harvest.
- If an entire framework is required, two free floating ribs are usually required for the helical rim and the antihelix.
  - The synchondrosis of two ribs is needed for the base of the framework, and sufficient additional cartilage is harvested to create the tragus-antitragus piece, small additional pieces to provide stabilization and projection, and a piece to be "banked" in the chest for the second stage of the procedure.

Pocket Dissection

- The operative field then shifts back to the temporal scalp.
- The incision is planned, with or without rotation of the lobule, and the pocket is dissected for placement of the framework. Hemostasis is obtained within the pocket.
- The dissection of the pocket is tedious but extremely important. More complications occur from soft tissue management than from management of the cartilage or an imperfect framework.
- When the pocket is created, the congenital cartilaginous remnant, which varies tremendously, is removed.
  - Care is taken not to injure the skin in the process of removing that cartilage.

Auricle Framework Construction

- On a sterile back table, the framework is assembled (**TECH FIG 1A,B**).
- The base is carved to match the template, and the details of the scapha and triangular fossa are created using sterilized gouges.
- The antihelix is attached as an onlay graft using nylon sutures on short, thin straight needles (**TECH FIG 1C**).
  - Some surgeons prefer wire sutures.
  - Creating a good framework is extremely difficult without these specialized sutures.
- The helical rim is then attached with another series of sutures of nylon or wire.
- The last piece of the main framework to be added is the tragus-antitragus piece with the intervening incisura, an important component of the aesthetically pleasing auricle (**TECH FIG 1D**).
- Additional small pieces are frequently attached to the deep surface of the framework for stabilization and projection.
  - The most important of these extends from the base to the tragus, fixing the latter in the correct position and adding to its projection. The tragus is a thin, floppy piece of cartilage, and it is important to keep it in precisely the correct position.

Insertion of the Framework and Wound Closure

- The framework is then inserted into the pocket along with two suction drains (**TECH FIG 2**).
  - The author prefers Axiom Petite Wound Drains (REF 201AT), which are silicone drains with perforations at one end and a 19G needle at the other end for insertion into the suction tubing or Vacutainer tubes.

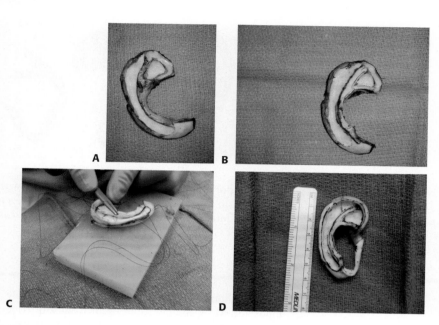

TECH FIG 1 • Construction of the framework. **A.** The base is carved from the synchondrosis of two rib cartilages. **B.** The antihelix and crura of the triangular fossa are attached as a single additional piece. **C.** Attachment of the helical rim. **D.** The completed framework after attachment of the tragus/antitragus piece.

- The drains are then attached to wall suction, and the overlying skin is sucked into the interstices of the framework.
- Only at this point can one decide which excess skin to excise.
- Excision of skin prior to the application of suction may result in over-resection of skin.
- The incisions are closed with interrupted nylon sutures.
- No dressing is placed.

Chest Wound Closure and Patient Transfer

- The chest incision is closed.
- Any holes in the parietal pleura are left alone without repair, and no chest tube or suctioning of the air in the pleural space is required.
  - Positive pressure ventilation pushes the air out with each breath, and if a small rim of pneumothorax remains, it is of no consequence.

- The cartilage chips that remain after the carving of the framework are wrapped in an absorbable mesh and used to create a "rib" to replace the caudal margin of the rib cage.
- The wound is closed in layers, and the piece of cartilage mentioned above is placed in a subdermal pocket so that it can easily be found and removed at the second stage.
- The suction drains are left attached to the tubing, which is in turn attached to wall suction.
- The recovery room is informed of the patient's imminent arrival, the suction tubing is temporarily disconnected from the wall, the patient is transported to the recovery room, and the tubing is reattached to wall suction.
  - Most wall suction units have a range for low, intermediate, and high suction.
  - The nurses are instructed to keep the suction exactly on the line that separates low from intermediate suction.

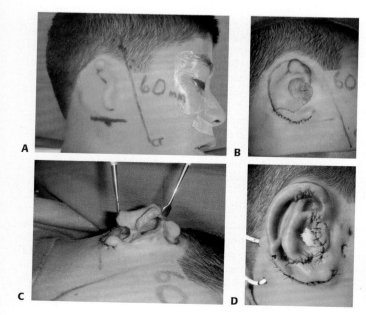

TECH FIG 2 • Dissection of the pocket. **A.** Preoperative markings. **B.** The lobule is rotated and the pocket is dissected. **C.** The pocket. **D.** After framework insertion and attachment of the drains to wall suction.

■ Stage Two

- Approximately 6 months later, the second stage is performed (**TECH FIG 3**).
- An incision is made around the posterior 180 degrees of the framework.
- The framework is elevated as far as the antihelix at the level of the temporalis fascia.
- A tunnel is created within the soft tissue, deep to the antihelix.
- The cartilage that had been left in the chest at the first stage is removed, shaped, and placed in the pocket, deep to the framework, to provide projection.

- The retroauricular skin is undermined and advanced into the sulcus.
- A full-thickness graft is taken from the inguinal crease and used to resurface the medial surface of the elevated framework.
  - Because the cartilage graft is in a soft tissue tunnel, the skin graft has an appropriate bed.
  - The alternative is to cover the graft with a temporoparietal fascial flap, but the author prefers to keep that option available in case of a complication with cartilage exposure. With that in mind, the dissection of the original skin pocket and the undermining at the second stage must avoid the superficial temporal artery pedicle.

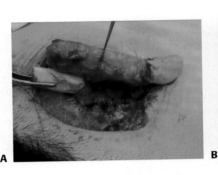
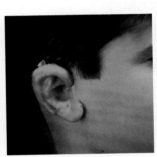

TECH FIG 3 • Second stage with elevation of the auricle. **A.** A cartilage graft that had been banked in a subdermal pocket below the original chest incision is inserted into a fascial pocket for projection of the auricle. **B.** Example after elevation. Xeroform is packed into the sulcus for 2 weeks after bolster removal.

PEARLS AND PITFALLS

Planning	■ Make sure the new auricle is in the best possible location and is the correct size and at the correct angle. A beautiful ear in the wrong place is ugly. The identification of the location is much more difficult in the patients with significant facial asymmetry where compromises may have to be made. Patients with microtia, especially those with more overt asymmetry, often have low hairlines. The management of the hairline is major topic unto itself. One choice is to excise the hair-bearing skin, either at the time of the initial operation or secondarily, and cover the framework with a temporoparietal flap and skin graft. Another choice is to place the framework under the hair-bearing skin and secondarily remove the scalp, leaving a thin layer of tissue over the framework to support the skin graft. This latter approach is tricky and requires both meticulous dissection and close postoperative observation. If the graft does not survive, the framework must be covered with vascularized tissue on an urgent basis.
Soft tissue management	■ More complications arise from errors in judgment regarding soft tissue management than from poor framework construction. Although tedious, the soft tissue dissection is a priority.
Cartilage framework	■ The imperfections of the framework, although hidden initially by swelling, will eventually show through the thin skin coverage. There are materials such as Styrofoam that can be used to practice the framework construction before attempting on a patient.
Exposed cartilage	■ Any skin necrosis/exposed cartilage requires immediate attention and coverage with a temporoparietal flap and skin graft.

POSTOPERATIVE CARE

- The two main issues with the postoperative care are pain management and making sure that suction is applied to the drains for the 1st day or so.
- Pain from the thoracotomy is severe and requires parenteral analgesics to be administered, at least for the first night. Pain pumps with agents such as bupivacaine have not proven to be helpful.
- The drains are left attached to wall suction until the following morning. At that point the wall suction is removed and

the drains are attached to red top Vacutainer tubes (or bulb suction if preferred).
- Patients are discharged on postoperative day 2 with the drains in place.
- The drains are then changed every 24 hours by the parents or caregivers, but not much fluid comes out after the 1st day, and it may be unnecessary to leave the drains after discharge.
- The patient is seen in the office on postoperative day 5 and the drains are removed.
- The sutures in the reconstructed auricle are usually left 10 to 14 days.

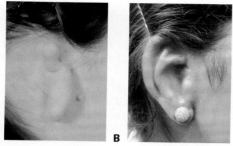

FIG 6 • Example of preoperative appearance **(A)** and postoperative result **(B)** after ear piercing.

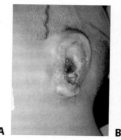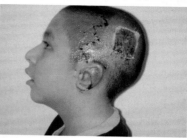

FIG 8 • **A.** The most common serious complication is necrosis of the overlying skin with impending exposure of framework. **B.** After salvage with temporoparietal flap and skin graft.

OUTCOMES

- Examples of reconstruction for microtia and for post-traumatic deformities are shown in **FIGS 6** and **7**.

COMPLICATIONS

- By far the most significant and important complication is necrosis of the skin with exposure of the underlying framework (**FIG 8**).

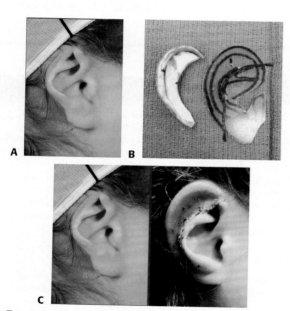

FIG 7 • **A.** Post-traumatic deformity. The remnant contains a normal concha, canal, and tragus, making an aesthetically pleasing result more likely. In this case, there was no scarring around the remnant as one might find in a burn patient or a victim of a motor vehicle accident. **B.** Framework constructed to replace the missing cartilage. **C.** Postoperative result.

- Small areas of necrosis (5 mm or less) over concavities will heal with conservative management.
- Anything larger or any necrosis over a convexity of the framework such as the helical rim or the antihelix will not and must be treated early and aggressively.
- If the wound is left to heal and does not do so, the area will become contaminated or infected and will require a more significant debridement.
  - The workhorse for closure is the temporoparietal fascial flap with a skin graft. The proximity of this tissue and its large size makes it possible to cover almost any area of necrosis.
  - In patients with craniofacial microsomia who have had other surgery and may have had the superficial temporal vessels injured by a coronal incision or a free tissue transfer, the situation becomes much more difficult. The occipital fascia can be used but tends to be thicker, and the aesthetics of the reconstruction tend to suffer more from the use of this flap.
  - In emergency situations, the exposed cartilage can be covered with a large scalping flap. The hair-bearing scalp is then returned to the scalp at a second stage, leaving skin-graftable tissue over the cartilage (crane principle).
  - In the absence of local tissue coverage, one may also consider a free temporoparietal fascial flap harvested from the contralateral side.

REFERENCES

1. Brent B. Technical advances in ear reconstruction with autogenous rib cartilage grafts: personal experience with 1200 cases. *Plast Reconstr Surg*. 1999;104(2):319-334.
2. Nagata S. A new method of total reconstruction of the auricle for microtia. *Plast Reconstr Surg*. 1993;92(2):187-201.
3. Firmin F. Ear reconstruction in cases of typical microtia: personal experience based on 352 microtic ear corrections. *Scand J Plast Reconstr Surg Hand Surg*. 1998;32(1):35-47.
4. Reinisch J, Li W. Medpor ear reconstruction: a 23-year experience with 1042 ears. *Plast Reconstr Surg*. 2014;133(4S):974.

Stahl Ear

CHAPTER 34

Akira Yamada and Arun K. Gosain

DEFINITION

- Stahl ear was first described by Binder in 1889.[1]
- Stahl ear is a congenital auricular malformation in which an abnormal third crus traverses the scapha, resulting in posterosuperior deformation of the helix.

ANATOMY

- Type 1: Obtuse bifurcation of antihelix: Superior crus of antihelix is missing, and third crus is present. Therefore, the superior and inferior crura make an obtuse angle (**FIG 1A**).
- Type 2: Trifurcation of antihelix (extra crus); this is classic Stahl ear. The third crus extends across the scapha from the antihelix (**FIG 1B**).
- Type 3: Broad superior crus, broad third crus (protruded scapha fossa) (**FIG 1C**).

PATHOGENESIS

- Etiology is unknown.
- Abnormal course of an intrinsic transverse muscle may be associated with Stahl ear.

PATIENT HISTORY AND PHYSICAL FINDINGS

- The third crus extends from the antihelix; the superior crus may or may not be present. The lower half of the auricle is usually normal.

NONOPERATIVE MANAGEMENT

- If the patient presents before 1 month of age, nonsurgical correction of the deformity with ear molding techniques may obviate the need for surgery.
- Ear molding techniques are most effective during the 1st month of life and are unlikely to work after the 2nd month of life.

SURGICAL MANAGEMENT

- There are three major types of normal helix-lobule curve (**FIG 2**). If the patient's helix-lobule curve falls into these three normal types, surgical correction of auricular shape may be directed toward deformities other than Stahl ear, such as prominent ear.

Preoperative Planning

- The possibility of ear molding is excluded if the patient presents after age 6 weeks. Ear shape analysis (especially helix type) is performed on the patient by applying an ear template for both auricles. Photographs are taken subsequent analysis. Based on photographic analysis, the patient shown has type A helix on both the normal (**FIG 3A**) and Stahl ear sides (**FIG 3B,C**).
- Two inflection points (abrupt change of the helix curve) are identified (**FIG 3D**), and the curve between the two inflection points is almost linear (**FIG 3E**).
- These two inflection points are the important landmark for wedge skin incision during surgery.

Positioning

- Supine position with slight head turn.
- Both auricles should be prepped in the sterile field, and the contralateral ear used as a reference in unilateral correction.

Approach

- Wedge excision is the simplest and most widely reported method.[2] Wedge excision is best indicated for type 2 Stahl ear. For type 1, excised cartilage may be transplanted to create the superior crus.[3] Other options for type 1 are to make parallel three cartilage cuts[4] or to place Mustarde sutures to accentuate the superior crus if there is adequate cartilage elasticity (**FIG 4A–D**).
- Cartilage turnover and rotation methods have been described but have mixed outcomes when used clinically.

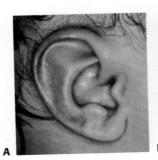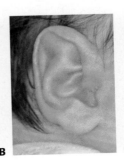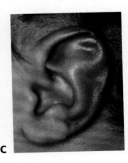

FIG 1 • A. Type 1 Stahl ear: Superior crus is missing. **B.** Type 2 Stahl ear: There are three crus (superior crus, inferior crus, and third crus). **C.** Type 3 Stahl ear: Wide third crus and protruded scapha fossa.

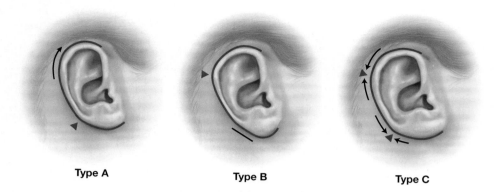

Type A   **Type B**   **Type C**

FIG 2 • The classification of helix-lobule curve.

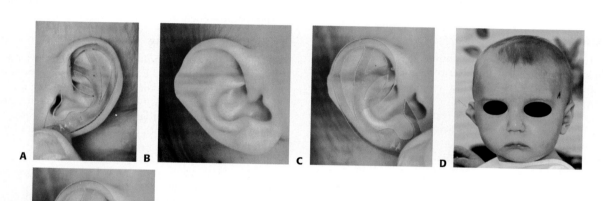

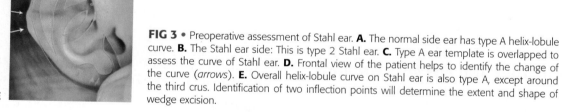

FIG 3 • Preoperative assessment of Stahl ear. **A.** The normal side ear has type A helix-lobule curve. **B.** The Stahl ear side: This is type 2 Stahl ear. **C.** Type A ear template is overlapped to assess the curve of Stahl ear. **D.** Frontal view of the patient helps to identify the change of the curve (*arrows*). **E.** Overall helix-lobule curve on Stahl ear is also type A, except around the third crus. Identification of two inflection points will determine the extent and shape of wedge excision.

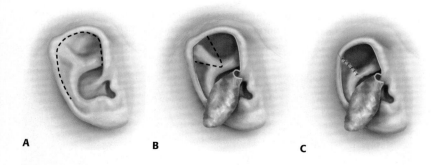

FIG 4 • Surgical approach for type 1 Stahl ear. **A.** Skin incision (*dotted line*) for type 1 Stahl ear. **B.** Wedge cartilage (third crus) is excised. **C.** Cartilage defect after wedge excision is closed primarily.

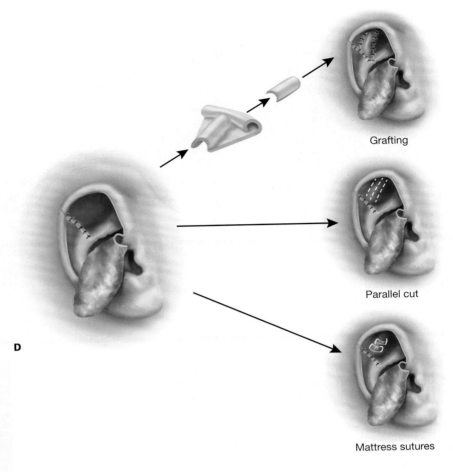

Grafting

Parallel cut

Mattress sutures

FIG 4 (Continued) • **D.** There are three options to create the superior crus: cartilage grafting, parallel cartilage incision, or mattress sutures.

■ Excision and Suturing

- Mark the wedge skin excision design between two inflection points (**TECH FIG 1A,B**).
- Cartilage (third crus) excision is expected to be longer than the skin wedge excision.
- Third crus excision is extended toward the antihelix, trying not to violate the antihelix (**TECH FIG 1C**).

- The cartilage is sutured together with 5-0 PDS (Ethicon Inc., Somerville, NJ). The focus is to align the curve of the helix (**TECH FIG 1D**).
- Suture the helix portion first and then move toward the antihelix (**TECH FIG 2A,B**).

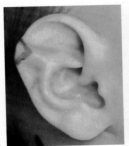

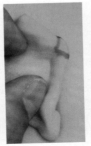

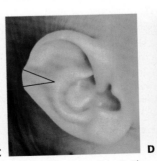

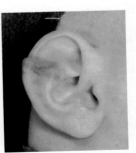

A **B** **C** **D**

TECH FIG 1 • The marking of the wedge skin excision. **A.** Anterior view. **B.** Posterior view. **C.** The marking for wedge cartilage excision. Note that cartilage excision is usually longer than the skin excision. Do not violate the antihelix. **D.** After wedge excision, the cartilage defect is closed primarily. The focus is to align the helix.

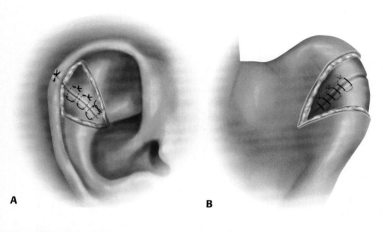

A   **B**

TECH FIG 2 • After aligning the cartilage of the helix, cartilage sutures are placed toward the antihelix. **A.** Anterior view. **B.** Posterior view.

■ Skin Closure

- Skin is closed in a single layer. Absorbable sutures can be used in children.

- We prefer 6-0 nylon suture for skin closure in adult patients, to be followed by suture removal in 2 weeks.

■ Bolster Sutures (TECH FIG 3)

- Bolster sutures are used to stabilize the helix and to prevent hematoma during the immediate post-op period.
- 4-0 Prolene is used to secure the bolster suture.
- Roll gauze is made with Xeroform plus Vaseline-based antibiotic ointments.
- Bolster sutures will be removed in 2 weeks. The wound is kept dry for 2 weeks.

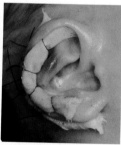

TECH FIG 3 • Bolster sutures are in place. Tie has to be very gentle to prevent pressure injury.

PEARLS AND PITFALLS

Identify inflection points.	■ This is the most important part of surgical planning. One must analyze the curve of the helix prior to surgery.
Photographic analysis	■ A slight oblique photo is best to capture the shape of the helix for analysis. Analysis of the ear on a true lateral profile is less useful for planning.
Bolster sutures	■ Tying very gently is the key. Even with a gentle tie, you will see tightness at the time of maximum swelling (48–72 h). ■ Check underneath the bolster suture with bright LED light for pressure injuries, especially 2–3 days postoperatively.
Keep the wound dry for 2 weeks	■ Avoid showering for 2 weeks postoperatively. The bolster must be kept clean to prevent infection.

POSTOPERATIVE CARE

- Periodic wound check for 2 weeks is mandatory to avoid complications.
- Keep the wound dry for 2 weeks to prevent infection. Showering may cause redness of the wound that may be difficult to differentiate from infection.
- Remove the bolster sutures in 2 weeks. During this time, periodic checks for pressure sore or tightness of the bolster sutures are important to prevent skin necrosis.

OUTCOMES

- Satisfactory outcomes are likely following the immediate wound healing process (**FIG 5**).

COMPLICATIONS

- Incomplete correction of helical deformities
- Infection
- Hematoma: Careful bolster suture helps to prevent hematoma and to stabilize the shape of the ear during the early wound healing process.

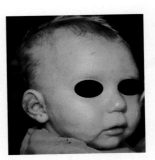

FIG 5 • Postoperative outcome.

REFERENCES

1. Binder H. Das morel'sche ohs: Eine psychiatrisch-anthroplogische studie. *Arch Psychiatr Nervenkr.* 1989;20:514.
2. Ono I, Gunji H, Terashita T. An operation for Stahl's ear. *Br J Plast Surg.* 1996;49:564.
3. Kaplan HM, Hudson DA. A novel surgical method of repair for Stahl's ear: a case report and review of current treatment modalities. *Plast Reconstr Surg.* 1999;103(2):566-569.
4. Ohmori S, Tange I, Fukuda O, et al. Operative procedure of Stahl's auricle. *Jpn J Plast Reconstr Surg.* 1962;5:212.

35
CHAPTER

Constricted Ear

Akira Yamada and Julia Corcoran

DEFINITION AND ANATOMY

- The concept of constricted ear was proposed by Tanzer.[1] The helix and scapha are hooded, and the body and crura of the antihelix are flattened in varying degrees.
  - Group 1 is the mildest form of constricted ear, often called lop ear, in which only the helix is involved (**FIG 1A**).
  - Group 2 is a moderate form of constricted ear that involves helix and scapha.
    - Group 2 is divided into 2A and 2B: 2A has only cartilage deficiency (**FIG 1B**); 2B has both skin and cartilage deficiencies (**FIG 1C,D**).
  - Group 3 is the most severe form of cupping and is characterized by a tubular structure (**FIG 1E**).
    - Differentiation between group 3 constricted ear and microtia can be difficult.

PATIENT HISTORY AND PHYSICAL FINDINGS

- Constricted ear is congenital, and the etiology is unknown.
- Ear height[2] is significantly shorter than normal.
- The helix tends to be cupped.
- The upper portion of the antitragus (superior and inferior crus) is difficult to see.
- The shape of the lower half of the auricle is likely to be normal, especially in mild to moderate constricted ear (see **FIG 1C,D**).

NONOPERATIVE MANAGEMENT

- Nonsurgical manipulation of the ear cartilage in infancy does not work for the constricted ear due to intrinsic deficiency of skin and/or cartilage.

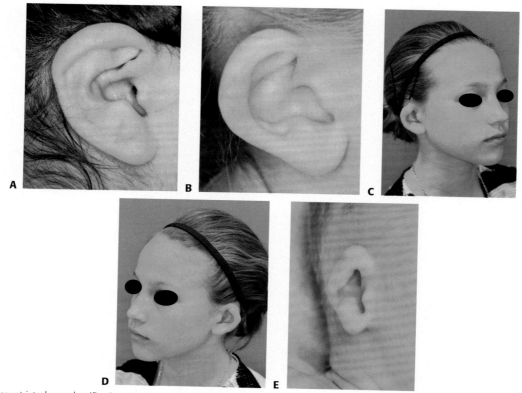

FIG 1 • Tanzer constricted ear classification. **A.** Group 1: Mild helix cartilage deformity without skin defect. **B.** Group 2A: Helix and scapha cartilage deformity without skin defect. **C,D.** Group 2B: Helix and scapha deformities with both cartilage and skin defects. **E.** Group 3: Most severe form of cupping; characterized by a tubular structure.

- Molding techniques in infancy may change the shape of the auricle but is unlikely to expand skin/cartilage.
- "Constricted" means there is cartilage and/or skin deficiencies that must be augmented by surgical procedures.

SURGICAL MANAGEMENT

Preoperative Planning

- Age-matched anthropometric data of ear dimension, especially vertical height, help to distinguish deviation of the patient's ear from norms (**FIG 2**).

Positioning

- Supine position with mild head turn. Both sides should be prepped, even with unilateral surgery, so that the contralateral ear can serve as a normal reference.

Approach

- If there is no skin defect and the cartilage defect is mild (Tanzer group 1), the Musgrave[4] procedure alone is effective to correct the deformities. If there is moderate skin and cartilage defect (Tanzer group 2B), a local skin/fascia flap plus floating rib cartilage grafting[5] is a good choice (presenting case).
- If the skin or cartilage defect is severe, microtia surgery[6] may be indicated.
- Recommended surgical options for skin envelope augmentation, based on the severity:
  - Mild: Grotting skin flap

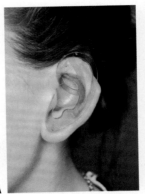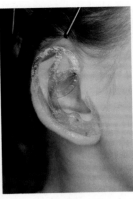

FIG 2 • A type A-2, 48-mm template is used to evaluate the degree of skin and cartilage defect of the upper half of the auricle of the left ear **(A)** and right ear **(B)**.[3] Although the left ear has more severe skin and cartilage defect, both auricles are diagnosed as Tanzer group 2B constricted ear.

  - Moderate: Park procedure (Grotting skin flap plus fascia flap)
  - Severe: Nagata microtia construction
- Recommended surgical options for cartilage defects, based on the severity:
  - Mild: Musgrave procedure
  - Moderate: floating rib (Park)
  - Severe: total framework (Nagata)

■ Markings

- The Grotting skin flap[7] measuring approximately 1.0 to 1.5 cm in width and 3.0 to 3.5 cm in length, is designed and elevated on the posterior surface of the superior auricle to drape the skin defects of the anterior and posterior helix and scapha.
- A bilobed flap is marked: the superior flap is a fascia flap, and the inferior flap is a Grotting skin flap. The fascia flap and the Grotting flap share a common base (**TECH FIG 1A,B**).

- A portion of the superficial temporal fascia will be attached beneath the proximal 1.5 cm of the Grotting flap to increase the vascularity of the Grotting flap (**TECH FIG 1C**).
- Three small, transverse skin incisions are marked at the helical crus, at or near the otobasion superius (the point of attachment of the superior helix to the temple), and at the descending helix (**TECH FIG 1D**).

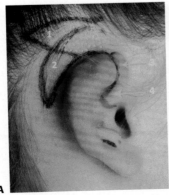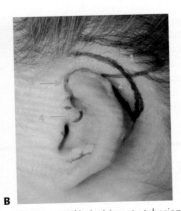

TECH FIG 1 • **A,B.** Design of the bilobed flaps. *1*: Fascia flap. *2*: Grotting skin flap. *3*: Skin incision at otobasion. *4*: Skin incision at crus helicis. *Dotted areas* indicate shared pedicle.

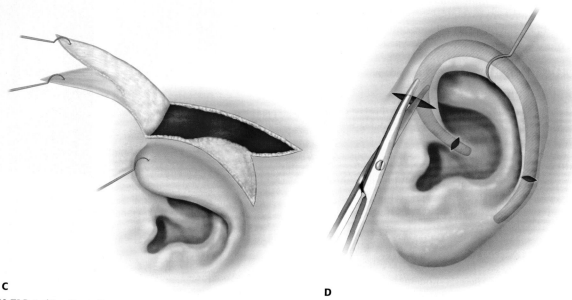

C   **D**

TECH FIG 1 (Continued) • **C.** The Grotting skin flap and the fascia flap are raised as a combined flap, sharing common pedicle at the base. **D.** Three small, transverse skin incisions are marked at the helical crus, at or near the otobasion superius (the point of attachment of the superior helix to the temple), and at the descending helix.

■ Harvesting the 8th Rib Cartilage

- A 3-cm traverse skin incision is marked at the right lower costal margin (**TECH FIG 2**). After local epinephrine injection, the skin is incised.
- After identifying the fascia of the external oblique muscle, the fascia is incised transversely. The course of the external oblique muscle is examined, and the muscle fibers are split along the course of the fibers and retracted to identify the costal cartilage.
- Care is taken to identify any perforator vessels that emerge from intercostal spaces. These vessels are coagulated with bipolar cautery well above the intercostal space.
- Prior to incising the perichondrium, a small amount of local anesthetics (eg, 0.125%–0.25% bupivacaine) is injected in the intercostal space as a nerve block.
- The anterior perichondrium of the 8th rib cartilage is gently incised with a no. 15 blade in the midline, beginning at the bone-cartilage junction.
  - A 360-degree subperichondrial dissection is performed to completely dissect the cartilage from the perichondrium.
- After 8th rib cartilage is cut at the bone-cartilage junction and removed, saline irrigation of the wound is performed.
- Once homeostasis is confirmed, the perichondrium is closed with 4-0 Vicryl. The wound is then closed in layers.

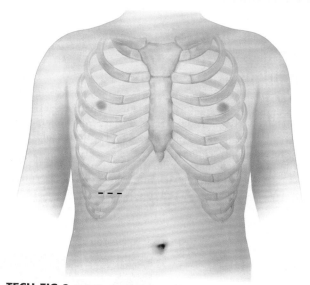

TECH FIG 2 • A 3-cm transverse skin incision at lower costal margin for harvesting 8th rib cartilage.

■ Splitting the Rib Cartilage and Creating the Skin Tunnel

- The cartilage is split longitudinally into two pieces (**TECH FIG 3A,B**).
- Splitting must be precisely in the middle for simultaneous bilateral constricted ear reconstruction.

- Through the three small skin incisions described above, a skin tunnel is created above the existing helix (see **TECH FIG 1C**).
- The split cartilage is inserted into the helical tunnel through the skin incision site at or near the otobasion superius (**TECH FIG 3C**).

TECHNIQUES

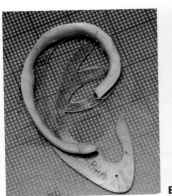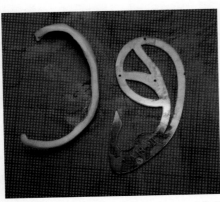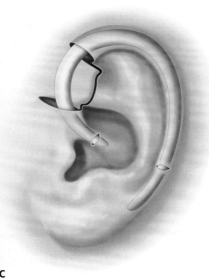

TECH FIG 3 • Split 8th rib cartilage for right **(A)** and left **(B)** ears is laid over a type A-2, 48-mm template.³ **C.** The split cartilage is inserted into the helical tunnel through the skin incision site at or near the otobasion superius.

■ Transpositioning the Fasciocutaneous Grotting Flap

■ After helix expansion with newly inserted helical cartilage, the skin envelope defect at or near the otobasion superius will be identified (the point of attachment of the superior helix to the temple). A bilobed skin/fascia flap will be transposed to fill the defect (**TECH FIG 4A**).

■ The size and location of the skin defect varies, depending on the severity and the nature of the constricted ear.
■ In the example case, both skin flap and fascia flap are transposed to cover the anterior helix and scapha on the left side (**TECH FIG 4B,C**), and only skin flap is used to cover anterior helix and scapha on the right side (**TECH FIG 4D**).

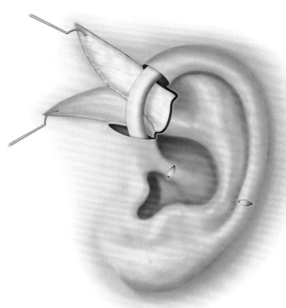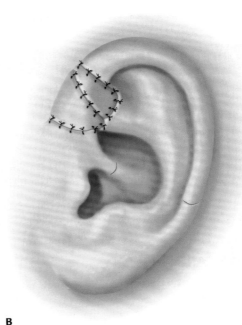

TECH FIG 4 • **A.** A bilobed skin/fascia flap will be transposed to fill the defect. **B,C.** Both skin flap and fascia flap are transposed to cover the anterior helix and scapha on the left ear. G, Grotting skin flap; F, fascia flap plus skin graft. **D.** Immediate postoperative view of the right ear showing a Grotting skin flap (*G*).

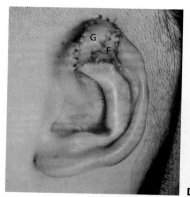
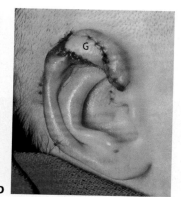

TECH FIG 4 (Continued)

■ Wound Closure and Bolster Sutures

- The skin incision is closed in a single layer.
- A small full-thickness skin graft is harvested from the back of the auricle and grafted above the fascia flap on the left side (see **TECH FIG 2**).
- Bolster sutures are used to stabilize the helix shape and to prevent hematoma during the immediate postoperative period (**TECH FIG 5**).
  - 4-0 Prolene (Ethicon, Somerville, NJ) is used to secure the bolster suture.
  - Roll gauze is made with Xeroform plus Vaseline-based antibiotic ointments.
- Bolster sutures will be removed in 2 weeks. The wound should be kept dry until removal of the bolsters.

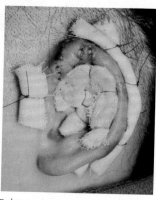

TECH FIG 5 • Bolster sutures are used to stabilize the construction and to prevent hematoma.

PEARLS AND PITFALLS

Template	■ A sterilized ear template helps to maintain precision during surgery.
Planning	■ Preoperative planning to assess the defects of skin and cartilage is critical. The ear template facilitates this process.
Costal cartilage harvesting	■ Harvesting rib cartilage while leaving the perichondrium behind is safer than harvesting cartilage with perichondrium. This helps to prevent pneumothorax and to minimize chest wall deformities.
Bolster sutures	■ A very gentle tie is the key. Even with a gentle tie, one will see tightness at the time of maximum swelling (48–72 h). Check underneath the bolster suture with bright LED light for pressure sores, especially by 2 or 3 days postoperatively. ■ The authors recommend not shampooing for 2 weeks postoperatively. Keeping the bolster dressing clean and dry helps to prevent infection.

POSTOPERATIVE CARE

- Periodic wound check for 2 weeks is strongly recommended to avoid complications.
- It is recommended to keep the wound dry for 2 weeks to prevent infection. Shampoo may cause redness of the wound and make it difficult to differentiate from infection.

- The bolster sutures will be removed in 2 weeks. Until then, periodic checks for pressure sores or tightness of the bolster sutures are important to prevent skin necrosis.

OUTCOMES

- If a balanced augmentation of the skin envelope and cartilage is achieved to expand the helix, a stable outcome is likely (**FIG 3**).

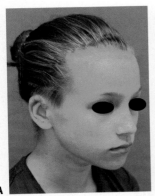 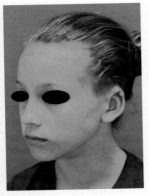

FIG 3 • Left **(A)** and right **(B)** ears are shown 3 months after surgery.

COMPLICATIONS

- Incomplete correction of the helix deformities
- Infection

- Hematoma: Careful bolster suture helps to prevent hematoma and to stabilize ear shape during the early wound healing process.

REFERENCES

1. Tanzer RC. The constricted (cup and lop) ear. *Plast Reconstr Surg.* 1975;55:406-415.
2. Farkas LG, Posnick JC, Hreczko TM. Anthropometric growth study of the ear. *Cleft Palate Craniofac J.* 1992;29(4):324-329.
3. Harada T, Yamada A, Sato A, Tomita I. Analysis of the characteristics of external ears' curves and the development of the templates. *Bull JSSD (Jpn)* 2011;57(5):21-26.
4. Musgrave RH. A variation on the correction of the congenital lop ear. *Plast Reconstr Surg.* 1966;37:394-398.
5. Park C. A new corrective method for the Tanzer's group IIB constricted ear: helical expansion using a free-floating costal cartilage. *Plast Reconstr Surg.* 2009;123(4):1209-1219.
6. Nagata S. Alternative surgical methods of treatment for the constricted ear. *Clin Plast Surg.* 2002;29:301-315.
7. Grotting JK. Otoplasty for congenital cupped protruding ears using a postauricular flap. *Plast Reconstr Surg.* 1958;22:164-167.

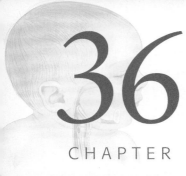

36
CHAPTER

Cryptotia

Akira Yamada and Arun K. Gosain

DEFINITION/ANATOMY

- Cryptotia is a relatively rare congenital ear deformity. The upper portion of the auricular cartilage is partially buried beneath the skin on the side of the head, hiding the upper portion of the ear. Cryptotia is often associated with helix-antihelix adhesion that results in a narrower helical arc in the upper pole. Cryptotia is also associated with upper helix deficiency that is a manifestation of constricted ear. Cryptotia is more frequent in Asian countries. In Japan, it has been reported in as many as 1 in 500 births.

PATHOGENESIS

- The cause of cryptotia is unknown. One theory is that cryptotia is the result of an anomaly of the intrinsic transverse and oblique auricular muscles.[1]

PATIENT HISTORY AND PHYSICAL FINDINGS

- The upper portion of the helix is buried underneath the skin (**FIG 1**). If one pulls the existing helix, the upper portion of the helix comes out easily. On releasing the helix, the upper helix returns to its initial position buried beneath the temporal skin.

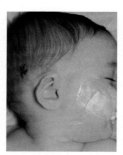

FIG 1 • Preoperative view of cryptotia; the upper pole of the helix is buried underneath the scalp.

DIFFERENTIAL DIAGNOSIS

- Helix-antihelix adhesion
- Constricted ear
- Microtia

NONOPERATIVE MANAGEMENT

- If the patient presents before 1 month of age, nonsurgical correction of the deformity with ear molding techniques may obviate the need for surgery.[2]
- Ear molding techniques are most effective during the first month of life and are unlikely to work after the 2nd month of life.
- Helix-antihelix adhesion associated with cryptotia or helix deficiency associated with constricted ear is less likely to resolve with molding techniques.

SURGICAL MANAGEMENT
Preoperative Planning

- It is important to check if the cryptotia is associated with other congenital anomalies, such as helix-antihelix adhesion or constricted ear. Pure cryptotia surgery will augment the skin deficiency but will not resolve helix-antihelix adhesion or cartilage defect of the helix associated with constricted ear.
- If cryptotia is not associated with cartilage deformities, surgery can be done in early childhood. However, if cryptotia is associated with helix deformities, the authors recommend delaying surgery until at least age 4 to 6 years because of the possible need to harvest rib cartilage.

Positioning

- Supine position with both ears prepped, including the temporal hair near the ears

■ Marking of Z-plasty

■ Z-plasty flaps are designed along the bandlike contracture above the auricle, while pulling outward away from head (**TECH FIG 1A**). The length of triangular flap depends on the degree of buried position of helix, but in this particular case, the tip of the triangular flap is located along the hairline margin (**TECH FIG 1B,C**).

■ Usually, the length of Z-plasty limb is 1.5 to 2 cm^3. The anterior limb of the Z (A–C) is usually placed 5 to 10 mm from the ascending margin of the helix. The posterior limb of Z-plasty (B–D) has a more obtuse angle than does the anterior limb, and the continuous extension of the skin incision is marked beyond the retroauricular sulcus (D–E). If more mobilization of the skin flap is needed, D–E can be extended further down, and a back cut may facilitate movement of the flap toward the skin deficiency behind the upper helix (**TECH FIG 2**).

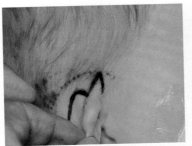
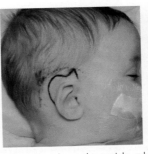
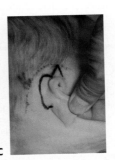

TECH FIG 1 • **A.** Triangular flap is designed along the bandlike contracture above the auricle, while pulling outward from head. **B.** The tip of the triangular flap is located along the hairline margin. **C.** If more mobilization of the skin flap is needed, the skin incision can be extended further down. A back cut may facilitate flap movement toward the skin deficiency behind the upper helix.

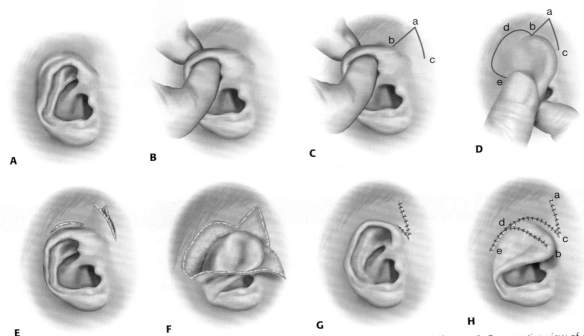

TECH FIG 2 • The diagram shows the basic design of the skin flaps, and the view after the wound closure. **A.** Preoperative view of cryptotia; upper helix is buried underneath the skin. **B.** The design of the skin incision is marked while buries portion of the upper helix is pulled out. **C.** AB lies along the line of traction. Point C must be located slightly anterior to the ascending margin of helix. **D.** CABD is a Z-plasty. The incision is extended further (as far as point E) in accordance with the requirement of cartilage plasty and the extent of skin advancement. 'de' curve is located posterior than intended retroauricular sulcus. **E.** Triangular skin flap 'cab' and skin flap 'bde' is raised. **F.** Upper ear cartilage is exposed with supraperichondrial skin flap dissection. **G.** Triangular skin flap is transposed posteriorly, and the wound is closed primarily: this maneuver eliminates the space for buried upper helix. **H.** Upper auricle is reflected anteriorly to demonstrate the completion of wound closure: Z-plasty plus advancement flap creates enough skin envelope for new helix.

TECHNIQUES

■ Skin Flap Dissection and Ear Cartilage Exposure

- Dissection of the skin flap is performed just above perichondrium to see if any cartilage modification is needed.

■ Skin Flap Transposition

- After skin flap preparation and careful hemostasis, the skin flaps are transposed toward the skin deficiency at the back of superior helix, filling residual defects.[3]

■ Wound Closure

- The skin is closed in single layer. In most cases, there is less skin tension after transposition of skin flaps to facilitate closure.

■ Bolster Sutures

- Bolster sutures (**TECH FIG 3**) are classic techniques, popularized by Tanzer more than 50 years ago. The bolster sutures have two purposes: (a) preventing hematoma formation and (b) to form an adhesion between the flap and cartilage. Nagata uses bolster sutures for almost all ear reconstruction. The key is to (a) use soft materials (eg, Xeroform gauze with additional soaking with ample Vaseline-based ointment) and (b) tie very gently to avoid any strain to the skin. The authors use 4-0 Prolene on a double-armed, SH needle (Ethicon Inc., Somerville, NJ). Periodic check, especially 2 days post-op when the swelling is maximum, is mandatory to prevent a pressure sore underneath the bolster sutures.

The temporal and mastoid skin is widely undermined to facilitate skin transposition so as to augment the posterior skin defect of the upper helix.

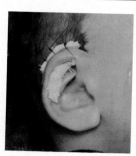

TECH FIG 3 • The view after the bolster sutures are placed.

PEARLS AND PITFALLS

Timing of surgery	■ If you are unsure about helix deformities, delay the surgery until 4–6 years of age when a floating rib graft becomes an option.
Associated ear anomalies	■ Look for helix-antihelix adhesion, and helix deficiencies associated with a constricted ear.
Design of skin flaps	■ Mark the hairline before shaving so as not to obscure the margin of the hairless posterior auricular skin.
Bolster sutures	■ Tie very gently. Use soft materials for a gauze pillow such as Xeroform soaked in Vaseline-based ointment.
Skin flap dissection	■ Skin dissection should be at uniform thickness in a plane just above perichondrium.

POSTOPERATIVE CARE

- Patients/parents should be instructed to keep the wound dry for 2 weeks. Early shampoo prior to 2 weeks may cause redness of the wound. Although this may not indicate an infection, redness is confusing for both physicians and patients. If bolster sutures are used, periodic check underneath the bolster is mandatory to prevent pressure sore.

OUTCOMES

- **FIG 2** shows the immediate outcome of surgery. If surgery is performed in early childhood, it is important to explain to the family that the child/family may notice recurrent deformities of the helix later in childhood. Families should understand that a second surgery may be considered should helix deficiencies recur. Mild helix deformities can be

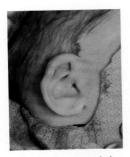

FIG 2 • The view immediately after wound closure.

addressed with the Musgrave procedure. For more severe helix deformities, floating rib graft (Park) may be indicated (see chapter on Constricted Ear).

COMPLICATIONS

- Infection: Infection can be caused by a break in proper sterile surgical technique or dehiscence secondary to excessive tension during closure. It can also be an untoward sequela of prior hematoma evacuation. A history of atopic dermatitis (eczema) is a warning sign. The ear canal could also serve as a reservoir of bacteria, especially in swimmers. Careful preparation of hairs near the surgical site is important to prevent infection.
- Postoperative hematoma: Hematoma is heralded by the acute onset of severe, persistent, and often unilateral pain.

If there is evidence of ongoing bleeding, reoperation and exploration are mandatory. Meticulous postoperative dressing, including bolster sutures, helps to prevent hematoma.
- Skin necrosis: When raising skin flap, it is important to raise the skin flap in the same plane and thickness to avoid irregular thickness of the skin flap. Small blunt straight scissors may be better than popular curved scissors in this respect. The proper plane of elevation for prominent ear is just above the perichondrium. A thinner dissection plane may result in skin necrosis. When using bolster sutures, it is mandatory to check for possible pressure sore beneath the bolster regularly until sutures removal 2 weeks postoperatively.
- Chondritis: Chondritis is a surgical emergency, which, if left untreated, can result in permanent deformity. Therefore, prompt debridement of devitalized tissue is necessary.
- Late sequelae of helix deformities of ear: These are mainly caused by unrecognized helix-antihelix adhesion or helix deficiencies associated with cryptotia. In order to avoid these complications, it is important to recognize the associated congenital ear deformities associated with cryptotia.

REFERENCES

1. Hirose T, Tomono T, Matsuo K, et al. Cryptotia: our classification and treatment. *Br J Plast Surg.* 1985;38(3):352-360.
2. Matsuo K, Hirose T, Tomono T, et al. Nonsurgical correction of congenital auricular deformities in the early neonate: a preliminary report. *Plast Reconstr Surg.* 1984;73(1):38-51.
3. Yanai A, Tange I, Bandoh Y, et al. Our method of correcting cryptotia. *Plast Reconstr Surg.* 1988;82(6):965-972.

CHAPTER 37

Prominent Ear

Akira Yamada and Arun K. Gosain

DEFINITION

- Prominent ears are a common abnormality, affecting about 5% of children. When observing other people's faces, the first thing we pay attention to is the facial triangle, eye–mouth–eye. The auricle is usually not the primary area of attention. However, if the auricle is projected more than 25 mm from the head, it tends to catch the attention of human eyes as "prominent."

ANATOMY

- The main components of the prominent ear are (1) loss of antihelical fold, (2) concha scapha angle greater than 90 degrees, and (3) conchal cartilage excess (**FIG 1**).
- Understanding ear shape anatomy, aesthetics of the ear, ear shape dimensions, and proper anatomical location of the ear is essential to achieving a natural result for the correction of prominent ear deformity.[1,2]

PATHOGENESIS

- The most common etiology of the prominent ear is effacement of the antithetical fold. Also a deep conchal bowl (greater than 1.5 cm) frequently contributes to the overall pathogenesis. Combination of these two is very common.

PATIENT HISTORY AND PHYSICAL FINDINGS

- Five parameters should be assessed systematically to ensure that all components of the prominent ear deformity are recognized: (1) auriculocephalic angle, (2) scapha-conchal angle, (3) relationship of the antihelix to the helix, (4) horizontal distance from the most lateral aspect of the helix to a point perpendicular to the skull, and (5) depth of the conchal bowl.

DIFFERENTIAL DIAGNOSIS

- Constricted ear
- Stahl ear
- Microtia

NONOPERATIVE MANAGEMENT

- If the patient presents in infancy, preferably less than 1 month of age, ear molding techniques may be indicated. Success of ear molding progressively diminishes after the first month of life, and after age 2 months, surgery is the only reliable option to correct the prominent ear.

SURGICAL MANAGEMENT

- If the distance from the head to the top of helix at any point is over 25 mm, it is considered to be a prominent ear.
  - Because the prominent ear could be the target of bullying and ridicule during school age, the most popular timing of surgery is before the start of primary school.
  - There seems to be a slightly different prominent ear concept among different cultures. Generally speaking, Asian countries are more tolerant to prominent ear, because the "big ear" is a good sign of luck and wealth.

Preoperative Planning

- Preoperative anthropometric measurement of the auricle is extremely important to achieve symmetry of the projection of the auricle postoperatively. The direct measurements also help to assess the nature of prominence. For example, if the patient has more prominence in the lower pole (25 to 30 mm), it is likely that conchal hypertrophy exists. To assess the degree of projection, the authors recommend measuring at least three points (eg, upper, middle, and lower) from the head to the top of helix. An otoplasty grid provides objective data of projection from the top to the tail of the helix (**FIG 2**). In case of unilateral prominent ear, otoplasty grid taken from normal data can be used as an intraoperative template to achieve symmetry (**FIG 3**).

Prediction of the Projection Reduction

- 20 mm distance from the mastoid to the peak of helix is acceptable projection, especially in Asian countries. In the United

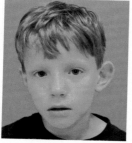

FIG 1 • Preoperative view of unilateral prominent ear (Case 2).

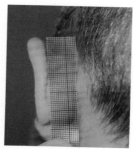

FIG 2 • Preoperative assessment of projection (Case 1).

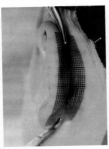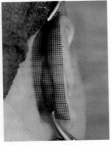

FIG 3 • Otoplasty grid is used to assess the postop helix-mastoid distance on the (**A**) left and (**B**) on the right.

States, somewhere between 15 to 20 mm is the reasonable goal to achieve. The trend of ear projection in the patient's family is a good indicator for the targeted height of projection.

Preoperative Quantification of Prominence by Otoplasty Grid

- After determining the goal of projection, the authors create a customized otoplasty grid for the patient, with a planned projection from the mastoid to the peak of the helix (15 mm in **FIG 2**). Upon placing the grid at the back of the auricle, one can visualize the amount of reduction needed for surgery.

Positioning

- Supine position with bilateral auricle preparation is recommended, even for the unilateral prominent ear, so as to check for symmetry (**FIGS 4** and **5**). One should also prepare the hair adjacent to the ears.

Approach

- Most cases need a combined approach to correct the deformities. Among numerous techniques reported in the literatures, Mustardé mattress sutures are the most commonly used method to create the antihelical fold.[3]
- Stenstrom-type anterior scoring[4] can be applied to more rigid cartilage in older children and adults to facilitate folding of the antihelix. One must be aware that adult cartilage is also fragile, and overly aggressive scoring can cause secondary deformities with irregularity of the antihelix, which are aesthetically unfavorable.
- To prevent recurrence of the prominent ear deformity, posterior skin excision is an effective adjunct that can be combined with the Mustardé techniques (**FIG 6**). The postauricular sulcus should not be markedly decreased; thus, the amount of skin excision should be conservative. Excessive skin excision

can cause tension in skin closure that may lead to hypertrophic scarring, especially in the dark-skinned population.
- If the patient has projection over 25 mm in the lower pole, conchal hypertrophy may exist and resection of conchal cartilage and/or conchal setback may be necessary. Conchal hypertrophy can cause two unwanted effects: (i) recurrence of projection, and (ii) unnatural bending with sharp angulation of the antihelix at the level of the antitragus.
- A prominent lobule not corrected by finger pressure on the helical rim will require an additional procedure.[5] Fishtail-type skin excision and a suture from the dermis to the scalp periosteum, identifying the point of control,[6] are techniques to address the prominent lobule (**FIG 7**).

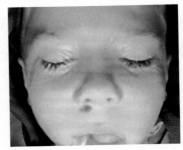

FIG 5 • Immediate postoperative view from the front. Symmetrical set back is achieved.

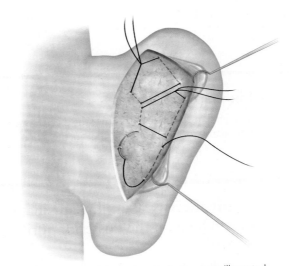

FIG 6 • Mustardé's radiated suture techniques are illustrated.

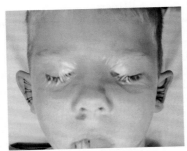

FIG 4 • The patient is placed in supine position to be able to assess bilateral projection.

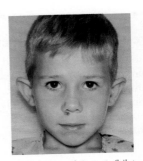

FIG 7 • Preoperative frontal view of Case 1 (bilateral prominent ears).

TECHNIQUES

■ Preoperative Marking After Intubation

- Visualizing the precise location to placing sutures: While using fingers to create ideal setback of the helix, the authors draw two curvilinear lines where the needle is planned to pass through the cartilage. Radiating direction of suture placement is also drawn (**TECH FIG 1**).

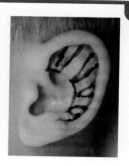

TECH FIG 1 • After intubation, curvilinear line (*red*) where sutures piercing cartilage and the direction of suture placement (*green*) are drawn on the anterior surface.

■ Deciding the Amount of Skin Incision

- Skin incision should be in the middle of posterior aspect of the auricle, so both helix and mastoid are accessible. The amount of skin excision should be conservative to preserve the postauricular sulcus. The skin closure should be tension free to prevent hypertrophic scarring (**TECH FIG 2**).

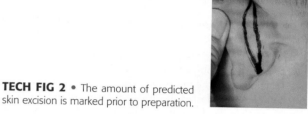

TECH FIG 2 • The amount of predicted skin excision is marked prior to preparation.

■ Local Injection

- 4 to 5 cc of half and half formula (mixture of 1% lidocaine with epinephrine, and 0.25% bupivacaine) is injected along the posterior skin incision, with pinpoint injection anteriorly where sutures are planned to penetrate cartilage. Injection is performed prior to skin prep to allow time for vasoconstriction.

■ Skin Flap Dissection

- The skin flap is dissected above the perichondrium. It is important to raise the skin flap in the same plane to create a skin flap of uniform thickness. The entire posterior cartilage surface can be exposed through this skin incision.

■ Identify the Two Curvilinear Lines and Draw Them on the Posterior Surface of the Auricle

- 25G needles are placed from the anterior surface through the posterior surface of the cartilage. These points are tattooed with blue ink (methylene blue). This maneuver is done for each point of insertion of the 25G needles, and the tattooed marks connected to create a curvilinear line on the posterior cartilage surface. Two curvilinear lines are drawn on the posterior surface.

■ Mattress Sutures Placement

- The authors use 4-0 double-armed needles (SH needle) for 4 points. A round needle is recommended because it is less likely to tear the cartilage. All four sutures are placed, but not tied, and held with mosquito forceps. The authors prefer to hand tie the sutures to visualize setback of the cartilage in creating the antihelix. The otoplasty grid helps to check the height of the helix from the skull (**TECH FIG 3A**). Sutures are tied sequentially from the top of the helix to the bottom. The lowest suture should be at the level of antitragus to avoid too much angulation or curve distortion of the antihelix due to the sutures. Care is taken to give a gentle curve to antihelix (**TECH FIG 3B**).

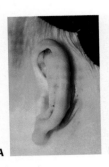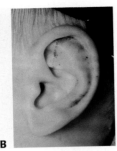

A   **B**

TECH FIG 3 • **A.** The view of projection immediately postoperatively on the left. **B.** The view of the anterior surface immediately after Mustardé suture placement.

■ Would Closure

- Two-layer skin closure is performed after confirmation of hemostasis and copious saline irrigation. The authors recommend lifting the helix very gently when closing the skin to minimize pull on the reshaped ear.

■ Bolster Sutures

- Use of bolster sutures (**TECH FIG 4**) is a classic technique popularized by Tanzer more than 50 years ago. Nagata also uses bolster sutures for most ear reconstructions. The key is to (1) use soft materials (eg, Xeroform gauze) amply soaked in vaseline-based ointment and (2) tie very gently to avoid excess pressure on the skin. The authors use 4-0 Prolene, double-armed, SH needles for the bolster sutures. Periodic checks, especially 2 days postoperatively when the swelling is maximum, are mandatory to prevent pressure sores underneath the bolster sutures.

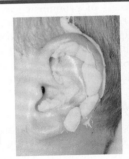

TECH FIG 4 • Bolster sutures are placed at the end.

PEARLS AND PITFALLS

Mustardé mattress sutures	■ Try to keep the natural curve of the antihelix. Do not destroy the curve by sutures.
Two curvilinear lines	■ Draw two curvilinear lines for suture placement on the posterior surface of the auricle before placing sutures.
Anterior cartilage surface scoring	■ Do not abrade the cartilage too aggressively, as this may cause late cartilage deformities.
Measurement of the projection	■ Check scalp-helix distance in at least three points bilaterally before and after surgery; the otoplasty grid can be used as a template.
Conchal hypertrophy	■ If the angle of the antihelix in the vicinity of the antitragus is too acute, consider excising a small amount of concha.

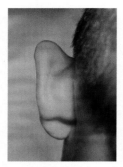

FIG 8 • Preoperative posterior left side view of Case 1 (bilateral prominent ears).

POSTOPERATIVE CARE

■ The authors ask patients/parents to keep the wound dry for 2 weeks. Early shampoo prior to 2 weeks may cause redness; this does not necessarily indicate infection, but it may confuse both the physician and the patient. If one uses bolster sutures, periodic check underneath the bolster is mandatory to prevent pressure sores.

OUTCOMES

■ Achieving symmetry is one of the key elements for the success of prominent ear correction (Case 1: **FIGS 8–10**). Measurement of the distance from mastoid to helix is a helpful guide. The authors use the otoplasty grid to help achieve symmetry. **FIG 11** shows the outcome of unilateral prominent ear correction (Case 2), for which the otoplasty grid was used as a guide to achieve symmetry.

COMPLICATIONS

■ Recurrence of prominent ear: Combined approaches instead of a single technique are better to prevent recurrence of the prominent ear. The use of resorbable sutures for the Mustardé techniques can contribute to recurrence.

■ Infection: Infection can be caused by a break in proper sterile surgical technique or dehiscence secondary to excessive tension during skin closure. Infection can also be an untoward sequela of prior hematoma evacuation. History of eczema, such as atopic dermatitis, is a warning sign. The external auditory canal could serve as a reservoir for bacteria, particularly in swimmers. Prepping the hair near the surgical site is important to prevent infection.

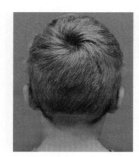

FIG 10 • Postoperative posterior view of Case 1 (bilateral prominent ears).

■ Postoperative hematoma: Hematoma is a dreaded immediate postoperative complication. It is heralded by the acute onset of severe, persistent, and often unilateral pain. If there is evidence of ongoing bleeding, reoperation and exploration are mandatory. Meticulous postoperative dressing is vital important to prevent hematoma. Compression dressings or bolster sutures are effective dressings and vary with surgeon preference.

■ Skin necrosis: It is important to raise the skin flap in the same plane and thickness to avoid irregularity of the skin flap. Small blunt straight scissors may be better than curved scissors in this respect. The proper plane of elevation for prominent ear is just above the perichondrium. A thinner skin flap is prone to skin necrosis. When using bolster sutures, it is mandatory to check for pressure sores beneath the bolster on a regular basis until the bolster sutures are removed 2 weeks postoperatively.

■ Chondritis: Chondritis is a surgical emergency. If left untreated, it can result in permanent deformity. Therefore, prompt debridement of devitalized tissue is necessary.

■ Dysesthesia: Dysesthesia is an uncommon, or less recognized, complication. The best way to avoid this complication is to use a single skin incision rather than multiple skin incisions.

■ Suture granuloma and extrusion: This is more common with permanent braided sutures.

■ Late sequelae of irregularities and deformities of the ear: These are mainly caused by too aggressive surgical techniques to modify the ear cartilage. In order to avoid these complications, less traumatic techniques and gentle manipulation of the ear cartilages are recommended.

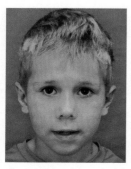

FIG 9 • Postoperative frontal view of Case 1 (bilateral prominent ears).

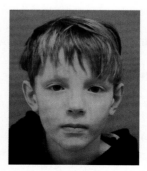

FIG 11 • Postoperative frontal view of Case 2 (unilateral prominent ear).

REFERENCES

1. Tolleth H. Artistic anatomy, dimensions, and proportions of the external ear. *Clin Plast Surg*. 1978;5:337.
2. Tolleth H. A hierarchy of values in the design and construction of the ear. *Clin Plast Surg*. 1990;17:193.
3. Mustardé JC. The correction of prominent ear susing simple mattress sutures. *Br J Plast Surg*. 1963;16:170.
4. Stenstrom SJ. A "natural" technique for correction of congenitally prominent ears. *Plast Reconstr Surg*. 1963;32:509.
5. Janis JE, Rohrich RJ, Gutowski KA. Otoplasty. *Plast Reconstr Surg*. 2005;115(4):60e-72e.
6. Gosain AK, Recinos RF. A novel approach to correction of the prominent lobule during otoplasty. *Plast Reconstr Surg*. 2003;112(2):575-583.

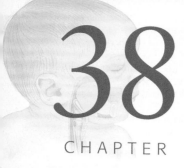

38

CHAPTER

Section IX: Eyelid Reconstruction

Eyelid Coloboma

Adam R. Sweeney and Christopher B. Chambers

DEFINITION

- Eyelid coloboma (plural: colobomata) is a congenital anomaly arising from developmental interruption of the eyelid folds causing an eyelid cleft in either the upper or lower eyelid.
- The defect may be isolated and incidental but is more commonly associated with craniofacial syndromes, ocular or periocular colobomata, or other facial clefts.[1,2]

ANATOMY

- The classic description of an eyelid coloboma is a full-thickness defect of a segment or an entire eyelid including absence of the conjunctiva, tarsus, orbicularis muscle, and skin.
- The term "pseudocoloboma" may be used to refer to a partial-thickness defect of the lid, usually involving the deeper structures with intact superficial layers.
- There is considerable variability in involvement including only a slight lid indentation to complete lid absence with underlying ocular abnormalities.
- The majority are found in the medial third of the upper lid.
- Approximately 75% of cases are unilateral.[2,3]

PATHOGENESIS

- The etiology of eyelid colobomata is not fully understood and likely varies.
- Variability in the formation of the eyelid folds early in embryogenesis vs later disruption of eyelid fusion/fissure may implicate the location of a coloboma defect and any associated facial clefts.[2,4]
- Attributed etiologies include intrauterine amniotic bands, abnormalities in vitamin A metabolism, intrauterine inflammation, decreased placental circulation, hamartomas, abnormal fetal vasculature, failure of eyelid fold fusion, or abnormal fetal migration of the neural crest cells.[5–7]
- Colobomata may occur in conjunction with Goldenhar syndrome (oculoauriculovertebral dysplasia),[1,8] Treacher Collins syndrome (mandibulofacial dysostosis),[3] frontonasal dysplasia, and Delleman syndrome.[9] Goldenhar syndrome is associated with unilateral upper lid coloboma, whereas Treacher Collins is associated with lower eyelid coloboma or pseudocoloboma.[2]

NATURAL HISTORY

- Untreated, an eyelid coloboma may lead to neonatal exposure keratopathy with corneal ulceration and perforation.

- A small coloboma associated with the appropriate amount of superior rotation of the eye upon eye closure, known as a Bell reflex, may be asymptomatic requiring only cosmetic surgery later in life.

PATIENT HISTORY AND PHYSICAL FINDINGS

- Careful physical examination should be performed to assess the thickness and extent of eyelid loss in both upper and lower eyelids of both eyes. Attention should be given to the degree of skin laxity for anticipated donor lids, integrity of anchor sites on the involved lid, and skin color/thickness.[10]
- Fornices of eyelids should be meticulously examined for adhesions (symblepharon) that may hint at underlying diagnosis of cryptophthalmos.
- Full ophthalmic examination with cycloplegic refraction, eye motility examination, external examination, slit-lamp examination and dilated fundus examination should be performed to identify other regions of adverse development.
- Both eyes should be closely examined.
- The most common finding is an upper eyelid medial full-thickness abnormality. The defect is typically a triangular or quadrangular lesion with the base toward the eyelid margin (**FIG 1**).[1,6,11]
- The defect may vary in severity from a small indentation to the full eyelid length.
- If present in the lower eyelid, partial-thickness defects are more common.

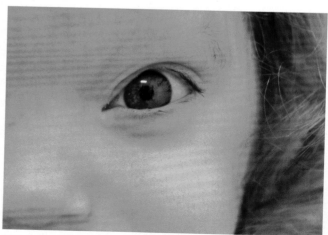

FIG 1 • Left upper eyelid coloboma with loss of lashes, eyelid notch, and irregular upper eyelid contour.

DIFFERENTIAL DIAGNOSIS

- Associated syndromes:
  - Goldenhar syndrome (epibulbar dermoids, preauricular appendages, blind pretragal fistulae, hemifacial atrophy, vertebral anomalies)[1,8]
  - Treacher Collins syndrome (lower eyelash irregularities, absence of lower puncta, iris coloboma, microphthalmos, midface hypoplasia, lateral downward slant of the palpebral fissures)[3]
  - Delleman syndrome (orbital cysts, intracranial cysts, skin appendages)[9]
  - Other facial clefting syndromes affecting the eyelids; as described by Tessier, facial clefts
- Eyelid trauma
- Entropion
- Cryptophthalmos

NONOPERATIVE MANAGEMENT

- A small eyelid coloboma with mild corneal exposure may be treated with lubrication, bandage contact lenses, or moisture chambers with surgery deferred until 6 months of age or later when pediatric eyelid tension has relaxed.[3]

SURGICAL MANAGEMENT

- Surgical correction is the preferred method of treatment.
- Surgery is required and urgently indicated in cases where exposure keratopathy is present or imminent.

Preoperative Planning

- General anesthesia is recommended for pediatric cases.
- Review the facial photos and examination including size, location, and shape of the lid defect to help determine the appropriate technique.

Positioning

- The patient is positioned supine on a surgical table with an adjustable headrest lowered to give the surgeon the best access. The patient should be prepped and draped leaving the full face exposed.

Approach

- Upper or lower eyelid lesions involving ¼ of the eyelid or less may be amenable to direct closure.
- Upper or lower eyelid lesions involving a quarter to half the eyelid are treated with Tenzel semicircular flap.
- Large lesions with significant tissue loss involving ½ or more of the eyelid may be managed via a one-stage graft technique involving a tarsomarginal graft from the ipsilateral lower intact lid or from the contralateral intact upper eyelid.[12]
- For lesions with greater than ½ eyelid tissue loss and not amenable to a one-stage closure, a two-stage lower lid rotation to the upper lid via a Cutler-Beard technique may be employed.[13]
- The vast majority of large colobomata involving greater than ½ of the eyelid involve the upper eyelid; thus, techniques specifically addressing upper eyelid repair are described below. One-stage and two-stage grafting for lower eyelid closures are routinely performed and described for other conditions; however, these are out of the scope of this chapter.

TECHNIQUES

■ Direct Closure

- Place topical tetracaine on the conjunctival surface.
- Inject 1 to 2 cc 2% lidocaine with 1:100 000 epinephrine into the subcutaneous space around the lesion and the lateral canthus.
- Unscroll the underlying tissue of the eyelid margin to explore the full depth of the defect.

- Using a no. 15 blade, trim the borders of the defect to prepare for a full-thickness, aligned graft site.
- Pull the defect edges together; if there is significant tension, consider a canthotomy and cantholysis (**TECH FIG 1**).
- Create a horizontal incision along the lid crease or intended lid crease from the border of the medial defect laterally along the lid crease. The extent of the lid crease incision should be lengthened to create the amount of

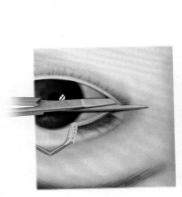
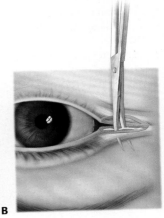

TECH FIG 1 • A,B. Upper eyelid coloboma with position of proposed canthotomy outlined in the *dotted line*.

A

B

laxity needed to approximate the lateral border of the defect to the medial border of the defect without tension.

- Using a 6-0 Vicryl suture, make a single pass at the eyelid margin from tarsus to tarsus spanning the defect. Ensure equal depth (2 mm deep to the margin) and horizontal distance from the defect (2 mm from the defect border) to create a perfectly reapproximated closure. Apply tension to the ends of the suture to assess the alignment of the closure, but do not tie a knot.
- Using 6-0 Vicryl suture, reapproximate the deep tarsus using a buried interrupted pass. This pass should be repeated for every 2 mm of vertical tarsus absent. Do not tie the knot.
- Using another 6-0 Vicryl suture, reapproximate the eyelash line using a single pass.
- Using another 6-0 Vicryl suture, make a third eyelid margin pass reapproximating the gray line (**TECH FIG 2A**). Ensure attention is paid to the same techniques as used to reapproximate the tarsus at the margin.
- Tighten all the sutures. The eyelid margin should realign with a slight eversion. If the eyelid has perfect reapproximation, tie all the knots with a 3-1-1 knot. Leave the suture tails 3 to 5 mm long (**TECH FIG 2B**).
- Close the superficial skin using 7-0 fast gut interrupted sutures. Tie the knots of the sutures with the tails of the Vicryl suture under the knot to keep the eyelid margin suture tails from rubbing against the cornea (**TECH FIG 2C**).
- Close the relaxation incision with 7-0 fast gut sutures in an interrupted fashion.
- Apply erythromycin ointment over the wound.

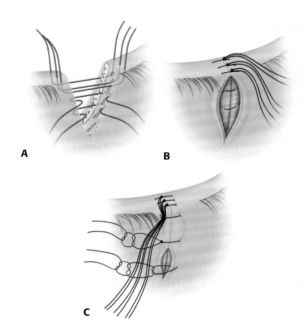

TECH FIG 2 • Margin involving defect closure. **A.** Simple closure of a small eyelid defect including three eyelid margin passes: one through the tarsus, one through the gray line, and one through the lash line. **B.** Deep nonmarginal tarsus passes are closed first in buried fashion. Tying of margin involving knots is then performed leaving suture tails 3 to 5 cm long. **C.** Close the superficial skin incorporating the marginal suture tails in the skin closure knots to detract the tails from the cornea.

■ Tenzel Semicircular Flap

- Place topical tetracaine on the conjunctival surface.
- Using a sterile marking pen, draw a semicircle at the lateral canthus inferiorly oriented for upper lid repair or superiorly oriented for lower lid repair (**TECH FIG 3A**).
- Inject 2% lidocaine with 1:100 000 epinephrine into the subcutaneous space around the defect extending to the frontozygomatic suture.
- Unscroll the underlying tissue of the eyelid margin to explore the full depth of the defect.
- Using a no. 15 blade, incise the skin and orbicularis tissue along the marked semicircle beginning at the lateral canthus.
- Undermine the musculocutaneous semicircular flap laterally using blunt dissection to create lid laxity (**TECH FIG 3B**).
- Complete a full-thickness canthotomy using Westcott scissors.

- Grasp the lateral aspect of the involved eyelid and gently apply anterior traction to expose the canthal tendon. For an upper eyelid coloboma, perform a superior arm cantholysis; and for lower eyelid coloboma, perform an inferior arm cantholysis (**TECH FIG 4A,B**).
- The cantholysis of the respective arm of the canthal tendon is performed by strumming the multiple attachments of the respective arm with closed scissors and then cutting each attachment, ensuring further laxity is felt with each cut (**TECH FIG 4B**). Avoid cutting conjunctiva by maintaining adequate visualization and hemostasis with handheld cautery.
- Full cantholysis is achieved when the respective eyelid can be distracted to reach the superior orbital rim for an inferior cantholysis or the inferior orbital rim for a superior cantholysis (**TECH FIG 4C**).
- Using a no. 15 blade, trim the borders of the defect to prepare a full-thickness, aligned graft site. This should be attempted to create a rectangle-shaped border to ensure easier closure.

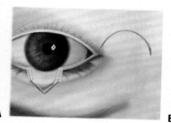 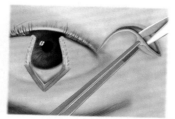

TECH FIG 3 • A,B. Diagram depicting inferiorly oriented semicircular orientation for large upper lid coloboma repair.

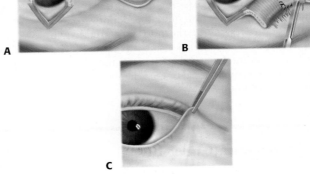

TECH FIG 4 • Lateral canthotomy and cantholysis. **A.** Following canthotomy, a lateral cantholysis is performed by grasping the eyelid margin and brought anteriorly to expose the multiple canthal tendon arms. For upper lid repairs, a superior cantholysis is performed; for lower lid repairs, an inferior cantholysis is performed **(B)**. **C.** Full lower lid cantholysis is achieved when the lower lid can be distracted superiorly to the superior orbital rim. Similarly, an upper lid cantholysis is achieved when the upper lid can be distracted to the inferior orbital rim.

- Using forceps, distract the loose eyelid margin to bring together the edges of the wound (**TECH FIG 5A**). Mark the temporal aspect of the distracted eyelid that aligns with the lateral canthus of the uninvolved/unaffected eyelid.
- Close the eyelid defect wound using the steps described in the "direct closure" technique above (**TECH FIG 3**).
- Using a single interrupted 5-0 Vicryl suture, make a pass through the deep tissues along the repaired eyelid where previously marked at the intended site of lateral canthus reconstitution. Secure this suture by passing it through the periosteum of the underlying lateral orbital rim exiting 1 to 2 mm superior to the entrance of the pass (**TECH FIG 5B**).

- Secure the lateral aspect of the flap using 5-0 Vicryl suture by making a single pass through the deep tissues of the flap, into the underlying prezygomatic fascia, and then out the deep tissue of the opposite side of the flap to create a buried suture adherent to the underlying fascia.
- Repeat this step with interrupted sutures to fully close the length of the flap.
- Reconstitute the lateral canthus by suturing the upper lid gray line to the lower lid gray line approximately 2 mm from the termination of the lateral gray line using 6-0 Vicryl suture.
- Close the superficial skin of the flap using 7-0 fast gut suture in an interrupted fashion.
- Apply erythromycin ointment over the wound.

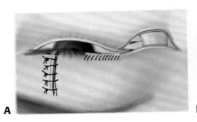
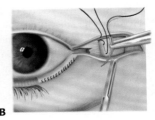

TECH FIG 5 • **A.** Align the tissue with minimal tension to the lateral canthus of the opposite eyelid. **B.** Secure the tissue with a 5.0 vicryl suture through the obicularis muscle to the orbital rim periosteum.

■ One-Stage Graft (Tarsomarginal Graft)

- Place topical tetracaine on the conjunctival surface.
- Using a sterile marking pen, draw an inferiorly oriented semicircle at the lateral canthus.
- Inject 2% lidocaine with 1:100 000 epinephrine into the subcutaneous space around the defect and the contralateral upper eyelid.
- Unscroll the underlying tissue of the eyelid margin to explore the full depth of the defect.
- Using a no. 15 blade, trim the borders of the defect for a full-thickness, aligned graft site.
- Using calibers, measure the dimensions of the missing underlying tarsus.
- Mark the contralateral (donor) upper eyelid with the calipers per the dimensions measured for the graft upper

lid using an inferior border that is superior to the eyelid margin (**TECH FIG 6**).
- On the contralateral (donor) upper eyelid, use Westcott scissors to dissect a plane at the level of the orbicularis

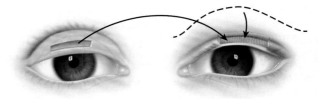

TECH FIG 6 • Scheme depicting one-stage contralateral upper eyelid graft using donor conjunctival/tarsus to host eyelid. Host upper eyelid anterior lamella is placed over the graft after undermining superiorly and laterally.

oculi, extending to the marked borders between the posterior lamella (conjunctiva and tarsus) and the anterior lamella (orbicularis muscle and skin).

- Using Westcott scissors, amputate the graft of tarsus and conjunctiva from the contralateral donor upper eyelid within the borders marked, sparing the eyelid margin.
- Bring the tarsomarginal graft into the donor site and suture the grafted tarsus to the host tarsus with two interrupted 6-0 Vicryl sutures per side leaving the eyelid margin free of suture. Ensure the knots are buried deep, avoiding potential conjunctival or corneal abrasion from posterior oriented knots.

Two-Stage Graft (Cutler-Beard)

- Place topical tetracaine on the conjunctival surface.
- Inject 2% lidocaine with 1:100 000 epinephrine into the subcutaneous space of the upper and lower eyelids.
- Unscroll the underlying tissue of the eyelid margin to explore the full depth of the defect.
- Using a no. 15 blade, trim the borders of the defect for a full-thickness, aligned graft site. This should be attempted to create a rectangle-shaped border to ensure easier closure.
- Using a sterile marking pen, make two vertical markings on the lower lid to outline the borders of the horizontal defect of the upper lid. Connect the vertical markings of the lower lid horizontal mark placed 4 mm inferior to the eyelid margin.
- Pass a 4-0 silk traction suture into the lower eyelid margin ensuring a tarsal bite is achieved.
- Using a no. 15 blade, incise the skin and orbicularis over the horizontal marking (**TECH FIG 7A**).
- Holding the silk suture by the tails, evert the lower lid over an eyelid retractor and make a horizontal conjunctival incision. This incision should be deep to the horizontal marking previously placed on the lower eyelid skin.
- Using Westcott scissors, incise through the conjunctival incision full thickness to connect to the anterior lamella incision.
- Using Westcott scissors, make deep orbicularis cuts through the vertical markings of the lower lid (**TECH FIG 7B**).
- With toothed forceps, grasp the superior edge of the flap created by the full-thickness horizontal incision already created. Bring this flap under the lower eyelid margin (through the blepharotomy) and place it into the region of the upper eyelid defect (**TECH FIG 7C**).
- Suture the lower lid grafted tarsus to the tarsus at the borders of the upper lid coloboma using 5-0 Vicryl suture with at least two passes per side ensuring anteriorly oriented knots to avoid conjunctival abrasion (**TECH FIG 7D**).
- Undermine around the lid defect until the anterior lamella is lax enough to close the anterior lamella directly and without tension using 5-0 Vicryl sutures (**TECH FIG 7E**).

- Using Westcott scissors, reconstruct the donor upper lid anterior lamella by undermining deep to the patient's adjacent orbicularis muscle using Westcott scissors. Advance the adjacent anterior lamella over the graft tissue ensuring no vertical tension is created. Close this tissue with interrupted 7-0 gut passes.
- Close the posterior lamella of the donor eyelid via the "direct closure" of deep horizontal eyelid lesion technique described above (**TECH FIG 3**).
- Apply erythromycin ointment over both eyelids.

- Close the superficial skin of the flap using 7-0 fast gut interrupted passes.
- Apply erythromycin ointment over the wound.
- The second stage is performed by releasing the flap with Westcott scissors at the intended eyelid margin. Excess conjunctiva and skin can be removed from the upper eyelid (**TECH FIG 8**).

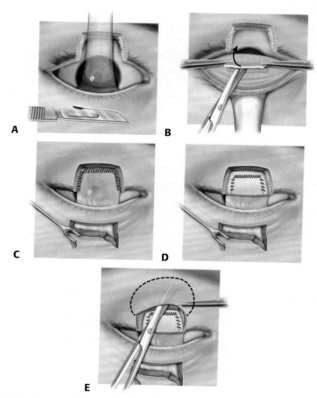

TECH FIG 7 • First stage of Cutler-Beard procedure. **A.** Incision is made through skin and orbicularis over the horizontal marking. **B.** Incision through the vertical markings is made revealing full tarsoconjunctival flap. This is dissected from the anterior lamellae. **C.** The flap is grasped and sutured into the graft position allowing laxity of tissue. **D.** The graft is sutured into position using 5-0 Vicryl suture ensuring anteriorly oriented knots. **E.** The anterior lamellae host tissue is then sutured into position using 7-0 fast gut.

TECHNIQUES

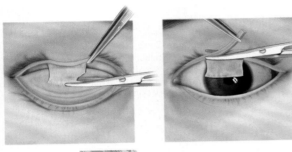

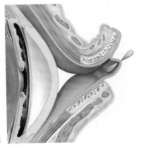

TECH FIG 8 • Second stage of Cutler-Beard procedure. **A.** Incise the graft tissue at the desired upper lid margin using a metal backing to protect the underlying cornea. **B.** Marginal and graft are then sutured ensuring no knots exposed to the cornea.

- The remaining conjunctiva is sutured into place to the anterior edge of the eyelid margin using 7-0 fast gut sutures with the knot placed away from the cornea (**TECH FIG 9**).
- In children between birth and 14 years old, the second stage is performed at 2 weeks, rather than the recommended 4 to 6 weeks, to minimize the risk of deprivation amblyopia.

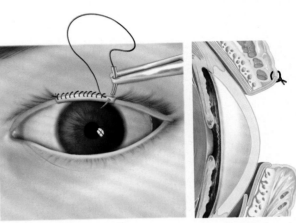

TECH FIG 9 • Suture the excess conjunctiva over the anterior edge of the eyelid margin with a fast gut suture.

PEARLS AND PITFALLS

Choosing a technique	■ Two-stage repairs for large colobomata incur a period of visual deprivation that can lead to amblyopia. Full consideration of one-stage technique, when applicable, is recommended. ■ Skin laxity and eyelid graft development must be considered when choosing a graft. There is tendency to underestimate the tension and required modifications to adequately close pediatric eyelid defects.
Timing of surgery	■ Children less than 3–6 months of age have less skin laxity, and when not contraindicated, postponement of surgery may achieve better outcomes. When early surgery is indicated, the lateral canthotomy and cantholysis described in the "direct closure" technique offers improved eyelid relaxation, decreasing horizontal tension.

POSTOPERATIVE CARE

- Prescribe topical application of antibiotic ointment over the wounds 3 times a day for 1 to 2 weeks.
- Recommend sun tan lotion to improve scar results.
- Comanagement with pediatric ophthalmologist is recommended for regular refraction and monitoring for development of primary or secondary strabismus or corneal scarring.

OUTCOMES

- Surgical success is dependent on the degree of the coloboma and the procedure type selected.
- Irregular postoperative eyelid contour may occur if the lid defect is closed under too much tension.[3]

COMPLICATIONS

- Exposure keratopathy from unintended vertical traction
- Loss of lashes from the graft or trichiasis

- Entropion or ectropion
- Ptosis secondary to poor levator function or postoperative horizontal traction
- Poor appearance

REFERENCES

1. Tawfik HA, Abdulhafez MH, Fouad YA. Congenital upper eyelid coloboma: embryologic, nomenclatorial, nosologic, etiologic, pathogenetic, epidemiologic, clinical, and management perspectives. *Ophthal Plast Reconstr Surg.* 2015;31(1):1-12.
2. Smith HB, Verity DH, Collin JR. The incidence, embryology, and oculofacial abnormalities associated with eyelid colobomas. *Eye (Lond).* 2015;29(4):492-498.
3. Grover AK, Chaudhuri Z, Malik S, et al. Congenital eyelid colobomas in 51 patients. *J Pediatr Ophthalmol Strabismus.* 2009;46(3):151-159.
4. Guercio JR, Martyn LJ. Congenital malformations of the eye and orbit. *Otolaryngol Clin North Am.* 2007;40(1):113-140, vii.
5. Roper-Hall MJ. Congenital colobomata of the lids. *Trans Ophthalmol Soc U K.* 1969;88:557-566.
6. Seah LL, Choo CT, Fong KS. Congenital upper lid colobomas: management and visual outcome. *Ophthal Plast Reconstr Surg.* 2002;18(3):190-195.

7. Miller MT, Deutsch TA, Cronin C, Keys CL. Amniotic bands as a cause of ocular anomalies. *Am J Ophthalmol.* 1987;104(3): 270-279.

8. Gorlin RJ, Jue KL, Jacobsen U, Goldschmidt E. Oculoauriculovertebral dysplasia. *J Pediatr.* 1963;63:991-999.

9. Delleman JW, Winkelman JE. [The significance of atypical colobomata and defects of the iris for the diagnosis of the hereditary aniridia syndrome (author's transl)]. *Klin Monbl Augenheilkd.* 1973;163(5):528-542.

10. Collin JR. Congenital upper lid coloboma. *Aust N Z J Ophthalmol.* 1986;14(4):313-317.

11. Nouby G. Congenital upper eyelid coloboma and cryptophthalmos. *Ophthal Plast Reconstr Surg.* 2002;18(5):373-377.

12. Hoyama E, Limawararut V, Malhotra R, et al. Tarsomarginal graft in upper eyelid coloboma repair. *J AAPOS.* 2007;11(5):499-501.

13. Cutler NL, Beard C. A method for partial and total upper lid reconstruction. *Am J Ophthalmol.* 1955;39(1):1-7.

Congenital Ptosis

Adam R. Sweeney and Christopher B. Chambers

DEFINITION

- Blepharoptosis, commonly referred to as ptosis, is eyelid positioning inferior to normal posture. Often, ptosis is defined as asymmetry of 1 mm or more between the two upper eyelids or a marginal reflex distance of less than 2.5 mm.[1]
- Congenital ptosis refers to cases presenting within the first year of life, as an isolated finding or as a manifestation of ophthalmic or systemic disorders.
- Typically, congenital ptosis results from fibrofatty degeneration of the levator complex.
- Congenital ptosis affects an estimated 1 in 842 births in the United States.[1]

ANATOMY

- The anterior lamella is made up of the skin and the preseptal orbicularis (**FIG 1**).
- The posterior lamella is made up of the tarsus and the palpebral conjunctiva.
- The tarsus is a fibrous plate located in the eyelid. It is 9 to 10 mm in height in the upper eyelid and 4 mm in height in the lower lid. The length of the tarsus is approximately 22 to 25 mm.
- Posterior to the orbital septum lies the preaponeurotic fat pad, an important surgical landmark.
- The levator aponeurosis is the primary retractor of the upper eyelid and is located just posterior to the preaponeurotic fat.
- The levator palpebrae originates above the annulus of Zinn and attaches to Whitnall ligament, a transverse facial suspensory structure. This attachment allows the levator muscle's horizontal vector to be redirected to the vertical vector created from its anterior extension, the levator aponeurosis, which terminates at the anterior tarsus.
- Muller muscle arises from the posterior layer of the levator muscle and inserts into the upper border of the tarsal plate.
- The lid crease is formed from levator aponeurosis fibers inserting into the fascicular bundles of the pretarsal orbicularis.
- In patients not of Asian descent, the lid crease is located between the upper border of the tarsus and the insertion of the orbital septum, which is approximately 3 to 5 mm superior to the upper border of the tarsus. The lid crease is approximately 9 to 11 mm and 8 to 9 mm superior to the eyelid margin in females and males, respectively.
- In Asians, the lid crease is much lower secondary to a more anterior preaponeurotic fat pad and low/absent attachment of the aponeurosis fibers to the fascicular bundles of the pretarsal orbicularis.

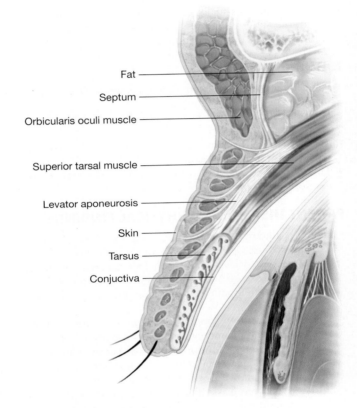

FIG 1 • Anatomy of the upper eyelid.

- The levator muscle is a striated muscle and is innervated by cranial nerve (CN) III, whereas Muller muscle is a smooth muscle innervated by the sympathetic chain.
- The frontalis muscle inserts into the orbicularis oculi at the inferior brow.

PATHOGENESIS

- There are multiple different etiologies of congenital ptosis.
- Approximately 80% of congenital ptosis arises from dysgenesis or fibrosis of the levator muscle with remaining integrity of the levator aponeurosis, termed myogenic ptosis or simple congenital ptosis.[1,2]
- Myogenic ptosis is more common unilaterally than bilaterally.
- Neurogenic etiologies are much less common and arise from innervation abnormalities during development such as abnormal motor nerve connections of the levator muscle

and branches of the trigeminal nerve innervating the external pterygoid muscle (Marcus Gunn jaw winking), interrupted sympathetic nervous chain (Horner syndrome), congenital cranial nerve III palsy, or congenital cranial dysinnervation disorders such as Duane retraction syndrome.

- Aponeurotic ptosis is caused by a defect in the tendon's ability to redirect the action supplied by the levator muscle. This is classically different from disinsertion of the aponeurosis from the levator muscle, as is commonly seen in advancing age or from trauma including childbirth.
- Mechanical ptosis is caused by a forced inferior excursion of the eyelid such as seen in tumor, eyelid inflammation/edema, cicatricial processes, or foreign body.
- Traumatic ptosis usually can be found to be inclusive in one of the above categories and may arise in utero or from trauma, such as during childbirth.

NATURAL HISTORY

- Congenital ptosis may be mild and benign with no impact on vision or function of the child.
- Severe congenital ptosis may cause amblyopia due to deprivation or astigmatism.
- Twenty to thirty percent with congenital ptosis have concurrent strabismus or astigmatism.[3,4]
- Twenty-five percent of patients with congenital ptosis develop amblyopia of the involved eye.[2]

PATIENT HISTORY AND PHYSICAL FINDINGS

- Hallmark findings distinguishing congenital myogenic ptosis from acquired ptosis: absence or irregular upper eyelid crease, decreased levator function (particularly prominent in upward gaze), eyelid retraction in downward gaze, and presence of lagophthalmos (a common finding in congenital ptosis).
- Marcus Gunn jaw-winking ptosis involves elevations of the eyelid with pterygoid muscle movement usually evident with sucking or chewing. Monitoring for association of lid height in various gazes and facial movements including jaw movement is important to rule out this condition.
- Horner syndrome classically manifests with ptosis, meiosis, and anhidrosis ipsilateral to the neurological defect. Ipsilateral lower lid inverse ptosis may also be seen. Heterochromia characterizes the congenital form from acquired Horner syndrome and necessitates systemic workup.
- Margin reflex distance (MRD) of the upper lid and vertical palpebral fissure height should be routinely assessed, when possible.
- MRD_1 in down gaze, evaluating chin, head, and brow position should be noted as compensatory mechanisms.
- Strength of Bell phenomenon (eye elevation and abduction on attempted lid closure) may indicate whether dysgenesis of the levator muscle includes the superior rectus muscle.
- Perform a pupil exam monitoring for symmetry.
- Test extraocular muscle movements assessing for partial CN III palsy or assessing for hypotropia-related pseudoptosis.
- Test the frontalis contribution by immobilizing the brow in primary position as children often will attempt to correct ptosis by recruiting the frontalis muscle.
- Assess corneal exposure issues with fluorescein staining.

- The phenylephrine test is performed by instilling one eye drop of 2.5% phenylephrine to the inferior cul-de-sac. This elevates the eyelids within 10 minutes via the sympathetic response on smooth muscles of the eyelid, principally Muller muscle. The MRD_1 should be assessed before and 10 minutes after instillation. Demonstration of adequate improvement of the ptosis after phenylephrine test may guide the surgical technique required, such as a Muller muscle resection. Unilateral phenylephrine dosing may reveal a contralateral ptosis masked by Hering law of equal bilateral innervation.
- Attaining visual acuity and fixation preferences may help detect amblyopia. Evaluation of these patients with a pediatric ophthalmologist is important.

IMAGING

- Quality full facial photographs should be obtained for preoperative planning and intraoperative reference.
- In older children or adults with congenital ptosis, visual field testing with taped and untaped eyelids should be performed.
- An A-scan may be performed if one is concerned about pseudoptosis, a term describing ptosislike appearance from pathology independent of the eyelid, such as microphthalmia or advanced hyperopia.
- Cycloplegic refraction or autorefraction may be performed to detect ptosis-induced astigmatism that may be amblyogenic.
- Congenital Horner syndrome should be evaluated with a tumor workup that may necessitate MRI investigation.

DIFFERENTIAL DIAGNOSIS

- Myogenic: myasthenia gravis, chronic progressive external ophthalmoplegia, muscular dystrophy, and oculopharyngeal dystrophy
- Myogenic etiology also seen in blepharophimosis-ptosis-epicanthus inversus syndrome (BPES), which also may have euryblepharon, telecanthus, ear deformities, and hypoplasia of the superior orbital rims and nasal bridge
- Neurogenic: Marcus Gunn jaw-winking ptosis, Horner syndrome, aberrant regeneration of the oculomotor nerve, Duane retraction syndrome
- Aponeurotic ptosis refers to slowly progressive ptosis from involutional changes in the levator aponeurosis with gradual stretching or dehiscence of this structure.
- Mechanical ptosis from excessive upper eyelid weight such as secondary to an eyelid mass, foreign body, or eyelid edema
- Pseudoptosis: Microphthalmia (underdevelopment of the orbit, lids, and socket) or advanced hyperopia with smaller anteroposterior globe length

NONOPERATIVE MANAGEMENT

- If ptosis is not cosmetically bothersome and does not appear to affect visual axis or lead to astigmatism, observation may be appropriate.

SURGICAL MANAGEMENT

- When potentially amblyogenic, prompt ptosis surgery is indicated.

- The timing of surgical correction in the absence of visually threatening ptosis is debated with many advocating for correction at approximately age 4 when structures are more defined and the child is more cooperative[5]; however, others suggest earlier treatment advocating ease of development and postoperative care.
- Consideration of the type of surgery should reflect the degree of ptosis, levator function, and emphasis on cosmetic outcomes.
- Surgeon preference often is considered when choosing a technique; however, surgeons should be comfortable with the major techniques including frontalis suspension, levator resection, and Muller muscle surgery.
- When levator function is less than 3 to 4 mm, frontalis suspension is typically preferred when possible.[2,5]
- External levator resection or advancement may be employed for patients with moderate levator function and mild to moderate ptosis.[2,5]
- A poor Bell phenomenon may require a temporary lower lid retraction suture, or Frost suture, to protect the cornea following ptosis surgery.
- Frontalis suspension may utilize a silicone, Mersilene mesh, Gore-Tex, Ptose-Up strips, or Supramid material. However, if the child is older than 3 or 4 years, autogenous fascia lata may be utilized, which some report yields better results.[6]

Preoperative Planning

- General anesthesia is recommended for pediatric cases.

- Review of the facial photos and exam including attention to the MRD_1, vertical fissure height, Bell phenomenon, and extraocular muscle
- For levator resection surgeries, the degree of levator function should be reviewed preoperatively. Unlike adult cases with intraoperative participation, pediatric cases under general anesthesia may require a preplanned amount of resection or intraoperative lid position. Berke offered guidelines for leaving the upper eyelid level 1 to 2 mm below the limbus if levator function is greater than 8 mm, at the limbus for levator function of 8 mm, and 1 to 2 mm above the limbus if levator function is less than 8 mm.[7]
- We recommend unilateral frontalis suspensions for unilateral congenital ptosis; however, some recommend bilateral surgery with extirpation of a functional levator muscle to offer improved symmetry.

Positioning

- Patient is positioned supine on a surgical table with an adjustable headrest lowered to give the surgeon the best access. The patient should be prepped and draped by leaving the full face exposed.

Approach

- Internal (posterior) approach: mullerectomy
- External (anterior) approach: levator resection
- Frontal approach: frontalis suspension

■ Frontalis Suspension

Markings and Eyelid Sutures

- Place topical tetracaine on the conjunctival surface.
- Mark the lid crease prior to injecting local anesthetic.
- Inject 1 to 2 cc 2% lidocaine with 1:100 000 epinephrine subcutaneously inferior to the brow.
- Mark desired lid crease with a sterile marking pen. This is typically 8 and 10 mm above the eyelid margin in males and females, respectively.
- Mark one midpupillary point on the eyelid skin. Mark two points 4 mm medial and lateral to the marked "central point" superior to the brow (**TECH FIG 1A**).
- Make one stab incision at each of the marked stab sites above the brow with a no. 15 blade.
- Make an incision with a no. 15 blade along the previously marked eyelid crease.
- Attach a free needle to the sling material. The authors prefer Supramid (polyfilament, cable-type 3-0 suture). Pass this needle laterally to medially along the eyelid crease beneath the orbicularis muscle and just anterior to the tarsus (**TECH FIG 1B**). If the skin puckers while doing this, the needle is being passed too superficially.

- Check the eyelid contour to ensure the tarsus pass does not create squared off lid (too broad of a pass) or a peaked eyelid (too narrow of a pass).
- Both medial and lateral ends of the sling material are then passed just deep to the dermis to the stab incision sites immediately superior to the brow (**TECH FIG 1C**).
- Close the eyelid crease incision with 6-0 fast gut running sutures (**TECH FIG 1D**).

Brow Sutures

- Pass the needle from the lateral brow stab incision to the medial stab incision deep to the dermis (**TECH FIG 2A**).
- Tighten the sling material with care not to break the sling elevating the lid to the height of the superior limbus or 1 mm below the superior limbus. Assess eyelid contour.
- If using synthetic material, pass a cuff around both sling ends (**TECH FIG 2B**).
- Secure the sling with two square knots.
- Close the stab incisions with a deep pass using 5-0 Vicryl suture on a P-2 needle and finally closing the eyelid crease and superficial tissues of the stab incisions with 5-0 fast gut interrupted sutures (**TECH FIG 2C,D**).

TECHNIQUES

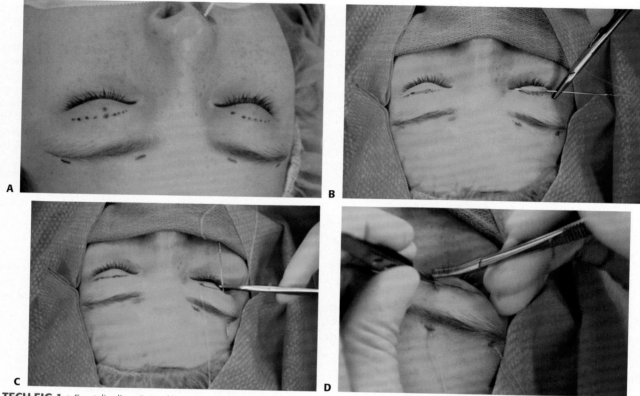

TECH FIG 1 • Frontalis sling. **A.** Markings are made, importantly including one midpupillary point on the eyelid skin and two points 4 mm medial and lateral to the marked midpupillary point superior to the brow. **B.** A free needle attached to the sling material of choice is passed laterally to medially beneath the orbicularis and anterior to the tarsus. **C.** Both medial and lateral ends of the sling material are passed just deep to the stab incision sites superior to the brow. **D.** The eyelid crease incision is closed in running fashion.

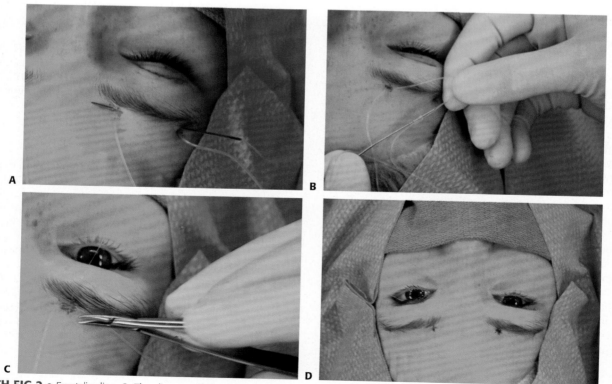

TECH FIG 2 • Frontalis sling. **A.** The sling needle is passed from the lateral brow stab incision to the medial stab incision deep to the dermis. **B.** Demonstration of passing a cuff around both ends of a silicone sling to be buried subcutaneously. **C.** Deep 5-0 Vicryl suture is placed underneath the sling prior to tying the sling. The Vicryl suture is then passed through subcutaneous tissue anterior to the enclosed sling. **D.** The stab incisions are closed with a deep pass using 5-0 Vicryl suture on a P-2 needle.

■ Levator Resection

Markings and Dissection

- Place topical tetracaine on the conjunctival surface.
- Mark the desired lid crease (8 to 10 mm) with a sterile marking pen aligning symmetry with the fellow eye.
- Inject 1 to 2 cc 2% lidocaine with 1:100 000 epinephrine into the subcutaneous space adjacent and superior to the tarsus. Take care not to infiltrate the levator muscle with local anesthetic or add too much volume to the lids, distorting surgical landmarks.
- Use a no. 15 blade to incise the marked eyelid crease deepening the incision with scissors to the level of the tarsus (**TECH FIG 3A**).

- Using Westcott scissors, make short cuts along the inferior edge of the incision to dissect to the superior tarsus (**TECH FIG 3B,C**).
- Tent up the eyelid septum by holding and gently retracting the tarsus and the superior septum away from each other. Carefully cut shallowly to dissect through the septal plane revealing the levator aponeurosis (**TECH FIG 3D**).

Suturing and Closure

- Pass 2 double-armed 5-0 Vicryl sutures through the anterior upper tarsus border via partial-thickness passes (**TECH FIG 3E**). Take care to avoid making full-thickness passes, checking the palpebral conjunctiva for suture by flipping the eyelid after each pass (**TECH FIG 3F**).

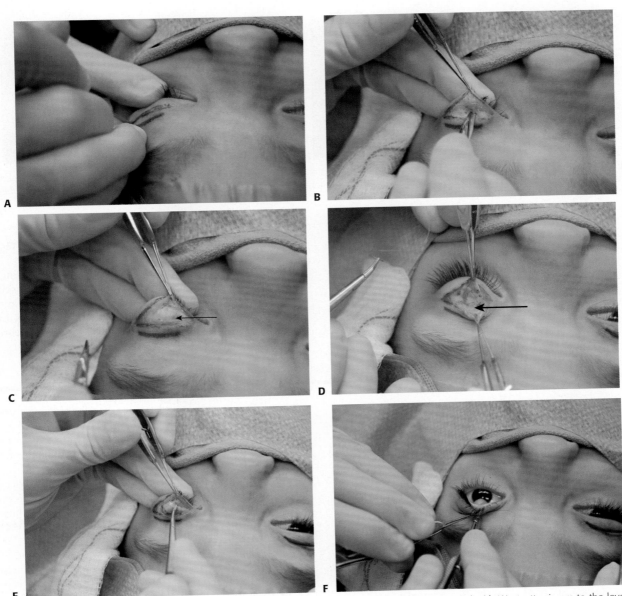

TECH FIG 3 • Levator resection. **A.** An incision is made along the marked eyelid crease and deepened with Westcott scissors to the level of the tarsus. **B.** Careful sharp dissection is made to dissect to the superior tarsus. **C.** The tarsus is seen by glistening white tissue (*arrow*). **D.** The tarsus and superior septum are retracted to allow a dissection through this pocket to the levator aponeurosis (*arrow*). **E.** Two double-armed 5-0 Vicryl sutures are passed through the anterior upper tarsus border via partial-thickness passes. **F.** The eyelid is flipped using a blunt needle driver to ensure full-thickness passes have been avoided.

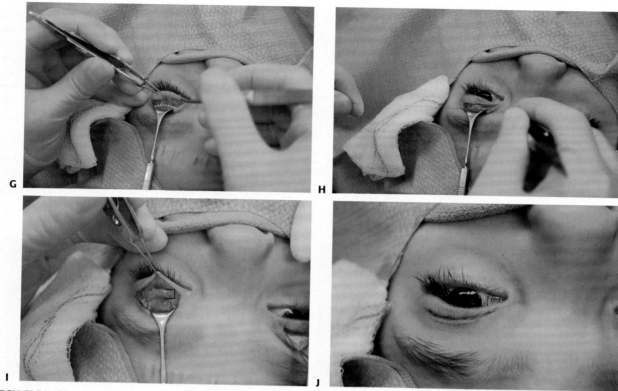

TECH FIG 3 (Continued) • **G.** Sutures are passed through the levator aponeurosis to the junction of Whitnall ligament, demarcated by a white linear band (*white dashes*). **H.** A temporary knot is tied, and the contour of the eyelid is checked. **I.** Excess levator aponeurosis (between *black brackets*) can be excised. **J.** The skin is closed in running fashion.

- Per the graded resection anticipated prior to the procedure, each suture is then passed through the levator aponeurosis, near the junction of Whitnall ligament (**TECH FIG 3G**).
- A temporary knot is tied and the contour of the eyelid is checked (**TECH FIG 3H**). If appropriate lid height is achieved, the sutures can be permanently tied using a surgeon's knot.
- Excess levator aponeurosis (**TECH FIG 3I**) can be excised if needed.

- Close the skin with 6-0 fast gut in running fashion (**TECH FIG 3J**).
- If interested in recreating the eyelid crease, make a single pass of 6-0 gut suture through the inferior edge of skin, orbicularis, passing partial thickness through the levator aponeurosis, and exiting via the superior orbicularis and skin. This effectively attaches it to the levator aponeurosis to recreate the skin crease.

■ Conjunctivomullerectomy

- Place topical tetracaine on the conjunctival surface.
- Place a subcutaneous eyelid block below the brow using 2 cc 2% lidocaine with 1:100 000 epinephrine. Evert the eyelid and inject 1 cc lidocaine into the superior tarsal border deep to the conjunctiva (**TECH FIG 4A**).
- Pass a 4-0 silk suture deeply through the gray line to serve as traction sutures (**TECH FIG 4B**).
- Evert the eyelid using a Desmarres retractor.
- Using a caliper, measure the amount of Muller muscle to resect and mark inside the lateral borders of the tarsus with handheld cautery (**TECH FIG 4C**).
- Pass a two 4-0 silk sutures through the conjunctiva and Muller muscle at the marked sites (**TECH FIG 4D**).
- Elevate Muller muscle and the conjunctiva via the silk sutures into a mullerectomy clamp at the marked sites (**TECH FIG 4E**).

- Lock the clamp. Cut and remove the silk traction sutures from the Muller muscle.
- Hold the clamp in the nondominant hand between the middle and index finger leaving the thumb and index finger to load suture.
- Holding this position, run a 6-0 double-armed Vicryl suture in running horizontal mattress fashion along the entire end of the locked clamp. Repeat the running horizontal mattress passes with the second suture arm (**TECH FIG 4F**).
- Tie the two Vicryl suture arms with a surgeon's knot.
- With slight upward tension, use a no. 15 blade to incise the tissue held by the clamp with attention to incising as close to the metal clamp edge as possible keeping a metal-on-metal feel to ensure the suture is not cut (**TECH FIG 4G**).
- Remove the mullerectomy clamp and retraction sutures (**TECH FIG 4H**).

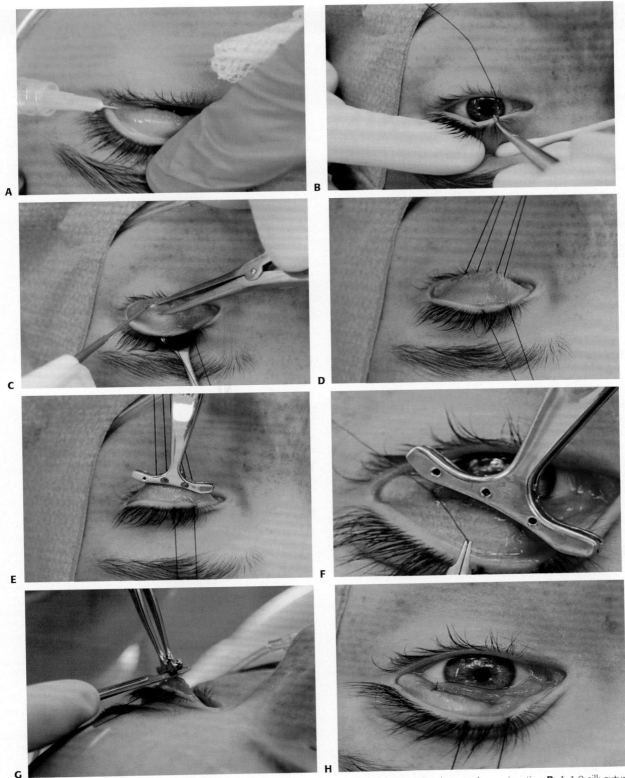

TECH FIG 4 • Conjunctivomullerectomy. **A.** Anesthetic is injected into the superior tarsal border deep to the conjunctiva. **B.** A 4-0 silk suture is passed deeply through the gray line to serve as traction sutures. **C.** The predetermined amount of Muller muscle to resect is measured with calipers inside the lateral borders of the tarsus and marked with handheld cautery. **D.** Two 4-0 silk sutures are passed through conjunctiva and Muller muscle at the marked sites. **E.** Grasping the sutures, Muller muscle and the conjunctiva are elevated into a mullerectomy clamp at the marked sites. **F.** Running horizontal mattress sutures passed below the clamp. **G.** Incision of Muller muscle and conjunctiva held in the clamp ensuring sutures are not cut. **H.** Final appearance after removal of clamp.

PEARLS AND PITFALLS

Creating an eyelid crease	▪ Gently push superiorly on the upper eyelid lashes. This will manifest an eyelid crease that may be otherwise underrepresented. ▪ If a natural eyelid crease is not present and is surgically desired, create a crease with an incision 8–10 mm superior to the upper eyelid margin for males and 10–12 mm for females.
Undercorrection	▪ Utilize the results from the phenylephrine test to plan for the degree of expected correction for mullerectomy procedures. ▪ Adjustable sutures may be used for early postoperative adjustment. ▪ Err on the side of undercorrection, unless performing levator resection, in which case aim for 1 mm overcorrection.
Irregular eyelid contour	▪ Avoid closing or removing levator aponeurosis with the mullerectomy by grasping conjunctiva with Muller muscle from the more posterior structures. ▪ Place or adjust sutures where the deformity is greatest after applying tension under this region. ▪ Postoperatively, lid massage may be of benefit in mild to moderate cases.
Ectropion/entropion	▪ Avoid suture tension at the inferior tarsus. ▪ Avoid applying too much tension to sutures.
Postoperative lagophthalmos	▪ Consider graded mullerectomy and tarsectomy in patients with significant preoperative lagophthalmos. ▪ If frontal sling is needed in a setting of significant preoperative lagophthalmos, place a temporal tarsorrhaphy at the end of the procedure. ▪ Place Frost sutures after levator resection procedures.

POSTOPERATIVE CARE

▪ Patients undergoing frontalis sling should be given an oral antibiotic for 7 days.

▪ Coordinate care with pediatric ophthalmologist to monitor for postoperative refractive error including induced amblyopia.

▪ Aggressive lubrication cannot be overstressed.

▪ If used, lower lid traction sutures should be removed at postoperative day 2.

▪ Topical antibiotic ointment should be applied 4 times a day for 1 week.

▪ If adjustable sutures are employed, the postoperative visit should be within 1 week.

OUTCOMES

▪ Overall, the reported successful outcome is 70% to 90% in pediatric ptosis cases with undercorrection accounting for the majority of poor results or failures.[2,8]

▪ Frontalis sling procedures using synthetic material historically have had recurrence rates as high as 29% to 40%; however, autogenous fascia lata grafts and newer graft materials used in a sling procedure may offer superior results.[5,6,9] Lee et al.[2] reported 5% to 10% poor outcomes with fascia lata grafts or Mersilene mesh.

▪ Anterior levator resection procedures result in poor outcomes in approximately 10% to 20%.[2,7]

▪ Although not generally agreed upon, some surgeons find external levator resection to be associated with less reoperation rate.[10]

▪ An asymmetry of greater than 1 to 2 mm between eyelids may be as common as 30% postoperatively.[8]

COMPLICATIONS

▪ Lagophthalmos
▪ Overcorrection
▪ Ectropion
▪ Exposure keratopathy
▪ Irregular eyelid contour or skin crease
▪ Implant infection or extrusion[6]
▪ Development or worsening of astigmatism postoperatively[4]
▪ Suture site granulomas over synthetic material

REFERENCES

1. Griepentrog GJ, Diehl NN, Mohney BG. Incidence and demographics of childhood ptosis. *Ophthalmology.* 2011;118(6):1180-1183.
2. Lee V, Konrad H, Bunce C, et al. Aetiology and surgical treatment of childhood blepharoptosis. *Br J Ophthalmol.* 2002;86(11):1282-1286.
3. Griepentrog GJ, Mohney BG. Strabismus in childhood eyelid ptosis. *Am J Ophthalmol.* 2014;158(1):208.e1-210.e1.
4. Merriam WW, Ellis FD, Helveston EM. Congenital blepharoptosis, anisometropia, and amblyopia. *Am J Ophthalmol.* 1980;89(3):401-407.
5. SooHoo JR, Davies BW, Allard FD, Durairaj VD. Congenital ptosis. *Surv Ophthalmol.* 2014;59(5):483-492.
6. Wasserman BN, Sprunger DT, Helveston EM. Comparison of materials used in frontalis suspension. *Arch Ophthalmol.* 2001;119(5):687-691.
7. Berke RN. Results of resection of the levator muscle through a skin incision in congenital ptosis. *AMA Arch Ophthalmol.* 1959;61(2):177-201.
8. Cates CA, Tyers AG. Outcomes of anterior levator resection in congenital blepharoptosis. *Eye (Lond).* 2001;15(Pt 6):770-773.
9. Elsamkary MA, Roshdy MM. Clinical trial comparing autogenous fascia lata sling and Gore-Tex suspension in bilateral congenital ptosis. *Clin Ophthalmol.* 2016;10:405-409.
10. Skaat A, Fabian D, Fabian ID, et al. Congenital ptosis repair-surgical, cosmetic, and functional outcome: a report of 162 cases. *Can J Ophthalmol.* 2013;48(2):93-98.

Epiblepharon

Adam R. Sweeney and Christopher B. Chambers

DEFINITION

- Epiblepharon is a congenital eyelid anomaly in which inward rotation of the normal lash line toward the globe results in eyelash approximation to the cornea and/or conjunctiva.

ANATOMY

- A horizontal eyelid fold composed of skin and orbicularis is evident inferior to the eyelid margin. This is caused by the absence of the adhesion between the thin smooth muscle contributing to lower eyelid retraction and the soft tissue immediately deep to the lower eyelid skin.[1,2]
- Often, the fold is more pronounced or isolated to the medial eyelid.
- The Asian lower eyelid has a higher attachment of the septum on the tarsus or inferior retractor. Additionally, there often is an absence or paucity of retractor septa attached to the overlying skin, similar to the Asian upper eyelid.[1]
- The tarsus is not rolled in, nor is there rotation of the eyelid muscle, separating this condition from entropion.[3]

PATHOGENESIS

- Epiblepharon is one of the most common eyelid abnormalities among Asian children, with majority demonstrating spontaneous resolution throughout childhood.[4]
- Up to 95% of Asian children with epiblepharon will have it bilaterally.[2,4,5]
- Epiblepharon much more commonly involves the lower eyelid than it does both upper and lower eyelids with a small minority of cases involving solely the upper eyelid.[2]
- There is no gender predilection.[2]
- Epiblepharon is less commonly seen in adults.
- Asian children with higher BMI are more likely to have epiblepharon.[6]
- Acquired epiblepharon is rare and often secondary to thyroid eye disease.[7]

NATURAL HISTORY

- The majority of patients will have spontaneous resolution with growth of the midface stretching and flattening the redundant fold.
- Patients with untreated epiblepharon may have a continuum of sequelae with some asymptomatic until development of thicker eyelashes, whereas others may develop conjunctival epithelial defects, corneal defects, recurrent corneal infections, and even corneal scarring.

PATIENT HISTORY AND PHYSICAL FINDINGS

- Patients may be asymptomatic or have inciting surface irritation evident by rubbing of eyes, photophobia, persistent tearing, or discharge.
- Eyelashes may be vertically oriented and may touch the cornea. This often is exacerbated in down gaze.
- Fluorescein staining may reveal epithelial defects.
- Epiblepharon may be associated with astigmatism.
- Diagnosis is by physical exam with the eyelashes directed vertically in the setting of normal eyelid position (**FIG 1**). Additionally, an eyelid fold may be found to be mechanically corrected with downward pressure applied on the skin away from the eyelid involved.

IMAGING

- Preoperative quality external photos documenting resolution of the epiblepharon with eyelid fold excursion are recommended prior to undergoing surgery.

DIFFERENTIAL DIAGNOSIS

- Entropion with or without epiblepharon
- Trichiasis, or misdirected growth of eyelashes toward the eye
- Epicanthus tarsalis
- Dermatochalasis with lash ptosis
- Ptosis
- Discharge in nonverbal children may be a sign of backflow from the tear drainage pathway, caused by nasolacrimal duct obstruction.

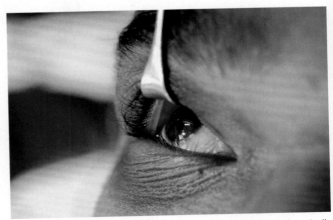

FIG 1 • Lower lid epiblepharon. Eyelashes are seen directed vertically with inferior eyelid fold.

NONOPERATIVE MANAGEMENT

- Monitoring is appropriate in asymptomatic cases without corneal eyelash apposition.
- Lubrication with scheduled artificial tears may suffice in asymptomatic cases with mild epiblepharon or conjunctival eyelash apposition.

SURGICAL MANAGEMENT

Preoperative Planning

- General anesthesia is recommended for pediatric cases.
- Surgical intervention is warranted in children whose lid abnormality causes keratopathy or conjunctivopathy, considerable irritation, or in cases where lubrication is not tolerated.
- Goals of surgical management are to achieve eyelid retractor tightening, removal of a strip of orbicularis and skin, and creation of a scar in a region between the preseptal and pretarsal orbicularis.

- In patients for whom a surgical eyelid crease is not desired, the standard technique for epiblepharon is used. If a surgical eyelid crease is desired, the modified Hotz technique is used.
- A noninvasive everting suture technique may be offered. This modality may be appropriate for mild cases of epiblepharon, parents wishing to avoid creation of an eyelid crease/scar, or avoidance of general anesthesia.

Positioning

- The patient is positioned supine on a surgical table with an adjustable headrest lowered to give the surgeon the best access. The patient should be prepped and draped, leaving the full face exposed.

Approach

- An external approach to the lower lid tarsus and eyelid retractors is classically used. Alternatively, a noninvasive suture technique may also be used.

■ Standard Technique

Markings and Incisions

- Place topical tetracaine on the conjunctival surface.
- Inject 1 to 2 cc 2% lidocaine with 1:100 000 epinephrine into the subcutaneous space adjacent to the eyelid margin of the lid involved.
- Using a sterile marking pen, outline the deficit nasally and temporally with a horizontal mark placed along the nonmarginal tarsus border (**TECH FIG 1A**).

- Use calipers to ensure the measured strip does not exceed 2 to 2.5 mm vertically (**TECH FIG 1B**).
- Use a no. 15 blade to incise a vertical semilunar-shaped strip of orbicularis and skin (**TECH FIG 1C**).
- Remove the incised skin using Westcott scissors (**TECH FIG 1D**).

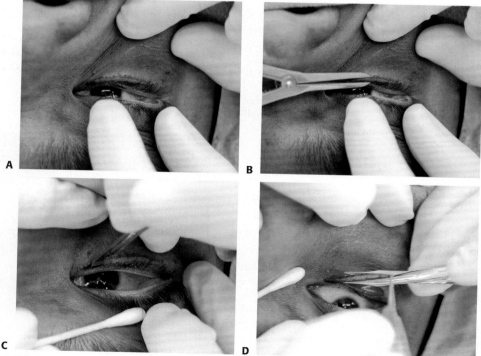

TECH FIG 1 • A. Epiblepharon with outlining markings including a horizontal marking along the nonmarginal tarsus border. **B.** Calipers are used to confirm less than 2 mm of vertical tissue to be excised. **C.** The outlining incision is made. **D.** Westcott scissors are used to excise outlined skin.

Suturing

- Maintain hemostasis with monopolar cautery.
- Remove the incised orbicularis using handheld cautery (**TECH FIG 2A**).
- Using a 5-0 Vicryl suture, make a pass through the orbital septum and through the lower eyelid retractors (**TECH FIG 2B**).
- Continue this pass through the inferior edge of the tarsus, rotating the needle to pass out through the septum (**TECH FIG 2C**).

- Rotate the eyelid to ensure a full-thickness eyelid suture has not been placed and tie this knot using a surgeon's knot (**TECH FIG 2D**).
- Pass two identical sutures separated by approximately 2 to 3 mm closing the horizontal length of the strip (**TECH FIG 2E–G**).
- Using 5-0 Vicryl suture, close the superior and inferior edges of the incised orbicularis tissue in buried subcutaneous-interrupted passes.
- Close the skin with 6-0 fast gut running sutures (**TECH FIG 2H**).

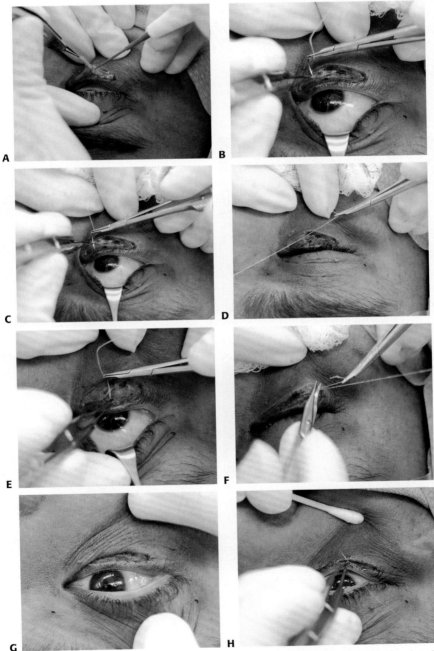

TECH FIG 2 • **A.** Handheld cautery is used to remove underlying orbicularis within the previously marked region. **B.** Vicryl suture is passed through the orbital septum and lower eyelid retractors. **C.** The pass is continued through the inferior edge of the tarsus. **D.** A surgeon's knot is used to reapproximate the sutured tissues. **E.** The retractors are reapproximated to the tarsus. **F.** Suture tails are cut just above the knot. **G.** Eyelashes are checked for resolution of corneal apposition. **H.** Skin is closed using 6-0 fast gut in a running fashion.

■ Modified Hotz Technique

Markings and Incisions

- Place topical tetracaine on the conjunctival surface.
- Inject 1 to 2 cc 2% lidocaine with 1:100 000 epinephrine into the subcutaneous space adjacent to the eyelid margin of the lid involved (**TECH FIG 3A**).
- Using a sterile marking pen, outline the eyelid crease prior to marking the epiblepharon deficit nasally and temporally with a horizontal mark placed along the nonmarginal tarsus border.
- Use a no. 15 blade to incise a 2- to 2.5-mm vertical semilunar-shaped strip of orbicularis and skin (**TECH FIG 3B**).
- Remove the incised skin using Westcott scissors (**TECH FIG 3C**).
- Maintain hemostasis with monopolar cautery.
- Remove the incised orbicularis using handheld cautery (**TECH FIG 3D**).

Suturing

- Using a 5-0 Vicryl suture, pass the needle externally through the skin inferior to the incision, through the orbital septum, and through the lower eyelid retractors (**TECH FIG 4A**).
- Proceed by passing this needle through the inferior edge of the tarsus (**TECH FIG 4B**), rotating the needle to pass out through the septum, the orbicularis, and the skin superior to the incision (**TECH FIG 4C**).
- Rotate the eyelid to ensure a full-thickness eyelid suture has not been placed.
- The suture can then be tied with an external surgeon's knot.
- Pass one identical suture both nasal and lateral to the central suture 2 mm from the nasal and lateral tarsal edge, respectively (**TECH FIG 4D**).

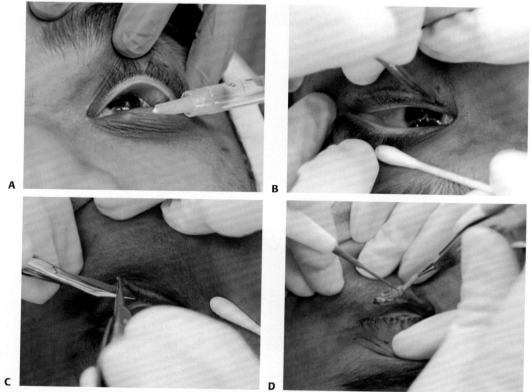

TECH FIG 3 • A. Anesthetic is injected into the subcutaneous space along the defect. **B.** The outlining incision is made. **C.** Westcott scissors are used to excise outlined skin. **D.** Handheld cautery is used to remove underlying orbicularis within the previously marked region.

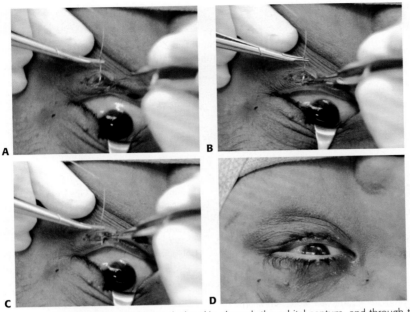

TECH FIG 4 • **A.** 5-0 Vicryl suture is passed externally through the skin, through the orbital septum, and through the lower eyelid retractors. **B.** The pass is continued through the inferior edge of the tarsus and out through the skin. **C.** Eyelashes are checked for resolution of corneal apposition. **D.** The final outcome and appearance of the surgically created lid crease.

■ Everting Sutures/Buried Sutures Technique

- Place topical tetracaine on the conjunctival surface.
- Inject 1 to 2 cc 2% lidocaine with 1:100 000 epinephrine into the subcutaneous space adjacent to the eyelid margin of the lid involved.
- Using a double-armed 3-0 silk suture, make a pass from the central cul-de-sac through the palpebral conjunctiva, orbicularis, and the eyelid skin (**TECH FIG 5**).

- The ideal exit of this suture is 3 mm below the eyelid margin for inferior epiblepharon repair and 3 to 4 mm above the eyelid margin for superior epiblepharon repair.[8,9]
- An identical suture is passed 2 to 3 mm medial to the central suture in the same fashion.
- The sutures are tied with long tails and the tails.
- Antibiotic ointment is applied over the suture site.
- The tails of the sutures are taped away from the eyelid margin.

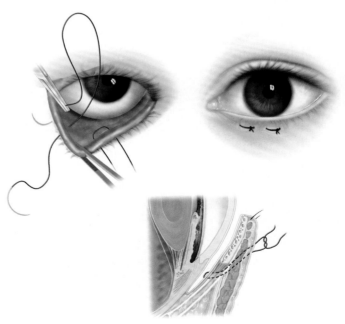

TECH FIG 5 • Illustration outlining the trajectory of the suture through the central cul-de-sac of the palpebral conjunctiva directed superiorly to exit 3 mm below the eyelid margin.

PEARLS AND PITFALLS

Technique	■ In very large epiblepharon cases, a modified Z-epicanthoplasty to tighten the lower eyelid to the medial canthus may be performed prior to the standard or modified Hotz procedure.[10]
Inadequate postoperative eversion	■ Overcorrect the eversion slightly to adjust for postoperative scarring.
Asymmetry	■ More orbicularis/skin may be taken medially to avoid recurrence and asymmetry.
Scar	■ Avoid tension on the skin. ■ Lubricate and protect the incision site from sun exposure postoperatively.

POSTOPERATIVE CARE

■ Apply antibiotic eye ointment to the operative site 4 times a day for 1 week.

■ Remove everting nonabsorbable sutures at 1-week follow-up, allowing for orbicularis scarring.

OUTCOMES

■ Following incisional epiblepharon repair, 80% to 90% of patients are either asymptomatic or anatomically repaired.[2,5]

■ The everting sutures/buried sutures technique may be associated with up to a 23% recurrence rate.[9]

■ There is no agreed-upon interval between surgical correction and possible recurrence.

COMPLICATIONS

■ Suture abscesses
■ Wound dehiscence
■ Lid retraction, ectropion
■ Canalicular trauma
■ Lagophthalmos

REFERENCES

1. Jordan R. The lower-lid retractors in congenital entropion and epiblepharon. *Ophthalmic Surg.* 1993;24(7):494-496.
2. Sundar G, Young SM, Tara S, et al. Epiblepharon in East Asian patients: the Singapore experience. *Ophthalmology.* 2010;117(1):184-189.
3. Bartley GB, Nerad JA, Kersten RC, Maguire LJ. Congenital entropion with intact lower eyelid retractor insertion. *Am J Ophthalmol.* 1991;112(4):437-441.
4. Noda S, Hayasaka S, Setogawa T. Epiblepharon with inverted eyelashes in Japanese children. I. Incidence and symptoms. *Br J Ophthalmol.* 1989;73(2):126-127.
5. Woo KI, Yi K, Kim YD. Surgical correction for lower lid epiblepharon in Asians. *Br J Ophthalmol.* 2000;84(12):1407-1410.
6. Hayasaka Y, Hayasaka S. Epiblepharon with inverted eyelashes and high body mass index in Japanese children. *J Pediatr Ophthalmol Strabismus.* 2005;42(5):300-303.
7. Chang EL, Hayes J, Hatton M, Rubin PA. Acquired lower eyelid epiblepharon in patients with thyroid eye disease. *Ophthal Plast Reconstr Surg.* 2005;21(3):192-196.
8. Quickert MH, Wilkes TD, Dryden RM. Nonincisional correction of epiblepharon and congenital entropion. *Arch Ophthalmol.* 1983;101(5):778-781.
9. Hayasaka S, Noda S, Setogawa T. Epiblepharon with inverted eyelashes in Japanese children. II Surgical repairs. *Br J Ophthalmol.* 1989;73(2):128-130.
10. Ni J, Shao C, Wang K, et al. Modified Hotz procedure combined with modified Z-epicanthoplasty versus modified Hotz procedure alone for epiblepharon repair. *Ophthalmic Plast Reconstr Surg.* 2017;33(2):120-123.

Canthopexy

Adam R. Sweeney and Christopher B. Chambers

DEFINITION

- Canthopexy is a resuspension of the canthus to the bony orbit used to treat eyelid laxity, ectropion, or misalignment.
- A common surgery in adult facial rejuvenation, canthopexy is an indispensable tool for treating children with eyelid positioning defects or deformities.

ANATOMY

- The canthal tendons maintain the shape of the palpebral fissure and also maintain lid apposition to the globe, important for proper corneal lubrication and tear drainage.
- The medial canthus has origins at the anterior and posterior lacrimal crests that *fuse temporal* to the lacrimal sac, enveloping the lacrimal sac. The medial canthus then divides into upper and lower segments that attach to the tarsus of the upper and lower lid.
- The medial canthus is involved in the lacrimal pump mechanism and intimately associated with the lacrimal sac.
- The lateral canthal tendon originates at the lateral orbital tubercle 4 to 5 mm posterior to the lateral orbital rim. This provides a posterior vector opposing the lid to the globe. The lateral canthal tendon then splits into superior and inferior segments that attach to the tarsal plates (**FIG 1**).

- The lateral canthal tendon inserts approximately 2 mm higher than does the medial canthal tendon. This creates a superior tilt to the palpebral fissure moving laterally.
- The orbital septum overlies the lateral canthus as it approaches the orbital rim and acts as a "superficial lateral canthus," which can be used for suspension in mild cosmetic defects.[1]

PATHOGENESIS

- Common conditions that may cause eyelid laxity or malposition including congenital facial clefting (ie, Tessier 2 to 12 clefts), amniotic band syndrome, congenital eyelid malposition, or deformities resulting from other etiologies including trauma and cancer resection or from craniofacial manipulation (iatrogenic)

NATURAL HISTORY

- Eyelid laxity is both a cosmetic and a functional problem.
- Uncorrected, lower lid laxity may cause exposure keratopathy, epiphora, or problems with the lacrimal pump mechanism.

PATIENT HISTORY AND PHYSICAL FINDINGS

- Lower eyelid laxity
- Canthal dystopia

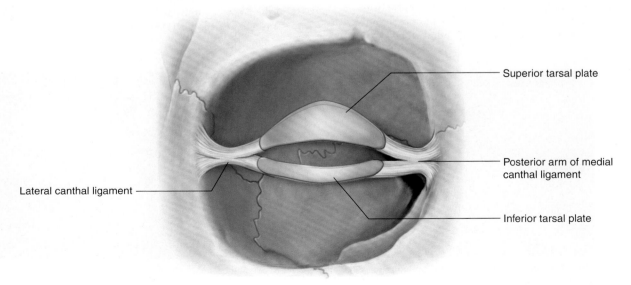

FIG 1 • Anatomy of the medial and lateral canthal tendons.

- Poor eyelid snap back test: This test refers to evaluating the time for the eyelid to return to normal position after pulling the lower lid down and away from the globe. It is graded from 0 (brisk snap back) to IV (severe laxity).
- Eyelid distraction—5 mm of eyelid distraction often considered excessively lax.
- Dry eye including exposure keratopathy or punctate epithelial erosions
  - Punctual stenosis from keratinization of the lid margin in medial ectropion[2]

IMAGING

- CT imaging of the face is appropriate in the evaluation of congenital craniofacial abnormalities. In the setting of orbital trauma, CT imaging is useful to assess for naso-orbital-ethmoid fractures.

NONOPERATIVE MANAGEMENT

- In patients not bothered by the cosmetic defect, scheduled application of lubricant artificial tears may provide the necessary corneal protection to defer or prevent surgery in mild cases.
- Careful attention must be made to prevent deprivation amblyopia by constant application of ointments, taping the eyelid shut, or patching of the eye.

SURGICAL MANAGEMENT

- If the cosmetic defect is bothersome or the patient is symptomatic, canthopexy, canthoplasty, or both may be performed to correct the eyelid abnormality.
- Medial canthopexy in the absence of nasal fractures may be performed either with or without wiring as adapted from Mustarde[3] and Callahan,[4] respectively.

Preoperative Planning

- General anesthesia is recommended for pediatric cases.
- Preoperative photos should be reviewed assessing the degree of malpositioning and marking of the face at the desired canthi position to create the proper slight superolateral contour of the eyelid with appropriate eyelid tightening achieved.

Positioning

- Patients should be positioned supine in an operating bed with adjustable head positioning. The contralateral eyelid may be temporarily taped shut or lubricated rather than covered to serve as a reference point during surgery.

Approach

- Medial, lateral, or a combination of approaches may be performed depending on the location of the lid abnormality or the desired results.

TECHNIQUES

■ Lateral Canthopexy

- The lateral canthopexy procedure tightens the canthal tendon with sutured reconstruction of the canthal tendon. This effectively tightens the eyelid.
- Place 2 drops of topical tetracaine on the conjunctival surface.
- Inject 1 to 2 cc 2% lidocaine with 1:100 000 epinephrine subcutaneously above and below the lateral canthus.
- Using a no. 15 blade, make a 1-cm horizontal subciliary incision at the lateral canthal angle (**TECH FIG 1A**).
- Retract the skin with skin hooks and bluntly dissect down to the periosteum using blunt-tipped scissors.

- Undermine and dissect in this plane to the lateral canthal tendon under the orbital septum (**TECH FIG 1B**).
- The lateral canthal tendon is identified by tension and the ability to "strum" if manipulated by closed blunt-tipped scissors. Grasping the lateral canthal tendon, vertically transect the lateral canthal tendon at its lateral insertion taking care to avoid the levator aponeurosis (**TECH FIG 1C**).
- Pass a double-armed 4-0 Vicryl suture on a P-2 needle (Ethicon, Somerville, NJ) entering anteriorly through the lateral canthus at its transected superior and inferior attachment points (**TECH FIG 1D**).

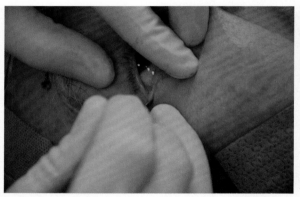
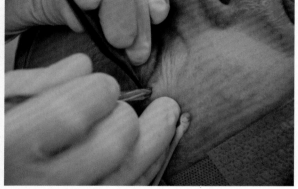

TECH FIG 1 • Lateral canthopexy. **A.** A 1-cm horizontal subciliary incision is made at the lateral canthal angle. **B.** Blunt-tipped scissors are used to dissect down to the periosteum.

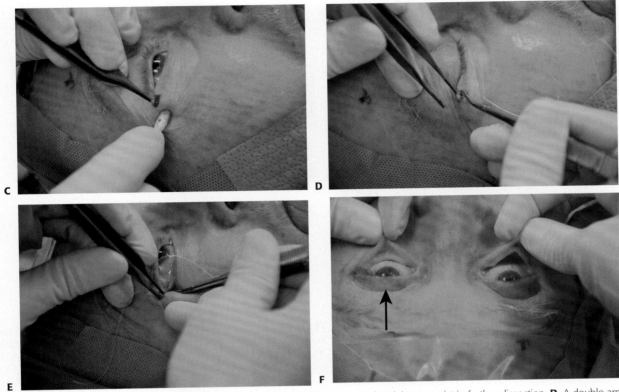

TECH FIG 1 (Continued) • **C.** The lateral canthal tendon is grasped following undermining to assist in further dissection. **D.** A double-armed 4-0 Vicryl suture on a P-2 needle is used to make two passes from anterior to posterior through the lateral canthal tendon. **E.** Deep suture placement ensuring a bite of periosteum is achieved at the (medial) aspect of the lateral orbital rim. **F.** The eyelid laxity in the operative eye (*arrow*) is assessed for appropriate tension.

- Pass each suture through the periosteum of the inner (medial) aspect of the lateral orbital rim approximately 1 cm superior to the medial canthus (**TECH FIG 1E**). Ensure tension is achieved with a strong bite.
- Check the tension of the eyelid to ensure slightly exaggerated tension, anticipating slight laxity after postoperative healing (**TECH FIG 1F**).

- Close with 2 deep passes to approximate soft tissues including the periosteum and orbicularis using 4-0 Vicryl suture.
- Close the skin with 6-0 fast gut suture.

■ Lateral Canthoplasty (Lateral Tarsal Strip)

- The terms lateral canthoplasty and lateral tarsal strip are interchangeable. This procedure involves reconstruction of the lateral canthal tendon with lysis and reattachment of the tendon.
- Place 2 drops of topical tetracaine on the conjunctival surface.
- Inject 1 to 2 cc 2% lidocaine with 1:100 000 epinephrine subcutaneously above and below the lateral canthus.
- Using a no. 15 blade, make a 2-cm partial-thickness skin incision at the lateral canthus (**TECH FIG 2A**).
- Use Westcott scissors to make a full-thickness cut at the site of the prior incision.
- Disinsert the inferior arm of the lateral canthus from the periosteum at the lateral incision site using Westcott scissors, strumming the canthal attachment points with

closed scissors to find remaining canthal tendon arms that need to be released (**TECH FIG 2B**).
- The lower eyelid should be freely mobile to the superior orbital rim once all canthal attachments have been cut.
- Grasping the lateral tarsus at the lateral most point with toothed forceps, use Westcott scissors to separate the anterior and posterior lamellae (**TECH FIG 2C,D**).

Creating the Lateral Tarsal Strip

- Remove the mucocutaneous junction prior along the length of the desired lateral tarsal strip (**TECH FIG 3A**).
- Using Westcott scissors, cut the grasped tissue inferior to the inferior border of the tarsus, 5 mm inferior to the lid margin (**TECH FIG 3B**).
- De-epithelialize the skin and conjunctiva off the strip using a scraping technique with a no. 15 blade (**TECH FIG 3C**).

TECHNIQUES

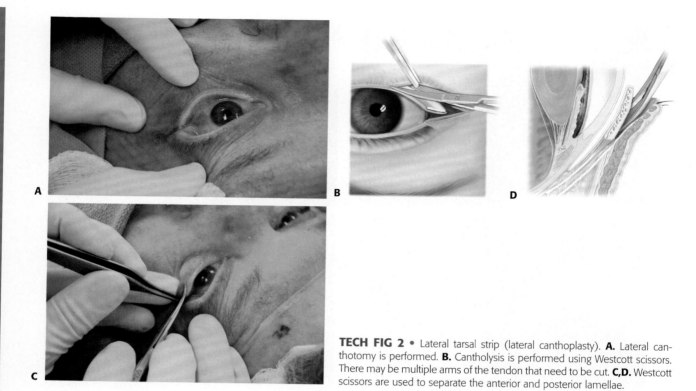

TECH FIG 2 • Lateral tarsal strip (lateral canthoplasty). **A.** Lateral canthotomy is performed. **B.** Cantholysis is performed using Westcott scissors. There may be multiple arms of the tendon that need to be cut. **C,D.** Westcott scissors are used to separate the anterior and posterior lamellae.

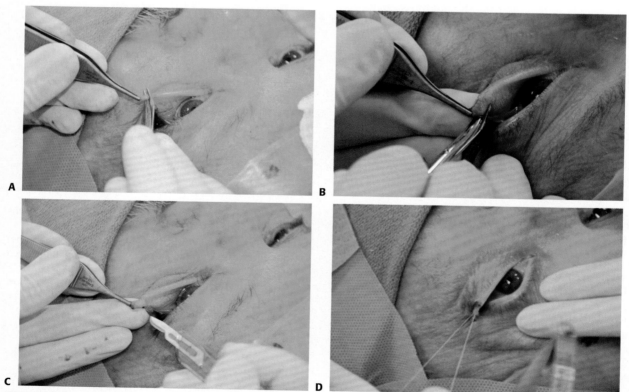

TECH FIG 3 • Lateral tarsal strip (lateral canthoplasty). **A.** The mucocutaneous junction is removed from the eyelid margin. **B.** Grasping the lateral canthus, the lateral tarsal strip is fashioned by cutting the inferior border of the tarsus 5 mm inferior to the lid margin. **C.** An ideal strip is created by de-epithelializing the skin and conjunctiva off the strip using a scraping technique with a no. 15 blade. **D.** Both arms of a double-armed suture are passed from posterior to anterior through the lateral end of the tarsal strip.

- Pass both arms of a double-armed 4-0 Vicryl suture on a P-2 needle from posterior to anterior through the lateral end of the tarsal strip, with one arm passing superiorly and one arm passing inferiorly (**TECH FIG 3D**).
- Pull the inferior lateral canthus superiorly into the desired position, generally 1 cm superior to the medial canthus.

Suturing

- Secure both arms of the suture by passing the needles deeply into the medial periosteum of the lateral orbital rim (**TECH FIG 4A**).

- Check the tension of the eyelid to ensure slightly exaggerated tension, anticipating slight laxity after postoperative healing (**TECH FIG 4B**).
- Using 6-0 fast gut suture, reform the lateral canthal angle with a circular stitch entering from the inferolateral wound, out the gray line of the lower lid, through the gray line of the upper lid, and out the superolateral wound (**TECH FIG 4C**).
- Close the skin using 6-0 fast gut suture.

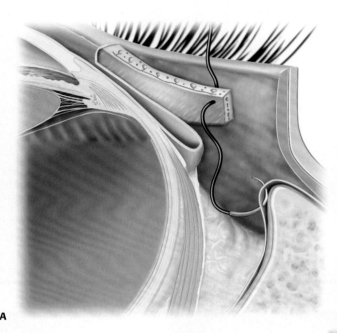

A

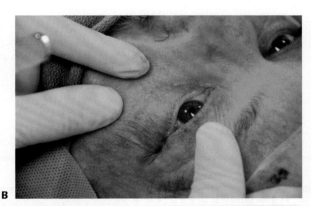

B

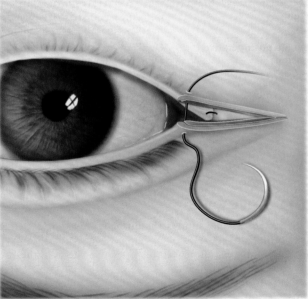

C

TECH FIG 4 • Lateral tarsal strip (lateral canthoplasty). **A.** Both arms of the suture are secured deeply in the medial aspect of the lateral orbital rim periosteum. **B.** Tension of the eyelid is checked. **C.** The lateral canthal angle is reformed with a circular stitch entering from the inferolateral wound, out the *gray line* of the lower lid, through the *gray line* of the upper lid, and out the superolateral wound.

TECHNIQUES

■ Y-V Medial Canthopexy

- Place 2 drops of topical tetracaine on the conjunctival surface.
- Inject 1 to 2 cc 2% lidocaine with 1:100 000 epinephrine subcutaneously above and below the medial canthus.
- With a sterile marking pen, draw a horizontal V terminating 5 mm medial to the medial canthal angle. Extend the marking with a 3-mm line horizontally from the tip of the V (**TECH FIG 5A**).
- Incise the skin and orbicularis using a no. 15 blade over the markings.
- Using Westcott scissors, bluntly dissect through the orbicularis and septum to the depth of the medial canthus ensuring to stay anterior to the nasolacrimal system (**TECH FIG 5B**).
- Pass both arms of a 4-0 double-armed silk suture underneath the lateral aspect of the medial canthus exiting anteriorly through the medial canthus. With each suture arm, make an additional pass through the medial canthus extending medially. Pull the suture arms to plicate the medial canthus (**TECH FIG 5C**).
- Tie the two suture arms with a surgeon's knot.
- Close the soft tissues using 6-0 Vicryl sutures in interrupted fashion and close the skin with 6-0 fast gut suture (**TECH FIG 5D**).

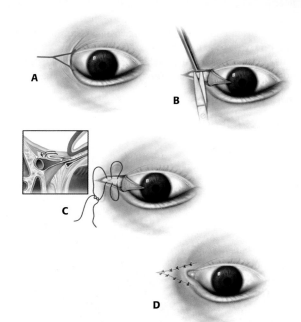

TECH FIG 5 • Y-V medial canthopexy. **A.** Markings of the V-Y with the point of the V terminating 5 mm medial to the medial canthal angle with a 3-mm horizontal extending line that is parallel to the palpebral fissure. **B.** Blunt dissection to the level of the medial canthus. **C.** Plication of the medial canthus with two throws of a double-armed suture extending medially. **D.** Soft tissue and overlying skin closed separately in interrupted fashion.

PEARLS AND PITFALLS

Technique	■ In children expected to have multiple facial surgeries, avoid a large amount of canthal tendon resection as this may render further procedures on these structures more difficult.
Inadequate postoperative suspension	■ Overcorrect the anatomic lateral canthopexy position slightly aiming for 1 cm superior to the medial canthus to allow for postsurgical laxity. ■ In procedures requiring a pass through periosteum, ensure the periosteum has indeed been grasped by applying a moderate amount of anterior tension on the suture after the pass. The tension felt on the suture should be firm. ■ When making a pass through the periosteum, aim to create a posterior vector to ensure the eyelid is approximated to the globes laterally.
Scar	■ Avoid tension on the skin. ■ Push on the inferior eyelashes to exaggerate the subciliary fold for accuracy of marking.

POSTOPERATIVE CARE

- If used, nonabsorbable sutures should be removed at 5 to 7 days postoperatively.
- Apply antibiotic eye ointment to the operative site until the suture absorbs.
- Sunscreen and lotion should be liberally applied over the operative region.

OUTCOMES

- Lateral canthoplasty is associated with an 83% reduction in discomfort by subjective grading scales and near universal improvement in objective eyelid position.[5]

COMPLICATIONS

- Improper positioning of fixation arm
- Loosening of the canthus
- Persistent pain lasting up to 3 months
- Eyelid contour abnormalities including rounding of the canthus
- Chemosis
- Eyelid imbrication can be seen if the inferior crus of the lateral canthal tendon is preferentially tightened or positioned too far cephalad.
- Epithelial inclusion cysts may occur in the lateral tarsal strip procedure if the tarsus is not denuded of epithelium prior to insertion.

REFERENCES

1. Knize DM. The superficial lateral canthal tendon: anatomic study and clinical application to lateral canthopexy. *Plast Reconstr Surg.* 2002;109(3):1149-1157.
2. Georgescu D. Surgical preferences for lateral canthoplasty and canthopexy. *Curr Opin Ophthalmol.* 2014;25(5):449-454.
3. Mustarde JC. Epicanthus and telecanthus. *Br J Plast Surg.* 1963;16:346-356.
4. Callahan A. Secondary reattachment of the medial canthal ligament. *Arch Ophthalmol.* 1963;70:240-241.
5. Moe KS, Linder T. The lateral transorbital canthopexy for correction and prevention of ectropion: report of a procedure, grading system, and outcome study. *Arch Facial Plast Surg.* 2000;2(1):9-15.

42
CHAPTER

Nasolacrimal Duct Obstruction

Emily M. Zepeda, Sarah M. Jacobs, and Christopher B. Chambers

DEFINITION

- Nasolacrimal duct obstruction (NLDO) is an obstruction that occurs within the duct of the nasolacrimal system, such that tears and mucus that have passed through the lacrimal sac are unable to appropriately drain into the nose.
- NLDO results in varying degrees of epiphora (tearing) and is often associated with mucopurulent discharge, swelling, and pain.

ANATOMY (LACRIMAL SYSTEM)

- The nasolacrimal duct is a part of the lacrimal drainage system that conveys tears from the ocular surface to drain into the nose (**FIG 1**).
- It is about 15 mm long, starting at the terminus of the nasolacrimal sac.
- The nasolacrimal duct passes inferiorly, posteriorly, and laterally within the canal formed by the maxillary and lacrimal bones. It travels into the inferior meatus and opens under the inferior turbinate. Its outflow is partially covered by the valve of Hasner.

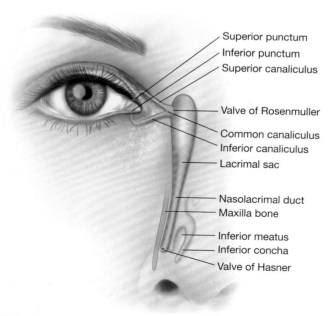

Superior punctum
Inferior punctum
Superior canaliculus

Valve of Rosenmuller

Common canaliculus
Inferior canaliculus

Lacrimal sac

Nasolacrimal duct
Maxilla bone

Inferior meatus
Inferior concha
Valve of Hasner

FIG 1 • Anatomy of the nasolacrimal system, which allows tears from the eye to pass through the puncta, canaliculi, and lacrimal sac, through the nasolacrimal duct to drain into the nasal cavity.

PATHOGENESIS

- NLDO can occur secondary to congenital or acquired disease.
- Congenital NLDO is usually secondary to a membrane blocking the valve of Hasner at the nasal end of the NLD.
  - Obstructions become clinically evident in only 2% to 6% of full-term infants at 3 to 4 weeks of age.
  - Conservative management options of congenital NLDO consist of observation, lacrimal sac massage, and topical/oral antibiotics. It is estimated that 90% of symptomatic congenital NLDO resolves in the first year of life with conservative management.
  - For the remaining 10% of these cases, probing of the NLD can be curative by creating an opening through the imperforate valve of Hasner.[1]
- Infants with craniofacial deformity or Down syndrome are also at higher risk of congenital NLDO. Dacryocystoceles can also create an obstructive process, leading to enlargement and potentially abscess of the lacrimal sac.
- Acquired NLDO may arise from numerous causes such as facial trauma, sinus disease, chronic allergy and inflammation, radiation treatment to the midface, toxicity from chemotherapeutic agents or radioactive iodine, or following sinonasal surgery. Involutional stenosis is the most common cause of NLDO in adults.
- Regardless of whether NLDO is congenital or acquired, any obstruction of the nasolacrimal outflow is capable of causing stagnation of bacteria leading to infection of the lacrimal sac known as dacryocystitis.

PATIENT HISTORY AND PHYSICAL FINDINGS

- In both congenital and acquired NLDO, the primary symptom is epiphora as a result of backflow of tears due to blockage of the duct.
  - At times, enough tear and mucous volume is accumulated within the lacrimal sac that there is a palpable or visible enlargement of the sac. Light pressure over the area of the lacrimal sac can often cause mucopurulent discharge to reflux through the lacrimal drainage system and out the puncta.
- Evaluation of a patient who presents with epiphora should focus on determining the underlying etiology of tearing, assessing for nonobstructive causes (eg, ectropion, reflex tearing, conjunctival infection or inflammation) and nonbenign entities (eg, nasolacrimal malignancy, granulomatosis with polyangiitis). Elements of the history and exam with this focus in mind include the following:
  - A history including duration since tearing onset, percentage of the day it occurs, how it interferes with activities of

daily living, and whether any particular activities provoke it (eg, cold, heat, wind, visual tasks such as computers or reading). Any history of facial trauma, prior episodes of dacryocystitis, radiation, or chemotherapy should be elicited. The patient should also be asked about bloody tears, which would be a concerning sign for underlying malignancy.

- Prior to instilling any eye drops, the tear meniscus height should be noted, and the tear breakup time should be measured, as a cue to whether dry eye–related reflex tearing is contributing to the patient's epiphora.

- Eyelid structures and position in relation to the globe should be assessed for concurrent disease states such as ectropion, entropion, and trichiasis. The upper and lower puncta should be examined for patency and position relative to the globe. Lower lid tone should be evaluated for degree of laxity.

- A dye disappearance test can be performed on patients of any age. A fluorescein eye drop is instilled in each eye. Normal nasolacrimal drainage will allow the dye to flow through the punctum, such that the yellow dye disappears from the ocular surface in a matter of minutes. Patients with nasolacrimal outflow obstruction show delayed clearance of fluorescein.

- In adults, the lacrimal system should be probed and irrigated. Passage of saline into the nose and throat with ease and no reflux signifies a patent system. Reflux of irrigant signifies obstruction, and the pattern of reflux can reveal where the obstruction is located within the system. Reflux from the same punctum that is being irrigated indicated obstruction within the canaliculus. Reflux from the opposite punctum without mucous indicates obstruction at the common canaliculus. Reflux from the opposite punctum with mucus indicates obstruction in the nasolacrimal sac or duct.

- Periocular skin may show erythema, edema, and breakdown of superficial tissues when the discharge or tearing is profuse and constant.

- Finally, nasal evaluation should be performed. This may reveal deviated septum, polyposis, or tumors as a cause of obstruction. Nasal mucosa may also show erythema and edema indicating chronic sinus inflammation.

DIFFERENTIAL DIAGNOSIS

- Congenital glaucoma: When the only symptom is epiphora in a child, one must always rule out congenital glaucoma. The classic triad for congenital glaucoma is blepharospasm (involuntary squeezing of the eyelids closed), photophobia (uncomfortable sensitivity to light), and epiphora. Other findings suggestive of glaucoma include buphthalmos (enlarged globe and corneal diameter) and Haab striae (breaks in the innermost layer of the cornea, leading to corneal haze). If concern for congenital glaucoma exists, the child should be referred to pediatric ophthalmology.

- Dry eye: Epiphora due to dry eye will typically occur when the patient is engaged in a visual task such as reading or computer usage, which decreases their blink rate and exacerbates the dryness of the ocular surface. The patient experiences blurring, burning or foreign body sensation,

and then tear flow. Symptoms are worse in hot, dry, or windy conditions.

- Trichiasis: Growth of eyelashes from malrotated lash follicles or metaplastic Meibomian oil gland orifices results in lashes rubbing and irritating the ocular surface, which provokes tearing. Penlight exam can locate these lashes, which can be treated with epilation or more permanent methods such as cryotherapy or radiofrequency ablation.

- Conjunctivitis: Infection or inflammation of the conjunctiva can cause epiphora and ocular discharge. On examination, patients with conjunctivitis will show injection and papillae or follicles, which appear as fine bumps on the normally smooth conjunctival surface.

- Eyelid ectropion or entropion: Poor eyelid position or lax lower eyelid tone can lead to epiphora. An eyelid with normal tone smoothly sweeps the tears across the ocular surface with each blink, pumping them down the punctal drains into the lacrimal sac. Lax eyelids that are rotated outward (ectropion) or inward (entropion) cannot serve this function effectively, so the unpumped tears spill over the lid margin onto the cheeks.

IMAGING

- The diagnosis of NLDO is based on patient history, elevated tear meniscus, and obstruction observed when the system is probed and irrigated. Imaging is not often needed for diagnosis.

- In select cases, maxillofacial computed tomography (CT) and magnetic resonance (MRI) scans are helpful to evaluate the anatomy after craniofacial injury, in patients with significant sinus or nasal disease, or to evaluate for neoplasia.

- Less commonly, two methods for specific mapping of the lacrimal drainage system itself can be employed:

- In contrast, dacryocystography, in which dye is injected into the punctum and CT or MRI imaging, is used to define the anatomic details of the lacrimal drainage system outlined by the contrast agent, allowing precise location of the obstructed site(s).

- Dacryoscintigraphy uses radionucleotide eye drops to follow tear flow as a gamma camera takes multiple pictures of the outflow system.

SURGICAL MANAGEMENT

- As mentioned, most congenital NLDO resolves with nonsurgical management.
  - Approximately 10% of children with congenital NLDO require probing of the duct. A small subset of those may require repeat probing with balloon dilation of the duct, infracture of the inferior turbinate, and/or placement of silicone stents within the nasolacrimal system to relieve their obstruction.
  - Because of the high success rate with these methods, dacryocystorhinostomy (DCR) is rarely needed in the pediatric population. It is reserved for children who have persistent tearing following intubation, recurrent dacryocystitis, or craniofacial abnormalities with bony obstruction of the duct.

- In adults, however, DCR is the preferred primary surgery for NLDO after the other causes of tearing have been eliminated or addressed.

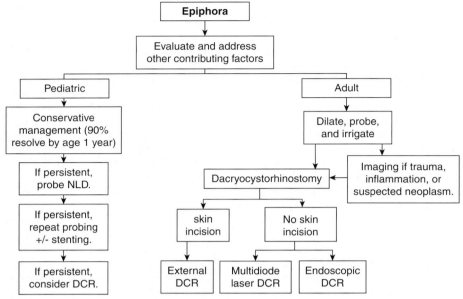

FIG 2 • Algorithm for management of epiphora due to nasolacrimal duct obstruction.

- The DCR operation can be performed in three ways (**FIG 2**):[2–4]
- External DCR: An incision is made through the skin overlying the lacrimal sac, allowing external access to the lacrimal sac fossa for bone removal, sac opening, and stent placement under direct visualization without the need for endoscopic camera equipment.
  - Literature reports a slightly higher success rate with the external approach in certain studies. When appropriately placed, the incision heals with a very subtle and cosmetically acceptable scar.
- Internal DCR (also known as endonasal or endoscopic DCR): Attention is brought to the middle meatus, which allows the most direct access to the lacrimal sac fossa so that the nasolacrimal duct can be bypassed. The middle meatus is visualized from within the nasal cavity, allowing removal of the nasal mucosa and the bone encasing the lacrimal sac from the inside, following by opening of the sac and retrieval of the stents.
  - The reported advantages of the internal approach include the lack of a visible incision, less discomfort, faster recovery, and lower risk of compromising the lacrimal pump mechanism.
- Transcanalicular diode laser: A diode laser probe is passed through the canaliculus with its tip resting within the lacrimal sac. The laser is used to ablate the tissue of the lacrimal sac, bone of the lacrimal fossa, and a localized zone of the underlying nasal mucosa. Silicone stents are then passed through these laser-cut openings and retrieved within the nose.
  - This method has no skin incision, and it enables a significantly faster operating time but reports a lower overall success rate.

Preoperative Planning

- For patients with dacryocystitis, active infection should be treated before DCR.[5] If concern is high for significant nasal septal deviation or other nasal abnormalities, which may need to be addressed intraoperatively, ENT evaluation should be considered prior to surgery. The risk of bleeding can be proactively addressed by ensuring perioperative blood pressure control and withholding anticoagulants if allowed by the patient's primary care physician or prescribing cardiologist.
- In the preoperative area, the patient is given oxymetazoline nasal spray to help vasoconstrict and decongest the nasal mucosa. For example, the spray is administered starting about 30 minutes prior to the procedure, with one dose every 5 minutes for a total of three doses.
- In the operating room after anesthesia induction, the middle meatus is injected with lidocaine with epinephrine, then packed with pledgets soaked in oxymetazoline to provide additional anesthesia and local vasoconstriction at the site.
- Moderate sedation or general anesthesia may be used for the procedure. The decision is based on surgeon and patient preference. General anesthesia is recommended for all pediatric cases and most adult cases.

Positioning

- The patient is positioned supine on a surgical table with an adjustable headrest. The headrest is lowered to extend the neck slightly which gives the surgeon the best access. The patient should be prepped and draped leaving adequate exposure of the eyelids and nose.

■ Internal/Endoscopic DCR

- The surgical site is accessed through the nose, using an endoscope for visualization of the middle meatus along the lateral sidewall of the nasal passage beneath the middle turbinate (**TECH FIG 1A,B**).
- If desired, a 23-gauge light pipe can be passed through the canaliculus, bringing the lit tip to rest in the lacrimal sac. This light pipe provides a point of illumination through the tissue to help localize the lacrimal fossa (**TECH FIG 1C,D**).
- A crescent blade is used to create a three-sided flap incision through the nasal mucosa down to the bone, starting just anterior to the uncinate process and extending inferiorly the height of the turbinate (**TECH FIG 1E**). A periosteal elevator is then used to push the mucosa and periosteum away, exposing bare bone.
- Rongeurs (typically 2- and 3-mm up-biting Kerrison punches) are used to remove the bone of the lacrimal fossa and the anterior process of the maxilla (**TECH FIG 1F**) to expose the entire lacrimal sac. If necessary, a DCR drill can be employed to bur away any bone that cannot be removed with the rongeurs.
- When bone removal is complete, the light pipe and/or a Bowman probe can be passed through the canalicular system to visibly put the lacrimal sac on stretch. A sickle blade is then used to open the lacrimal sac vertically from its superior to inferior pole, allowing the probe to pass freely into the nasal cavity (**TECH FIG 1G,H**). A ball-tipped seeker probe can be used to break any adhesions within the sac, which are commonly present in patients with a history of dacryocystitis. An antimetabolite such as mitomycin C can be applied to the sac to decrease the potential formation of scar adhesions.[6]
- Nasolacrimal stents, such as the silicone Crawford bicanalicular stent, are then passed through the upper and lower puncta and retrieved in the nose (**TECH FIG 1I,J**). The stents remain in place for several weeks postoperatively to maintain patency of the openings during the healing process.

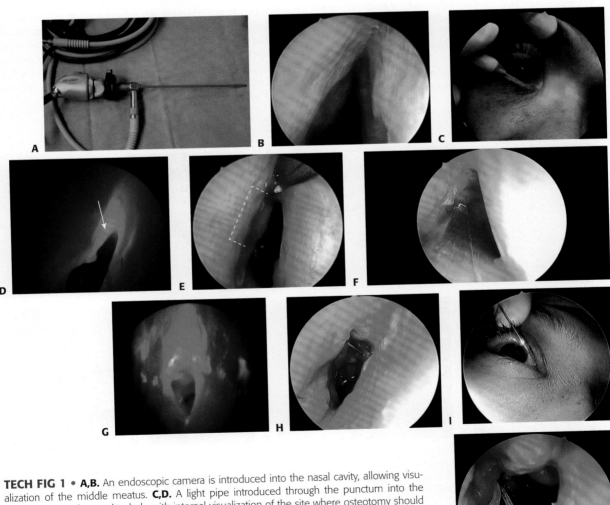

TECH FIG 1 • A,B. An endoscopic camera is introduced into the nasal cavity, allowing visualization of the middle meatus. **C,D.** A light pipe introduced through the punctum into the lacrimal sac can be used to help with internal visualization of the site where osteotomy should be placed. **E.** Incision is made through the mucosa down to bone along the *white dotted line*. **F.** Kerrison rongeurs are used to remove bone from the site to create the osteotomy. **G,H.** The site is confirmed with a light pipe, then the sac is incised open, and a Bowman probe is passed. **I,J.** Silicone stent tubes are passed through the upper and lower puncta and then visualized and within the nose.

■ External DCR

- A local anesthetic is injected, then the skin incision is made 3 to 4 mm from the medial canthus, starting 2 to 3 mm above the medial canthal tendon and extending over the lacrimal sac, following the direction of the nasojugal fold (**TECH FIG 2A**).
- A hemostat is used to bluntly spread the subcutaneous tissue apart, taking care to visualize the angular artery and cauterize it if necessary. Blunt dissection is carried down to the periosteum, which is scored with a blade or Bovie cautery needle. A periosteal elevator is then used to reflect the periosteum away from the bare bone, working in a posterolateral direction to access the bone of the lacrimal sac fossa (**TECH FIG 2B**).
- The periosteal elevator or hemostats are used to break through the lacrimal bone into the nose, and then the osteotomy is enlarged with rongeurs (typically 2 mm and 3 mm up-biting Kerrison punches) (**TECH FIG 2C**). Care is taken to punch through the bone cleanly, rather than rocking the pieces to break them away. This helps avoid propagating cracks along the skull base, which can result in cerebrospinal fluid (CSF) leak. An opening of 1 to 1.5 cm should be created through the bone, spanning the entire vertical height of the lacrimal sac.
- A Bowman probe is passed through the canaliculus, and its tip is used to tent the lacrimal sac (**TECH FIG 2D,E**).

While holding the sac on stretch with the probe, a sickle blade is used to open the lacrimal sac vertically from its superior to inferior pole and then to make a horizontal cutback at the superior and inferior ends of the sac incision to create an anteriorly based lacrimal sac flap. A corresponding anteriorly based flap is then opened through the nasal mucosa using Bovie or a blade. A ball-tipped seeker probe can be used to break any adhesions within the sac, which are commonly present in patients with a history of dacryocystitis. An antimetabolite such as mitomycin C can be applied to the sac and the nasal mucosa to decrease the potential formation of scar adhesions.[6]

- Nasolacrimal stents, such as the silicone Ritleng monocanalicular stent, are then passed through the upper and lower puncta, through the opened sac, and across through the opening in the nasal mucosa and retrieved in the nose (**TECH FIG 2F**). The stents remain in place for several weeks postoperatively to maintain patency of the openings during the healing process.
- The anterior flap of the lacrimal sac is sutured to the nasal mucosal flap with interrupted absorbable sutures (eg, 5-0 polyglactin), to hold both tissues tented above the stents (**TECH FIG 2G**). The skin incision is closed with buried absorbable sutures within the orbicularis muscle (**TECH FIG 2H**) and skin sutures of choice (eg, 6-0 fast gut, skin adhesive, or 6-0 nylon to be removed at 1 week).

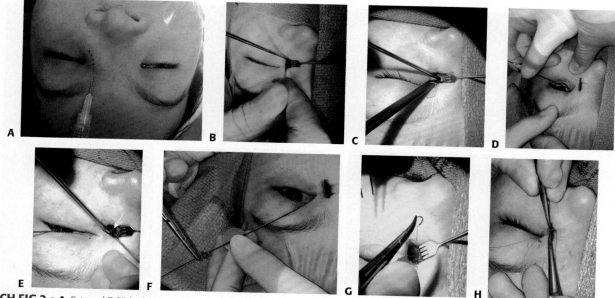

TECH FIG 2 • A. External DCR incision marking and injection of local anesthetic. **B.** Incision is retracted open, allowing use of a periosteal elevator to lift the lacrimal sac from its fossa. **C.** An osteotomy is created with Kerrison rongeurs. **D,E.** A Bowman probe is advanced through the canaliculus into the sac, resulting in tenting of the lacrimal sac (*white arrow*). **F.** A monocanalicular stent is placed. **G,H.** The lacrimal sac flap is sutured to nasal mucosa with absorbable sutures, and then the skin incision is closed.

PEARLS AND PITFALLS

Internal vs external approach	■ Most patients have good outcomes with either approach, determined by patient and surgeon preference. ■ External approach is recommended for reoperations, patients with inflammatory disease, tight internal anatomy (eg, deviated septum toward the operative side), and patients with bleeding disorders or blood thinners that cannot be stopped.
Intraoperative bleeding	■ External DCR: visualize and cauterize the angular artery if it crossed the incision site, prior to opening the osteotomy. ■ Internal DCR: epinephrine-soaked pledget packing helps slow intraoperative bleeding. Suction Bovie cautery is also of use, but take care to avoid too much heat exposure to the internal site, as overlying skin burns can result.
Stent duration	■ Classically, stents are kept in place for 12 wk after surgery. If two monocanalicular stents are used, one can be removed at 6 wk and the other retained until 12 wk. This gives the patient earlier relief from epiphora during the recovery phase.

POSTOPERATIVE CARE

DCR is an outpatient surgery. Once the patient is deemed stable postoperatively, he/she may be discharged home with a responsible adult. Postoperative instructions should include the following:

- Avoid straining, bending, heavy lifting, or strenuous activity for at least 1 week.
- Ice pack or cold compresses can be used for the first 1 to 2 days to limit swelling and bruising.
- Nose blowing should be avoided for the first week to decrease the risk of bleeding. To reduce the risk of nose bleed from nasal vasodilation, hot drinks and food should be avoided for the first 1 to 2 days.
- At the 1 week postoperative visit, the surgical site is evaluated for any signs of impaired healing or infection, and any nonabsorbable sutures may be removed. At 6 to 12 weeks after surgery, the silicone stent is removed in the clinic, and the lacrimal drainage system is irrigated to confirm patency.

OUTCOMES

The DCR surgery is considered successful when the patient experiences total or near-total relief from epiphora. Patients often still experience tearing under circumstances in which reflex tears are normally expected (ie, emotion, ocular surface irritation, etc.), as would any eye, which is not considered a surgical failure. Surgeries fail for a variety of reasons, most relating to formation of adhesions that block the drainage tract and prevent tears from flowing freely into the nose.[7]

- The reported success rates for external DCR range from 90% to 95%. The success rate is improved by ensuring a large enough osteotomy, suturing the lacrimal and nasal mucosal flaps to keep them from obstructing the healing tract, and keeping the stents in place for several weeks postoperatively.
- There is a wider range of reported success rates for endonasal (internal) DCR. In the hands of an experienced surgeon, the success rate has been shown to be statistically equivalent to the external approach. The success rate is improved by ensuring a large enough osteotomy, avoiding excessive soft tissue maceration of the nasal mucosa and lacrimal sac, limiting thermal injury with cautery, and keeping the stents in place for several weeks postoperatively.

Intraoperative usage of the antimetabolite mitomycin-C has been shown to decrease scar formation and thereby increase success rate of the surgery, regardless of whether an external or endoscopic approach is used.[6,8] Postoperative mitomycin C eye drops have also been tried but with less compelling effects.[9]

COMPLICATIONS

Intraoperative

- Hemorrhage. To decrease this risk, hold blood thinners preoperatively, utilize a block that contains epinephrine, and carefully visualize the anatomy to protect major vascular structures.
- Canalicular injury. Improper probing of the canaliculi can create a false passage and damage the common canaliculus when opening the sac. This risk can be decreased by using blunt probes and only advancing them along the existing canalicular lumen where there is minimal resistance.
- Orbital tissue injury. The use of drills and rongeurs can damage the structures of the orbit. Care must be taken to establish the anatomic location of the instrument with certainty prior to engaging it for bone removal. If fat is encountered in the surgical field, that is an indication that the orbit has been entered inadvertently.
- Skull base fracture and CSF leak. This risk can be decreased by carefully studying the preoperative imaging and taking note of the skull base contours across the ethmoid sinuses. Endoscopic DCR surgeons must avoid bone removal too far superiorly, to avoid breaching the fovea ethmoidalis or breaking the cribriform plate. External DCR surgeons must avoid rocking or twisting the rongeurs during bone removal, so that the skull base does not crack. The operative site should be inspected for leakage of CSF, which will be a clear fluid slightly more viscous than saline, which tests positive for beta-2-transferrin. Appropriate postoperative neuroimaging and consultation with neurology should be pursued if there is concern that a CSF leak has occurred.

Postoperative

- Bleeding can occur postoperatively, typically from the nasal mucosal vessels. Following the postoperative care instructions outlined earlier in the chapter decreases this risk. Most postoperative bleeding is self-limited and can be stopped by holding pressure against the nose for 5 to 10 minutes. For severe or persistent bleeding, patients should be seen emergently.

- Infection. It is rare to have postoperative infection after DCR, occurring only about 1% of the time even without the use of systemic antibiotics.[10] If an infection does occur, the patient should be given a course of oral antibiotics with broad coverage of typical skin and mucosal flora.
- Extrusion/loss of the silicone stent tubing. The patient should be instructed not to pick or pull at the tubing within the nose or at the eyelid puncta. If it partially extrudes, it can sometimes be carefully advanced back into place. If it fully extrudes, most surgeons advise allowing the patient to heal without the tubing rather than returning to the operating room to place a new stent.
- Lacrimal sump syndrome. Despite a patent osteotomy and normal results on probing and irrigation, patients with sump syndrome continue to experience tearing and mucous discharge due to an intact inferior pole of the lacrimal sac, which collects a pool of drainage. The chance of this complication can be decreased by creating a large osteotomy (at least 1 cm in diameter), ensuring the bone is opened all the way down to the level of the nasolacrimal duct entrance, and fully opening the lacrimal sac down to its inferior pole so that no pocket remains to collect fluid.
- Scarring of the ostium. After DCR, the bone or soft tissue can grow closed over the osteotomy site. When this occurs, the patient's epiphora returns and surgical revision is necessary to reopen the drainage tract. The risk of this complication can be decreased by creating a large enough osteotomy, clearing away soft tissue around the lumen, and applying mitomycin C to the tissue intraoperatively.

REFERENCES

1. Ali MJ, Joshi SD, Naik MN, Honavar SG. Clinical profile and management outcome of acute dacryocystitis: two decades of experience in a tertiary eye care center. *Semin Ophthalmol.* 2015;30(2):118-123.
2. Balikoglu-Yilmaz M, Yilmaz T, Taskin U, et al. Prospective comparison of 3 dacryocystorhinostomy surgeries: external versus endoscopic versus transcanalicular multidiode laser. *Ophthal Plast Reconstr Surg.* 2015;31(1):13-18.
3. Cheng SM, Feng YF, Xu L, et al. Efficacy of mitomycin C in endoscopic dacryocystorhinostomy: a systematic review and meta-analysis. *PLOS One.* 2013;8(5):e62737.
4. Dave TV, Mohammed FA, Ali MJ, Naik MN. Etiologic analysis of 100 anatomically failed dacryocystorhinostomies. *Clin Ophthalmol.* 2016;28:10:1419-1422.
5. Do JR, Lee H, Baek S, et al. Efficacy of postoperative mitomycin-C eyedrops on the clinical outcome in endoscopic dacryocystorhinostomy. *Graefes Arch Clin Exp Ophthalmol.* 2016;254(4):785-790.
6. Dulku S, Akinmade A, Durrani OM. Postoperative infection rate after dacryocystorhinostomy without the use of systemic antibiotic prophylaxis. *Orbit.* 2012;31(1):44-47.
7. Huang J, Malek J, Chin D, et al. Systematic review and meta-analysis on outcomes for endoscopic versus external Dacryocystorhinostomy. *Orbit.* 2014;33(2):81-90.
8. Jawaheer L, MacEwen CJ, Anijeet D. Endonasal versus external dacryocystorhinostomy for nasolacrimal duct obstruction. *Cochrane Database Syst Rev.* Feb 24, 2017;(2):CD007097.
9. Mukhtar SA, Jamil AZ, Ali Z. Efficacy of external dacryocystorhinostomy (DCR) with and without mitomycin-C in chronic dacryocystitis. *J Coll Physicians Surg Pak.* 2014;24(10):732-735.
10. Qian Z, Tu Y, Xiao T, Wu W. A lacrimal sump syndrome with a large intranasal ostium. *J Craniofac Surg.* 2015;26(5):e386-e388.

Management of the Microphthalmic or Anophthalmic Orbit

Sarah M. Jacobs and Christopher B. Chambers

43

CHAPTER

DEFINITION

A spectrum exists ranging from small eyes to complete absence of any ocular tissue:

- Nanophthalmos is defined as a small eye with otherwise normal internal structures. The axial length of the eye is ≥2 standard deviations shorter than average.
- Microphthalmos is an eye with axial length less than 20 mm and additional structural abnormalities.[1]
- Clinical anophthalmos describes some cases of microphthalmia in which the eye is so small that the patient appears anophthalmic. However, histopathologic examination of the tissue does identify products of optic vesicle formation.
- True anophthalmos involves the complete failure of primary optic vesicle outgrowth resulting in the absence of any detectable eye tissue.[1,2]

ANATOMY

- Nanophthalmos: In addition to short axial length, the sclera is thickened relative to the eye, the anterior chamber angles are narrow, and the refractive error is highly hyperopic. The small eye may or may not result in a hypoplastic orbit.[3,4]
- Microphthalmos: In addition to short axial length, the internal structures of the eye are abnormal. Microphthalmic eyes can be associated with coloboma of the uvea and/or lens, persistent fetal vasculature, Peters anomaly, glaucoma, and anterior polar cataracts. An uncommon variant, microphthalmia with cyst results from failure of the ocular embryonic fissure to close, leading to a small rudimentary eye joined to a larger cystic cavity along the colobomatous inferonasal sclera.[5] The orbit on the affected side is hypoplastic.
- Anophthalmos: There is complete absence of any ocular tissue. The eyelids have a small palpebral fissure, and beneath the lids a rudimentary conjunctival membrane is present covering the hypoplastic orbit.

PATHOGENESIS

- Embryologic failure of the optic vesicle to develop normally from the cerebral vesicle during the 4th to 8th week of gestation can lead to congenital absence or malformation of one or both eyes.
- Because the globe influences orbital growth, these ocular anomalies can result in orbital and facial maldevelopment as well.
- Nanophthalmos is typically sporadic, but autosomal recessive or autosomal dominant forms have been described (NNO1 on chromosome 11p and NNO3 on chromosome 2q). It can occur as an isolated disorder, or as part of a syndrome such as oculo-digital-dental syndrome (ODD), or autosomal dominant vitreoretinochoroidopathy with nanophthalmos (ADVIRC).[6]

- Microphthalmos occurs in approximately 10 per 100 000 live births. It can occur sporadically, with some suspected association to fetal alcohol syndrome or maternal infections during gestation, especially rubella, cytomegalovirus, and herpes simplex virus. It is estimated that over half of cases occur in conjunction with systemic abnormalities, including those occurring in the setting of chromosomal anomalies, including Trisomy 13 (Patau syndrome), Trisomy 18 (Edwards syndrome), or Wolf-Hirschhorn syndrome.[7] In inherited cases, mutations of the SOX2 gene on chromosome 3q are frequently encountered.[7] This condition can be associated with CHARGE syndrome (Coloboma, Heart defect, Atresia choanae, Retarded growth, Genital abnormality, and Ear abnormality), and PHACE syndrome (Posterior fossa anomalies, Hemangioma, Arterial lesions, Cardiac abnormalities, and Eye anomalies).
- Anophthalmos occurs approximately 2 per 100 000 live births. It is most often sporadic but can be associated with autosomal dominant defects of the SOX2 or RBP4 genes. Maternal deficiency of vitamin A during pregnancy can also pose a risk of anophthalmia.

NATURAL HISTORY

- Ocular volume drives the growth of the eyelids, fornices, and bony orbit. In turn, hemifacial development parallels orbital development. Thus, a small or absent eye leads to a hypoplastic orbit that can result in deformity of the hemifacial skeleton (**FIG 1**).
- At birth, the normal newborn eye is approximately 70% of its adult size. In contrast, the newborn face is only 40% of its adult size. Rapid growth of the facial skeleton and soft tissues occurs during early childhood, with the face reaching 70% adult size by 2 years and 90% adult size by 5.5 years.[8] The degree of orbital and facial maldevelopment is different for each microphthalmic child, depending on the amount of ocular tissue present and the trophic influence that tissue exerts.

PATIENT HISTORY AND PHYSICAL EXAMINATION

As part of the initial assessment, the following questions should be considered as they will guide further management throughout childhood:

- Is the eye present or absent?
- Is this a seeing eye?

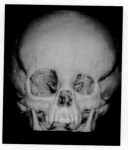 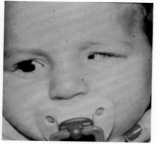

FIG 1 • A,B. Hypoplastic orbit and hemiface secondary to left microphthalmia.

- Is the other eye present? If so, is it normal?
- Are the orbits symmetric and appropriate in size?
- Are the periocular and facial soft tissues symmetric and appropriate in size?

A coordinated multidisciplinary approach is needed for evaluation of the microphthalmic or anophthalmic child, as approximately 50% have associated systemic abnormalities and 25% have defined systemic syndromes. This approach should include:

- Comprehensive assessment by a pediatrician is needed, with particular attention to the face, ears, and palate; feeding difficulties, which can indicate neurologic or esophageal abnormalities; the cardiac system and genital anatomy (due to association with CHARGE); and metabolic disturbances, which may indicate pituitary dysfunction due to midline brain abnormalities.
- Referral to subspecialists such as neurologist, cardiologist, endocrinologist, nephrologist, and audiologist should be arranged if indicated.
- In cases with systemic findings or a syndromic diagnosis, evaluation and counseling by a pediatric geneticist is also recommended.

Ophthalmologic exam is recommended as soon as possible within the first 2 to 3 weeks of life. This should involve:

- Complete anterior and posterior assessment of both eyes to assess orbital and ocular anatomy as well as visual function. In unilateral cases, the fellow eye may have subtle findings such as coloboma, cataract, retinal dystrophy, or optic nerve hypoplasia.[9]

- Full cycloplegic refraction should be prescribed to maximize visual acuity of seeing eyes. Eyeglasses with polycarbonate lenses should be used in order to protect the globes from trauma.

IMAGING AND OTHER DIAGNOSTIC STUDIES

- Preferential gaze testing (eg, Teller cards) or pattern visual evoked potential (pattern VEP) can assess basic visual acuity in preverbal patients.
- Flash visual evoked potential (VEP) testing can evaluate for any visual-cortical function in patients with severe microphthalmia or apparent anophthalmia.[9]
- Facial photographs should be taken, including a ruler in the photo for scale.
- Imaging with ultrasound of the eye and orbit to evaluate its structure and detect ocular remnants or cysts.
- MRI for detailed assessment of the soft tissues of the orbit and brain
- Maxillofacial CT for assessment of the orbital and facial bones

NONOPERATIVE MANAGEMENT

- Management focuses on utilizing the remaining vision in one or both eyes, promoting appropriate growth of the orbit and face, and optimizing ocular appearance.
- **FIG 2** outlines a treatment algorithm to accomplish these goals according to varying degrees of severity. Parents should be counseled that a series of procedures and/or devices will be needed over time to help the orbit expand in parallel to the growth of the rest of the face.
- Certain cases can be managed nonoperatively with placement of progressively larger conformers:
  - Children with useful vision in the affected eye(s) should be fitted with a series of clear conformers to progressively expand the lids, fornices, and orbit while still allowing the eye to see through the device so that visual development can occur (**FIG 3**).
- Blind eyes measuring greater than 16 mm in length can be fitted with a series of ocular prostheses to maintain the socket while also improving the appearance of the eye.
- If an eye is unable to tolerate wearing a prosthetic shell due to mechanical irritation of the corneal surface, a graft can be placed to cover the cornea (**FIG 4**).

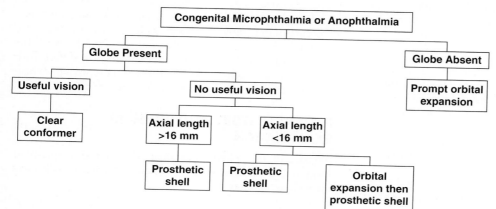

FIG 2 • Management framework for the microphthalmic or anophthalmic orbit.

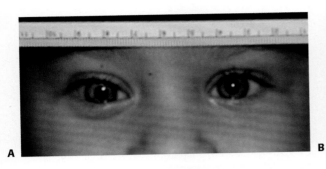
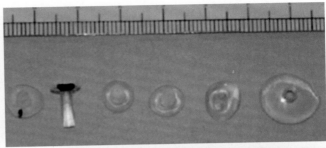
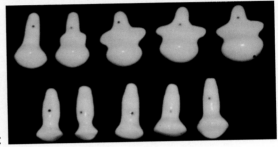

FIG 3 • A–C. A series of progressively larger conformers can be made to maintain the socket, exerting pressure to help the orbit expand and promote appropriate facial growth. For eyes with meaningful vision, clear material is used in order to avoid deprivational amblyopia.

- More severe cases can be managed with expandable devices placed into the conjunctival sac that are then inflated or exchanged for larger devices over time:
- Inflatable chambers. A flexible chamber with an anterior port that is nonsurgically seated into the conjunctival sac (**FIG 5**). A conformer holds the implant in place. Every 2 to 3 weeks in the clinic, additional saline volume is injected through the port into the chamber.
- Self-expanding hydrogels. Hydrophilic osmotic expanders (polymethyl methacrylate/polyvinylpyrrolidone), absorb up to 2000% their weight in water, resulting in expansion of 8 to 10 times the original volume (**FIG 6**).[10] Hydrogel hemispheres or spheres are placed beneath the eyelids onto the conjunctival surface and secured in place with a temporary tarsorrhaphy.[10–12] The gel is removed and exchanged for a larger-volume insert every 2 to 3 months, usually requiring a series of 2 to 4 hydrogels over the course of 4 to 12 months for adequate expansion depending on the initial size of the orbit (**FIG 7**).

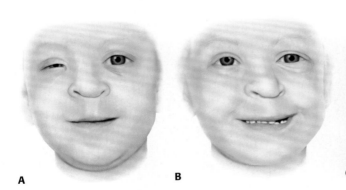
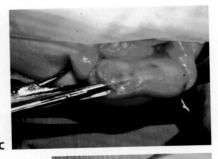
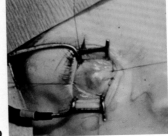

FIG 4 • A–D. To improve tolerance of the scleral shell prosthesis over the microphthalmic right eye, a mucous membrane graft is harvested from the lower lip and placed onto the ocular surface to protect the cornea.

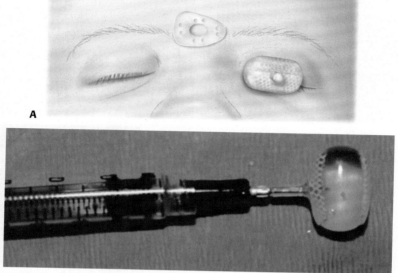

FIG 5 • A,B. A noninvasive inflatable orbital expander. The flexible chamber is seated into the conjunctival sac with its port facing anteriorly. A conformer (shown here resting on the glabella prior to insertion) is inserted over the chamber to maintain it in place. The port can be accessed with a needle and syringe to inject saline for progressive expansion of the chamber volume.

SURGICAL MANAGEMENT

■ Most cases of microphthalmia or anophthalmia require surgical management for orbital expansion. There are four goals of orbital expansion:

■ Stretch the periocular soft tissue to reduce the phimosis of the palpebral fissure and enlarge the fornices. This stretching makes it possible to wear a more appropriately sized conformer or prosthesis.[13]

■ Stimulate orbital bone growth. Animal models and human cases repeatedly demonstrate that anophthalmic orbital volume does not increase at a normal growth rate.[14] Placing a device that exerts pressure within the orbit is effective in stimulating expansion of the bony orbital walls.

■ Promote symmetric facial growth because the craniofacial skeleton is cued by the bony orbit.[15]

■ Create space for a more permanent orbital implant. Having a larger orbital implant enables wearing of a smaller-volume prosthetic, which often improves the comfort and appearance for the patient.

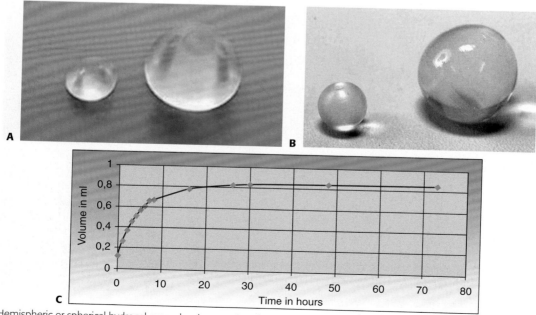

FIG 6 • A–C. Hemispheric or spherical hydrogel expanders increase in volume as they absorb water, with the potential to reach full volume within about 30 hours after implantation.

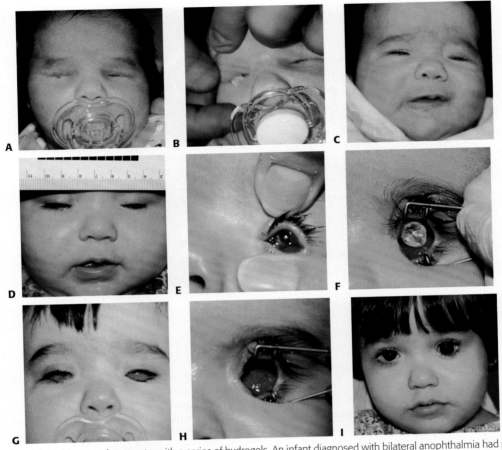

FIG 7 • A–I. Orbital growth and improved symmetry with a series of hydrogels. An infant diagnosed with bilateral anophthalmia had placement of 0.9 mL hydrogel spheres at 21 days of age. Progressive expansion of the orbit can be seen in photos from 3 to 5 months of age. At 5 months, the hydrogel was exchanged for a 1.5 mL volume. At 9 months, it was exchanged for a 2 mL volume. By 14 months of age, the orbital expansion was sufficient for placement of a dermis fat graft and subsequent fitting with ocular prostheses. Ongoing symmetric orbital and facial growth can be appreciated at 2 years of age.

- There are multiple surgical methods for achieving expansion:
  - Rigid spherical implants within the orbit. Although these have the advantage of creating direct pressure within the deep orbit to stimulate growth, they are limited by the need for multiple surgeries to place serially larger implants to promote progressive orbital growth (**TECH FIG 1**)
  - Injectable fillers. These substances allow placement of added volume into the retrobulbar orbit without significant violation of the conjunctiva. Hydroxyapatite (HA) fillers are commercially available and long-lasting, making them a viable option for socket augmentation.[16] An infraciliary skin incision is made, the filler cannula is introduced and advanced to the retrobulbar space and HA is then injected along the inferolateral orbital wall. The cannula is withdrawn, and the incision is closed with absorbable suture (**TECH FIG 2**). Serial injections can be performed to add more volume as the child grows.
  - Hydrogel pellets can be injected into the retrobulbar orbit (**TECH FIG 3**).[17]

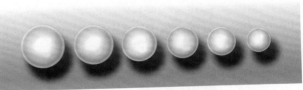

22 mm   20 mm   18 mm   16 mm   14 mm   12 mm

TECH FIG 1 • Rigid spherical orbital implants—shown here in silicone, ranging 12 to 22 mm in diameter—can be placed in the anophthalmic orbit to maintain space and promote volume expansion. The implants must be surgically exchanged for progressively larger sizes to keep pace with facial growth as the child grows.

TECHNIQUES

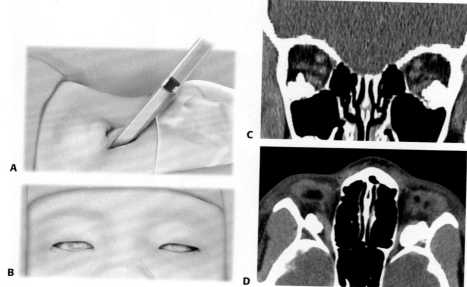

TECH FIG 2 • A–D. Retrobulbar injection of hydroxyapatite granules for orbital volume expansion through an infraciliary incision. Postprocedural CT scan demonstrates the radio-opaque filler along the inferolateral deep orbit.

- Inflatable orbital expanders. These devices are implanted into the orbit and then accessed through an external port to progressively add volume over time, thereby avoiding the need for serially exchanged conformers or implants. Early designs had a port placed beneath the scalp connected to an inflatable chamber in the orbit.[18] A later design for an integrated orbital expander design involved a globe-shaped chamber with an anterior injection port implanted into the orbit and secured to the lateral orbital rim via screw-fixated titanium plate (**TECH FIG 4**). Saline injections through the anterior port inflate the chamber to accomplish gradual orbital expansion.[15,19]

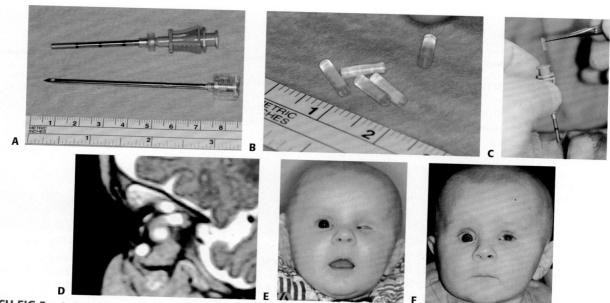

TECH FIG 3 • A–F. Hydrogel pellets are injected into the retrobulbar space under anesthesia. Sagittal CT scan shows their location and expansion. Clinical photos demonstrate orbital growth and improved hemifacial symmetry.

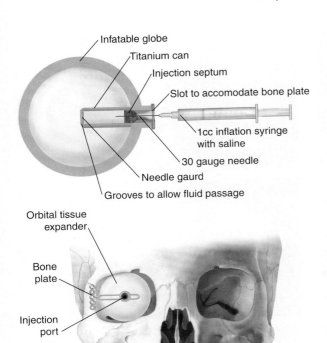

TECH FIG 4 • The integrated orbital expander is an inflatable globe placed as an orbital implant, screw-fixated with a bone plate to the lateral orbital rim. Serial injections with saline through the anterior port inflate the globe to promote orbital expansion.

- The device is surgically removed when sufficient volume has been achieved.
- When sufficient orbital expansion has been achieved by one of the above methods, a dermis fat graft (DFG) should be placed as an autologous long-term orbital expander.[20]
- In infants and young children, the graft is harvested from the buttock (**TECH FIG 5**).
- An ellipse is outlined on the skin, first with ink and then reinforced with stab incisions. The marked area should correspond to the surface area of the socket where it will be implanted.
- Dermabrasion is performed to remove the epithelium down to the level where punctate bleeding is observed from the dermal vessels.
- The graft perimeter is then incised with a scalpel. Dissection is carried down through the fat in a wide cone, such that the harvested fat area is broader than the dermal surface.
- Hemostasis is obtained with bipolar cautery and then the incision is closed in 3 layers (fat, dermis, skin) with absorbable sutures.
- The orbit is prepared with an orbitotomy incision, typically oriented horizontally aligning with the palpebral fissure.
- The DFG is tucked into the orbit through this incision and then the dermis is sutured edge to edge with the conjunctiva using absorbable sutures (**TECH FIG 6**).
- After the graft is secured along its entire perimeter, a conformer is placed and the lids are closed with temporary tarsorrhaphy.

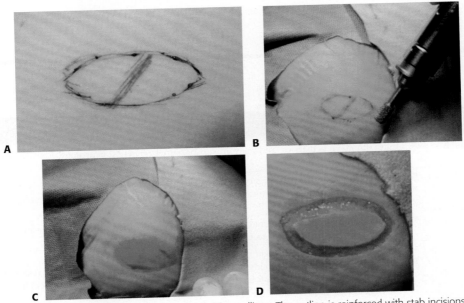

TECH FIG 5 • **A–D.** Dermis fat graft harvest. Buttock is marked with an ellipse. The outline is reinforced with stab incisions and then dermabrasion is performed to remove epithelium. The dermis is incised with a blade and then broader dissection is carried down through fat.

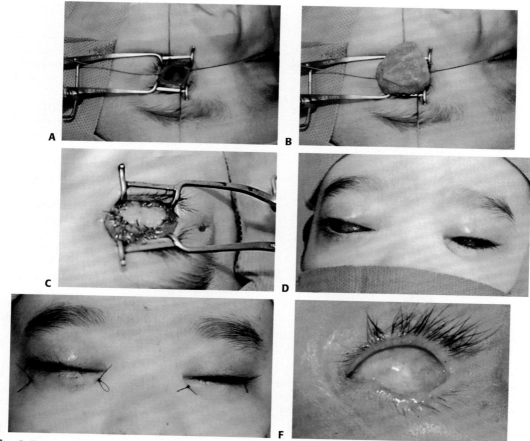

TECH FIG 6 • A–F. Dermis fat graft implantation. An orbitotomy is made through the conjunctiva, allowing insertion of the dermis graft into the orbit. The graft is secured edge to edge with conjunctiva to reform the socket surface. A conformer is placed over the graft and then the lid is closed with a temporary tarsorrhaphy. The dermis conjunctivalizes as it heals, creating a stable surface for prosthetic wear.

PEARLS AND PITFALLS

Multidisciplinary approach	■ Ophthalmology, pediatrics, and relevant subspecialties (genetics, neurology, ENT) work together to optimize care outcomes.
Minimize surgical encounters	■ Repeated transconjunctival surgery creates traumatic conjunctival scarring, which impedes good results. ■ The risks of repeated general anesthesia to the neurocognitive development of young children are still uncertain.[21,22]
Retaining hydrogels	■ Conjunctival hydrogel placement can be performed in the office with topical anesthesia, using cyanoacrylate glue rather than sutures to tarsorrhaphize the lids (**FIG 8**).
Dermis fat grafts	■ For bilateral cases, a single larger ellipse can be harvested then divided in two. ■ As the fat volume can be unwieldy during graft placement, placing the sutures systematically at the cardinal points first (12 o'clock and 6 o'clock and followed by 3 o'clock and 9 o'clock) helps retain the graft in the orbit during insertion. ■ In contrast to DFG in adults, fat atrophy does not occur to a significant degree in pediatric dermis fat grafts.
Trends in treatment	■ Management of the microphthalmic or anophthalmic orbit is moving toward goals of fewer invasive procedures, less exposure to anesthesia, and maximum symmetric growth. ■ At present these goals are best accomplished via serially larger conjunctival hydrogels, followed by dermis fat graft after sufficient expansion is achieved.

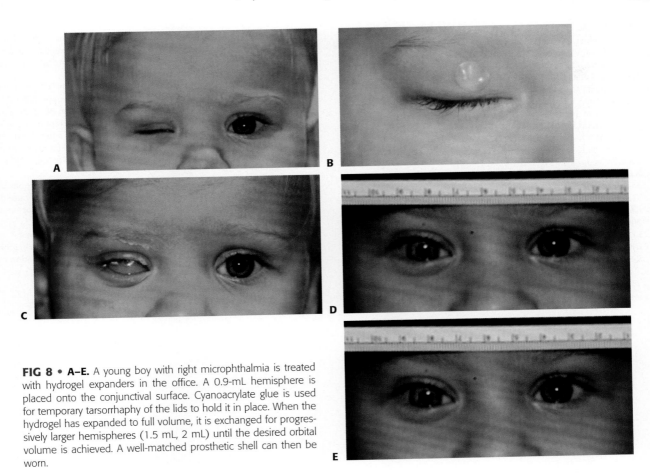

FIG 8 • A–E. A young boy with right microphthalmia is treated with hydrogel expanders in the office. A 0.9-mL hemisphere is placed onto the conjunctival surface. Cyanoacrylate glue is used for temporary tarsorrhaphy of the lids to hold it in place. When the hydrogel has expanded to full volume, it is exchanged for progressively larger hemispheres (1.5 mL, 2 mL) until the desired orbital volume is achieved. A well-matched prosthetic shell can then be worn.

OUTCOMES

- Expansion of the bony orbit by surgical or nonsurgical means can enable near-normal facial growth, thereby improving cosmesis.
- Expansion of the eyelids and conjunctival fornices can enable wearing of an ocular prosthesis, which further improves cosmesis.
- Serial conformer therapy only directly expands the anterior orbital soft tissues, but the pressure created does induce some secondary expansion of the bony orbit. In one series of 61 microphthalmic eyes in 44 children, satisfactory symmetry was achieved in 21 cases with conformer therapy alone.[13]
- The sequence and timing of treatments must be tailored to each child to achieve the best outcome.

COMPLICATIONS

- Inadequate expansion, with residual hemifacial hypoplasia.
- Contracted conjunctival fornices, with inability to wear prosthesis.
- Infection, exposure, or extrusion of orbital implant.
- Secondary hypertrophy of dermis fat graft, requiring later debulking.

REFERENCES

1. Shaw GM, Carmichael SL, Yang W, et al. Epidemiologic characteristics of anophthalmia and bilateral microphthalmia among 2.5 million births in California, 1989-1997. *Am J Med Genet A*. 2005;137 (1 suppl):36-40.
2. Williamson KA, Fitzpatrick DR. The genetic architecture of microphthalmia, anophthalmia, and coloboma. *Eur J Med Genet*. 2014;57 (8 suppl):369-380.
3. Nouri-Mahdavi K, Nilforushan N, Razeghinejad M, et al. Glaucoma in patients with nanophthalmos. *J Ophthalmic Vis Res*. 2011;6 (3 suppl):208-214.
4. Singh OS, Simmons RJ, Brockhurst RJ, Trempe CL. Nanophthalmos: a perspective on identification and therapy. *Ophthalmology*. 1982;89 (9 suppl):1006-1012.
5. Weiss AM, Koussef BG, Ross EA, Longbottom J. Complex microphthalmos. *Arch Ophthalmol*. 1989;107:1619-1624.
6. Yardley J, Leroy BP, Hart-Holden N, et al. Mutations of VMD2 splicing regulators cause nanophthalmos and autosomal dominant vitreoretinochoroidopathy (ADVIRC). *Invest Ophthalmol Vis Sci*. 2004;45:3683-3689.
7. Verma AS, Fitzpatrick DR. Anophthalmia and microphthalmia. *Orphanet J Rare Dis*. 2007;2:47.
8. Farkas LG, Posnick JC, Hreczko TM. Growth patterns in the orbital region: a morphometric study. *Cleft Palate Craniofac J*. 1992;29: 315-318.
9. Ragge NK, Subak-Sharpe ID, Collin JRO. A practical guide to the management of anophthalmia and microphthalmia. *Eye*. 2007;21: 1290-1300.

10. Maxxoli RA, Raymond WR, Ainbinder DJ, Hansen EA. Use of self-expanding, hydrophilic osmotic expanders (hydrogel) in the reconstruction of congenital clinical anophthalmos. *Curr Opin Ophthalmol.* 2004;15(5 suppl):426-431.

11. Quaranta-Leoni FM. Congenital anophthalmia: current concepts in management. *Curr Opin Ophthalmol.* 2011;22(5 suppl):380-384.

12. Hou Z, Yang Q, Chen T, et al. The use of self-inflating hydrogel expanders in pediatric patients with congenital microphthalmia in China. *J AAPOS.* 2012;16(5 suppl):458-463.

13. Wavereille O, Francois Fiquet C, Abdelwahab O, et al. Surgical and prosthetic treatment for microphthalmia syndromes. *Br J Oral Maxillofac Surg.* 2013;51(2 suppl):e17-e21.

14. Kennedy RE. Growth retardation and volume determination of the anophthalmic orbit. *Trans Am Ophthalmol Soc.* 1972;70:278-297.

15. Tse DT, Pinchuk L, Davis S, et al. Evaluation of an integrated orbital tissue expander in an anophthalmic feline model. *Am J Ophthalmol.* 2007;143(2 suppl):317-327.

16. Kotlus BS, Dryden RM. Correction of anophthalmic enophthalmos with injectable calcium hydroxylapatite (Radiesse). *Ophthal Plast Reconstr Surg.* 2007;23(4 suppl):313-314.

17. Schittkowski MP, Guthoff RF. Injectable self-inflating hydrogel pellet expanders for the treatment of orbital volume deficiency in congenital microphthalmos: preliminary results with a new therapeutic approach. *Br J Ophthalmol.* 2006;90(9 suppl):1173-1177.

18. Gossman MD, Mohay J, Roberts DM. Expansion of the human microphthalmic orbit. *Ophthalmology.* 1999;106(10 suppl):2005-2009.

19. Tse DT, Abdulhafez M, Orozco MA, et al. Evaluation of an integrated orbital tissue expander in congenital anophthalmos: report of preliminary clinical experience. *Am J Ophthalmol.* 2011;151(3 suppl):470-482.

20. Heher KL, Katowitz JA, Low JE. Unilateral dermis-fat graft implantation in the pediatric orbit. *Ophthal Plast Reconstr Surg.* 1998;14(2 suppl):81-88.

21. Graham MR, Brownell M, Chateau DG, et al. Neurodevelopmental assessment in kindergarten in children exposed to general anesthesia before the age of 4 years: a retrospective matched cohort study. *Anesthesiology.* 2016;125(4 suppl):667-677.

22. Davidson AJ, Disma N, de Graaff JC, et al. Neurodevelopmental outcome at 2 years of age after general anaesthesia and awake-regional anaesthesia in infancy (GAS): an international multicentre, randomised controlled trial. *Lancet.* 2016;387(10015 suppl):239-250.

Section X: Nasal Reconstruction

Nasal Tip Hemangioma

Terence Kwan-Wong and Jugpal S. Arneja

44

CHAPTER

DEFINITION

- Infantile hemangiomas is a benign, proliferative, vascular tumor of infancy that has a defined, although unpredictable natural history.
- Infantile hemangiomas is the most common pediatric benign tumor, affecting between 4% and 10% of children in their 1st year of life.[1]
- Approximately 60% of infantile hemangiomas involve the head and neck regions,[2] and of these, a small percentage affect the nose.
- Nasal tip hemangioma can cause significant deformity, affecting the psychological and emotional well-being of the patient and the family.

ANATOMY

- Nasal contour is determined by draping of the nasal skin over a framework formed by the nasal bones in the cephalic third, by the upper lateral cartilages in the middle third, and by the paired lower lateral cartilages and the caudal septum in the caudal third.
- Nasal tip hemangioma usually resides in a subcutaneous plane—although cutaneous manifestations are not uncommon—and can extend between the medial crura of the lower lateral cartilages and occasionally into the columellar region as well.[3,4]
  - Hemangioma extending between the lower lateral cartilages tends to splay the medial and middle crura of the lower lateral cartilages from each other and can occasionally dislocate the lower lateral cartilages, by displacing the cephalic edge of the cartilage into the nasal passage.

PATHOGENESIS

- Infantile hemangiomas is histologically characterized by proliferating endothelial cells with varying luminal sizes, which tend to be smaller during the proliferative phase, becoming larger during the involutional phase.
- Involution is reflected by slowing of endothelial proliferation, apoptosis of existing endothelial cells, and replacement of vascular tissue with adipocytes and connective tissue.

NATURAL HISTORY

- Infantile hemangiomas is not present at birth but becomes apparent within the first few weeks of life.

- The initial presentation of an infantile hemangioma may manifest as a localized telangiectasia, blanched spot, or area of ecchymosis.[1,2,5,6]
- The natural course of infantile hemangioma is relatively predictable:
  - The proliferative phase (0 to 1 year) is characterized by rapid growth.
  - The involutional phase (until 7 to 10 years) when the hemangioma shrinks and fades
    - Complete involution in 50% of children at 5 years of age, 70% by 7 years[5,7]
    - Nasal tip hemangiomas is slower to regress than those in other parts of the body.
  - Involutional phase (greater than 10 years) when the involutional process has completed
    - Even after involution, there are often residual stigmata such as residual fibrofatty tissue, atrophic/redundant/telangiectatic skin, and persistent deformity of nasal cartilage in about 50% of patients.[3-7]

PATIENT HISTORY AND PHYSICAL FINDINGS

- A thorough history should be obtained, including information about onset, progression, prior treatments, and symptoms of the nasal tip hemangioma.
- Physical examination (**FIG 1**)
  - Local—size, location, distortion of nasal cartilages, involvement of nasal vault, skin quality, presence of any scars, signs of active infection, ulceration.

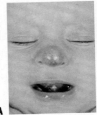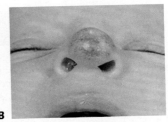

FIG 1 • **A,B.** A bulbous, pigmented hemangioma is evident at 6 months of age. (Reprinted from Arneja JS, Chim H, Drolet B, Gosain AK. The "Cyrano nose": refinements in surgical technique and treatment approach to hemangiomas of the nasal tip. *Plast Reconstr Surg.* 2010;126:1291, with permission.)

- Regional—determine presence of any other lesions. Assess for any airway, visual, or auditory involvement that may necessitate earlier intervention.
- Systemic—rare with isolated infantile hemangioma of the nasal tip
  - Beardlike distribution may indicate airway involvement.
  - Large plaquelike distributions may suggest PHACES syndrome.

IMAGING

- Imaging is usually not required.
- Ultrasound may be useful to delineate flow within and the depth of the lesion.
- MRI may be used to delineate the extent of the hemangioma and its relation to the underlying nasal framework.

DIFFERENTIAL DIAGNOSIS

- Hemangioma
- Vascular malformation (lymphatic, venous, arteriovenous)
- Dermoid cyst

NONOPERATIVE MANAGEMENT

- Nonoperative options are usually considered as adjunctive rather than definitive treatments.
- Mainstay of nonoperative management is propranolol and corticosteroid therapy.[1-3,8]
  - Propranolol is first-line medical therapy, and many practitioners feel this medication to be superior to oral corticosteroid treatment alone.
    - Dosing—1 to 3 mg/kg/d divided into TID dosing
    - Rare complications include hypoglycemia and limb cyanosis, while almost never bronchospasm and hypotension.
  - Oral or intralesional steroid therapy ideally is used during proliferative phase (**FIG 2**). Steroid therapy can be administered for up to three treatment cycles.

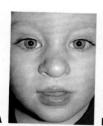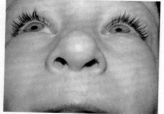

FIG 2 • A,B. After completion of treatment with intralesional steroids and pulsed dye laser therapy, the lesion has decreased in size and cutaneous manifestations have resolved in the patient in FIG 1, shown here at age 3 years. (Reprinted from Arneja JS, Chim H, Drolet B, Gosain AK. The "Cyrano nose": refinements in surgical technique and treatment approach to hemangiomas of the nasal tip. *Plast Reconstr Surg.* 2010;126:1291, with permission.)

- Can slow and sometimes arrest growth, but has little effect on regression. Response is usually seen within 1 week of initiating treatment.
- Oral corticosteroid—2 to 3 mg/kg/d of prednisolone for 8 weeks
- Intralesional corticosteroid—20 mg of triamcinolone directly into the lesion

SURGICAL MANAGEMENT

- Although precise timing of surgery is controversial, several principles exist:
  - Children begin experiencing psychosocial stigma from their peers around the age of 5 to 7 years. Consequently, surgical correction is usually timed prior to school age.[3,4,6,7]
  - Surgical correction is usually preceded by adjuvant medical therapy to reduce the size.
  - Surgery is usually not undertaken prior to the involutional phase unless the hemangioma causes significant airway obstruction and normal skin quality is important (see **FIG 1 & 2**).[1]

Preoperative Planning

- Type of approach is determined based on the location of the lesion to be debulked or resected and orientation of the skin redundancy to be resected.
- Determine if any lower lateral cartilage or columellar reorientation or reconstruction is needed.

Positioning

- The patient is positioned supine on the operating table with a shoulder roll and neck hyperextension. Limbs and pressure points are adequately padded and protected.

Approach

- Techniques differ principally with respects to scar placement and ability to control transverse and vertical skin excess.
  - The open tip rhinoplasty is the generally preferred technique because it permits good visualization of the entire nasal tip, as well as excellent control of both horizontal and vertical dimensions.
  - The nasal subunit approach attempts to hide the incisions within the junctions of the nasal subunits, providing good control of horizontal skin redundancy but with limited vertical control.
  - The Rotterdam (extended L rhinotomy) trades more extensive scarring for excellent access to the nasal tip and dorsum and is useful in controlling extreme cutaneous redundancy.
- Epinephrine containing local anesthetics should be used prior to skin incision. It provides hydrodissection, hemostasis, and postoperative analgesia.

■ Open Tip Rhinoplasty Approach

- A transverse transcolumellar incision is made at the junction of the middle and distal thirds of the columella (**TECH FIG 1**).
  - This incision may be adjusted proximally toward the columellar-lip junction if the hemangioma extends into the columella.
- Extended rim incisions are made, connecting to the columellar incision medially and proceeding along the length of the alar rim laterally.
  - The rim incision should be kept close to the nasal skin of the alar rim to avoid resection of vestibular lining, which can cause rim retraction.

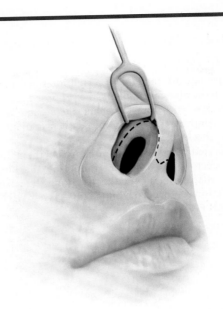

TECH FIG 1 • Markings for an open tip rhinoplasty approach. The transcolumellar incision is connected to alar rim incisions to provide access to the nasal tip and dorsum.

■ Nasal Subunit Approach

- An incision is planned along the lateral aspect of the nasal dorsum, curving around the junction between the nasal tip and ala before proceeding medially and inferiorly around the medial aspect of the soft tissue triangle and into the lateral columellar region (**TECH FIG 2**).
  - Depending on the size and location of the hemangioma, it may not be necessary to use the full length of the incision.

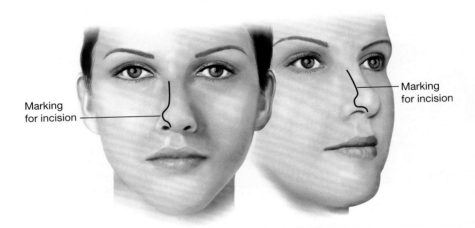

Marking for incision

Marking for incision

TECH FIG 2 • Markings for the nasal subunit approach. The full incision may not be needed depending on what areas of the nose need to be accessed.

■ Rotterdam/Extended L Rhinotomy Approach

- Markings are made for an inferior rhinotomy. Starting from the alar-cheek sulcus, the proposed incision follows the alar rim before traversing the columella and across the contralateral alar rim and then cranially along the alar-cheek sulcus.
- The extended L component is then marked by connecting the inferior rhinotomy markings with a line that courses cephalically along the nasomaxillary junction before curving medially across the nasion (**TECH FIG 3**).

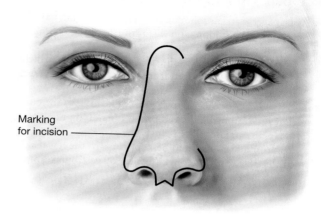

Marking for incision

TECH FIG 3 • Markings for the Rotterdam/extended L rhinotomy.

■ Elevation and Resection of the Hemangioma (Open Tip Rhinoplasty Approach)

- Using tenotomy or sharp-tipped scissors, the hemangioma with its overlying skin is dissected free from the lower lateral cartilages (**TECH FIG 4A**).
  - If the hemangioma invades the nasal columella, dissection should proceed between the medial crura of the lower lateral cartilages.
- Using sharp scissors or a no. 15 blade scalpel, hemangioma and fibrofatty tissue is sharply resected from the nasal skin in a subdermal plane (**TECH FIG 4B**).

- Caution should be taken throughout to ensure that sufficient thickness of nasal skin remains for flap perfusion and to avoid inadvertently "button holing" through the skin.
  - A finger may be placed on the superficial surface of the nasal skin to provide constant tactile feedback regarding the depth of resection.
- If the hemangioma involves vestibular lining, it is preferable to allow it to naturally involute to avoid alar rim retraction, which can result from overaggressive resection in this area.

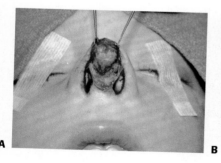
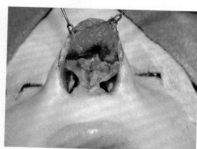

A
B

TECH FIG 4 • **A.** Dissection of the hemangioma begins in a plane between the hemangioma and nasal cartilage. **B.** Sharp excision of the hemangioma from the overlying nasal skin, ensuring uniform and adequate skin flap thickness, with lower lateral cartilage reconstruction.

■ Lower Lateral Cartilage Reconstruction

- The shape and position of the lower lateral cartilages are assessed.
- If the lower lateral cartilage has been dislocated by the hemangioma, it should be resuspended to the upper lateral cartilage using sutures.[5]

- Interdomal sutures using 6-0 polydioxanone (PDS) are placed to reapproximate the medial and middle crura of the lower lateral cartilages if they have been splayed apart by the hemangioma (**TECH FIG 4A**).
- Transdomal sutures are placed using 6-0 PDS to restore domal projection if the intercrural angle has been flattened by mass effect of the hemangioma (**TECH FIG 4B**).

■ Skin Resection and Closure (Open Tip Rhinoplasty Approach)

- The nasal skin is redraped over the cartilaginous framework, and the redundant skin is marked out and sharply trimmed (**TECH FIG 5A**).
  - Skin resection should be conservative to avoid undue tension, which can produce nasal distortion, blunting of the nasal tip, or alar rim retraction.
  - With the open rhinoplasty approach, vertical skin excess can be corrected by adjusting the resection at the tip of the columellar flap, whereas horizontal skin excess can be controlled by adjusting the margin of resection at the columellar-rim flap.[5]
- The skin is approximated using rapid absorbing 5-0 polyglactin 910 (Vicryl Rapide), and if alar rim incisions were used for access, the vestibular lining is closed using 5-0 polyglactin 910 (Vicryl) (**TECH FIG 5B**).
  - If alar rim incisions were used, a silicone-conforming stent is inserted into the nares and secured using tape.

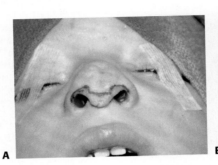 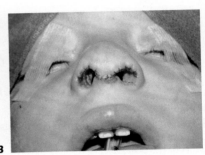

TECH FIG 5 • A. The nasal skin is loosely redraped over the nasal framework, and the skin excision is marked. Markings should err toward being more conservative to avoid undue tension during closure, which can cause nasal distortion. **B.** The final result after hemangioma excision, reconstruction of the lower lateral cartilages, and excision of resultant skin excess. Following this, Silastic-conforming stents are inserted and secured with tape.

PEARLS AND PITFALLS

Timing	■ Surgery should be delayed until involution is completed and/or cutaneous manifestations are resolved, unless there is airway/visual axis obstruction or life-threatening symptoms. ■ Surgery should be completed prior to school age to minimize the psychosocial impact experienced by the patient and parents.
Nonsurgical therapies	■ Propranolol should be considered for first-line medical therapy. Reduction in volume and color is often seen within 24–48 hours of initiating therapy. ■ Adjunctive corticosteroid therapy may be used in an intralesional or oral fashion. ■ Pulsed dye laser can be used to treat telangiectatic skin changes.
Surgical access	■ Location of the hemangioma and the vectors of skin excess will help determine the type of incision used. The authors prefer the open tip rhinoplasty approach for its exposure and ability to control both horizontal and vertical skin excess. ■ Use of local anesthetic with epinephrine provides hemostatic, analgesic, and hydrodissective benefits.
Hemangioma resection	■ If the hemangioma involves vestibular lining, it is preferable to leave residual hemangioma in these areas and to allow it to involute naturally. ■ Overaggressive resection of tumor can cause nasal tip blunting, nostril-tip disproportion, or a "skeletonization" appearance of the lower lateral cartilages.
Lower lateral cartilage reconstruction	■ Reconstruction and reapproximation of the lower lateral cartilages using domal creation and/or interdomal sutures may be necessary, especially if the hemangioma is large and/or involves the columellar region.
Minimize risk of alar rim retraction	■ If alar rim incisions are to be used, stay close to the cutaneous rim to avoid resecting vestibular lining. ■ Skin resection should be conservative, with closure being done under virtually no tension. ■ Silicone intranasal conforming stents should be used for 3 months post-operatively.

POSTOPERATIVE CARE

- If alar rim incisions are made, silicone intranasal stents should be placed intraoperatively and left in place for at least 3 months to minimize the effects of scar contraction.
  - Sutures should not be used to hold the stent in due to the risk of inadvertent columellar trauma if the suture is pulled through.
- Parents should be taught how to remove the stents for cleaning of the surgical site and how to replace and resecure the stents using tape.
- Scar massage may be started approximately 4 weeks following surgery.

OUTCOMES

- Good cosmetic results with high patient and parental satisfaction can be expected following resection of nasal tip hemangiomas (**FIG 3**).[3,4,7]
- There is rarely a risk of recurrence if the resection is performed after the proliferative phase has passed.
- Families should be prepared for the possibility of secondary procedures such as repeat resection, scar revision, and laser therapy for cutaneous sequelae or secondary rhinoplasty.

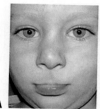 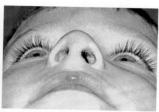

A **B**

FIG 3 • Surgical correction was performed on the patient in FIGS 1 and 2 at 5 years of age and served to "sculpt" the final appearance of the nose. **A,B.** The postoperative result is shown 1 year later. Combined medical and surgical management resulted in an optimal aesthetic result in this patient. (Reprinted from Arneja JS, Chim H, Drolet B, Gosain AK. The "Cyrano nose": refinements in surgical technique and treatment approach to hemangiomas of the nasal tip. *Plast Reconstr Surg.* 2010;126:1291, with permission.)

COMPLICATIONS

- Infection
- Hematoma
- Necrosis of skin flap margins
- Alar rim retraction and/or stenosis
- Poor nasal tip definition
- Nasal tip distortion
- Hypertrophic/keloid scarring

REFERENCES

1. Drolet B, Esterly N, Frieden I. Hemangiomas in children. *N Engl J Med.* 1999;341:173-181.
2. Chen T, Eichenfield L, Friedlander S. Infantile hemangiomas: an update on pathogenesis and therapy. *Pediatrics.* 2013;131(1):99-108.
3. Arneja J, Gosain A. The Cyrano nose: refinements in surgical technique and treatment approach to hemangiomas of the nasal tip. *Plast Reconstr Surg.* 2010;126(4):1291-1299.
4. Waner M, Kastenbaum J, Scherer K. Hemangiomas of the nose: surgical management using a modified subunit approach. *Arch Facial Plast Surg.* 2008;10(5):329-334.
5. Jackson I, Sosa J. Excision of nasal tip hemangioma via open rhinoplasty—a skin sparing technique. *Eur J Plast Surg.* 1998;21(5):265-268.
6. Warren S, Longaker M, Zide B. The subunit approach to nasal tip hemangiomas. *Plast Reconstr Surg.* 2002;109(1):25-30.
7. Van der Meulen J, Gilbert P, Roddi R. Early excision of nasal hemangiomas: the L-approach. *Plast Reconstr Surg.* 1994;94(3):465-473.
8. Drolet B, Frommelt P, Chamlin S, et al. Initiation and use of propranolol for infantile hemangioma: report of a consensus conference. *Pediatrics.* 2013;131(1):128-140.

Nasal Septal Hematoma

Whitney Laurel Quong and Jugpal S. Arneja

DEFINITION

- Hematoma of the nasal septum is a relatively rare, yet potentially serious consequence of trauma to the nose where blood accumulates between the cartilaginous/bony portion of the septum, and its overlying mucoperichondrium/mucoperiosteum. Any degree of craniofacial trauma should urge evaluation for the condition.
- Without prompt recognition and intervention, a septal hematoma may precipitate future cosmetic distortion, including secondary infection, resulting in septal abscess and/or ultimately a saddle nose deformity.
- Incision and drainage is the mainstay of treatment, but immediate reconstruction with autograft or homograft is an option if there is structural defect in the nasal septum.

ANATOMY

- The nasal septum comprises cartilaginous, membranous, and bony components (perpendicular plate of the ethmoid, vomer, premaxilla, maxillary crest, and palatine crest) covered by mucoperichondrium and mucoperiosteum layers (**FIG 1**). The septum is typically 2 to 4 mm thick.
- The blood supply of the nasal septum is derived from the sphenopalatine and the anterior and posterior ethmoid arteries, along with contributions from the superior labial artery (anteriorly) and the greater palatine artery (posteriorly). These vessels travel in the overlying mucous membrane and penetrate the mucoperichondrium through vascular canals. It is through diffusion that the cartilaginous septum receives its blood supply. The Kiesselbach plexus (Little area) is a region where the chief blood supplies to the internal nose converge and is found in the anteroinferior third of the nasal septum.
- Bleeding into the potential space between the cartilage and its overlying mucoperichondrium leads to a septal hematoma (**FIG 2**), whereas external bleeding from Kiesselbach plexus results in epistaxis.

PATHOGENESIS

- Nasal septal hematoma typically results from trauma to the nasal complex, with even minor trauma causing the condition. Rarely, chronic irritation of the septum by nasogastric tube has also been found to precipitate the condition.[1]
- Children are particularly prone to developing septal hematomas, as the pediatric cartilage is soft and prone to buckling,[2] and the mucoperichondrium is only loosely adherent to the underlying cartilage.[1]
- The precise mechanism for development of nasal septal hematoma has not been defined, but has been proposed to occur when mechanical force to the nasal cartilage precipitates leakage or rupture of the mucoperichondrial vessels in the septum.
- If the mucosa remains intact, extravasated blood strips the mucoperichondrium and/or mucoperiosteum from cartilage/bone as it accumulates within a closed space.
- Where vessel compromise is coincident with fracture of the septal cartilage or bony components, blood may dissect through the fracture and form a hematoma.

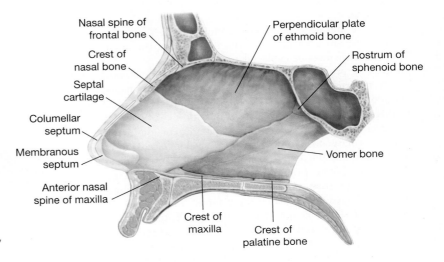

FIG 1 • The nasal septum is formed by cartilaginous, membranous, and bony components.

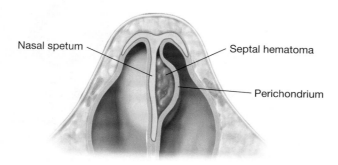

FIG 2 • A septal hematoma is formed when there is accumulation of blood into the potential space between the cartilaginous septum and the overlying mucoperichondrium.

NATURAL HISTORY

■ When not promptly recognized, extravasated blood continues to expand between the perichondrium and cartilage. Eventually, the increased pressure causes collapse of the vessels supplying the septal cartilage. Pressure-induced ischemia, avascular necrosis, and liquefaction can result rapidly within 24 to 72 hours.

■ Where there is significant necrosis and destruction of the septal cartilage, the structural integrity of the septum is compromised, and a saddle nose deformity may be the end result.

■ Necrosed tissue may also act as a nidus for infection and abscess development. Bacteria isolated from septal abscesses are predominantly those species of the normal nasal flora, which include *Staphylococcus aureus*, *Streptococcus pneumonia*, group A β-hemolytic streptococcus, and *Haemophilus influenzae*.[3] Collagenases produced by these bacteria serve to accelerate cartilage liquefaction.

■ Meningitis, cerebral abscess, subarachnoid empyema, and cavernous sinus thrombosis have also been reported as complications of septal hematomas.[3]

■ Because the development of septal hematoma may be delayed up to 48 to 72 hours from initial trauma,[1] sequential evaluation is recommended.

PATIENT HISTORY AND PHYSICAL FINDINGS

■ Though relatively rare—occurring as a consequence to only 0.8% to 1.6% of nasal traumas[1]—one should be suspicious for septal hematoma when there is any history of craniofacial trauma.

■ A full head and neck examination should be performed to evaluate for any coincident injuries. In children, the possibility of abuse must be explored.

■ On history, progressive nasal obstruction is the most commonly reported symptom. Report of facial pain/headache, epistaxis, and fever are also common symptoms. Clinical features elucidated on physical examination that increase the pretest probability include hyperemia of the nasal mucosa, enlargement of the septum, swelling/ecchymoses of the nasal dorsum, external nasal deformity, and purulent rhinorrhea.[1] Presence of any of these features should prompt further history about preceding nasal trauma, upper respiratory tract infections, or dental procedures.

■ With nasal septal hematoma on the differential diagnosis, focused intranasal examination of the nasal septum is required. Direct anterior rhinoscopy to evaluate the nasal septum may be performed with nasal specula. In addition to the septum, the inferior turbinate, a portion of the middle turbinate, and possibly the nasopharynx should be visualized. Both sides of the nasal septum must be evaluated.

■ The nasal mucosa is normally pink, without ulcerations, crusting, or bleeding. The septal hematoma is visualized as a lateral bulging (unilateral, or bilateral), with purple/dusky fluctuance. Palpation of the septum, by inserting a gloved finger into the nostril, may aid identification of a fluctuance. If such fullness persists even after topical administration of a vasoconstrictive agent such as oxymetazoline, the diagnosis of septal hematoma is highly likely.

IMAGING

■ If the diagnosis is an isolated nasal septal hematoma, without other indication, no further imaging studies are required.

■ If the septal hematoma has further developed into a nasal septal abscess, computed tomography scanning of the head and neck region with contrast enhancement should be considered to evaluate for intracranial extension. Particularly, where there is extensive facial cellulitis, focal neurologic defects, altered consciousness, meningismus, severe headache, failure to improve with treatment, delay in diagnosis and treatment, or isolation of an unusual/virulent microorganism, further radiologic imaging is recommended.[4]

DIFFERENTIAL DIAGNOSIS

■ Nasal septal abscess
■ Deviated nasal septum
■ Nasal septal polyp
■ Nasal fracture

NONOPERATIVE MANAGEMENT

■ In a cooperative patient presenting soon after injury and where necrosis and infection are not suspected, the hematoma may be evacuated in the clinic or emergency department. Under local anesthetic, a simple aspiration with needle (**FIG 3**) and syringe can be performed, and the nose subsequently packed and reassessed 48 to 72 hours later.

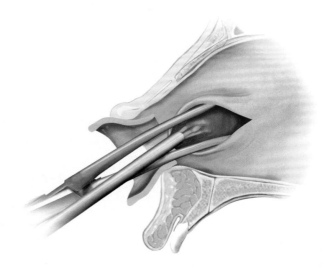

FIG 3 • A needle and syringe can be used to enter the hematoma and evacuate the accumulated clot.

- For a more organized hematoma, incision and drainage in the operating room is suggested.
- In a pediatric patient, if significant necrosis is suspected, or if immediate reconstruction is likely to be required, management in the operating room with incision and drainage under general anesthetic is recommended.

SURGICAL MANAGEMENT

- Antibiotics should be administered upon identification of a septal hematoma. Coverage should include the common upper respiratory tract microorganisms, with amoxicillin-clavulanate recommended for uncomplicated cases, and clindamycin used where abscess is suspected or known.
- If there is compromise to the structural integrity of the nasal septum, as is commonly seen with delayed identification of a hematoma or abscess, immediate reconstruction can be considered. This is particularly supported in the pediatric population, for whom loss of portions of the cartilaginous septum may ultimately have a long-term effect on the growth of the facial skeleton.[5]

Preoperative Planning

- To anesthetize the septum, pledgets soaked in an equal part mixture of 4% lidocaine and 0.05% oxymetazoline should be packed into the nares. Adequate contact of the pledgets with the septum should be ensured. After 10 minutes, a small amount of 1% or 2% lidocaine with epinephrine can be injected into the septum.

Positioning

- Place the patient supine, ensuring adequate access, visualization, and lighting of the nasal septum.

Approach

- After the septum is anesthetized, thorough examination of septum should be permissible. With a nasal speculum, the full extent of the hematoma should be evaluated, and both sides of the septum visualized.

■ Aspiration

- With a needle attached to a syringe, pierce the hematoma and aspirate the cavity. Blood should be amenable to being withdrawn with little force. If there is concern regarding infection, send the aspirate for culture and sensitivity. This step may also be performed in the clinic/emergency department if the diagnosis is unclear, or as a temporizing measure prior to operative management.

■ Hemitransfixion Incision

- A hemitransfixion incision is made at the junction of the membranous septum and the lower border of the nasal septal cartilage to further explore and evacuate the hematoma. Residual clot should be suctioned, and the cavity irrigated with saline. Necrotic cartilage should also be debrided. Subsequently, any defect in the cartilage can be assessed, and the need for reconstruction considered.

■ Septum Reconstruction

- Defect in the septal cartilage following debridement of the necrotic tissue can be reconstructed immediately. In this case, the surgeon may consider converting to an open tip approach for direct access to the nasal base and septum; the precise amount of the cartilage defect can be evaluated, and approach for reconstruction considered.
- Three principal methods of cartilage reconstruction are advocated: the "exchange technique" using posterior septal components to reconstruct the anterior defect, a "mosaicplasty" piecing together residual cartilage with fibrin glue, and reconstruction with a cartilage autograft or homograft.[7]
- An "exchange technique" is suitable where larger pieces of cartilaginous/bony septum remain in the posterior septum.
    - From the dorsal portion of the septum, a portion of the cartilage can be harvested and implanted into the defect as an autogenous septal graft.
    - Guide sutures may be used to position the graft into anatomic position, and transverse mattress sutures used for fixation.
- If a defect still exists, and there is insufficient cartilage, a graft from the osseous septum may also be taken.
- This exchange technique is not recommended in children, however, because disruption of the posterior septum may ultimately affect septal and midface growth.
- For multiple small cartilaginous septal components underlying the hematoma—that is the septum has fractured but not necrosed—a "mosaicplasty" can be performed. In this technique, the septal fragments are held together with fibrin glue and used to patch the defect. Although relatively simple, it has been suggested that this technique may not be the most effective in preventing or treating a saddle nose deformity.[6]
- A cartilage autograft or homograft is possibly the most preferred method of reconstruction. Cartilage is typically consistent, appropriately elastic, amenable to shaping, and typically heals uneventfully. There is debate as to its ideal source, with conchal, tragal, costal, or preserved donor cartilage being options.
    - When using preserved donor cartilage, there is typically not as significant limitation in size or volume as in

comparison to employment of an autograft. Although different constructions including the "L-shaped" and "angular-shaped" types have been described, possibly the "boomerang-shaped" (**TECH FIG 1**) design is the most preferred. The boomerang shape is proposed to best resist mechanical stress, as it provides supports to both the Little area, as well as the anterior nasal spine.[6] Ultimately, if a graft is used, it should be fit to the size of the defect and provide support to the nose.

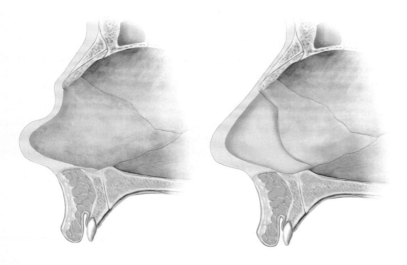

TECH FIG 1 • The boomerang-shaped cartilage graft provides support to the anterior spine and Kiesselbach plexus area and is resistant to mechanical stress.

Preventing Reaccumulation: Drain, Wick, or Quilt

- A few different measures are available to prevent reaccumulation of the hematoma. Into the hemitransfixion incision, an iodoform wick can be inserted, or a penrose drain may be stitched in place (**TECH FIG 2A**). Alternatively, and preferred, a quilting stitch (with an absorbable suture) can be performed, which runs back and forth across the septum in a random pattern to firmly press the mucoperichondrium against the cartilage and eliminate dead space (**TECH FIG 2B**).

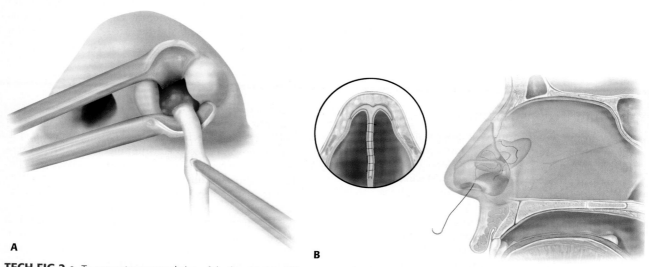

A   B

TECH FIG 2 • To prevent reaccumulation of the hematoma, **(A)** a penrose drain may be stitched into place temporarily, or **(B)** a quilting stitch (with an absorbable suture) can be performed to firmly press the mucoperichondrium against the cartilage and eliminate dead space.

Nasal Packing

- Vaseline gauze packing is placed with or without suturing of the mucosa to the septum.

PEARLS AND PITFALLS

Bilateral hematoma incisions	■ For bilateral septal hematomas, the hemitransfixion incisions should be staggered/nonopposing, as to avoid a through-and-through perforation of the septum.
Securing the cartilage graft	■ To further secure the cartilage graft into the defect in an effort to avoid migration, silicone sheets can be placed on the mucosa, and mattress sutures used through the silicone sheet, mucosa, perichondrium, and cartilage graft. The sheets may be kept in place for up to 10 days.

POSTOPERATIVE CARE

■ If infection was present, the patient should be monitored for fever, worsening facial cellulitis, increasing pain, and changes in mentation in the immediate postoperative period. Emergence of any of these features should prompt re-exploration of the hematoma and drainage of fluid, alteration on the antibiotic regimen, or CT scan to evaluate for intracranial involvement as necessary.

■ The head of the bead should remain elevated to reduce edema and pain.

■ For noninfected patients, the nasal packing and drain/wick should be kept in place for 72 hours before removal. At that time, re-evaluation is recommended to ensure no recurrence of the hematoma.

■ Follow-up at 1 year is recommended to evaluate for saddle nose deformity. In children, ongoing follow-up may be necessary to assess growth of the nose.

OUTCOMES

■ Large outcome studies of nasal septal hematoma treatment are not available. However, the data seem to suggest a significant rate of long-term complications.

■ One study of 16 pediatric patients (7 with nasal septal hematoma, 9 with nasal septal abscess) with a mean follow-up period of 3 years found minor sequelae in 6 patients (minor cosmetic deformity, minor septal/vault alterations without airway compromise), and major sequelae in 10 patients (dorsum/tip/pyramid deformation with important cosmetic impairment, deviation of the septum with nasal obstruction, swelling of the septal cartilage, functional vault deformity, septal perforation).[7] Another study using this classification system found a long-term complication rate of 63% patients with nasal septal hematoma and 89% in patients with septal abscess.[1]

■ One review of 8 articles discussing outcomes of early nasal septal reconstruction in the management of nasal septal abscess reported sequelae in 11 of the total 28 patients.[5] These complications included underdevelopment of the nasal tip and premaxilla in one patient undergoing homologous reconstruction, minimal saddle deformity in one patient with homologous reconstruction, nonobstructing deviation of the nasal septum in four patients with homologous/exchange reconstruction, columellar retraction in one patient with autologous reconstruction, and three patients with over-rotation of the nasolabial angle after autologous reconstruction. One patient also developed saddle nose deformity, upward displacement of the anterior maxilla, diminished vertical development of the nasal cavity, and a retrognathically positioned maxilla after reconstruction with homologous tissue.

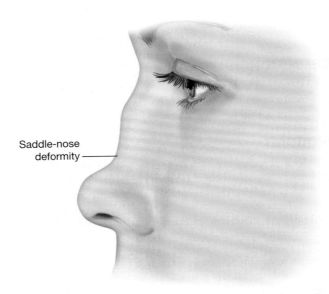

Saddle-nose deformity —

FIG 4 • The saddle nose deformity is one long-term cosmetic complication of cartilage collapse post-untreated septal hematoma.

COMPLICATIONS

■ Nasal septal abscess, leading to meningitis, orbital cellulitis, intracranial abscess, cavernous sinus thrombosis, or oronasal fistula

■ External deformity of the nose: saddle-nose type (**FIG 4**), tip over-rotation

■ Growth inhibition of the midface in children, leading to underdevelopment of the nose and maxilla, midface retroposition, or retracted columella

■ Nasal obstruction

■ Septal deviation

■ Septal perforation

REFERENCES

1. Sayin I, Yazici ZM, Bozkurt E, Kayhan FT. Nasal septal hematoma and abscess in children. *J Craniofac Surg.* 2011;22(6):e17-e19. doi:10.1097/SCS.0b013e31822ec801.
2. Wright RJ, Murakami CS, Ambro BT. Pediatric nasal injuries and management. *Facial Plast Surg.* 2011;27(5):483-490. doi:10.1055/s-0031-1288931.
3. Canty PA, Berkowitz RG. Hematoma and abscess of the nasal septum in children. *Arch Otolaryngol Head Neck Surg.* 1996;122(12):1373-1376.
4. Thomson CJ, Berkowitz RG. Extradural frontal abscess complicating nasal septal abscess in a child. *Int J Pediatr Otorhinolaryngol.* 1998;45(2):183-186.
5. Alshaikh N, Lo S. Nasal septal abscess in children: from diagnosis to management and prevention. *Int J Pediatr Otorhinolaryngol.* 2011;75(6):737-744. doi:10.1016/j.ijporl.2011.03.010
6. Hellmich S. Reconstruction of the destroyed septal infrastructure. *Otolaryngol Head Neck Surg.* 1989;100(2):92-94.
7. Alvarez H, Osorio J, De Diego JI, et al. Sequelae after nasal septum injuries in children. *Auris Nasus Larynx.* 2000;27(4):339-342.

Section XI: Pediatric Neck Masses

46

CHAPTER

Branchial Cleft Sinuses and Cysts

Mark Felton, Jugpal S. Arneja, and Neil K. Chadha

DEFINITION

- Spectrum of congenital sinuses and cysts due to developmental anomalies in the branchial system.[1,2]
- Account for up to 17% of cervical neck masses.[3]

ANATOMY

- Branchial arches are akin to ancient gill apparatus (**FIG 1**).
- Humans have five branchial/pharyngeal arches, 1 to 4 and 6 (there is no 5th branchial arch), which form craniocaudally from week 4.
- Membrane ectoderm externally and endoderm internally covers the arches.
- Cleft externally separates each arch.
- Pouch internally separates each arch.
- Each arch forms an artery, cartilaginous structure, nerve and muscle.
- Arches 1 and 3 mainly form the face, and arches 3, 4, and 6 form the neck, with 4 and 6 fusing.
- Ectodermal clefts obliterate except for the 1st branchial cleft, which forms the external auditory canal with outer side of the tympanic membrane forming the medial limit.
- Branchial pouches form various head and neck organs (Tables 1 and 2).

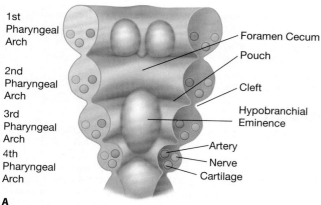

1st Pharyngeal Arch

2nd Pharyngeal Arch

3rd Pharyngeal Arch

4th Pharyngeal Arch

Foramen Cecum

Pouch

Cleft

Hypobranchial Eminence

Artery

Nerve

Cartilage

A

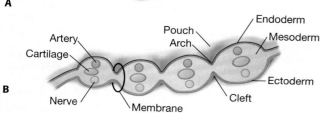

Pouch Arch

Artery

Cartilage

Endoderm

Mesoderm

Ectoderm

Cleft

B

Nerve

Membrane

FIG 1 • Branchial arch and pouches.

PATHOGENESIS

- Failure of branchial pouch or cleft to obliterate during embryonic development can lead to fistula, sinus, or cyst formation:
  - A cyst is an epithelial-lined fluid-filled sac.
  - A sinus is a blind-ended epithelial lined tract opening on to skin or mucosa.
  - A fistula is an epithelial-lined tract connecting two surfaces (skin/mucosa).
- The resultant anomaly from failure of this process relates to the specific arch, pouch or cleft derivatives.
- The main branchial anomalies associated with sinuses and fistulae are 1st and 2nd cleft anomalies and 3rd and 4th pouch anomalies.
- Type 1 branchial anomalies are rare anomalies resulting in duplication of the external ear canal and are classified as Work's type 1 or 2.
- Branchial cleft cysts are regarded as 2nd branchial anomalies. Several theories exist as to their origin including[3]:
  - Lymph node inclusion theory—cystic transformation of lymph nodes
  - Branchial cleft remnant theory—remnant of branchial cleft/pouch
  - Thymopharyngeal duct theory—remnant of the connection between the thymus and 3rd pouch
  - Cervical sinus of His theory—cyst is formed by remains of the cervical sinus.

PATIENT HISTORY AND PHYSICAL FINDINGS

- Branchial sinuses and fistulas may present as a discharging neck punctum +/– neck swelling.
- Type 1 branchial anomaly is rare.
  - Often a late diagnosis
  - May present with a mass in parotid or submandibular region
  - Discharging neck punctum or discharging ear
- Type 2 branchial anomalies are the most common branchial anomaly.
  - Often present at or just after birth
  - External opening in the skin (punctum) along anterior border sternocleidomastoid muscle +/– discharge
- Type 3 and 4 brachial sinus
  - Neonates—lateral neck cyst/abscess +/– airway obstruction
  - Child/young adult—thyroiditis/recurrent neck abscess
  - Most commonly diagnosed in childhood (delayed diagnosis)
- Branchial cysts
  - May present as a cystic neck swelling +/– infection/abscess

Table 1 Branchial Arch and Pouch Derivatives

	Arch Derivatives				Pouch Derivatives
	Artery	**Cartilage**	**Cranial Nerve**	**Muscle**	
1	Part of terminal branches maxillary artery	Meckel cartilage: malleus and incus, anterior malleolar ligament, mandible template, maxilla, zygomatic bone and squamous temporal bone, mandible	V—trigeminal	Muscles of mastication, mylohyoid, tensor tympani, anterior belly digastric	Tubo-tympanic recess, tympanic cavity, mastoid antrum, Eustachian tube
2	Stapedial arteries	Reichert cartilage: stapes, styloid process, stylohyoid ligament, lesser cornu, and superior body of hyoid	VII—facial	Muscles of facial expression, stapedius, stylohyoid, posterior belly digastric	Tonsils
3	Common carotid arteries, internal carotid arteries	Greater cornu and inferior part of hyoid	IX—glossopharyngeal	Stylopharyngeus	Inferior parathyroid glands and thymus
4	Left forms part of aortic arch, right forms part right subclavian artery	Laryngeal	X—vagus, superior laryngeal	Cricothyroid, pharynx constrictors	Superior parathyroid glands and possibly the calcitonin-producing cells of thyroid
6	Pulmonary arteries, ductus arteriosus	Laryngeal	X—vagus, recurrent laryngeal	Intrinsic muscles of larynx	

- Peak age 3rd decade
- Most are located anterior to the upper part of the sterno-cleidomastoid muscle
- Branchio-oto-renal syndrome is an autosomal dominant syndrome with a prevalence of 1 in 40 000 people. It is caused by mutations in the *EYA1*, *SIX1*, and *SIX5* genes.[4]
- Children born with this typically have branchial anomalies, ear abnormalities (including pits, tags, atresia, hearing loss) and kidney abnormalities (including hypoplastic/absent kidneys). If suspected, these children require audiometry, an ultrasound of the renal tract, and genetic counseling.

IMAGING

- Imaging varies depending on the branchial anomaly.
- Cysts—ultrasound (USS) is obtained usually, but an MRI may be helpful when the diagnosis is not clear on USS.
- Type 1—CT to image middle ear and MRI for soft tissues and course of sinus/fistula (**FIG 2A**).
- Type 2—clinical diagnosis; usually no imaging required.
- Types 3 and 4—barium swallow/and direct laryngoscopy to assess for sinus/fistula entrance at the pyriform fossa; USS +/– MRI to assess thyroid involvement and any cystic component (**FIG 2B**).

Table 2 Pathophysiology and Sinus/Fistula Course

	1st Branchial Anomaly (Work's Type 1)	1st Branchial Anomaly (Work's Type 2)	2nd Branchial Anomaly	3rd Branchial Anomaly	4th Branchial Anomaly
Pathogenesis	1st cleft anomaly, derived from ectoderm	1st cleft anomaly, derived from ectoderm and mesoderm (cartilage and adnexal features).	2nd cleft anomaly	3rd pouch anomaly, persistence of thymobranchial canal	4th pouch anomaly, derived from pharyngobranchial canal, which connects the pharynx to the ultimobranchial body and superior PT gland
Course	Tract runs parallel to external auditory canal, opening medial, inferior or posterior to conchal cartilage and pinna.	Tract runs from lower more anterior in the neck than type 1, is always superior to hyoid bone, coursing over the angle of the mandible, through the parotid gland, terminating at or near the bony cartilaginous junction of the EAC, and often entering the middle ear. Has a close relationship to the facial nerve.	Fistula, sinus or cyst along SCM anterior border, pass superiorly between ICA and ECA, over the hypoglossal nerve (3rd Arch) and open into the posterior pillar of tonsillar fossa (2nd pouch)	Tract runs through the thyrohyoid membrane and above superior laryngeal nerve. Opens in upper/lateral wall piriform fossa	Tract runs through the cricothyroid membrane below the superior laryngeal nerve. Opens into the apex of piriform fossa

SCM, sternocleidomastoid muscle; ICA, internal carotid artery; ECA, external carotid artery; PT, parathyroid; EAC, external auditory canal.

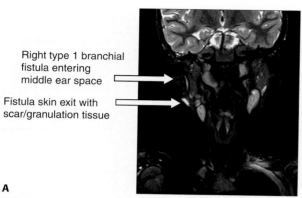

Right type 1 branchial fistula entering middle ear space

Fistula skin exit with scar/granulation tissue

A

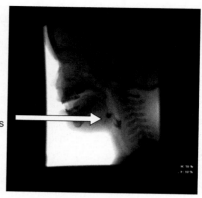

Contrast pooling in pyriform fossa and passing in to sinus

B

FIG 2 • A. MRI of type 1 branchial fistula. **B.** Sinogram of type 3 branchial sinus.

DIFFERENTIAL DIAGNOSIS

- Type 1 anomaly—parotitis, parotid tumor.
- For an infected/discharging type I branchial fistula, atypical mycobacterium is a differential to be considered.
- For neck swelling associated with type 3/4 branchial anomaly—lymphatic malformation, thyroiditis, abscess, lymph nodes.
- Branchial cysts—lymph nodes, abscess, lymphatic malformation, dermoid.

NONOPERATIVE MANAGEMENT

- Watchful approach may be opted for initially in very young children and those who are asymptomatic or have only minor symptoms.
- Treat any infections with antibiotics and avoid incision and drainage because this may lead to a persistent discharging fistula and/or make future surgical excision more challenging due to scarring.
- The majority will require surgical treatment.

SURGICAL MANAGEMENT

Preoperative Planning

- Review relevant imaging.

- Examine the patient preoperatively to check if the swelling/sinus/fistula is still present.
- Antibiotics are not routinely required for noninfected cases.
- Facial nerve monitoring should be used for type 1 branchial anomaly excisions.

Positioning

- Supine on head ring, with shoulder roll to extend neck
- Table in reverse Trendelenburg for hemostasis (head 30 degrees above feet)

Approach

- For branchial fistulas, type 2 branchial sinuses, and branchial cysts, the treatment of choice is open excision.
- Type 1 fistulas should be removed by a superficial parotidectomy approach. Type 1 branchial cleft fistulas may enter the middle ear or external auditory canal and therefore should be managed in conjunction with an otolaryngologist.
- For types 3 and 4 sinuses with a piriform sinus opening, the mainstay of treatment is now endoscopic sinus ablation via suspension laryngoscopy, usually performed by an otolaryngologist.[5] If initial endoscopic treatment fails, open resection with possible hemithyroidectomy may be required.

■ Excision of Type 1 Branchial Fistula

- The facial nerve monitor is used throughout the procedure.
- Rotate the neck away from the lesion.
- The neck is prepped with aqueous Betadine. Drape the patient, leaving the ear, angle of mandible, and operated side of face exposed. The temple and side of mouth should be left exposed so as to see the facial muscles twitch, and a clear sterile drape can be used to cover the face.
- A modified parotidectomy incision (cervico-mastoid-facial incision) is marked out, descending from the anterior to the tragus, around the earlobe, continuing down the neck toward the fistula site and finishing by making an ellipse around the fistula punctum/wound.
- The incision site is infiltrated with 1% lidocaine with 1 in 100 000 epinephrine (**TECH FIG 1A**).

- The skin is then incised with a no. 15 blade, and the ellipse of the skin around the punctum is removed.
- Subplatysmal flaps are raised inferiorly and superiorly and retracted using silk stay sutures. A further stay suture is also used retract the earlobe back (**TECH FIG 1B**).
- Dissect around the fistula punctum and any inflamed tissue to reveal a fistula tract.
- Using a fine artery clip, carefully dissect the parotid gland from the tragal cartilage and mastoid tip, exposing the tympanomastoid suture.
- Next attention should be turned to finding the facial nerve by dissecting with an artery clip and microbipolar forceps over the tragal cartilage toward the tragal pointer. The fascia over the sternocleidomastoid muscle is also freed and the posterior belly of the digastric muscle is found deep to the sternocleidomastoid muscle. When dissecting over the upper 1/3 of the sternocleidomastoid muscle, the greater auricular nerve will be encountered

and the posterior branch of this nerve may need to be sacrificed (**TECH FIG 1C,D**).

- Note that the facial nerve may be displaced inferiorly and medially by the fistula. Use the facial nerve stimulator to aid in finding the facial nerve. The nerve is usually found:
  - 5 mm deep to the tympanomastoid suture
  - 1 cm deep and inferior to the tragal pointer
  - At the level of the posterior belly of digastric muscle
- This main branch of the facial nerve is traced to the bifurcation of upper and lower branches, using a fine artery clip and microbipolar forceps (or a blade) to remove the tissue superficial to the nerve. The artery clip is advanced along the nerve with blades open when dividing parotid tissue above the nerve for good visualization of the nerve. The upper and lower branches of the nerve are traced in same manor to free them from the fistula tract as required. The fistula tract will run in close proximity to the nerve, with the possibility of branches going both lateral and medial to the fistula.
- If it is difficult to find the facial nerve trunk, retrograde dissection may be performed, initially by tracing the fistula tract from the punctum and finding the nerves overlying the tract and then tracing them back to the main trunk in a retrograde fashion.

- Once facial nerve branches are dissected from both above and below the fistula, the surgery progresses to removing the fistula tract, slowly elevating the tract from over the inferior branches of the facial nerve and carefully sliding the tract from beneath any overlying branches.
- The fistula tract is dissected from surrounding tissue using microbipolar forceps and traced to its origin, which may be into tragal cartilage, the cartilaginous part of the outer external auditory canal, the bony part of the external ear canal, middle ear, or a combination of these (**TECH FIG 1E**).
- If the fistula ends at the tragus or cartilaginous canal, it can be separated from the cartilage and the area allowed to heal by secondary intention.
- If the fistula enters the bony ear canal and middle ear, which will be evident on CT scanning and preoperative examination, the case should be performed with someone skilled in Otologic surgery. Middle ear exploration, tympanoplasty, and possible bony canalplasty may need to be performed to fully remove the tract.

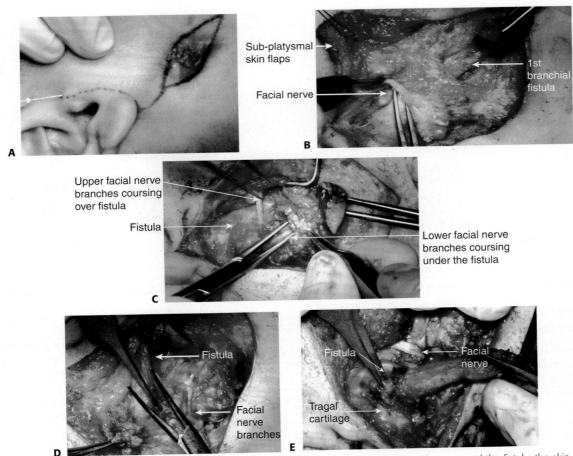

TECH FIG 1 • Excision of type 1 branchial fistula. **A.** Incision planned to excise scar/granulation tissue around the fistula; the skin in infiltrated with 1% lidocaine with 1 in 100 000 epinephrine. **B.** Subplatysmal skin flaps are raised, and then the priority is to locate the main trunk of the facial nerve and follow its branches. **C.** Facial nerve branches are seen coursing both over and under the fistula and are traced and freed from the fistula. **D.** The fistula is dissected from lower facial nerve branches on its undersurface. **E.** Once free from the facial nerve, the fistula is traced to its origin at the tragal cartilage and external ear canal/middle ear. The neck component of the fistula is excised prior to removing the middle/external ear component of the fistula.

- Once the fistula is fully removed, the wound is closed. Exposed facial nerve may be covered by loosely apposing parotid tissue with 4/0 Vicryl sutures. Platysmal muscle edges are also apposed with interrupted buried 4/0 Vicryl sutures. No drain is required.
- The skin can be closed with a continuous running sub-cuticular 5-0 Prolene suture. Both ends of the Prolene suture should be left 1 to 2 cm long outside of the skin to facilitate removal. ¼ in. 3M Steri-Strips (St. Paul, MN) are applied to the wound with the cut ends of the suture hidden beneath.
- The patient can be discharged the same day once they are eating and drinking.
- No postoperative antibiotics are required.

■ Excision of Type 2 Branchial Sinus/ Fistula (TECH FIG 2)

- The neck is prepared with aqueous Betadine.
- Drape the neck so as to square off the operative site, leaving the neck exposed from below the punctum to the mentum and lateral to the sternocleidomastoid muscle.
- Mark a small horizontal ellipse around the punctum.
- Inject 1% lidocaine with 1 in 100 000 epinephrine around the incision site.
- Use a lacrimal probe placed gently through the punctum to identify the sinus/fistula tract and confirm that it runs upward in the classic pattern toward the tonsillar fossa.
- Incise an ellipse of the skin around the punctum and dissect on to the tract using the microbipolar forceps. The lacrimal probe can be left in the tract to help follow the tract. Dissect along the tract superiorly using the microbipolar forceps. Keep close to the tract as it

may course over the hypoglossal nerve and between the internal and external carotid arteries. If access is restricted, an endoscope or further separate superior "step-ladder" incision may be used to improve visualization of the tract.
- The tract is traced through the defect in the mylohyoid muscle. An artery clip and a 3-0 Vicryl tie are applied above the level of mylohyoid; the tract is then cut and sent for histology.
- The skin can be closed with a continuous running sub-cuticular 5-0 Prolene suture. Both ends of the Prolene suture should be left 1 to 2 cm long outside of the skin to facilitate removal. ¼ in. 3M Steri-Strips (St. Paul, MN) are applied to the wound with the cut ends of the suture hidden beneath.
- The patient can be discharged the same day once they are eating and drinking.
- No postoperative antibiotics are required.

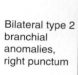
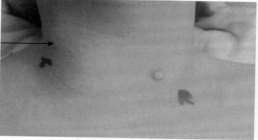

Bilateral type 2 branchial anomalies, right punctum

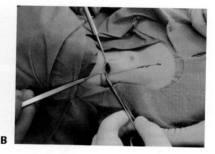

TECH FIG 2 • Excision of type 2 branchial anomaly.

■ Endoscopic Management of Type 3/4 Branchial Sinuses

- The patient is intubated.
- Suspension laryngoscopy is performed using an age-appropriate Parsons laryngoscope. The laryngoscope is positioned to visualize the pyriform fossa (**TECH FIG 3A,B**).
- If a sinus is identified then a flexible bugbee monopolar cautery needle (size 4/5 French) is placed into the sinus and used to ablate the tract (set at 4–6 watts). Two

to three passes of the cautery tip are usually required (**TECH FIG 3C,D**).
- The laryngoscope is then removed and the surgery complete.
- The patient is observed for any signs of airway compromise on the day unit and discharged once they are eating and drinking.
- If endoscopic ablation fails initially, it may be repeated. If revision endoscopic surgery fails, the patient will typically require open excision of the cyst/sinus/fistula with possible hemithyroidectomy.

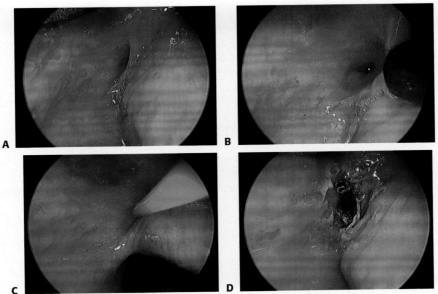

TECH FIG 3 • Endoscopic ablation of type 3 branchial anomaly. **A,B.** Endoscopic photograph of the left pyriform fossa showing start of type 3 sinus tract. **C,D.** Ablation of the tract with Bugbee cautery (4–6 watts).

■ Excision of Branchial Cyst

- Rotate the neck away from the side of the cyst.
- The neck is prepared with aqueous Betadine.
- Drape the neck so as to square off the operative site, leaving the neck exposed from below the supraclavicular notch to the angle of the mandible and lateral to the sternocleidomastoid muscle.
- Mark a horizontal incision over the swelling but at least 2 cm below the angle of the mandible. This will avoid damage to the marginal mandibular nerve as it runs superficially.
- Inject 1% lidocaine with 1 in 100 000 epinephrine around the incision site.
- Incise the skin, through platysma and raise upper and lower subplatysmal flaps. The flaps are retracted back using either a self-retaining retractor or silk sutures.
- Identify the anterior edge of the sternocleidomastoid muscle and instruct your assistant to retract this posteriorly.

- You should then identify the cyst. Dissect the cyst from the surrounding tissue using microbipolar forceps, being careful not to damage or puncture the cyst wall. The hypoglossal nerve, accessory nerve, jugular vein and carotid arteries may be in close proximity to the cyst and therefore dissecting on the cyst wall will avoid damage to these structures.
- Once all edges of the cyst are freed the cyst can be removed. Bipolar cautery should be used for hemostasis.
- The platysmal muscle edges are apposed with interrupted buried 4-0 Vicryl sutures. No drain is required.
- The skin can be closed with a continuous running subcuticular 5-0 Prolene suture. Both ends of the Prolene suture should be left 1 to 2 cm long outside of the skin to facilitate removal. ¼ in. 3M Steri-Strips (St. Paul, MN) are applied to the wound with the cut ends of the suture hidden beneath.
- The patient can be discharged the same day once they are eating and drinking.
- No postoperative antibiotics are required.

PEARLS AND PITFALLS

Diagnosis	■ Given the number of differential diagnoses for and complex surgical anatomy of branchial anomalies, a combination of imaging methods may be required to formulate a diagnosis. ■ The standard for diagnosing a type 3 or 4 branchial anomaly is direct laryngoscopy of the pyriform fossa under general anesthetic.
Incision	■ For type 1 fistulas use a modified cervico-mastoid-facial incision, excising the skin punctum and surrounding inflamed tissue in the same incision. ■ Place incisions parallel to or over skin creases where possible.
Hemostasis	■ Use of microbipolar forceps for cutting tissues allows accurate dissection with effective hemostasis. ■ Prior to skin closure, place patient in Trendelenburg position and ask anesthetist to perform a Valsalva maneuver on the patient to raise venous pressure and assist identification of any potential bleeding sites.
Dissection	■ In performing open branchial sinus/fistula or cyst excisions, stay close to and dissect on the cyst/tract to minimize damage to surrounding structures.
Closure	■ Closing the final skin layer with interrupted subcuticular 5-0 Prolene and 3M Steri-Strips (St. Paul, MN) removed at 10–14 days after surgery minimizes tissue reaction seen through use of absorbable skin sutures.

POSTOPERATIVE CARE

■ Surgery is performed as outpatient surgery with discharge on the same day.

■ Advice to keep wound dry.

■ Postoperative antibiotics are not usually required, unless there is active infection at the time of surgical excision.

■ Review with patient at 10 to 14 days with histology results and for removal of subcuticular Prolene skin suture and 3M Steri-Strips (St. Paul, MN).

■ Follow up as an outpatient 3 months postoperatively.

OUTCOMES

■ Recurrence rates:
  ■ Type 1—less than 2% although greater for middle ear involvement
  ■ Type 2—less than 2%
  ■ Type 3—The success rate for endoscopic management of pyriform fossa sinus tracts was 89.3% overall in a recent review (90.5% in primary cases and 85.7% in revision cases).[5]

COMPLICATIONS

■ General—bleeding, infection

■ Type 1—risk of injury to facial nerve (temporary/permanent) and potential complications from middle ear exploration (perforation tympanic membrane, hearing loss, temporary altered taste due to damage to chorda tympani nerve)

■ Type 2—risk of injury to hypoglossal nerve, accessory nerve, lingual nerve

■ Type 3—risk of injury to recurrent laryngeal nerve (endoscopic or open); external laryngeal nerve, parathyroid injury, hypothyroidism (open)

■ Branchial cyst—vascular injury, nerve damage; marginal mandibular, vagus, hypoglossal, accessory, greater auricular

REFERENCES

1. LaRiviere CA, Waldhausen JH. Congenital cervical cysts, sinuses, and fistulae in pediatric surgery. *Surg Clin North Am.* 2012;92(3):583-597, viii.
2. Prosser JD, Myer CM III. Branchial cleft anomalies and thymic cysts. *Otolaryngol Clin North Am.* 2015;48(1):1-14.
3. Jarvis S, Pal AR, Al-Qudehy ZA, et al. Branchial anomalies in children. *The Otorhinolaryngologist.* 2012;4:148-154.
4. Morisada N, Nozu K, Iijima K. Branchio-oto-renal syndrome: comprehensive review based on nationwide surveillance in Japan. *Pediatr Int.* 2014;56:309-314.
5. Lachance S, Chadha NK. Systematic review of endoscopic obliteration techniques for managing congenital piriform fossa sinus tracts in children. *Otolaryngol Head Neck Surg.* 2016;154:241-246.

Thyroglossal Duct Cysts

Mark Felton, Jugpal S. Arneja, and Neil K. Chadha

DEFINITION

- The most common congenital midline neck cyst[1]
- Caused by embryological remnants of thyroid gland formation

ANATOMY

- These cysts can exist anywhere from the base of tongue to the level of the thyroid gland as they form in remnants of the thyroglossal duct (**FIG 1**).
- 75% are at the level of the hyoid bone.

PATHOGENESIS

- During week 4 of embryological development, the thyroid develops between the 1st and 2nd pharyngeal pouches from floor of the pharynx at the level of the foramen cecum (posterior 1/3 tongue) (**FIG 2**).
- This becomes a bilobed diverticulum and descends through the neck to reach final position anterior to the tracheal cartilages. As it descends through the neck, it leaves a tract.
- The tract usually atrophies after 5 to 10 weeks.
- Caudal attachment of the tract may remain as the pyramidal lobe of the thyroid.
- Failure of the tract to obliterate can lead to cyst formation at any point throughout the tract length (**FIG 3**).

NATURAL HISTORY

- Thyroglossal duct cysts are present at birth but may not be clinically apparent until enlarged secondary to infection.
- They present as a midline neck swelling most commonly in childhood and adolescents.
- 90% present as midline neck swellings only, but infection and formation of a secondary discharging sinus are possible (10%).

PATIENT HISTORY AND PHYSICAL FINDINGS

- Midline neck cyst.
- May elevate on swallowing and tongue protrusion.
- With a history of infection, there may be signs of an abscess or sinus formation with discharge.

IMAGING

- Ultrasonography of the neck and thyroid to evaluate the swelling and confirm a normal thyroid is present (**FIG 4**).
- In the absence of a thyroid gland, a thyroglossal duct cyst (TGDC) may contain the only functioning thyroid tissue.
- Nuclear imaging in the form of radioactive iodine scan can be used if there is doubt regarding normal functioning thyroid.
- Thyroid function blood tests are only required if presence of normal thyroid tissue is in question.

DIFFERENTIAL DIAGNOSIS

- Midline dermoid cyst
- Sebaceous cyst
- Midline branchial cleft cyst
- Lymph node
- Ectopic thyroid tissue
- Laryngocele
- Thyroid carcinoma within TGDC

NONOPERATIVE MANAGEMENT

- Conservative watchful waiting in children until over age 12 months
- Advise there is a risk of infection with possible sinus formation if conservative approach is taken.
- Antibiotics with possible aspiration if the cyst becomes infected and forms an abscess. It is not recommended to

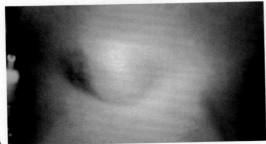
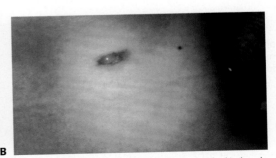

FIG 1 • Clinical photographs of anterior neck showing TGDC. **A.** Scar tissue is from previous site of infection with skin breakdown. **B.** TGDC with central discharging sinus.

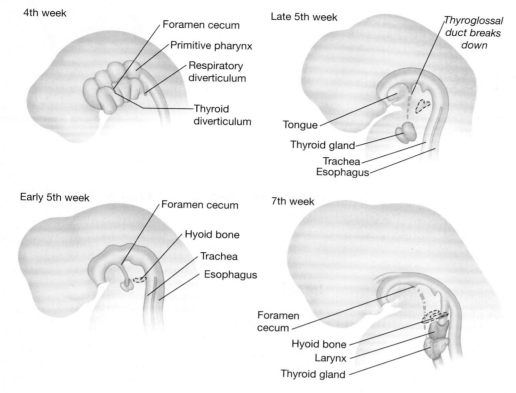

FIG 2 • Thyroid development.

incise and drain an infected TGDC because this risks sinus formation with chronic discharge.

- Uncommonly infection and inflammation may actually lead to closure of the residual duct and resolution of symptoms.
- Theoretical risk of malignant change of thyroid tissue within TGDC if left indefinitely, with less than 1% of excised TGDCs having a primary carcinoma on histology.[2]

SURGICAL MANAGEMENT
Preoperative Planning
- Review ultrasound scan result to confirm that normal thyroid tissue is present in the usual location.

- Examine preoperatively to check that swelling is still present.
- Assess ideal level for placement of a transverse incision that will provide exposure from the level of the suprahyoid muscles to the superior border of the thyroid gland for removal of the TGDC (typically approximately midway between the palpable landmarks of the hyoid and upper thyroid notch).

Positioning
- Supine on head ring, with shoulder roll for neck extension
- Table in reverse Trendelenburg for hemostasis (head 30 degrees above feet)

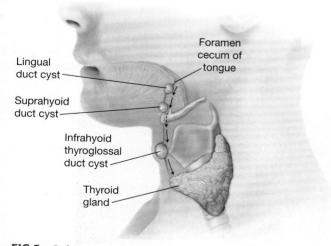

FIG 3 • Pathogenesis of TGDC development.

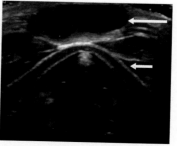

FIG 4 • Ultrasound scan of TGDC (*long arrow*) overlying thyroid cartilage (*short arrow*).

■ Modified Sistrunk Procedure

Preparation of the Neck and Wound Incision

- Antibiotics are not indicated for routine noninfected cases.
- The neck is prepared with aqueous Betadine.
- Drape the neck so as to square off the operative site, leaving the neck exposed from the mentum to below the sternoclavicular notch and the sternocleidomastoid muscles laterally.
- Mark the site of horizontal incision over the cyst, ideally midpoint between the hyoid and thyroid notch so as to allow adequate access to both the suprahyoid muscles and the pyramidal lobe of the thyroid. Initially, plan to incise skin to incorporate the width of the cyst only in case it is identified to be a dermoid cyst, in which case following a tract superiorly and inferiorly is not required and cystectomy is adequate (**TECH FIG 1A,B**)
- Inject 1% lidocaine with 1 in 100 000 epinephrine around the incision site.
- An incision is made through the skin and subcutaneous tissue. Subplatysmal flaps are elevated both superiorly to above the level of the hyoid and inferiorly to below the level of the cricoid cartilage (**TECH FIG 1C**). Take care with this step as the cyst can be superficial, making it easy to puncture, which is more likely if the cyst is large and under pressure. If a cyst is punctured, the dissection can continue with a clip on the cyst capsule at the puncture site.

Exposure of Thyroglossal Cyst and Tract

- Once the cyst is exposed, if clinically it is a dermoid and there is no obvious tract or surrounding attachments, the cyst can be removed and skin closed. Otherwise, the cyst can be left alone and dissection of the tract performed next, with widening the skin incision for better access if required (**TECH FIG 2A**).
- Identify the infrahyoid strap muscles, usually below the cyst. Identify the midline and carefully separate the right and left strap muscles, the more superficial muscle being sternohyoid and deeper muscle being sternothyroid (**TECH FIG 2B,C**).

- Carefully dissect along the medial edge of the sternohyoid and sternothyroid muscles if necessary, separating them from the cyst. Carefully expose the medial border of the length of the infrahyoid strap muscles from their hyoid attachment superiorly as far inferiorly as the superior border of the thyroid gland. Any tissue between the infrahyoid strap muscles will be removed in continuity with the cyst and will contain the inferior tract if present.
- Look for an inferior component of the thyroglossal duct extending inferiorly from the cyst, which extends to the pyramidal lobe of the thyroid gland. If the duct extends down to the thyroid gland, remove a small cuff of pyramidal lobe with the specimen. Even if the tract is not clearly visible, it will be safely removed by removing all the tissue between the strap muscles from the cyst down to the pyramidal thyroid lobe inferiorly.

Hyoid and Tongue Base Dissection, With Specimen Excision

- After completion of this inferior dissection, ensure that the medial borders of the infrahyoid strap muscles are identified and exposed up to their attachments to the hyoid bone. The infrahyoid strap muscles are often adherent to the cyst just inferior to the hyoid bone. When there has been previous infection, a small portion of infrahyoid strap muscle may need to be left attached to the cyst and removed with the cyst and specimen. A tract arising from the superior aspect of the cyst may be seen passing into the hyoid bone, although the whole cyst may be adherent to the hyoid mid-portion.
- The superior muscular attachments of the hyoid bone (predominantly the mylohyoid and geniohyoid) are then detached from the midportion of the hyoid bone superiorly, using the medial borders of the infrahyoid strap muscle attachments as a guide to how far to laterally dissect superiorly, thereby avoiding the hyoid lesser horns and the hypoglossal nerve.
- The central portion third of the hyoid bone is resected by cutting through the hyoid. It is imperative that this cut is precisely vertical and level with the medial borders of the infrahyoid strap muscles, lateral to the cyst or cyst tract if identified. An Allis forceps holding the central

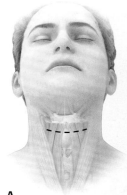
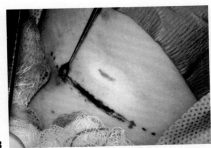
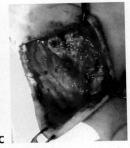

A   **B**   **C**

TECH FIG 1 • A. Position of TGDC, relations of the duct and position for surgical incision (midline collar incision), with the duct running through the hyoid bone and ending at pyramidal lobe of thyroid. **B.** Midline collar skin crease incision. **C.** Subplatysmal skin flaps are raised.

TECHNIQUES

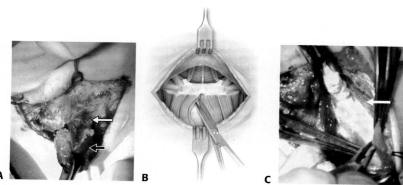

TECH FIG 2 • A. Midline dissection on the TGDC (*black arrow*) and tract (*white arrow*). **B.** Dissecting out the TGDC. **C.** The strap muscles are separated in the midline. *Arrow* indicates sternohyoid muscle.

portion of the hyoid bone can help stabilize the bone. In small children, bipolar forceps are often sufficient to cut through the noncalcified hyoid, but in older children/adolescents/adults, straight Mayo scissors or even bone cutting forceps may be required cut through the hyoid bone. Cautery and bone wax can be used to stop any bleeding from the cut edges of the hyoid (**TECH FIG 3A,B**).

- Now the inferior tract, cyst, and hyoid bone are free of the surrounding tissue; a superior tract arising from the superior

and posterior aspect of the hyoid may be seen running into the tongue base. If present, the tract should be dissected from the surrounding tissue and followed up to the tongue base. A cuff of tongue muscle (genioglossus muscle) should always be taken with the midportion of the hyoid and the specimen to complete the excision and minimize risk of a residual superior tract. There is no need to excise tongue muscle in complete thickness through to the oropharynx, as originally described by Sistrunk (**TECH FIG 3C,D**).

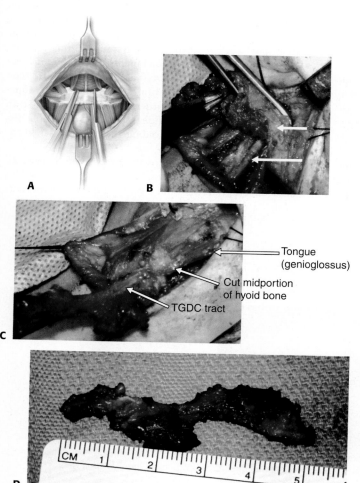

Tongue
(genioglossus)

Cut midportion
of hyoid bone

TGDC tract

TECH FIG 3 • A. Division of mid third of hyoid bone. **B.** The tract is traced to the hyoid and the hyoid (*short arrow*) is cut either side of tract in line with the medial edge of the thyrohyoid muscles (*long arrow*). **C.** A cuff of tongue muscle is taken with the specimen. **D.** Specimen.

TECHNIQUES

- Attention should then be focused on ensuring meticulous hemostasis. The patient should be placed in the Trendelenburg position (30 degrees head down) and saline wash poured in to the wound. A prolonged Valsalva maneuver by the anesthetist will reveal any further bleeding points for cauterization.

Wound Closure

- The operating table is then placed in a neutral position for wound closure.
- The strap muscles are apposed with 4-0 Vicryl and the skin flaps closed with interrupted buried 4-0 Vicryl sutures. No drain is required (**TECH FIG 4A,B**).
- The skin can be closed with a continuous running subcuticular 5-0 Prolene suture. Both ends of the Prolene suture should be left 1 to 2 cm long outside of the skin to facilitate removal. ¼ in. Steri-Strips are applied to the

wound with the cut ends of the suture hidden beneath (**TECH FIG 4C**).

- The patient can be discharged the same day once they are eating and drinking.
- No postoperative antibiotics are required.

Modifications of the Procedure

- Skin sinus tract—A skin ellipse around the sinus and ellipse of tissue around the sinus tract is taken, which should be taken in continuation with the rest of the dissection of the thyroglossal cyst. This may lead to the horizontal incision site being more superior than ideal, and the incision therefore is lengthened to facilitate the inferior access.
- Recurrent cysts—En-bloc wide local of excision around the recurrent cyst, taking a core of strap muscle on either side down to pretracheal fascia.

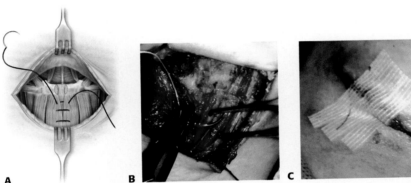

TECH FIG 4 • A. Suturing of infrahyoid muscles. **B.** Strap muscles reapposed with 4-0 Vicryl sutures. **C.** Skin is closed with 5-0 Prolene and Steri-Strips.

PEARLS AND PITFALLS

Incision	▪ Initially only make your incision the width of the swelling until the diagnosis is confirmed in case it is a dermoid cyst, for which a smaller incision will suffice. Once a dermoid cyst is excluded, the incision can be widened.
Hemostasis	▪ Use of microbipolar forceps for cutting tissues allows accurate dissection with effective hemostasis. ▪ Prior to skin closure, place patient in Trendelenburg position and ask anesthetist to perform a Valsalva on the patient to raise vascular pressure and assist identification of any potential bleeding sites. Bone wax can help oozing from edges of cut hyoid bone.
Dissection	▪ Actively look for any extension of the cyst/duct toward the pyramidal lobe and remove a cuff of the pyramidal lobe if the duct is in continuation. ▪ Dissect along the medial aspect of strap muscles on to the hyoid bone. Remove the hyoid at the level of the medial aspects of the strap muscles to avoid damage to the hypoglossal nerve. ▪ Look for a tract extending from the hyoid to the tongue base, dissect along this, and remove a cuff of tongue base with the specimen.
Closure	▪ Closing final skin layer with interrupted subcuticular 5-0 Prolene and Steri-Strips removed at 10–14 days after surgery minimizes tissue reaction seen through use of absorbable skin sutures

POSTOPERATIVE CARE

- Day case surgery
- Advice to keep wound dry
- Review 10 to 14 days with histology and for removal of Prolene skin suture and Steri-Strips
- Follow up outpatients 3 months

OUTCOMES

- Recurrence rate of 0% to 3% for modified Sistrunk as described above may be much higher with other techniques such as cystectomy only.[1,3]

COMPLICATIONS

- Bleeding, infection, hypertrophic/keloid scar
- Accidental pharyngostomy
- Hypoglossal nerve injury
- Recurrence—treat with en-bloc wide local excision

REFERENCES

1. Oomen KP, Modi VK, Maddalozzo J. Thyroglossal duct cyst and ectopic thyroid: surgical management. *Otolaryngol Clin North Am.* 2015;48(1):15-27.
2. Heshmati HM, Fatourechi V, van Heerden JA, et al. Thyroglossal duct carcinoma: report of 12 cases. *Mayo Clin Proc.* 1997;72(4):315-319.
3. Ibrahim FF, Alnoury MK, Varma N, Daniel SJ. Surgical management outcomes of recurrent thyroglossal duct cyst in children—a systematic review. *Int J Pediatr Otorhinolaryngol.* 2015;79(6):863-867.

Sural Nerve Harvest

Andre P. Marshall, Jeffrey R. Marcus, and Michael R. Zenn

DEFINITION

- The sural nerve is a lower limb sensory nerve that provides sensation to the lateral and posterior distal third of the leg, lateral calcaneal region, lateral foot, and small toe.[1]
- The sural nerve is easily accessible, has several large fascicles, and is the donor nerve most commonly used in peripheral nerve reconstructive surgery.[2,3]
- Unilateral sural nerve harvests can provide up to 40 cm of autogenous nerve graft.

ANATOMY

- The sural nerve is a sensory nerve that begins in the lateral aspect of the foot and coalesces from branches between the Achilles tendon and lateral malleolus.
- The nerve splits into the medial and lateral cutaneous nerves of the leg along the posterior leg.
- The larger contributor, the medial sural cutaneous nerve, arises from the tibial nerve in the popliteal fossa between the medial and lateral heads of the gastrocnemius.[4]
- The sural nerve runs deep to the investing fascia down the posterior calf between the two heads of the gastrocnemius muscle and then subcutaneously in the distal third of the leg.
- It can be found close to, but deep to, the lesser saphenous vein to the ankle.
- It is consistently found in the space between the lateral malleolus and the calcaneus tendon.[2-5]

PATIENT HISTORY AND PHYSICAL FINDINGS

- Any history of prior lower extremity operation, either open or endoscopic, should be elicited from the patient.

- Physical exam should note any scars or prior incisions on the lower extremities, or numbness or paresthesias in the distribution of the sural nerve.

IMAGING

- Prior to sural nerve harvesting, no imaging of the lower extremities is necessary.

SURGICAL MANAGEMENT

Preoperative Planning

- Preoperatively, a comprehensive history and physical exam should be performed. It is imperative to note any prior lower extremity trauma, fractures, or previous operations.
- Patients should be counseled on the expected postoperative outcomes of cutaneous sensory loss in the sural nerve distribution.

Positioning

- The donor limb is placed in flexion at the knee.
- A bump, sandbag, or roll under the ipsilateral buttocks provides additional access to the posterior leg.
- In children, prone positioning is usually preferred and well tolerated.

Approach

- Open
- Endoscopically assisted

■ Stair-Step Incisions

- The patient is placed in supine or prone position (**TECH FIG 1A**).
- An endoscope can be used to facilitate dissection.[6]
- A pneumatic tourniquet (optional) is placed around the thigh and the leg exsanguinated in the usual fashion prior to incision.
- A 2- to 3-cm transverse or vertical incision is made in the groove made by the lateral border of the Achilles tendon at the level of the lateral malleolus.
- The lesser saphenous vein is seen, retracted, and preserved.
- Blunt dissection is used to identify the nerve.
- The nerve is dissected of all surrounding tissue moving superior along the posterior calf.

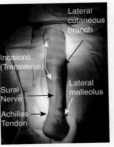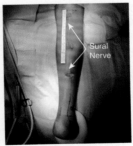

TECH FIG 1 • A. Preoperative markings and an outline of the sural nerve and its lateral cutaneous branch are shown. The proposed transverse incisions are shown in addition to the Achilles tendon and lateral malleolus. **B.** The sural nerve is shown following harvest along the transverse incisions.

T E C H N I Q U E S

- At approximately 10 cm, an additional 2- to 3-cm transverse incision is made more proximally along the course of the nerve.
- Proximal and distal dissection of the nerve is made through each incision.
- Up to two additional transverse incisions are made along the course of the nerve until adequate length is obtained.

- The nerve is transected at the popliteal fossa and removed from the leg (**TECH FIG 1B**).
- Incisions are closed in standard fashion, in a minimum of two layers with absorbable sutures.
- No drain tubes are necessary.

■ Harvest With a Tendon Stripper[4,7]

- A pneumatic tourniquet is placed around the thigh and the leg exsanguinated in the usual fashion.
- A 2- to 3-cm transverse or vertical incisions is made in the groove made by the lateral border of the Achilles tendon at the level of the lateral malleolus.
- The lesser saphenous vein is seen, retracted, and preserved.
- Blunt dissection is used to identify the nerve, and then transecting it up to 5 cm distal to the incision to gain additional length.

- The cut end of the nerve is passed through a tendon stripper.
- Mild traction is placed on the nerve, and the tendon stripper is passed proximally until its tip can be felt in the subcutaneous tissues near the popliteal fossa.
- The stripper is twisted and counter-pressed until the nerve is felt to give way and able to slide out of the ankle wound.
  - Optionally, the leading edge of the tendon stripper is tented against the skin, a stab incision is made, across the end of the stripper to divide the nerve.

PEARLS AND PITFALLS

Anatomy	■ The sural nerve has many variations during its course. ■ The surgeon must be aware of the variable sural anatomy, particularly the branches of the medial and lateral cutaneous nerves.
Positioning	■ Sural nerve harvest can be done in either supine or prone position. In children, prone positioning is well tolerated and can better facilitate exposure and shorten harvest time.
Dissection	■ Avoid excessive circumferential dissection, which may place the nerve at greater risk of injury. ■ Superficial dissection is usually adequate to facilitate release from the overlying subcutaneous tissues.
Graft processing	■ In most cases, the graft is used intact. ■ Splitting of the graft into multiple grafts and preserving fascicles longitudinally has been described but is not practiced in our unit.

POSTOPERATIVE CARE

- Elastic bandages from the foot to the knee are placed and used to provide compression and help decrease hematoma formation. They are left in place for 48 hours and used thereafter for control of swelling as needed.
- Patients are encouraged to begin ambulation on postoperative day 1 to help reduce the risk of deep venous thrombosis. Full activity restrictions are kept in place for 2 weeks or dictated by the concurrent grafting procedure at the recipient site.
- Pain is minimal and managed with a combination of narcotic and non-narcotic analgesic medications.

OUTCOMES

- Scars should be expected at the donor site and are permanent. Regular scar management is recommended.
- The area of paresthesia and numbness in the ankle and foot is likely permanent but may decrease in size over time due to contributions from surrounding intact nerves.[1]

COMPLICATIONS

- Postoperative complications are infrequent but include proximal neuroma formation, hematoma, and deep venous thrombosis. We have not seen cellulitis in our patient cohort, but it is possible.
- The iatrogenic sensory nerve deficit along the lateral foot should be expected and is not considered a complication. It is generally well tolerated by patients and should be discussed preoperatively.

REFERENCES

1. Lapid O, Ho ES, Clarke HM. Evaluation of the sensory deficit after sural nerve harvesting in pediatric patients. *Plast Reconstr Surg.* 2007;119:670.
2. Riedl O, Koemuercue F. Sural nerve harvesting beyond the popliteal region allows a significant gain of donor nerve graft length. *Plast Reconstr Surg.* 2008;122:798.
3. Garcia R, Hadlock H. Contemporary solutions for the treatment of facial nerve paralysis. *Plast Reconstr Surg.* 2015;135:1025e.
4. Hill HL, Vasconez LO, Jurkiwicz MJ. Method for obtaining a sural nerve graft. *Plast Reconstr Surg.* 1978;61:2.
5. Dellon AL, Coert JH. Clinical implications of the surgical anatomy of the sural nerve. *Plast Reconstr Surg.* 1994;94:850.
6. Capek L, Clarke HM. Endoscopically assisted sural nerve harvest in infants. *Semin Plast Surg.* 2008;22:25-28.
7. Hankin FM, Jaeger SH, Beddings A. Autogenous sural nerve grafts: a harvesting technique. *Orthopedics.* 1985;8:9.

Cross Face Nerve Graft

Michael J. A. Klebuc

DEFINITION

- Cross face nerve graft—interposition nerve graft utilized to transmit facial nerve motor axons from a neurologically intact to a paralyzed/paretic, contralateral hemiface.
- Utilized to restore motor innervation to denervated muscles of facial expression and to neurotized free, functional muscle flaps, also can be employed for sensory restoration.
- Frequently utilized sources of nerve graft (sural nerve, saphenous nerve, medial antebrachial cutaneous nerve).
- Approximately 50% of a facial nerve's zygomatic and buccal branches can be selectively transected and their function redirected to the paralyzed hemiface without producing significant donor weakness (functional reserve).
- The facial nerve is the only donor nerve that can consistently restore spontaneous, emotionally mediated facial motion.

ANATOMY

- Facial nerve (somatic motor efferent component)—innervates the muscles of facial expression, auricular muscles, occipitalis, posterior belly digastric, stylohyoid, and stapedius.
- The facial nerve main trunk emerges from the skull base via the stylomastoid foramen where it can be identified coursing 1 cm deep to the tragal pointer and medial to the posterior belly of the digastric muscle.[1]
- Within the parotid gland, the facial nerve divides into a temporofacial and cervicofacial trunk.
- Distal branches exit the parotid on its anteromedial surface.
- The following branches innervate the corresponding muscles of facial expression[2]:
  - Frontal branch—frontalis muscle
  - Zygomatic branches—orbicularis oculi, zygomaticus major, zygomaticus minor, levator labii superioris, levator labii superioris alaeque nasi, corrugator supercilii, procerus
  - Buccal branches—buccinator, risorius, orbicularis oris
  - Marginal mandibular branches—depressor anguli oris, depressor labii inferioris, mentalis
  - Cervical branches—platysma
- Muscles of facial expression are innervated on their deep surface with the exception of the levator anguli oris, buccinator, and mentalis.
- Zuker point describes the approximate location of the facial nerve branch supplying the zygomaticus major (**FIG 1**):
  - Midway point of a line drawn from the root of the helix to the lateral commissure.
  - Preferentially divided and coapted to a cross facial nerve graft (CFNG) as the first step in a two-staged free, functional muscle flap reconstruction.[3]

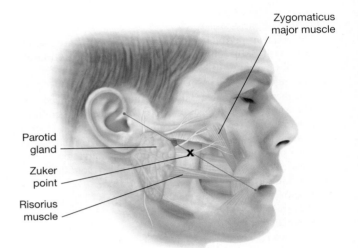

FIG 1 • The facial nerve branch supplying the zygomatic major is typically found at a point halfway between the root of the helix and the commissure (Zuker point).

- Pitanguy line describes the course of the frontal branch of the facial nerve. The line extending 0.5 cm below the tragus to 1.5 above the lateral brow with the nerve running on the undersurface of the temporoparietal fascia.[4]
- The marginal mandibular branches—consistently lie on top of the facial artery and vein 1 to 3 cm below the mandibular border.[5]

NATURAL HISTORY

- Axonal growth through the cross face graft proceeds at approximately 1 mm/d.
- Ten to twelve months is typically required for the axons to traverse the graft.
- After 18 months of denervation, mimetic muscles undergo significant atrophy and poor functional outcomes are associated with nerve grafting.
- A narrow time window is present for the use of cross face nerve grafts as an isolated procedure to restore innervation to the paralyzed muscles of facial expression.
- The therapeutic window of CFNG is enhanced by the addition of a nerve "babysitter."[6]
  - Transfer of an adjacent cranial nerve to the injured facial nerve to achieve rapid reinnervation and motor end plate preservation.

- Partial hypoglossal-to-facial nerve transfer with an inter-position jump graft and secondary selective facial nerve branch transection and distal end-to-end repair to CFNG.
- Masseter-to-facial nerve transfer with immediate CFNG and distal end-to-end and/or end-to-side coaptation.[7]

PATIENT HISTORY AND PHYSICAL FINDINGS

- Etiology of the facial paralysis:
  - Developmental
  - Traumatic
  - Post-tumor extirpation
  - Bell palsy
  - Ramsay Hunt syndrome
- Duration of paralysis:
  - Denervation periods greater than 18 months are associated with poor functional recovery (irreversible muscle atrophy) without utilization of a muscle flap.
- Patient age:
  - Peripheral nerve regeneration declines with advanced age.
  - There is no definitive age cut off for cross face nerve grafting; however, after the age of 50 to 55 years, the ipsilateral motor nerve branch to masseter or other adjacent cranial nerves often provide a more reliable source of innervation to free muscle flaps with more powerful muscle flap contraction.
- Comorbidities impairing nerve regeneration:
  - Smoking—higher risk of skin flap necrosis
  - Diabetes
  - Vascular disease
  - Previous radiation
  - Neurologic disorders
- History of hypercoagulable state:
  - Patient or family history of pulmonary emboli or deep venous thrombosis signal the need for a hematologic workup if a subsequent free, functional muscle flap is planned.
- Physical Examination
  - A strong smile, normal blink, forceful eye closure, good lip pucker, and depression without synkinesis should be present on the donor hemiface.
  - Perform a complete cranial nerve exam to look for additional deficits.
  - Examine the eye on the paralyzed side for signs of exposure keratitis.
  - Look for previous incisions that could compromise perfusion to the cheek flaps elevated during facial nerve exploration.
  - Palpate and Doppler the superficial temporal and facial artery and veins on the paralyzed hemiface if a subsequent free, functional muscle flap is planned.
  - Palpate lower extremity pulses if sural or saphenous nerve grafts are to be harvested to rule out peripheral vascular disease.
  - The progressive growth of axons through the CFNG can be monitored by eliciting a Tinel sign.
  - An active Tinel sign at the distal end of the cross face nerve graft suggests signals readiness for the next phase of the reconstruction.

IMAGING

- MRI of brain and facial nerve
  - High-resolution multiplanar T1 and T2 images, gadolinium-enhanced, fat-suppressed, and internal auditory canal (IAC) protocol
  - Used to evaluate injury to the facial nerve (ie, Bell palsy, tumors, stroke)

- Computed tomography
  - 0.625-mm or thinner axial images, reconstructions in coronal plane
  - Valuable for imaging temporal bone fractures
- CT angiogram
  - Useful for evaluating possible sites for microvascular anastomosis in patients with multiple head-neck surgeries or developmental differences including hemifacial microsomia.
- EMG of the facial nerve
  - Look for signs of early facial nerve recovery.
  - Look for signs of reversible muscle atrophy.

SURGICAL MANAGEMENT

Preoperative Planning

- Facial nerve EMG is obtained to evaluate for irreversible mimetic muscle atrophy.
- Facial nerve imaging as guided by the etiology of the paralysis (MRI, CT, CT angiogram).
- Determine the number of cross face nerve grafts to be utilized and evaluate the potential nerve graft donor sites.
- Discontinue smoking and nicotine products.
- Discontinue anticoagulants.

Positioning

- Supine on the operating table with narrow head extension.
- Head on foam or gel-filled headrest.
- Nasotracheal intubation with endotracheal tube sutured to nasal columella and supported on the hair-bearing scalp with foam, silk tape and staples (**FIG 2**) or an Oral RAE tube secured to the lower dentition with a 2-0 silk Ivy loop suture.
- Oral cavity cleansed with chlorhexidine gluconate mouth wash.
- Sterile tourniquet applied to the thighs.
- Sterile calf sequential compression devices.

Approach

- Preauricular approach is most frequently employed.
  - Aesthetically favorable access incision especially in children and young adults
  - Permits dissection of all facial nerve braches facilitating nerve stimulation, creating of a functional map and optimal donor nerve selection
  - Allows retrograde dissection of selected facial nerve branches into the parotid gland to enhance axonal concentration
- The nasolabial fold approach is infrequently used.
  - Unaesthetic scarring in children and young adults.
  - Limited ability to select the optimal donor nerve branch.
  - Access to only distal nerve branches with more limited axon counts.

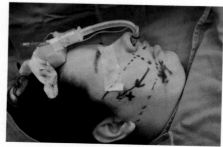

FIG 2 • Nasotracheal intubation with head positioned on a narrow head-rest. Endotracheal tube sutured to columella and supported with foam to prevent pressure on the nasal alae.

▪ Exposure and Flap Elevation

- The anterior border of the masseter muscle is palpated and marked.
- A pretragal, incision with an extension into the sideburn is now marked with a surgical pen.
- An additional point is marked half way between the root of the helix and the commissure to indicate the general location of the facial nerve branch to the zygomaticus major muscle (Zuker point) (**TECH FIG 1**).[3]
- A petrolatum gauze dressing is used to occlude the external auditory canal.
- The subcutaneous tissues in the preauricular, zygomatic, and buccal regions are infiltrated with a 1:100 000 epinephrine, hemostatic solution (local anesthetics should be avoided).

- The preauricular incision with the sideburn extension is made and a skin and subcutaneous tissue flap is elevated in the preauricular, zygomatic, and buccal regions caring the medial aspect of the dissection approximated 3 cm past the medial border of the masseter muscle.
- An SMAS flap is now elevated with scissor dissection and bipolar cautery.
  - The flap is mobilized to the anteromedial border of the parotid gland where the zygomatic and buccal branches of the facial nerve are identified.
  - The SMAS flap is released transversely along the inferior zygomatic border and reflected to facilitate exposure (**TECH FIG 2**).

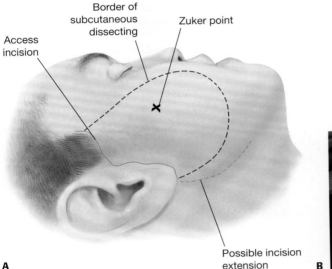
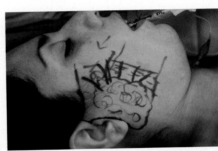

TECH FIG 1 • Operative markings. **A.** Preauricular incision with a possible submandibular extension (*X*) marks Zuker point and the *dashed lines* represent the region of skin flap elevation. **B.** Markings shown on the patient in the sample case.

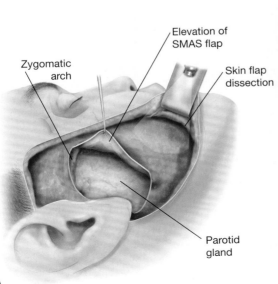
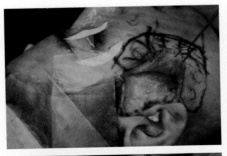
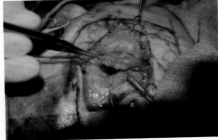

TECH FIG 2 • **A,B.** Extent of the skin-subcutaneous flap elevation and initial SMAS flap dissection. **C.** SMAS flap elevation.

■ Nerve Mobilization and Graft Harvest

- The operating microscope is brought onto the field to enhance visualization and microsurgical dissection is used to further explore and mobilized the facial nerve branches.
- During the dissection, the transverse facial artery is often encountered. This is a useful landmark as the zygomatic branches above and below this structure often produce an excellent smile with little activation of the orbicularis oculi.
- The facial nerve branches are encircled with thin segments of microvascular background to facilitate later identification.
- Electrical stimulation is now performed. The facial nerve branches are stimulated at 0.5 to 1 mA at 40 Hz and a functional map of their activity is created.
- The largest and most powerful zygomatic branch that produces activation of the zygomatic major and levator anguli oris muscles without associated eye closure is identified.
  - It is traced in a retrograde fashion into the parotid gland to maximizing its caliber (**TECH FIG 3**).
  - Selective nerve branch transection at this site will be performed later in the case for smile restoration.

- If the surgical goals include restoration of eye closure, pucker and lip depression, then approximately 50% of the facial nerve branches to the orbicularis oculi, orbicularis oris, and depressor anguli oris and depressor labii inferioris are selected for eventual transection.[8]
- A submandibular extension of the initial access incision may be required to reach the marginal mandibular branches.
- Gowns and gloves are changed and new instruments are used to harvest the nerve grafts under tourniquet control.
- The sural nerve is approached via a limited access incision approximately 2 cm posterior to the lateral malleolus (**TECH FIG 4**).
- The sural nerve is separated for the lesser saphenous vein, ligated with 4-0 silk ties, and divided. A nerve stripping device (Aesculap TEK784, Aesculap Inc., Center Valley, PA) is used with a gentle back and forth twisting motion to mobilize the nerve from distal to proximal. If significant resistance is encountered, an additional counter incision is made and the tethering side branch released. Grafts measuring 25 to 30 cm are reliable harvested.

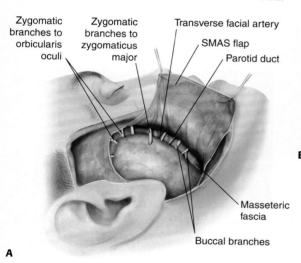

Zygomatic branches to orbicularis oculi

Zygomatic branches to zygomaticus major

Transverse facial artery

SMAS flap

Parotid duct

Masseteric fascia

Buccal branches

A

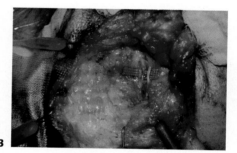

B

TECH FIG 3 • A. The facial nerve branches bordering the transverse facial artery are frequently selected for transfer as they often produce an isolated smile with little or no activation of the orbicularis oculi or orbicularis oris. **B.** Isolation of zygomatic facial nerve branches.

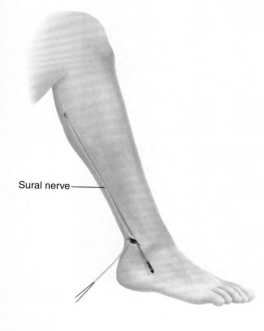

Sural nerve

TECH FIG 4 • Sural nerve harvested via a limited access incision utilizing a nerve-stripping device.

■ Graft Passage and Completion

- If more than one nerve graft is to be passed through an adjacent tunnel, they are marked in increments with different colored sutures to facilitate identification.
- An alligator, tendon passing clamp is inserted through limited incision in the contralateral hairline and preauricular region. The clamp is now tunneled through either the subcutaneous or deep supraperiosteal plane, traversing the upper lip, lower lip, and submental region as determined by the number of cross face nerve grafts (**TECH FIG 5**).
- Small access incisions may be required in the upper and lower lip to successfully create the tunnels.
- These incisions can be used to identify branches of the infraorbital and mental nerves that can be selectively transected and eventually coapted to the cross face nerve graft (end-to-side) if desired in an effort to enhance axonal growth.[9]
- The nerve grafts are reversed and the proximal nerve end is ligated with a colored 4-0 nonabsorbable, monofilament suture (facilitates delayed identification).

- The tendon passing clamps are used to gently draw the graft across the face.
- The donor facial nerve branches are selectively divided, and an end-to-end nerve repair is made between the facial nerve branch and corresponding nerve graft with 10-0 nylon suture in an interrupted, epineurial fashion (**TECH FIG 6**).
- The SMAS flap is returned to its native position and secured with 4-0 absorbable suture.
- The subcutaneous pocket is treated with spray thrombin or fibrin glue, and the incision is repaired over a closed suction drain.
- The nerve graft donor site access incisions in the extremities are closed in layers with absorbable, monofilament suture and covered with cyanoacrylate tissue adhesive. The incisions are covered with ABD pads and elastic bandages are utilized to support the feet and calves.
- Antibiotic ointment is applied to the head and neck incisions and no dressings are applied.
- A deep, atraumatic, extubation is then coordinated with the anesthesiologist.
- Foot sequential compression devices are applied for deep venous thrombosis prophylaxis.

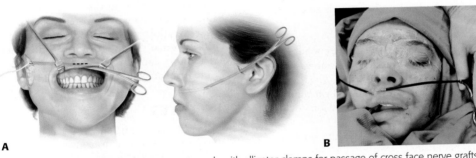

TECH FIG 5 • Creating of subcutaneous tunnels with alligator clamps for passage of cross face nerve grafts.

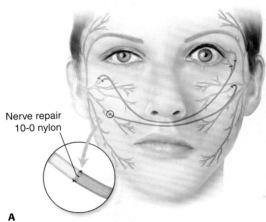

Nerve repair
10-0 nylon

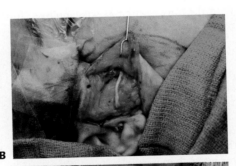

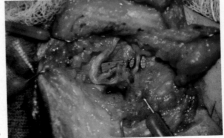

TECH FIG 6 • **A.** Cross face nerve grafts for restoration of eye closure and smile with proximal and distal end-to-end nerve repairs. **B.** Cross face nerve graft in situ. **C.** End-to-end nerve repair between sural cross face nerve graft and a zygomatic branch of the facial nerve.

PEARLS AND PITFALLS

Facial nerve branch selection	■ For smile restoration, select the largest facial nerve branch that produces isolated activation of the zygomaticus major without associated eye closure. ■ Trace the nerve branch into the parotid gland to increase the axon density.
Nerve graft injury	■ If significant resistance is met when harvesting the graft with a nerve-stripping device, an additional incision should be created. ■ The obstructing side branch is then transected to prevent accidental nerve graft avulsion. ■ Failure to do this may result in a graft of inadequate length with disruption of the internal architecture.
Hemostatic solutions	■ Avoid local anesthetics that contain epinephrine as they will impair nerve conduction and the ability to create a functional map. ■ A solution of 1:100 000 epinephrine will achieve good vasoconstriction without impairing nerve conduction.
Avoid aesthetic complications	■ Short-acting muscle relaxants are only permitted on induction, if essential. ■ The need to avoid muscle paralysis must be communicated during changes of anesthesia providers. ■ Deep, atraumatic, extubation without compressive, face mask ventilation.

POSTOPERATIVE CARE

- Patient is maintained a clear liquid diet for 48 hours followed by a soft diet for 4 weeks.
- The oral cavity is rinsed with chlorhexidine gluconate mouth wash twice a day for 7 days, after which an electric tooth brush is utilized for oral hygiene.
- Pressure on the cheeks is strictly avoided.
- Incentive spirometry is avoided and patients are encouraged to deep breathe. A pinwheel can be used to encourage pediatric patients to breathe deeply.
- Ambulation with assistance is usually initiated on the first postoperative day and pedal sequential compression devices are utilized while in bed.
- Anticoagulation is generally avoided due to the potential increased risk of facial hematoma.
- No strenuous exercise or heavy lifting for 6 to 8 weeks following surgery.
- Elastic bandaging of the lower extremities is employed for 2 to 3 weeks to reduce edema and improve patient comfort.

OUTCOMES

- The ability of cross face nerve grafts to successfully innervate free, functional, muscle flaps for smile restoration has been demonstrated in multiple publications over the past two decades.[7]
- Although the reconstructed smile is spontaneous, it is frequently weaker than that achieved with a muscle flap innervated by the motor nerve to masseter.[10]
- The ability of CFNGs to deliver an adequate axonal load decreases with age, and alternate strategies are often employed for individuals in the sixth and seventh decades of life.
- Cross face nerve grafting as an isolated technique rarely produces adequate strength to achieve symmetric facial motion.
- Cross face nerve grafts can be used with a distal end-to-side coaptation to enhance the power of paretic muscles of facial expression.[11]

COMPLICATIONS

- Potential weakening of the unaffected hemiface following selective transection of facial nerve branches.
- Hematoma formation requiring evacuation and potential disruption of the nerve grafts.
- Cheek skin flap necrosis (patients should be counseled on smoking cessation and avoiding nicotine).
- Neuroma formation at the nerve graft donor site.
- Failure of adequate nerve regeneration.
- Sialocele, salivary fistula, and parotitis.
- Otitis external resulting from blood collecting in the external auditory canal.
- Compartment syndrome after sural nerve graft harvest.

REFERENCES

1. Sharma R, Sirohi DJ. Proximal and distal facial nerve exploration during superficial parotidectomy. *J Maxillofac Oral Surg.* 2010;9(2):150-154.
2. Tzafetta K, Terzis J. Essays on the facial nerve: part I. microanatomy. *Plast Reconstr Surg.* 2010;125(3):879-889.
3. Dorafshar AH, Borsuk DE, Bojovic B, et al. Surface anatomy of the middle division of the facial nerve: Zuker's point. *Plast Reconstr Surg.* 2013;131(2):253-257.
4. Pitanguy I, Ramos AS. The frontal branch of the facial nerve: the importance of its variations in face lifting. *Plast Reconstr Surg.* 1966;38:352-356.
5. Dingman RO, Grabb WC. Surgical anatomy of the mandibular ramus of the facial nerve based on the dissection of 100 facial halves. *Plast Reconstr Surg* 1962;29:266-272.
6. Terzis J, Tzafetta K. The "babysitter" procedure: minihypoglossal to facial nerve transfer and cross-face nerve grafting. *Plast Reconstr Surg.* 2009;123(3):865-876.
7. Garcia RM, Hadlock TA, Klebuc MJ, et al. Contemporary solutions for the treatment of facial nerve paralysis. *Plast Reconstr Surg.* 2015;135(6):1025e-1046e.
8. Conley J. Search for and identification of the facial nerve. *Laryngoscope.* 1978;88(1 Pt 1):172-175
9. Placheta E, Wood MD, Lafontaine C. Enhancement of facial nerve motoneuron regeneration through cross-face nerve grafts by adding end-to-side sensory axons. *Plast Reconstr Surg.* 2015;135(2):460-471.
10. Bae YC, Zuker RM, Manktelow RT, et al. A comparison of commissure excursion following gracilis muscle transplantation for facial paralysis using a cross-face nerve graft versus the motor nerve to the masseter nerve. *Plast Reconstr Surg.* 2006;117(7):2407-2413.
11. Frey M, Giovanoli P, Michaelidou M. Functional upgrading of partially recovered facial palsy by cross-face nerve grafting with distal end-to-side neurorrhaphy. *Plast Reconstr Surg.* 2006;117(2):597-608.

Motor Branch of Masseter for Innervation of Free Muscle Flap

Michael J. A. Klebuc

DEFINITION

- The descending branch of the motor nerve to the masseter muscle (CN V) can be selectively divided and employed to innervate free muscle flaps, utilized for smile restoration.

ANATOMY

- The masseter nerve branches from the mandibular nerve and passes above the lateral pterygoid muscle where it runs through the mandibular notch to enter the substance of the masseter muscle.
- Along its intramuscular path, the main trunk liberates a series of small proximal branches and terminates in a long descending branch that courses obliquely in posteroanterior, proximal-distal trajectory.
- The main trunk of the masseter nerve can be identified at a point 3 cm in front of the tragus, 1 cm below the zygomatic arch, and 1.5 cm deep to the SMAS (**FIG 1**).[1]
- The masseter muscle has three lobes (superficial, middle, and deep).
- The motor nerve to the masseter (CN V) lies on the superficial surface of the deep lobe.[2]
- The main trunk and descending branches contain approximately 2700 and 1550 myelinated motor fibers, respectively.[1,3]

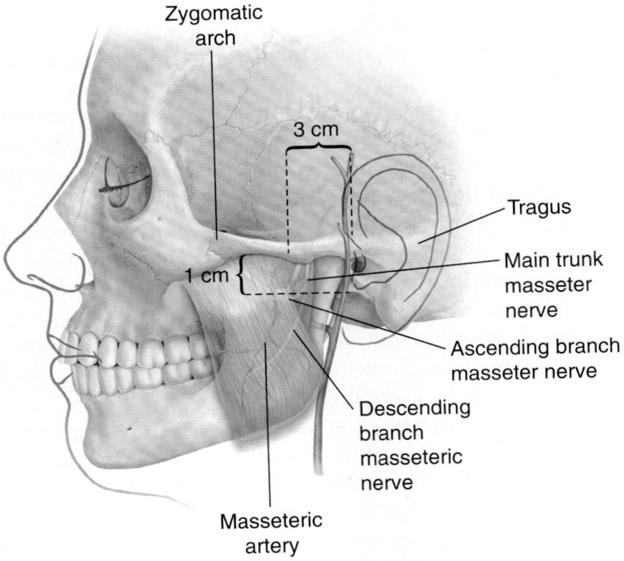

FIG 1 • Topographic landmarks for masseter nerve isolation. Main nerve trunk located 3 cm in front of the tragus, 1 cm below the zygomatic arch, and 1.5 cm deep to the SMAS.

- The descending branch of the masseter nerve is usually selectively transected and employed to innervate free muscle flaps utilized for facial reanimation.

PATHOGENESIS

- The masseter nerve is frequently selected as a source of innervation in cases of bilateral facial paralysis and when the facial nerve is unavailable as a donor (ie, Moebius syndrome, Lyme disease, bilateral temporal bone fractures, brainstem cavernous malformation, Guillain-Barré).[4]
- Often selected over cross face nerve grafts in older patients where the potential for nerve regeneration is diminished.[5]

PATIENT HISTORY AND PHYSICAL FINDINGS

- Etiology of the facial paralysis:
  - Developmental
  - Traumatic
  - Post-tumor extirpation
  - Bell palsy
  - Ramsay Hunt syndrome
- Patient age:
  - Peripheral nerve regeneration declines with advanced age.
  - There is no definitive age cutoff for cross face nerve grafting; however, after the age of 50 to 55 years, the ipsilateral motor nerve branch to masseter or other adjacent cranial nerves often provide a more reliable source of innervation to free muscle flaps with more powerful muscle flap contraction.
- Comorbidities impairing nerve regeneration:
  - Smoking—higher risk of skin flap necrosis
  - Diabetes
  - Vascular disease
  - Previous radiation
  - Neurologic disorders
- History of hypercoagulable state:
  - Patient or family history of pulmonary emboli or deep venous thrombosis signals the need for a hematologic workup prior to free, functional muscle flap reconstruction.
- The patient's level of motivation and willingness to comply with postoperative physical therapy is also important to ascertain.
- History of temporomandibular joint dysfunction—consider alternative technique.

Physical Examination

- Active, forceful, contraction of the masseter and temporalis muscles is confirmed by palpation.

- The face is examined for previous access incisions and signs of trauma or injury to the muscles of facial expression.
- Dental occlusion and mouth opening are evaluated to rule out temporomandibular joint dysfunction.
- A cranial nerve examination is performed to identify additional neurologic deficits.
- Palpate and Doppler the superficial temporal and facial artery and veins on the paralyzed hemiface to verify patency.

IMAGING

- Imaging studies are seldom required in the presence of a normal physical examination.

SURGICAL MANAGEMENT

Preoperative Planning

- Smoking cessation and avoidance of nicotine
- Discontinuation of oral anticoagulants
- EMG
  - Concomitant activation of the masseter muscle with attempted smiling (may predict development of an effortless smile)[6]
- Mark the nasolabial folds and smile vectors prior to entering the operating room.

Positioning

- Supine on the operating table with arms tucked
- Narrow head extension with foam- or gel-filled headrest.
- Nasotracheal intubation with nasal ray endotracheal tube sutured to the columella and supported on the hair-bearing scalp with foam, silk tape, and staples (**FIG 2**)

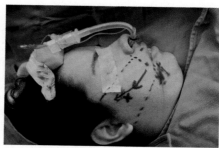

FIG 2 • Nasotracheal intubation with head positioned on a narrow headrest. Endotracheal tube sutured to columella and supported with foam to prevent pressure on the nasal alae.

- Oral cavity cleansed with chlorhexidine gluconate mouthwash
- Preoperative intravenous antibiotic coverage for oral flora (ie, clindamycin)
- Contralateral lower extremity prepped if a free gracilis muscle flap will be utilized
- Sequential compression devices (sterile SCD on the donor leg)
- Foley catheter

Approach

- In the standard approach, the masseter nerve is explored via a preauricular incision after elevation of a cheek skin flap.
- When a limited preauricular approach is used, the neurorrhaphy is performed prior to the microvascular anastomosis to facilitate exposure.

TECHNIQUES

■ Standard Preauricular Approach

- The external auditory canal is occluded with a petrolatum gauze dressing.
- A preauricular incision with a sideburn extension is made if the superficial temporal artery and vein will be used as recipient vessels. A submandibular extension is incorporated if the facial vessel will be used.
- A skin and subcutaneous tissue flap is elevated in the preauricular, zygomatic, and buccal regions, extending the medial aspect of the dissection to the lateral border of the orbicularis oris muscle.
- A point is marked on the SMAS, 3 cm in front of the tragus and 1 cm below the zygomatic arch. This landmark reliably corresponds to the general location of the underlying masseter nerve (**TECH FIG 1A**).[1]
- The operating microscope is brought onto the field to enhance visualization and microsurgical dissection is utilized to identify zygomatic branches of the facial nerve that traverse this site.
- In cases of incomplete facial paralysis, these facial nerve branches are mobilized and gently retracted to provide access to the deeper tissues. Facial nerve branches are often absent in cases of developmental paralysis. This significantly simplifies the dissection (**TECH FIG 1B**).

- With the aid of bipolar cautery, the cephalic border of the parotid is released from its attachments to the zygomatic arch and the gland is reflected inferiorly exposing the masseteric fascia.
- A window of the masseteric fascia is excised below the zygomatic arch exposing the superficial lobe of the masseter muscle.
- A right angle clamp and bipolar cautery are now utilized to release the muscle in layers by propagating the dissection through the superficial and middle lobes of the masseter muscle (**TECH FIG 1C**).
- In the deeper portion of the dissection, an electrical stimulator set at 0.5 to 1 mA at 40 Hz is employed to help identify the masseter nerve that usually resides in the zone of maximal muscle contraction.
- Small branches of the masseter nerve are frequently encountered and can be traced in a retrograde fashion back to the main trunk.
- The main nerve trunk is usually identified resting on the superficial surface of the deep lobe of the masseter muscle approximately 1.5 cm deep to the SMAS. Once identified, the main trunk of the masseter nerve is encircled with a vessel loop and the descending branch is further mobilized with microsurgical dissection (**TECH FIG 1D**).

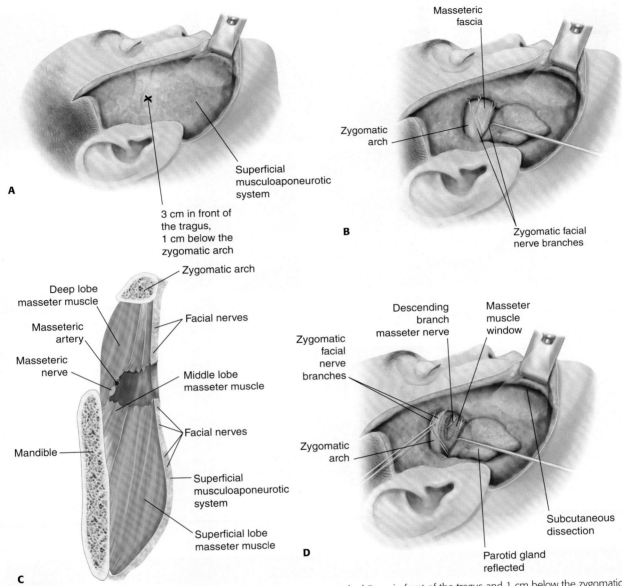

TECH FIG 1 • A. Skin flap elevated and location of the masseter nerve marked 3 cm in front of the tragus and 1 cm below the zygomatic arch. **B.** Regional zygomatic facial nerve branches mobilized and reflected. May be absent in cases of developmental paralysis. **C.** Cross-sectional view of masseter nerve dissection with the main nerve trunk resting on the superficial surface of the deep muscular lobe. **D.** Masseter nerve identified within the muscle. The descending branch will be mobilized and selectively transected. The ascending branch will be preserved to prevent atrophy.

- The masseter nerve is accompanied by a sizable artery, and microvascular clips can prove beneficial in achieving hemostasis and avoiding frustrating hemorrhaging that impaired visualization.
- Once the maximal length of the descending branch has been dissected, it is selectively transected and transposed into a more superficial plane to facilitate later nerve repair. It is important to preserve the integrity of the proximal branches to prevent muscle atrophy and the development of a cosmetic deformity.
- With the aid of the operating microscope, an end-to-end microsurgical nerve repair is made in an interrupted, epineurial fashion with 10-0 nylon between the masseter nerve and the motor nerve of the free muscle flap.

■ **Limited Preauricular Approach**

- When a limited preauricular approach is used, the neurorrhaphy is performed prior to the microvascular anastomosis to facilitate exposure (**TECH FIG 2A**).

- **TECH FIG 3** shows an extended submandibular dissection to access the facial artery and vein for recipient vessels.

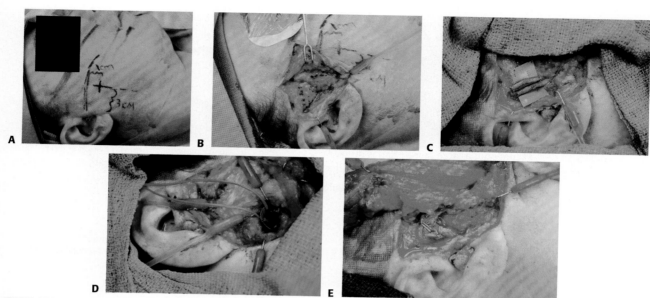

TECH FIG 2 • A. Preoperative markings. **B.** Skin flap elevation for limited, preauricular approach. **C.** Superficial temporal vessels isolated. **D.** Descending masseter nerve branch isolated and transected. **E.** Nerve repair followed by microvascular anastomosis to facilitate exposure.

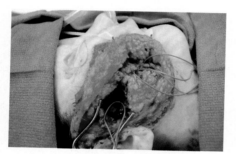

TECH FIG 3 • Extended submandibular dissection to access the facial artery and vein for recipient vessels.

PEARLS AND PITFALLS

Selective masseter nerve transection	▪ The descending branch is frequently divided and used to innervate free muscle flaps. Proximal branches are left intact to prevent muscle atrophy and development of a cosmetic deformity.
Excessive power	▪ Small muscle flaps should be utilized to avoid excessively powerful muscle contraction and exaggerated commissure excursion. The decreased bulk in the midface enhances the cosmetic result.
Inadequate resting tone	▪ Free muscle flaps innervated by the masseter nerve often produce inadequate facial tone to achieve symmetry in repose. Consider additional static support with fascia and or tendon grafts.
Patient motivation	▪ Selection of well motivated patients with a strong commitment to postoperative physical therapy is essential.
Facial motion with mastication	▪ Some individuals may notice significant facial motion with chewing. This is often improved by favoring the contralateral cheek region when eating.
Single-stage procedure	▪ Facial reanimation can be achieved in a single operative setting.

POSTOPERATIVE CARE

- The patients are maintained on a clear liquid diet for 48 hours and then transitioned to a soft mechanical diet for 4 weeks.
- Please refer to Chapter 52 for additional postoperative care after free muscle flap facial reanimation.

OUTCOMES

- Single-stage procedure
- Produces greater commissure excursion than cross face nerve grafts[7]
- More reliable motion in the older patient, as compared to cross face nerve grafts[8]

- Dense innervation permits the use of small muscle flaps with less midface bulk.
- Potential for cerebral adaptation[9]
- In longer-term follow-up, greater than 80% can make a smile without clenching and more than 50% develop an effortless smile.[10]

COMPLICATIONS

- Thrombosis and flap loss (rare)
- Excess commissure excursion if a large muscle flap is utilized
- Masseter muscle atrophy if the main nerve trunk is divided with development of a sharp mandibular angle
- Separation of the muscle flap from orbicularis oris with retraction into the midcheek
- Adhesion of the muscle flap to the dermis if excessively thin skin flaps are elevated
- Asymmetry in repose if additional static support is not provided
- Unwanted facial motion with mastication

REFERENCES

1. Borschel GH, Kawamura DH, Kasukurthi R, et al. The motor nerve to the masseter muscle: an anatomic and histomorphometric study to facilitate its use in facial reanimation. *J Plast Reconstr Aesthet Surg.* 2012;65:363-366.
2. Hwang K, Kim YJ, Chung IH, et al. Course of the masseteric nerve in masseter muscle. *J Craniofac Surg.* 2005;16:197-200.
3. Coombs CJ, Ek EW, Wu T, et al. Masseteric-facial nerve coaptation: an alternative technique for facial nerve reinnervation. *J Plast Reconstr Aesthet Surg.* 2009;62:1580-1588.
4. Gaudin RA, Jowett N, Banks CA et al. Bilateral facial paralysis: a 13-year experience. *Plast Reconstr Surg.* 2016;138(4):879-887.
5. Garcia RM, Hadlock TA, Klebuc MJ, et al. Contemporary solutions for the treatment of facial nerve paralysis. *Plast Reconstr Surg.* 2015;135(6):1025e-1046e.
6. Schaverien M, Moran G, Stewart K, Addison P. Activation of the masseter muscle during normal smile production and the implications for dynamic reanimation surgery for facial paralysis. *J Plast Reconstr Aesthet Surg.* 2011;64:1585-1588.
7. Bae YC, Zuker RM, Manktelow RT, Wade S. A comparison of commissure excursion following gracilis muscle transplantation for facial paralysis using a cross-face nerve graft versus the motor nerve to the masseter nerve. *Plast Reconstr Surg.* 2006;117(7):2407-2413.
8. Klebuc M, Shenaq SM. Donor nerve selection in facial reanimation surgery. *Semin Plast Surg.* 2004;18:53-60.
9. Lifchez SD, Matloub HS, Gosain AK. Cortical adaptation to restoration of smiling after free muscle transfer innervated by the nerve to the masseter. *Plast Reconstr Surg.* 2005;115:1472-1479.
10. Manktelow RT, Tomat LR, Zuker RM, Chang M. Smile reconstruction in adults with free muscle transfer innervated by the masseter motor nerve: effectiveness and cerebral adaptation. *Plast Reconstr Surg.* 2006;118:885-899.

51

CHAPTER

Masseter-to-Facial Nerve Transfer

Michael J. A. Klebuc

DEFINITION

- The descending branch of the masseter nerve can be transferred to selected zygomatic-buccal branches of the facial nerve (V–VII) to restore motion in the midface and perioral region.
- The V to VII nerve transfer is utilized when intracranial and/or intratemporal segments of the facial nerve are irreversibly damaged in the presence of intact distal facial nerve branches and viable muscles of facial expression.

ANATOMY

- The masseter nerve branches from the mandibular nerve and passes above the lateral pterygoid muscle where it runs through the mandibular notch to enter the substance of the masseter muscle.
- Along its intramuscular path, the main trunk liberates a series of small proximal branches and terminates in a long descending branch that courses obliquely in a posterior-anterior, proximal-distal trajectory.
- The main trunk of the masseter nerve can be identified at a point 3 cm in front of the tragus, 1 cm below the zygomatic arch, and 1.5 cm deep to the SMAS (**FIG 1**).[1]
- The masseter muscle has three lobes (superficial, middle, and deep).
- The motor nerve to masseter (CN V) lies on the superficial surface of the deep lobe.[2]

- The main trunk and descending branches contain approximately 2700 and 1550 myelinated motor fibers, respectively.[1,3]
- The descending branch of the masseter nerve is usually selected for the V to VII transfer.
- Facial nerve (somatic motor efferent component) innervates the muscles of facial expression, auricular muscles, occipitalis, posterior belly digastric, stylohyoid, and stapedius.
- The facial nerve main trunk emerges from the skull base via the stylomastoid foramen where it can be identified coursing 1 cm deep to the tragal pointer and medial to the posterior belly of the digastric muscle.[4]
- Within the parotid gland, the facial nerve divides into a temporofacial and cervicofacial trunk.
- Distal branches exit the parotid along its anteromedial border.
- The following branches innervate the corresponding muscles of facial expression[5]:
  - Frontal branch—frontalis muscle
  - Zygomatic branches—orbicularis oculi, zygomaticus major, zygomaticus minor, levator labii superioris, levator labii superioris alaeque nasi, corrugator supercilii, procerus
  - Buccal branches—buccinator, risorius, orbicularis oris
  - Marginal mandibular branches—depressor anguli oris, depressor labii inferioris, mentalis
  - Cervical branches—platysma
- Zuker point-midway point of a line drawn from the root of the helix to the lateral commissure (**FIG 2**)[6]:

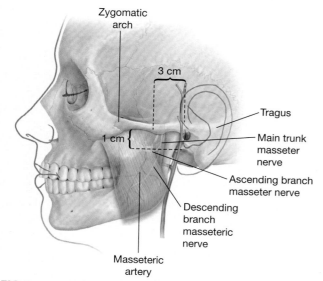

FIG 1 • Topographic landmarks for isolation of the motor nerve branch to masseter. The main trunk is identified 3 cm in front of the tragus, 1 cm below the zygomatic arch, and 1.5 cm deep to the SMAS.

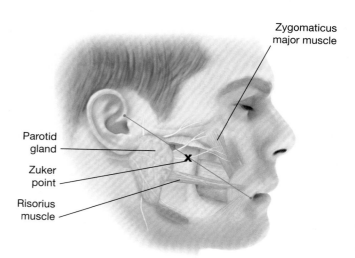

FIG 2 • The facial nerve branch supplying the zygomatic major is typically found at a point half way between the root of the helix and the lateral commissure.

- Describes the approximate location of the facial nerve branch supplying the zygomaticus major muscle.
- At this location, the zygomatic facial nerve branches coursing above and below the transverse facial artery are often selected for the V to VII transfer.

PATHOGENESIS

- Employed when intracranial and/or intratemporal segments of the facial nerve are irreversibly damaged in the presence of intact distal facial nerve branches and viable mimetic muscles.
- Commonly utilized after ablative oncologic surgery or trauma involving the brainstem and skull base.
- Etiology of facial nerve injury includes resection of acoustic neuroma, facial nerve schwannoma, cerebellopontine angle tumors, AVM, cholesteatoma, and skull base tumors. Unrecovered Bell palsy, mastoiditis, and skull base fractures are other common causes of facial nerve injury.[7]

PATIENT HISTORY AND PHYSICAL FINDINGS

- The duration of the paralysis is one of the most important pieces of information garnered from the patient's history, as the masseter-to-facial nerve transfer must be performed before the muscles of facial expression have undergone irreversible atrophy.
- The V to VII transfer is optimally employed immediately at the time of tumor extirpation yet remains a viable option up to 18 months after the onset of the paralysis.
- The patient's age is also of consequence in surgical planning. Generally, in the older patient population (greater than 55 years), the V to VII transfer is used in isolation with fascia lata grafts for additional static support. In younger patients, the V to VII transfer is often combined with cross face nerve grafts (CFNG) in a single operative setting. This is performed in an effort to create a marriage of power (V–VII) and spontaneity (CFNG).[8,9]
- A history of diabetes, coronary artery disease, chronic obstructive pulmonary disease, smoking, underlying neurologic disorders, previous head-neck radiation, and temporal mandibular joint dysfunction should be noted and accounted.
- The patient's level of motivation and willingness to comply with postoperative physical therapy is also important to ascertain.
- On physical examination, active, forceful contraction of the masseter and temporalis muscles is confirmed by palpation.
- The face is examined for previous access incisions and signs of trauma or injury to the muscles of facial expression.
- Dental occlusion and mouth opening are evaluated to rule out temporomandibular joint dysfunction.
- A cranial nerve examination is performed to identify additional neurologic deficits.
- The eye is examined for signs of exposure keratitis as adjunctive eye procedures may be performed with the V to VII transfer to maintain corneal health.
- A vascular examination of the lower extremities is undertaken to rule out significant peripheral vascular disease if fascia lata or sural nerve grafts are to be harvested.

IMAGING

- MRI of the brain and facial nerve
  - High-resolution multiplanar T1 and T2 images, gadolinium enhanced, fat suppressed, and internal auditory canal (IAC) protocol
  - Used to evaluate injury to the facial nerve (ie, Bell palsy, tumors, stroke)
- Computed tomography
  - 0.625 mm or thinner axial images, reconstructions in coronal plane
  - Valuable for imaging temporal bone fractures
- EMG of the masseter muscle and mimetic muscles innervated by the facial nerve
  - Look for signs of early facial nerve recovery.
  - Look for signs of reversible muscle atrophy.
  - Look for signs of coordinated activity between the mimetic muscles and the masseter.

SURGICAL MANAGEMENT

Preoperative Planning

- Smoking cessation and avoidance of nicotine
- Discontinuation of oral anticoagulants
- Facial nerve imaging as guided by the etiology of the paralysis (MRI, CT)
- EMG
  - Presence of muscle fibrillation (suggests potential, positive response to reinnervation)
  - Concomitant activation of the masseter muscle with smiling (may predict development of an effortless smile)

Positioning

- Supine on the operating table with arms tucked
- Narrow head extension with foam or gel-filled headrest
- Nasotracheal intubation with nasal RAE endotracheal tube sutured to the columella and supported on the hair-bearing scalp with foam, silk tape, and staples (**FIG 3**)
- Oral cavity cleansed with chlorhexidine gluconate mouthwash
- Lower extremities prepped if nerve or fascia grafts are to be utilized

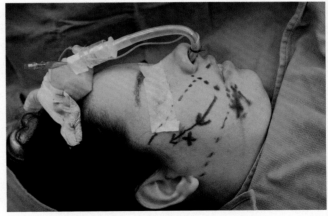

FIG 3 • Nasotracheal intubation with head positioned on a narrow headrest. Endotracheal tube sutured to columella and supported with foam to prevent pressure on the nasal alae.

- Sterile calf sequential compression devices
- Foley catheter

Approaches

- V to VII retrograde approach with adjacent branch preservation
- V to VII anterograde approach with distal, selective, facial nerve branch transection
- V to VII with fascia lata static suspension
- V to VII with CFNG

■ Retrograde Masseter-to-Facial Nerve Transfer

- The anterior border of the masseter muscle is palpated and marked.
- A pretragal incision with an extension into the sideburn is now marked with a surgical pen.
- An additional point is marked half way between the root of the helix and the commissure to indicate the general location of the facial nerve branch to the zygomaticus major muscle (Zuker point).[6]
- The topographic location of the masseter nerve is also marked 3 cm in front of the tragus and 1 cm below the zygomatic arch (**TECH FIG 1A**).
- A petrolatum gauze dressing is utilized to occlude the external auditory canal.
- The subcutaneous tissues in the preauricular, zygomatic, and buccal regions are infiltrated with a 1:100 000 epinephrine, hemostatic solution (**local anesthetics should be avoided to preserve nerve stimulation**).

- The preauricular incision with the sideburn extension is made, and a skin and subcutaneous tissue flap is elevated in the preauricular, zygomatic, and buccal regions extending the medial aspect of the dissection approximated 3 cm past the medial border of the masseter muscle (**TECH FIG 1B**).
- A SMAS flap is now elevated with scissor dissection and bipolar cautery. The flap is mobilized to the anteromedial border of the parotid gland where the inferior zygomatic and buccal branches of the facial nerve are identified. The SMAS flap is released transversely along the zygomatic border and reflected to facilitate exposure.
- The operating microscope is brought onto the field to enhance visualization, and microsurgical dissection is utilized to further explore and mobilize the facial nerve branches.
- During the dissection, the transverse facial artery is often encountered. This is a useful landmark, as the zygomatic branches above and below this structure often produce an excellent smile with little activation of the orbicularis oculi (**TECH FIG 1C**).

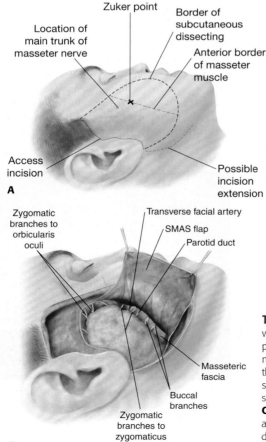

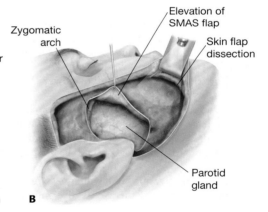

TECH FIG 1 • A. Operative markings: preauricular incision with a possible submandibular extension (X) marks Zuker point and (*asterisk*) identifies the general location of the motor nerve branch to masseter. The *dashed lines* represent the anterior border of the masseter muscle and the region of skin flap elevation. **B.** Demonstrates the extent of the skin-subcutaneous flap elevation and initial SMAS flap dissection. **C.** The facial nerve branches bordering the transverse facial artery are frequently selected for transfer as they often produce an isolated smile with little or no activation of the orbicularis oculi or orbicularis oris.

- These facial nerve branches often merge into a larger common branch. This is dissected in a retrograde fashion through the parotid gland until it dives into a deep plane in the preauricular region. At this point, adequate nerve length is usually present to achieve a primary nerve repair. However, the facial nerve is left undivided until this can be confirmed.
- Once the selected facial nerves have been mobilized, attention is focused on identifying the motor nerve branch to the masseter.

Identifying the Motor Nerve Branch

- A point 3 cm in front of the tragus and 1 cm below the zygomatic arch is again marked. The masseter fascia is released from the inferior border of the zygomatic arch with the bipolar cautery exposing the superficial surface of the masseter muscle.
- A right-angle clamp and bipolar cautery are now utilized to release the muscle in layers, propagating the dissection through the superficial and middle lobes of the masseter muscle (**TECH FIG 2A**).

- In the deeper portion of the dissection, an electrical stimulator set at 0.5 to 1 mA at 40 Hz is employed to help identify the masseter nerve that usually resides in the zone of maximal muscle contraction.
- Small branches of the masseter nerve are frequently encountered and can be traced in a retrograde fashion back to the main trunk (**TECH FIG 2B**).
- Once identified, the main trunk of the masseter nerve is encircled with a vessel loop, and the descending branch is further mobilized.
- The masseter nerve is accompanied by a sizable artery, and microvascular clips can prove beneficial in achieving hemostasis and avoiding frustrating hemorrhaging and impaired visualization.
- Once the maximal length of the descending branch has been dissected, it is selectively transected and transposed into a more superficial plane to facilitate later nerve repair. It is important to preserve the integrity of the proximal branches to prevent muscle atrophy and the development of a cosmetic deformity.

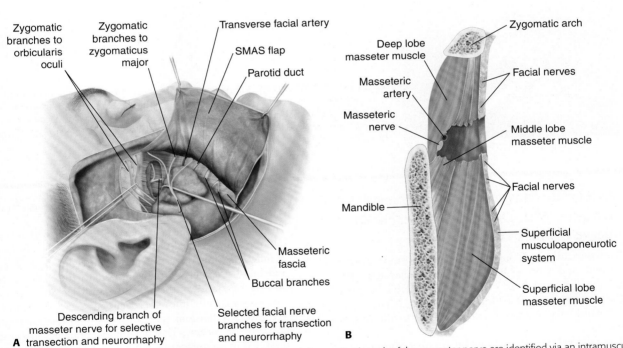

TECH FIG 2 • A. The main trunk, proximal ascending branches, and descending branch of the masseter nerve are identified via an intramuscular window. **B.** Cross-sectional view of masseter nerve dissection with the main nerve trunk resting on the superficial surface of the deep muscular lobe.

Dividing the Nerve Branch

- After verifying adequate length, the previously mobilized facial nerve branch is divided. With the aid of the operating microscope, an end-to-end microsurgical nerve repair is made in an interrupted, epineurial fashion with 10-0 nylon (**TECH FIG 3**).
- The SMAS flap is now returned to its native location and secured with absorbable monofilament sutures.

- The plane of subcutaneous dissection is treated with fibrin glue, and a 10-French closed suction drain is inserted.
- A layered closure of the access incisions is now performed, and the incisions are covered with antibiotic ointment. Stickers cautioning the need to avoid pressure are applied to the cheek.
- A deep, atraumatic extubation is then coordinated with the anesthesia provider.

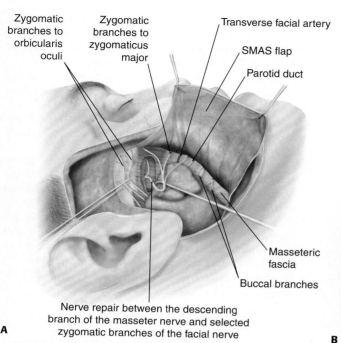

Zygomatic branches to orbicularis oculi

Zygomatic branches to zygomaticus major

Transverse facial artery

SMAS flap

Parotid duct

Masseteric fascia

Buccal branches

Nerve repair between the descending branch of the masseter nerve and selected zygomatic branches of the facial nerve

A

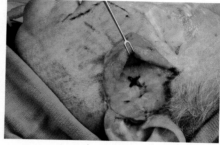

B

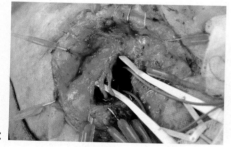

C

TECH FIG 3 • A. Microsurgical neurorrhaphy between the descending branch of the masseter nerve and selected zygomatic branches of the facial nerve. **B.** Masseter nerve location marked on SMAS 3 cm in front of the tragus and 1 cm below the zygomatic arch. **C.** Zygomatic facial nerve branches and the descending branch of the masseter nerve isolated for transfer.

Antegrade Masseter-to-Facial Nerve Transfer With Distal, Selective, Facial Nerve Branch Transection

- A preauricular incision with a subsideburn extension is created, and a broad based skin flap is elevated carrying the dissection 2 to 3 cm past the anterior border of the parotid gland. If additional exposure is required, a submandibular extension can be added to the original incision.

- The relatively avascular interval between the posterior border of the parotid gland and tragal cartilage (cartilaginous portion of the external auditory canal) is dissected with the aid of bipolar cautery and self-retaining Weitlaner retractors.

- The dissection is propagated deeply into the mastoid and retromandibular region. The main trunk of the facial nerve is identified exiting the skull base via the stylomastoid foramen approximately 1 cm deep to the tragal pointer and medial to the posterior belly of the digastric muscle.[4] The main trunk of the facial nerve emerges from the skull base approximately 5 cm from the skin surface (**TECH FIG 4**). The depth of this structure is significant, and a submandibular extension of the access incision can

be made to facilitate exposure, although it detracts from the overall aesthetics of the result.

- The main trunk of the facial nerve is encircled with a vessel loop and electrically stimulated to verify the absence of function. Blunt dissection with a fine right-angle clamp and bipolar cautery is then utilized to trace the nerve into the substance of the parotid gland. The nerve often transitions rapidly into a vertical course before separating into two divisions (temporofacial and cervicofacial) at the pes anserinus. The facial nerve branches are now dissected in an antegrade manner in a fashion akin to a superficial parotidectomy. The facial nerve branch mobilization is terminated approximately 1 to 2 cm from the anterior border of the parotid (**TECH FIG 4B**).

- In cases of complete facial paralysis, the main trunk of the facial nerve is transected at the stylomastoid foramen and transposed anteriorly to provide unobstructed access for the masseter nerve dissection (**TECH FIG 4C**).

- In cases of incomplete paralysis, isolation of the masseter nerve is significantly more complicated, as the main trunk of the facial nerve is left intact and the dissection must be propagated between the zygomatic branches to the eye, without injuring these structures.

- In cases of complete paralysis, the frontal branch, zygomatic branches innervating the orbicularis oculi, and the cervical branches are selectively transected to prevent development of synkinesis.

- The descending branch of the masseter nerve is now mobilized and selectively transected (as described above in the retrograde approach). An end-to-end neurorrhaphy is now created with the aid of the operating microscope and 10-0 nylon (**TECH FIG 4D–F**).

- The parotid fascia is repaired with absorbable monofilament sutures, the region of subcutaneous dissection is treated with fibrin glue, and the access incision is closed over a 10-French closed suction drain.

- "No pressure" stickers are applied to the cheek, and an atraumatic extubation is coordinated with the anesthesia provider.

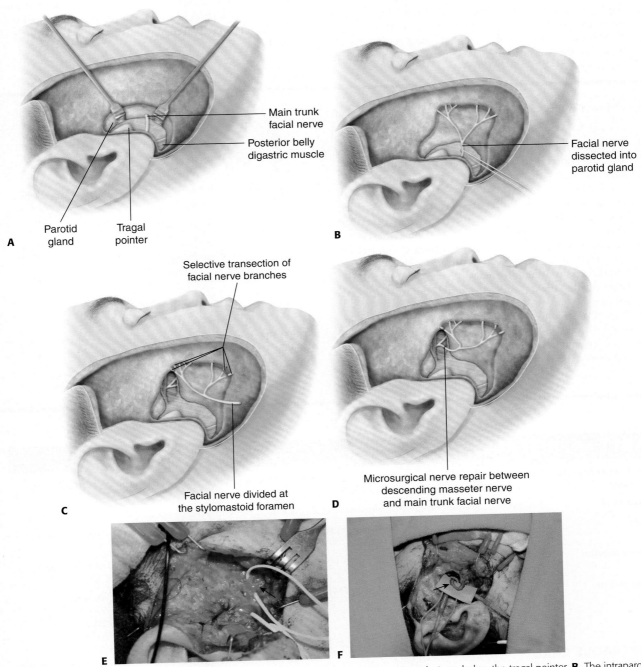

TECH FIG 4 • A. Facial nerve trunk identified exiting the stylomastoid foramen approximately 1 cm below the tragal pointer. **B.** The intraparotid portion of the facial nerve dissected in a fashion analogous to a superficial parotidectomy. **C.** Facial nerve trunk selectively transected to enhance exposure and frontal, selected zygomatic, marginal mandibular and cervical branches of the facial nerve divided to prevent synkinesis. Masseter nerve identified resting on the deep lobe of the masseter muscle. **D.** Microsurgical neurorrhaphy between the masseter and facial nerve in an end-to-end fashion utilizing the operating microscope. **E.** Clinical example of the facial nerve mobilized within the parotid gland. *Arrow* and vessel loop identify the facial nerve branches to zygomaticus major and levator anguli oris. **F.** *Arrow* identifies the descending branch of the masseter nerve coapted to facial nerve trunk with 10-0 nylon in an interrupted epineurial fashion.

T E C H N I Q U E S

■ Masseter-to-Facial Nerve Transfer With Fascia Lata Grafts

- Isolated V to VII transfers in adult patients often lack adequate resting tone.
- In elderly patients, the V to VII transfer is often combined with fascia lata grafts for provision of additional, static support.
- The fascia lata graft is harvested from a proximal, lateral thigh incision with the aid of a lighted retractor. A graft measuring approximately 15 to 17 cm in length and 3 cm in width is obtained, and the fascial defect repaired with 0 polydioxanone suture. A layered closure is performed over a 15-French closed suction drain, as the donor site is prone to seroma formation.
- The graft is frequently divided into three segments that can be used independently to support the upper lip, commissure, and lower lip.
- The grafts can be positioned in the subcutaneous plane or delivered through Bichat-fat pad via a retrozygomatic tunnel.
- Only mild overcorrection is required as the reinnervated muscles of facial expression will provide additional support, and limited stretching of the fascia lata graft will develop.

■ Masseter-to-Facial Nerve Transfer With Cross Face Nerve Grafts

- In the younger patient population, the V to VII transfer is frequently combined with cross face nerve grafts (single-stage operation) in an effort to enhance spontaneity and resting tone.[9]
- The cross face nerve grafts are performed as described in Chapter 49 and the V to VII transfer as described above.
- Electrical stimulation of the unaffected, contralateral facial nerve branches is utilized to create a functional map, and the information is extrapolated to the "electrically silent" side to guide the distal nerve repairs.
- Typically, three to four cross face nerve grafts are combined with the V to VII transfer and target the orbicularis oculi, zygomatics major, orbicularis oris, and lower lip depressors (**TECH FIG 5**).

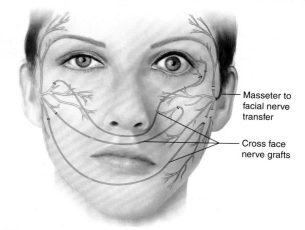

Masseter to facial nerve transfer

Cross face nerve grafts

TECH FIG 5 • Three to four cross face nerve grafts are combined with the V to VII transfer and target the orbicularis oculi, zygomatics major, orbicularis oris, and lower lip depressors.

PEARLS AND PITFALLS

Proximal nerve branch preservation	■ Only the descending branch of the masseter nerve should be transferred. Proximal branches are left intact to prevent irreversible atrophy and a cosmetic deformity.
Static support	■ Fascia lata grafts are frequently required in older patients as the V to VII may not create adequate resting tone.
Sialocele	■ When extensive intraparotid dissection is performed, salivary collections can develop. This is reduced with the application of fibrin glue in the subcutaneous plain and usually responds to glycopyrrolate.
Patient motivation	■ These techniques are best suited to highly motivated individuals who are strongly committed to participate in postoperative therapy.
TMJ dysfunction	■ There is a potential for exacerbation of TMJ dysfunction, and therefore one should consider an alternate technique.

POSTOPERATIVE CARE

- No surgical dressings employed; apply antibiotic ointment to incisions for 48 to 72 hours.
- Avoid pressure on the surgical site (only one thin pillow under the head).
- Avoid incentive spirometry, and encourage deep breathing.
- IV antibiotic coverage for skin organisms and anaerobic oral flora (ie, clindamycin)
- Sequential Compression Devices (SCDs) and early mobilization
- Chlorhexidine mouthwash for 5 to 7 days and then electric toothbrush
- Soft mechanical diet for 4 weeks

- Once motion develops, the patient must practice smiling in front of a mirror (visual feedback) for a minimum of 30 min/d.

OUTCOMES

- Facial tone usually starts to develop at 3 to 4 months and facial motion at 5 to 6 months.[7,10]
- In longer-term follow-up (greater than 2 years), 75% of patients can create a smile without clenching their teeth.
- Average commissure excursion achieved is 90% of the normal side.
- Many patients fail to develop adequate resting tone. Static suspension and cross face nerve grafts are frequently employed to counteract this problem.
- Donor site problems are rare due to the duplication of function between the masseter and temporalis muscles and the selective transection of only the descending branch of the masseter nerve.[11]

COMPLICATIONS

- Sialocele formation that usually responds to glycopyrrolate
- Otitis externa from collection of sanguineous material in the external auditory canal
- Masseter muscle atrophy and development of a sharp mandibular angle if the entire masseter nerve is transected
- Oral-ocular, synkinetic dysfunction that usually responds favorably to botulinum toxin injections and is preferable to paralytic ectropion

REFERENCES

1. Borschel GH, Kawamura DH, Kasukurthi R, et al. The motor nerve to the masseter muscle: an anatomic and histomorphometric study to facilitate its use in facial reanimation. *J Plast Reconstr Aesthet Surg.* 2012;65:363-366.
2. Hwang K, Kim YJ, Chung IH, et al. Course of the masseteric nerve in masseter muscle. *J Craniofac Surg.* 2005;16:197-200.
3. Coombs CJ, Ek EW, Wu T, et al. Masseteric-facial nerve coaptation: an alternative technique for facial nerve reinnervation. *J Plast Reconstr Aesthet Surg.* 2009;62:1580-1588.
4. Conley J. Search for and identification of the facial nerve. *Laryngoscope.* 1978;88(1 Pt 1):172-175.
5. Tzafetta K, Terzis J. Essays on the facial nerve: part I. Microanatomy. *Plast Reconstr Surg.* 2010;125(3):879-889.
6. Dorafshar AH, Borsuk DE, Bojovic B, et al. Surface anatomy of the middle division of the facial nerve: Zuker's point. *Plast Reconstr Surg.* 2013;131(2):253-257.
7. Klebuc MJ. Facial reanimation using the masseter-to-facial nerve transfer. *Plast Reconstr Surg.* 2011;127:1909-1915.
8. Faria JC, Scopel GP, Ferreira MC. Facial reanimation with masseteric nerve: babysitter or permanent procedure? Preliminary results. *Ann Plast Surg.* 2010;64:31-34.
9. Garcia RM, Hadlock TA, Klebuc MJ, et al. Contemporary solutions for the treatment of facial nerve paralysis. *Plast Reconstr Surg.* 2015;135(6):1025e-1046e.
10. Spira M. Anastomosis of masseteric nerve to lower division of facial nerve for correction of lower facial paralysis: preliminary report. *Plast Reconstr Surg.* 1978;61:330-334.
11. Klebuc M, Shenaq SM. Donor nerve selection in facial reanimation surgery. *Semin Plast Surg.* 2004;18:53-60.

52
CHAPTER

Pediatric Facial Reanimation Using a Functional Gracilis Muscle Transfer

Brad M. Gandolfi, Jeffrey R. Marcus, and Michael R. Zenn

DEFINITION

- *Facial paralysis* does not describe a disease but instead the sequelae of denervation resulting from a spectrum of diseases, congenital defects, and acquired defects with a similar effect on the facial musculature.
- Facial nerve paralysis can involve the entire facial nerve distribution or only certain branches of the facial nerve. The facial nerve may be affected symmetrically or asymmetrically. The extent of the paralysis may be complete or incomplete relative to residual motor capacity.
- The pathogenesis of facial paralysis is complex and dependent on the etiology of the disease.[1,2] That discussion is beyond the scope of this chapter but briefly can be divided into congenital and acquired facial paralysis (Table 1). An accurate diagnosis is crucial to selecting the proper surgical (or nonsurgical) intervention.
- *Facial reanimation* is a general term to describe restoration of facial movement. There are two main distinctions based on the status of native facial muscles:
  - Nerve transfers—When the denervating event is such that existing native facial musculature can be amenable to reinnervation with a functioning nerve, a nerve transfer is warranted. In this setting, the goal may be to restore multiple facial nerve targets—ie, multiple separate but coordinated movements.
  - Functional muscle transfer—In long-standing or congenital facial paralysis, native muscles are not present to perform the function. Therefore, a transfer of functioning muscle provides reanimation. In such cases, only one facial movement, rather than multiple, is the goal of the procedure. One muscle provides one movement.
- This chapter focuses on free muscle transfer for restoration of smile in the pediatric population.

ANATOMY

Facial Nerve

- The facial nerve exits the stylomastoid foramen and enters the posterior parotid gland, dividing the gland into superficial and deep components.
- The facial nerve divides into two main branches within the parotid gland: the frontozygomatic and the cervicofacial trunks. These branches further divide before exiting the parotid gland.
- Five branches are classically described as exiting the parotid (frontal/temporal, zygomatic, buccal, marginal mandibular, and cervical). However, the branching pattern for each individual is unique, and many of the abovenamed nerves exist in multiples.[3] The average number of branches exiting the parotid is 7 (**FIG 1**).
- Buccal and zygomatic branches begin to arborize and cross within and beyond the parotid, resulting in redundancy in the functional territory of these buccal-zygomatic branches.[3,4] It is difficult to separate the activity of these branches as purely buccal or zygomatic because stimulation often results in a mixed response. Due to mixed nerve function, sacrifice of one nerve for end-to-end coaptation does not result in functional loss.
- The target for reanimation of smile is a buccal or zygomatic branch, selected based on targeted muscle stimulation. Stimulation should ideally identify a branch that produces vertical and horizontal movement of the commissure and upper lip consistent with the patient's natural smile, with minimal extraneous movement.
- Zuker point describes a relatively consistent buccal-zygomatic branch that meets the needs for facial reanimation.[4] It is found at the center of a line drawn from the oral commissure to the helical root.

Nerve to the Masseter

- The nerve to the masseter arises as a branch of the trigeminal nerve (V3), passing posterior to the temporalis muscle en route to the deep surface of the masseter (**FIG 2**).[5,6]

TABLE 1 Causes of Facial Paralysis

Congenital		Acquired			
Syndromic	**Nonsyndromic**	**Traumatic**	**Tumor**	**Inflammatory**	**Neuromuscular Disease**
Developmental	Developmental	Intracranial	Benign	Bacterial	Bacterial
Genetic	Genetic	Extracranial	Malignant	Viral	Viral
Intrapartum	Intrapartum			Toxic	Toxic
Idiopathic	Idiopathic			Genetic predisposition	Genetic predisposition

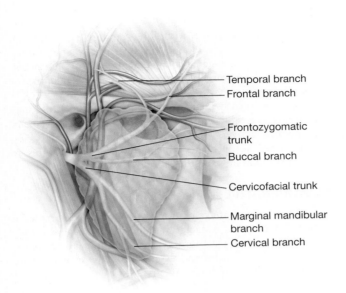

FIG 1 • The anatomy of the facial nerve.

Temporal branch
Frontal branch
Frontozygomatic trunk
Buccal branch
Cervicofacial trunk
Marginal mandibular branch
Cervical branch

- The nerve is reliably found 3 cm anterior to the tragus, 1 cm inferior to the zygomatic arch, and 1.5 mm deep to the SMAS.[5,6]

Gracilis Muscle

- The gracilis muscle originates along the body and inferior ramus of the pubis, just below the pubic tubercle.[7] It runs along the medial thigh and inserts into the medial tibial condyle, immediately deep to the sartorius muscle (**FIG 3A**).
- The gracilis lies immediately posterior to the much larger adductor longus, which is easily palpated on most patients.

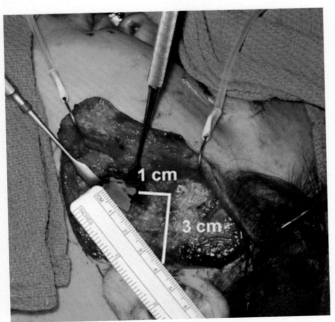

FIG 2 • The nerve to the masseter is found by splitting the temporalis and masseter muscles, under the zygoma. (Reprinted from Borschel GH, et al. The motor nerve to the masseter muscle: an anatomic and histomorphometric study to facilitate its use in facial reanimation. *J Plast Reconstr Aesthet Surg.* 2012;65(3):363-366, with permission from Elsevier.)

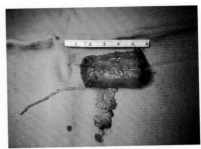

FIG 3 • Gracilis muscle with the pedicle ex vivo. Note the length of obturator nerve (left side of image).

- The muscle is supplied by the medial circumflex femoral artery, a branch of the deep femoral artery. The pedicle runs underneath the adductor longus en route to the gracilis.
- The artery enters the muscle 5 to 12 cm inferior to the pubic tubercle. It is generally 1 to 2 mm in diameter and may have two or three branches at the level of the muscle (**FIG 3B**).
- The artery is accompanied by two vena comitantes.
- The artery and the accompanying vein are 5 to 6 cm when dissected to the deep femoral vessels.
- The muscle has a minor pedicle at its distal aspect that is not appropriate for microvascular transfer.
- A branch of the obturator nerve supplies the gracilis muscle. It splits from the anterior branch of the obturator behind the pectineus and runs with the branch to the adductor longus. The nerve joins the muscle from its lateral aspect, generally at a 45-degree angle to the vascular pedicle. The nerve pierces the muscle and arborizes within it.
- The gracilis muscle has a tendinous origin from the pubis, which can be included with the flap. The muscle can be 3 to 4 cm wide at the level of the pedicle, requiring some muscle splitting to avoid bulky reconstructions.

PATIENT HISTORY AND PHYSICAL FINDINGS

- The most important initial distinction in the preoperative evaluation of pediatric patients with facial paralysis is whether the condition is congenital or acquired. For those with congenital paralysis, the condition may have been apparent at birth or recognized shortly thereafter (**FIG 4**). For those with acquired paralysis, the circumstances and details of the inciting event(s) should be carefully noted. The timing of functional loss is the most critical detail.

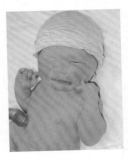

FIG 4 • Photo taken shortly after birth, depicting a left-side congenital facial nerve paralysis.

- Functional impairment, including the following, should be noted:
  - Excessive tearing and/or dryness requiring frequent use of lubricating drops
  - Inability to close the eyes fully at night requiring the use of viscous eye lubricant
  - Oral incompetence (drooling) or speech articulation difficulties
  - Presence and extent of dental caries, which are predisposed on the affected side
- Any prior treatments should be noted as well as any progression or improvement in the condition.
- Prior medical, neurologic, or surgical history that would potentially be associated with the condition or the potential surgical treatments that may be considered should be noted.
- A focused examination of the function of the facial nerve is performed, taking care to document both static and dynamic deficiencies. The motor territory associated with each branch should be graded relative to the completeness of the paralysis. We prefer the Toronto Facial Grading System to track our progress.[2] If etiology of paralysis is unclear, level of injury can be elucidated using the Schirmer test, stapedius reflex test, salivary flow test, and taste examination.
- Photographs and video of the following should be included in the initial evaluation:
  - Repose
  - Brow elevation
  - Eye closure (gentle)
  - Eye closure (strong)
  - Smile (lips together)
  - Smile (natural dental display)
  - Full dental display
  - Pucker
- The ability to close the eyelids such that the cornea is protected must be assessed. Those who are unable to close fully and require viscous lubrication should be identified early and treated with priority ahead of smile reanimation.
- Amblyopia may be seen in as many as 50% of patients with facial nerve palsies, and thus a thorough ophthalmologic examination is warranted.[1] The eye examination should also assess for corneal pathology due to exposure.
- The presence of the facial artery should be confirmed. It is palpable in most patients regardless of age.
- The temporalis and masseter muscles should be palpated, particularly if considering the motor nerve to the masseter as a potential donor nerve. Normal strength and mass should be present.
- Syndromic associations can be seen in congenital facial paralysis and can include hemifacial microsomia, Mobius syndrome, and Poland syndrome among others. Therefore, the examination should include an evaluation of the facial bones (orbits, zygoma, maxilla, and mandible), soft tissues, and ear. Mobius syndrome includes the presence of a cranial nerve VI deficit and can also be associated with a Poland deformity and congenital hand anomalies. Thus, cranial nerves VI, VII, IX, X, and XII should be evaluated for disability.

IMAGING

- For candidate patients with long-standing or congenital paralysis, a radiographic workup is generally unnecessary. For those with associated congenital anomalies, such as craniofacial microsomia, craniofacial CT may be valuable for the comprehensive workup.
- In cases of recently acquired facial paralysis, an EMG may be useful to establish a baseline, demonstrate improvement, or predict recovery. In congenital or long-standing cases, EMG does not provide information that contributes to treatment planning and therefore is not necessary.

NONOPERATIVE MANAGEMENT

- Nonoperative management plays an important role in partial paralysis. A facial rehabilitation specialist may be able to obtain a more symmetric smile by strengthening weaker muscles and de-emphasizing stronger, more active muscles. Such treatment requires participation of the child.
- In certain instances of incomplete paralysis, neurotoxins can be used on the unaffected side as an adjunct to obtain symmetry.
- Long-standing, complete, and near-complete paralysis in the pediatric population generally requires surgical management.

SURGICAL MANAGEMENT

- For the pediatric patient with congenital or long-standing complete paralysis affecting smile, our preferred treatment is microvascular free functional gracilis transfer. Using the gracilis, we can obtain satisfactory, and often outstanding, static and dynamic symmetry of smile.
- For unilateral facial paralysis, we prefer to use a branch of the facial nerve from the contralateral (functional) side to power the gracilis by way of a cross face nerve graft (CFNG). This allows a spontaneous, emotion-driven smile.
- In cases of bilateral facial paralysis, the nerve to the masseter is coapted to the obturator nerve, powering the functional gracilis. This nerve is powerful, is located in the field of dissection, and does not cause a functional deficit. Although jaw clenching (masseter activation) is required to stimulate activity in the transferred muscle, with postoperative psychomotor training, the patient can learn to use this muscle spontaneously. However, in contrast to CN VII (CFNG), the masseter nerve—which arises from CN V—lacks baseline tone. Therefore, even a strong smile powered by the masseter nerve will lack baseline tone in repose and therefore will potentially still be associated with repose asymmetry including facial shift.

Preoperative Planning

- As with any operation, the patient and parents should be thoroughly informed of risks, benefits, and expected outcomes of the procedure. Free flaps in any population may be lengthy in duration and carry a rare but present risk for early failure. Even when technically successful, achievement of a long-term symmetric smile cannot be guaranteed.

- Families must be briefed on the nature of nerve coaptations, timing of functional results, and postoperative care necessary. In general, the timing of nerve regeneration is as follows:
  - Two-stage repair:
    - Cross face nerve graft: 6 to 9 months
      - In older children, a Tinel sign may be followed. In younger children, it may not be elicited.
    - Free gracilis transfer: 6 to 12 months
  - Nerve to masseter: 2 to 4 months
  - Lack of activity (visible or palpable) beyond the later time limits suggests a poor prognosis relative to success of the procedure.
- Preoperatively, the patient is asked to smile, and the vectors of commissure and upper lip elevation are marked on the normal side (if present). These will be used to guide the reconstruction. It is important to do this with the patient in the upright position. Care must be taken not to wash these marks off during the procedure.
  - In cases of bilateral paralysis, two sequential single-stage procedures using the nerve to masseter are performed. The vectors of desired pull to obtain a smile are also marked in these patients, guided by the typical appearance and location of the nasolabial fold.
- Given the substantial recovery process required, it is helpful to schedule the muscle transfer in the summer for school-aged children.
- As noted, a Tinel sign may or may not be present over the distal aspect of the CFNG. In the event that the Tinel sign cannot be elicited, intraoperative frozen section of the CFNG may confirm a normal fascicular pattern, thus confirming nerve regeneration and readiness for free muscle transfer.
- The functional muscle transfer of the gracilis is best accomplished with two surgical teams, minimizing anesthetic time and allowing the procedure to be accomplished in a safe and efficient manner. One team focuses on the recipient site preparation, whereas the other harvests the gracilis muscle and prepares it for transfer.

Positioning

- Stage 1 of two-stage procedure (CFNG):
  - A discussion with anesthesia team is important. The following needs must be conveyed:
    - No paralytic agents after induction
    - Choice of endotracheal tube and method of stabilization should not distort facial features or interfere with assessment of stimulation during surgery. The authors prefer nasal or oral RAE for stage 1 procedures.

- The bed is turned 90 degrees to allow all surgeons access to the field. The circuit must be long enough to accommodate the positioning.
  - Corneal protection and lubrication must be provided and accommodated at each step of the operation.
- The surgery starts in the prone position, with harvest of the sural nerve.
- Once the nerve is harvested and the leg incisions closed, the patient is turned supine for the facial nerve dissection and nerve coaptation.
- Stage 2 of two-stage procedure or single-stage gracilis transfer (CNV masseter):
  - The patient is placed in the supine position.
  - The bed is positioned so the anesthesiologist is at the ipsilateral hip (turned 90 degrees), which allows both teams to operate freely.
  - For gracilis harvest, the legs are placed in a frog-leg position, with the hips and knees gently flexed. The ipsilateral gracilis is used for the following reasons:
    - The direction of the nerve and vascular pedicle are appropriate to allow muscle to be positioned in line with the facial artery and nerve and with maximal available obturator nerve length.
    - Two teams may operate simultaneously without interference.

Approach

- First stage (CFNG):
  - The sural nerve is harvested first. We prefer stair-step incisions (3) with a lighted retractor and direct visualization of the nerve during dissection. The proximal portion of the sural nerve is preferred due to size match and limited branching.
  - The facial nerve exploration is accomplished through a preauricular (face-lift) incision with a 3- to 5-cm extension along the mandibular angle to facilitate exposure (**FIG 5A**).
- The gracilis harvest is accomplished through a 10-cm incision placed over the medial aspect of the upper thigh.
  - The incision is placed on a line drawn from the inferior ramus of the pubis to the medial tibial condyle, centered approximately 10 cm below the pubic tubercle (**FIG 5B**).
- Recipient site (paralyzed face) and nerve to masseter
  - Similar to first-stage CFNG, the incision follows a preauricular face-lift design with an extension 3 to 5 cm along the angle of the mandible.
  - The incision stops 2 cm anterior to the palpable facial artery, which limits the length of incision while providing adequate microsurgery exposure.

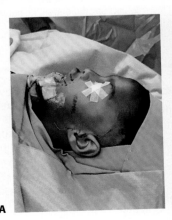
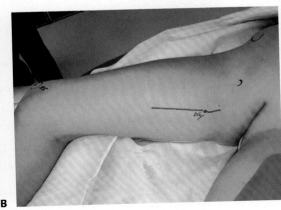

FIG 5 • A. Incision pattern for a first-stage cross face nerve graft. **B.** The incision for the gracilis is centered on the presumed location of the pedicle on the medial thigh. **A** **B**

■ Cross Face Nerve Graft

- The field is copiously infiltrated with a dilute solution of epinephrine (without any local anesthetic). This decreases blood loss, enhancing visibility, and facilitates the skin flap elevation.
- A modified face-lift–style incision is made on the normal (nonparalyzed) side as described above (see **FIG 5A**).
- Sharp dissection proceeds in a superficial plane until the border of the parotid is reached. Skin hooks are used for retraction.
- Once the border of the parotid is reached, the SMAS is incised, and the dissection continues in the sub-SMAS plane (**TECH FIG 1A**).
- The branches of the facial nerve are identified exiting the parotid with the help of a nerve stimulator (**TECH FIG 1B**).
- A proper donor nerve is identified. The donor nerve should supply the zygomaticus muscles and the levator labii. Nerves that simultaneously supply portions of the orbicularis should be avoided, if possible. The goal is to find a nerve that produces the patient's natural smile in relative isolation. The candidate nerves are then followed distally. Stimulation of two or three candidate branches ensures that enough redundancy exists to preclude functional loss with sacrifice of the ideal donor selection.

- A preperiosteal tunnel is then created from the medial extent of the dissection plane to the superior buccal sulcus. A small incision is made at the level of the contralateral canine to aide in the dissection.
- A vessel loop is then passed from the buccal sulcus incision into the edge of the face-lift dissection site (**TECH FIG 1C**).
- The sural nerve is harvested at this time.
- The nerve graft is reversed and then secured to the end of the vessel loop. The vessel loop is then pulled back through the subcutaneous tunnel, delivering the distal end of the nerve graft to the upper buccal sulcus atraumatically.
- The distal end of the graft is tagged with a hemoclip and secured to the periosteum lateral to the canine with a 4-0 nylon suture. This aids in identification at the second stage.
- The upper buccal sulcus incision is then closed.
- The proximal nerve graft is coapted to the donor facial nerve end to end under the surgical microscope.
- The cheek flap is then closed using 4-0 Vicryl dermal sutures, followed by 4-0 nylon skin suture. A short Penrose drain segment is placed for 24 hours.
- No compressive dressings or head wraps are used.

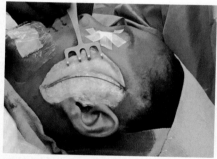

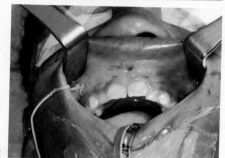

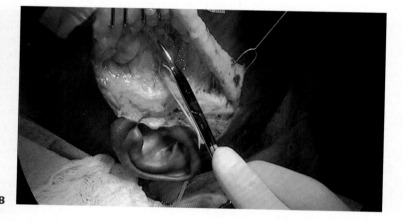

TECH FIG 1 • A. Incision of SMAS to enable donor nerve dissection. **B.** Nerve branches are identified on the nonparalyzed side. **C.** The sural nerve is passed through a preperiosteal tunnel across the maxilla using stepped incisions. Tunneling is facilitated by securing the end of the nerve to a vessel loupe and sliding the loupe through the tunnel.

■ Identification of Nerve to Masseter

- The nerve to the masseter is identified after cheek flap elevation (described below in the gracilis muscle inset).
- An incision is made in the SMAS anterior to the temporomandibular joint, parallel to the zygomatic arch and just below the arch (**TECH FIG 2A**).
- Dissection proceeds through the superficial and intermediate muscle bellies of the masseter, and a nerve crossing

obliquely from zygomatic arch to commissure is sought. The nerve can be found 3 cm anterior to the helical root and 1 cm below the arch. A nerve stimulator may be used to help identify the nerve (**TECH FIG 2B**).
- The nerve is traced to its entrance into the undersurface of the masseter, where it is transected and transposed superficially (**TECH FIG 2C**).
- Any excess obturator nerve is trimmed prior to coaptation to the masseteric nerve to decrease reinnervation time.

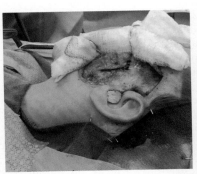
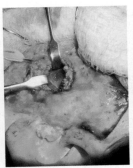
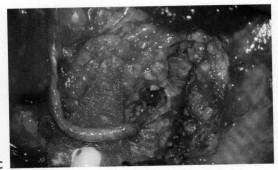

TECH FIG 2 • A. The incision to find the nerve to the masseter is anterior to the TMJ, just below the arch. **B.** The nerve to the masseter is identified. **C.** The nerve is superficially translocated and coapted to the obturator nerve.

■ Recipient Site Preparation

- The field is copiously infiltrated with a dilute solution of epinephrine (without any local anesthetic). This decreases blood loss, enhancing visibility, and facilitates the skin flap elevation (**TECH FIG 3A**).
- A pretrichial, retrotragal incision is made on the paralyzed face. The incision follows the pattern of a basic face-lift incision with an extension inferiorly that allows access to the facial vessels (**TECH FIG 3B**).
- The area from the zygomatic arch to the mandible is elevated in a sub-SMAS plane toward the oral commissure.
- The buccal fat pad is resected to decrease cheek bulk in anticipation of muscle placement (**TECH FIG 3C**). Additionally, deep fat of the cheek is excised as necessary or available.
- The facial vessels are identified and isolated. The vessels are dissected to the level of the commissure to provide length and different diameter choices for anastomosis (**TECH FIG 3D**).
- Using preoperative vector marks as guides, three to four no. 2 Vicryl inset sutures are placed internally in the upper lip, commissure, and occasionally at the lower lip. One suture is always placed at the commissure.
  - Generally, two sutures are placed for the upper lip.
  - Depth of suture placement is key, as too shallow a bite will cause lip eversion and too deep lip inversion.
  - If orbicularis muscle is present, sutures can be placed through the muscle. In many cases, no muscle is present, and sutures are placed in the submucosa (**TECH FIG 3E**).
- As sutures are placed, traction is placed on the suture to replicate smile. Suture placement is modified until the vectors of pull and the nasolabial fold mimics the anticipated smile (**TECH FIG 3F**).

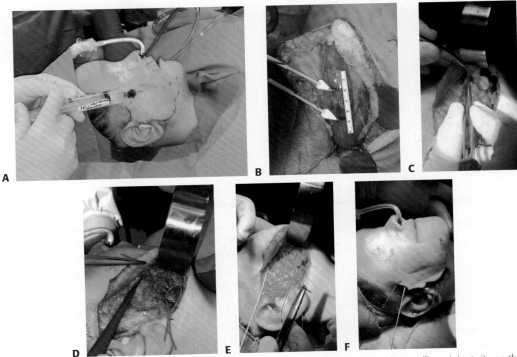

TECH FIG 3 • A. The dissection plane is copiously injected with dilute epinephrine. The incision for the gracilis recipient site on the face mimics a face-lift with an inferomedial extension along the mandible to access the facial vessels. **B.** The gracilis muscle is measured for size and cut to length in situ. **C.** The ipsilateral buccal fat pad is resected to decrease the bulk deformity of the gracilis muscle. **D.** The facial vessels are identified at the border of the mandible. **E.** A series of sutures are placed at commissure in preparation for securing the muscle. **F.** The location of the commissure sutures is checked by placing traction on them and assessing the smile produced.

Determination of the Length of Muscle Needed for the Reconstruction

- This is done with slight traction applied to the inset sutures such that a slight smile is created.
- For purposes of semantics, we refer to the distal inset at the commissure as the insertion and the proximal inset along the zygoma as the origin.
- The muscle is positioned along the proposed vector of the smile—a reflection of the same vector estimated and drawn on the normal side.
- The distances from the commissure to the proposed medial and lateral points of origin along the zygoma are determined (**TECH FIG 4A**).
  - The distance along the medial point of origin is shorter than that to the lateral point of origin (**TECH FIG 4B**).
- The muscle is taken at the greater length, with an additional 2 cm of length added (1 cm per side) to accommodate a row of sutures at each end. These help prevent

pull-through of the subsequent inset sutures. The muscle is then cut on a bias at the proximal end to account for the medial/lateral length discrepancy.

- If pedicle position and required muscle length are ideal, the proximal tendinous portion of the gracilis may be used at the inset origin.
- Once the segmental length is determined, it must be properly centered over the pedicle.
- Three measurements must be made:
  - Total length of muscle (described above, generally around 8 cm)
  - Length of muscle proximal to the facial vessels (approximately 5 cm)
  - Length of muscle distal to the facial vessels (approximately 3 cm)
  - In this way, the dimensions can be transferred to the donor site.
- The dimensions are conveyed to the donor site surgical team.

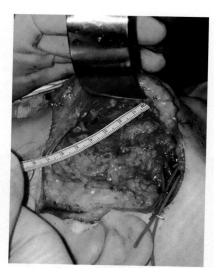
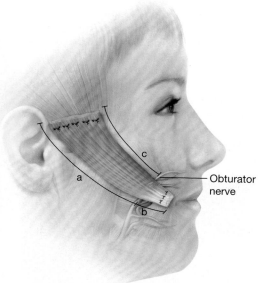

TECH FIG 4 • A. Measurements are taken from the proposed origin to the insertion of the gracilis in preparation for harvest. **B.** The gracilis muscle measurements are measured precisely using the proposed origins and insertions and their relation to the facial vessels. Most times, the anterior border of the muscle (measurement *c* in the diagram) will be shorter than the posterior border of the muscle (measurement *a*) because the origin is secured parallel to the zygoma. Measurement *b* is the length of the gracilis caudal to the vessel insertion.

◼ Gracilis Muscle Harvest

- The patient is placed in the supine position. The hip and knees are slightly flexed (frog-leg position).
- The course of the gracilis muscle is marked out on the patient using anatomic landmarks as guides, and an incision is made above the course of the gracilis as described above (see **FIG 5B**).
- The incision is taken straight down toward the adductor longus. The saphenous vein will be encountered and preserved if possible.
- The adductor longus fascia is incised (**TECH FIG 5A**).
- The pedicle is identified approximately 5 to 10 cm below the pubic tubercle. It can be identified by its course: it

travels below the adductor longus, entering the muscle at a 90-degree angle, at the posterolateral aspect of the muscle (**TECH FIG 5B**).

- The obturator nerve is identified as the pedicle enters the muscle, at a 45-degree angle to the muscle belly.
- The pedicle and nerve are traced under the adductor longus muscle to obtain the most length and size possible. A lighted retractor facilitates this dissection.
- A neurolysis is done to obtain greater length on the nerve pedicle. This can be taken back to the anterior and posterior division of the obturator nerve (**TECH FIG 5C**).
- Distal minor pedicles of the gracilis are ligated, and the muscle is isolated on all sides.

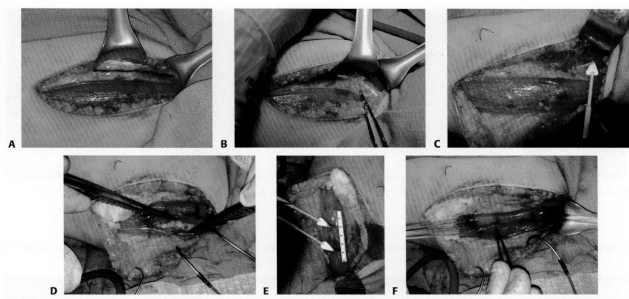

TECH FIG 5 • A. The adductor longus fascia (marked in *blue*) is incised to reveal the gracilis pedicle. **B.** The gracilis pedicle (*blue arrow*) and obturator nerve (*yellow arrow*) in situ below the adductor longus. **C.** The dissection of the obturator nerve (seen over the WECK-CEL) extends under the adductor longus to its branch point. **D.** The gracilis muscle is split longitudinally to decrease bulk. **E.** The length of gracilis to be used is measured, while the muscle is still in situ. **F.** Mattress sutures are placed on the edges of the gracilis to prevent suture pull-through.

- Once isolated, a nerve stimulator is used to assess the contractile units of the muscle. The gracilis can usually be split into medial and lateral components (**TECH FIG 5D**).
  - This split occurs along a natural cleavage plane. Spanning vessels between the muscle segments should be preserved until nerve contraction has been tested.
  - The nerve is stimulated, and the best contractile segment is prepared for transfer.
  - In general, no more than one-third to one-half of the muscle is required for transfer, depending on the size of the child and muscle. Any muscle not harvested is left in situ.
- The length of the gracilis needed is then determined using measurements obtained from the recipient site (described above).

- A total length measurement (a + b), length proximal to the pedicle (a), and length distal to the pedicle (b) will be relayed.
  - An additional 1 cm is added to each side to allow for a layer of bolster sutures to be placed at either end (**TECH FIG 5E**).
- A row of mattress sutures of 0-0 Vicryl are placed 1 cm from each end of the muscle to prevent suture pull-through (**TECH FIG 5F**).
- The proximal and distal muscle bellies are severed using bipolar electrocautery.
- Once the recipient site is ready, a heparin bolus is given. After 10 minutes, the vascular pedicle is clipped, and the muscle is transferred to the face.

■ Gracilis Muscle Inset

- The orientation of the muscle is then determined with consideration of microvascular anastomosis and the nerve coaptation.
- The previously placed inset sutures are then placed in the gracilis, just central on the gracilis to the row of mattress sutures. The muscle is then parachuted into position at the commissure (**TECH FIG 6A**).
- The obturator nerve is then passed through a previously created tunnel to the upper lip (if using a CFNG) or placed in position to coapt to the nerve to the masseter.
- The muscle is then temporarily placed and secured in its final inset position in preparation for a tension-free anastomosis that will not change after the final muscle inset.
- The microvascular anastomosis is then performed, generally vein before artery.

- The epineural nerve coaptation is performed. The buccal sulcus incision is closed at this time.
- The inset origin of the muscle is secured to the deep tissues and periosteum of the zygoma using mattress sutures of no. 1 Vicryl again behind the row of mattress sutures on the gracilis. The muscle should be spread over the inset origin to prevent excess bulk (**TECH FIG 6B**).
- When the muscle is inset, proper tension must be set. If the measurements have been properly made, the resting position will appear as a slight (20%–30% of max) smile.
- A Penrose drain is placed behind the ear by way of a separate stab wound.
- The cheek flap is closed using 4-0 Vicryl sutures in the dermis and a 5-0 Monocryl plus skin closure (**TECH FIG 6C**).

TECHNIQUES

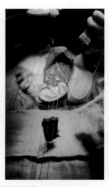 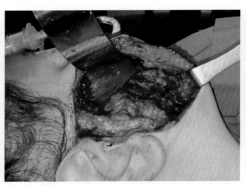 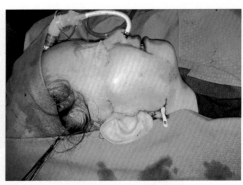

TECH FIG 6 • A. The gracilis muscle is parachuted into position at the commissure. **B.** The gracilis in the final position. **C.** The skin is closed and the area drained with a Penrose drain.

PEARLS AND PITFALLS

Donor nerve evaluation	▪ Selection of an appropriate donor nerve for the CFNG is crucial to the overall success of the operation. ▪ The donor nerve should supply the zygomaticus muscles and the levator anguli oris, with minimal (if any) contributions to the orbicularis oris. ▪ The donor nerve branch taken must have redundancy with other nearby branches and therefore can (and should) be divided relatively proximally. This should be determined with a nerve stimulator to avoid any donor-site weakness.

Muscle inset	▪ An incorrectly inset muscle is nearly impossible to correct. Unfortunately, this may not be noticed until the muscle starts to function, months after the initial procedure. Care must be taken to avoid potential issues by concentrating on the following:
	  ▪ Determine the desired vector of pull, and focus on adequate vertical orientation during inset.
	  ▪ Use a row of mattress sutures to prevent pull-through.
	  ▪ Avoid excess bulk by splitting the muscle in situ before transfer and by removing buccal fat.
	  ▪ The muscle should be inset with tension to simulate 20%–30% of a natural smile.
	  ▪ Avoid excess bulk by coursing the muscle posterior to the malar eminence and fanning the muscle out in the temple area.

Inset insertion suture placement	▪ Preoperative smile vector analysis is key to creating a pleasing smile and should be done in the upright position in the holding area. ▪ Time and care should be taken to place each suture in the appropriate position on the upper lip and commissure, avoiding inversion, eversion, and dimpling. ▪ A symmetric nasolabial fold should be created.
Gracilis harvest	▪ Identification of the gracilis is best done by visualizing the obturator nerve and the medial femoral circumflex vessels traversing underneath the adductor longus muscle en route to the medial aspect of the gracilis. ▪ The pedicle size can be small but can be followed below the adductor longus to its origin on the profunda for additional length and diameter. ▪ The pedicle is best found by scoring the fascia of the adductor longus exposing the space below the adductor that contains the medial femoral vessels and obturator nerve. ▪ Donor site seromas are less common in facial reanimation than when the gracilis is used in breast reconstruction but still warrant placement of a drain. ▪ Lidocaine should not be used as a vasodilator during this portion of the procedure to avoid any effects on nerve stimulation. Papaverine is preferred.

POSTOPERATIVE CARE

▪ Free muscle transfers are monitored via implantable Doppler probes. Postoperative flap checks are performed on an hourly basis for 2 days, followed by every 4 hours for the next 2 days.
▪ Our postoperative management follows a gradual increase in activity:
  ▪ Bed rest for 1 day
  ▪ Gradual and slow mobilization thereafter

▪ No pressure on the operated side of the face for 6 weeks
▪ Perioperative antibiotics are given.
▪ Signs of reinnervation are followed in the clinic and can generally be expected at 2 to 4 months when the nerve to the masseter is used and 6 to 12 months when a CFNG is used.
▪ Once reinnervation is noted on examination, therapy is started. Patients work with therapists specifically trained in facial reanimation rehabilitation. We believe this to be critical to success.

- Exercises done in front of a mirror are useful to provide a feedback mechanism and improve symmetry. This should be done 2 or 3 times a day for 4 to 5 minutes at a time.
- Therapy should be continued for a period of 6 months.

OUTCOMES

- The goal of a functional gracilis transfer is smile recreation using a single vector pull of the muscle. Thus, limitations exist. A pure symmetric smile is a lofty goal, but with attention to detail and therapy, dramatic results can be obtained (**FIG 6**).
- Studies have shown improved speech outcomes in patients with Mobius syndrome after undergoing bilateral gracilis transfers.

COMPLICATIONS

- Garcia et al. in a pooled data analysis reported a complication rate of 9.6%.[7]
- Complications included the following:
  - Postoperative hematoma (3.6%)
  - Infection (3.5%)
  - Vascular compromise (1.4%)
  - Salivary leak (1%)
  - Seroma (0.4%)
- Long-term failure of the muscle to reinnervate was reported at 1.8%

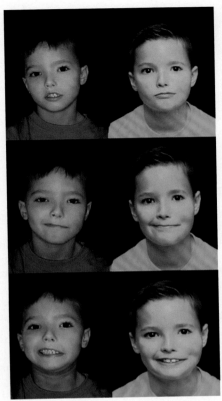

FIG 6 • Preoperative and 2-year postoperative pictures of the patient in **FIG 4**, who underwent a two-stage free gracilis transfer for a congenital facial nerve palsy.

REFERENCES

1. Garcia RM, Hadlock TA, Klebuc MJ, et al. Contemporary solutions for the treatment of facial nerve paralysis. *Plast Reconstr Surg.* 2015;135(6):1025e-1046e.
2. Westin LM, Zuker R. A new classification system for facial paralysis in the clinical setting. *J Craniofac Surg.* 2003;14(5):672-679.
3. Proctor B. The anatomy of the facial nerve. *Otolaryngol Clin North Am.* 1991;24(3):479-504.
4. Dorafshar AH, Borsuk DE, Bojovic B, et al. Surface anatomy of the middle division of the facial nerve: Zuker's point. *Plast Reconstr Surg.* 2013;131(2):253-257.
5. Fisher MD, Zhang Y, Erdmann D, Marcus J. Dissection of the masseter branch of the trigeminal nerve for facial reanimation. *Plast Reconstr Surg.* 2013;131(5):1065-1067.
6. Borschel GH, Kawamura DH, Kasukurthi R, et al. The motor nerve to the masseter muscle: An anatomic and histomorphometric study to facilitate its use in facial reanimation. *J Plast Reconstr Aesthet Surg.* 2012;65(3):363-366.
7. Garcia RM, Gosain AK, Zenn MR, Marcus JR. Early postoperative complications following gracilis free muscle transfer for facial reanimation: a systematic review and pooled data analysis. *J Reconstr Microsurg.* 2015;31(8):558-564.

53
CHAPTER

Corneal Neurotization

Joseph Catapano, Ronald Zuker, Asim Ali, and Gregory H. Borschel

DEFINITION

- Neurotrophic keratopathy is a degenerative corneal disease caused by impairment of corneal innervation.[1]
- Corneal neurotization involves using functioning sensory nerves from elsewhere on the face as donor nerves to reinnervate the cornea and restore corneal sensation and improve ocular surface health.

ANATOMY

- The cornea is the most densely innervated part of the body.[1,2]
- Corneal innervation derives from the ophthalmic branch (V1) of the trigeminal nerve (CN V).[3]
- Lesions may occur anywhere along the course of the corneal innervation pathway including the pons, the trigeminal (gasserian) ganglion, the ophthalmic branch, the nasociliary nerves, and the long ciliary nerves.
- Despite corneal nerve density, the cornea is supplied by relatively few trigeminal neurons as a single neuron may support hundreds of individual nerve endings.[4–6]
- The corneal innervation is divided into three networks: stromal, sub-basal, and epithelial.[7,8]

PATHOGENESIS

- Corneal sensation is a necessary component of reflexive tearing and blinking, which prevent corneal injury.
- Pain ordinarily would prompt patients to seek appropriate treatment after corneal injuries; however, an insensate cornea leaves patients unaware of their corneal injury.
- Repetitive corneal epithelial injury and ulceration cause corneal scarring and vision loss.[9–11]
- Corneal nerves also contain neuromediators that promote corneal epithelial maintenance and repair.[3,11]
- Immediately following corneal denervation, animal models show decreases in epithelial cell vitality and mitosis, resulting in thinning, breakdown, and ulceration of the corneal epithelium.[12–15]

NATURAL HISTORY

- Neurotrophic keratopathy is one of the most difficult ocular diseases to treat.[1]
- Prognosis is dependent on the severity of corneal hypoesthesia and the presence of other concomitant ocular disorders such as dry eye disease, exposure keratopathy, and corneal limbal stem cell deficiency.
- Patients require lifelong treatment and even with optimal management many develop vision loss and blindness in the affected eye.
- Inflammation and repeated corneal injury may also result in neovascularization of the cornea, further impeding vision.

PATIENT HISTORY AND FINDINGS

- Patients typically present with persistent asymptomatic corneal epithelial defects.
- Neurotrophic keratopathy is classified into three stages depending on clinical findings based on the Mackie classification[1]:
  - Stage 1: epithelial irregularity with punctate keratopathy and minimal stromal scarring.
  - Stage 2: epithelial ulceration surrounded by a rim of loose epithelium +/– stromal swelling.
  - Stage 3: corneal ulceration involving the stroma with risk of corneal perforation.

IMAGING AND OTHER DIAGNOSTIC STUDIES

- Diagnosis is based on clinical findings and a patient history of corneal hypoesthesia or anesthesia with delayed healing and persistence of corneal epithelial defects.[16,17]
- Slit lamp: identifies corneal epithelial abnormalities, including diffuse staining with fluorescein, epithelial sloughing, and stromal neovascularization.
- Corneal esthesiometry: measures corneal sensation. This can be performed with a Cochet-Bonnet aesthesiometer (Luneau, France) by a skilled ophthalmologist.
- Schirmer test: used to diagnose concomitant dry eye disease, when needed.
- In vivo corneal confocal microscopy (IVCCM): documents the absence of corneal nerve fibers.

DIFFERENTIAL DIAGNOSIS

- Hallmark for diagnosis is the presence of a corneal ulcer and the absence of corneal sensation.
- Possible etiologies of corneal anesthesia and hypoesthesia are as follows:[9,16]
  - Viral infection (herpes simplex and zoster keratoconjunctivitis)
  - Chemical burns
  - Physical injury to the trigeminal innervation (such as intracranial surgery)
  - Corneal surgery
  - Diabetes

- Leprosy
- Topical anesthetic abuse
- Congenital (such as trigeminal agenesis, cerebellar hypoplasia, brainstem hypoplasia)
- Certain disease may also exacerbate neurotrophic keratopathy:
  - Dry eye disease
  - Exposure keratopathy; facial nerve paralysis
  - Corneal limbal stem cell deficiency

NONOPERATIVE MANAGEMENT

- The goals of treatment are to prevent corneal ulceration and promote epithelial healing when ulcerations occur.[1,16,17]
  - Preservative-free topical artificial tears
  - Punctal occlusion
  - Therapeutic contact lenses (eg, the "Boston lens")
  - Topical antimicrobials
  - Protective tarsorrhaphy
- If a corneal perforation is suspected, then cyanoacrylate glue or keratoplasty (cornea transplant) may be indicated.
- Exacerbating conditions, such as exposure keratopathy and limbal stem cell deficiency, should be treated.
- Experimental treatments for persistent ulcerations include topical IGF-1, substance P, or nerve growth factor (NGF).[18–21]

SURGICAL MANAGEMENT

- Surgical management to restore corneal sensation in patients with corneal anesthesia or hypoesthesia has been described.[22–24]
- Samii first decribed a surgical technique to reinnervate the cornea using an intracranial approach through an osteoplastic frontal craniotomy to guide regenerating axons directly into the ophthalmic nerve using a long sural nerve graft and the occipital nerve as donor.
- Avoiding an intracranial approach, Terzis[22] described a technique using the peripheral nervous system to reinnervate the cornea by directly transferring the supraorbital and supratrochlear nerves to neurotize the cornea.
  - This technique necessitates a coronal incision and extensive dissection to access the supratrochlear and supraorbital nerves distally.
- This technique was then modified by Borschel, Ali, and Zuker,[23,24] who were able to avoid a coronal incision by guiding axons from the proximal supratrochlear nerve into the anesthetic cornea via a sural nerve graft.
  - This technique uses two small supraorbital incisions.
  - This approach is described in detail in this chapter.

Preoperative Planning

- Thorough facial sensory nerve examination and mapping must be done in order to identify potential donor nerves for reconstruction. The authors use an occupational therapist and Semmes-Weinstein monofilaments to document facial sensation.
- All patients should be evaluated by an ophthalmologist to document visual acuity, overall ocular health, and corneal sensation using Cochet-Bonnet aesthesiometry.

Positioning

- The patient is placed in the supine position on the operating table, and the entire face is prepped and draped (**FIG 1**).
- The leg to be used for sural nerve harvest is also prepped and draped.

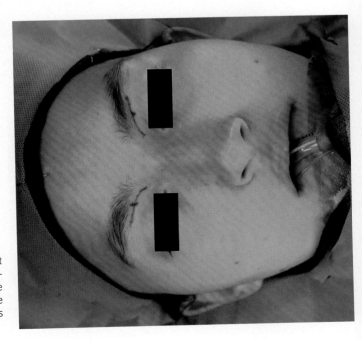

FIG 1 • We prefer to operate from the head of the bed with the patient in the supine position. Even with a thorough sensory examination documenting normal sensation in the contralateral face, we have found the donor supratrochlear or supraorbital nerves to be insufficiently large enough for coaptation on occasion. For this reason, we prep the patient's entire face in case we use the infraorbital nerve as a donor.

■ Sural Nerve Harvest

- This can be performed using the surgeon's preference. We prefer using a nerve stripper device that permits harvesting of the proximal tibial component of the sural nerve, which usually provides a branch-free graft of sufficient length.

Identification of the Contralateral Supratrochlear Nerve

- Any functioning sensory nerve in the face can be used for corneal neurotization.
- Many patients have hemifacial sensory deficits associated with neurotrophic keratopathy. Our preferred technique is to use the contralateral supratrochlear nerve as a donor. If the ipsilateral supratrochlear or supraorbital nerves are normal and available, they may be used instead of the contralateral nerves.
- Two- to three-centimeter supraorbital incisions are made on the medial lower border of the eyebrows over each eye (**TECH FIG 1A**).
- The donor supratrochlear or supraorbital nerve is then identified through this incision on the donor side (**TECH FIG 1B**).
- The supratrochlear nerve is identified deep to the origin of the frontalis muscle, on the surface of the corrugator

supercilii muscle traveling cephalad from the supratrochlear notch.
- The supratrochlear notch can often be palpated to guide dissection.
- Some supratrochlear nerves divide distal to the notch. Both branches can be incorporated as donors.

Tunneling of the Sural Nerve Graft to the Affected Cornea

- Once the supratrochlear or supraorbital nerve has been identified, the contralateral incision over the affected eye is deepened to the level of the subcutaneous tissue.
- A fine hemostat is used to bluntly dissect a subcutaneous plane between the two incisions to provide a passage for the sural nerve graft.
- With the distal portion of the hemostat through the incision on the affected eyelid, the distal end of the sural nerve graft is grasped and pulled through the subcutaneous pocket so that the nerve graft is traversing the incisions, reversing the direction of the nerve graft for coaptation.
- A superonasal perilimbal incision is made in the conjunctiva using blunt scissors, and a small pocket is made in the potential space between the sclera and Tenon capsule (**TECH FIG 2A**).

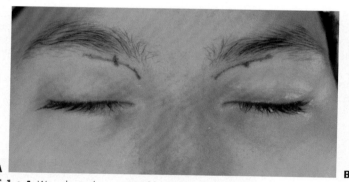 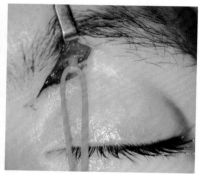

TECH FIG 1 • A. We palpate the supratrochlear notch to mark two incisions over the ipsilateral and contralateral supratrochlear nerves. As most patients with corneal anesthesia have hemifacial sensory abnormalities, we most frequently use the contralateral supratrochlear nerve as a donor sensory nerve for corneal neurotization. **B.** The supratrochlear nerve is identified below the level of the frontalis muscle at the location of the supratrochlear notch and is secured with vessel loop.

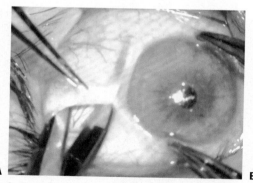 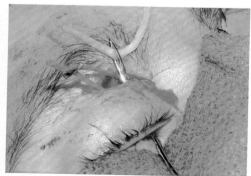

TECH FIG 2 • A. Once the sural nerve graft has been tunneled to the ipsilateral supraorbital incision, an incision is made into the perilimbal conjunctiva and a potential space is expanded between the conjunctiva and sclera. This permits the Wright needle to be passed from the perilimbal conjunctiva to the ipsilateral supraorbital skin incision. **B.** The Wright needle is passed from the perilimbal conjunctival incision into the ipsilateral supraorbital skin incision. The sural nerve graft is then placed within the eye of the needle, tunneling the sural nerve graft into the orbit as the needle is withdrawn through the perilimbal conjunctival incision.

- A Wright needle (curved ophthalmologic trocar with eyelet) is then used to pass the sural nerve graft from the supraorbital incision over the affected eye, below the conjunctiva and Tenon capsule, to be delivered to the perilimbal incision (**TECH FIG 2B**).

Dissection of the Sural Nerve Fascicles

- Under the operating microscope and on the surface of the affected eye, the sural nerve graft is divided into separate fascicles so that they may be evenly distributed around the eye to reinnervate the cornea (**TECH FIG 3A**).
- We aim to produce three to four fascicles from the sural nerve graft; however, in many patients, we have used only two fascicles, with good results.
- The fascicles are then distributed around the cornea to evenly distribute the location of regenerating axons into the cornea (**TECH FIG 3B**).

Tunneling of Fascicles Into the Corneal Stroma

- Separate perilimbal incisions are then made for each of the fascicles, and again a small perilimbal pocket is made between the sclera and Tenon capsule. Each fascicle in then tunneled below the conjuctiva into these incisions to lie adjacent to the cornea.
- A corneal scalpel blade is used to make a small scleral tunnel incision 1.0 to 1.5 mm from the limbus and approximately 1.5 mm wide (about twice the width of the fascicle) into the clear peripheral cornea so that each fascicle can be tunneled directly into the cornea (**TECH FIG 4A**).
- The nerve graft fascicle is then gently placed directly into the stromal pocket (**TECH FIG 4B**), and 10-0 absorbable (Vicryl) stitch is placed through the sclera and the epineurium of the fascicle to keep the fascicle in place.
- This is then done for each of the fascicles individually.
- Each of the perilimbal conjunctival incisions are then closed with 10-0 absorbable stitch (**TECH FIG 4C**) being careful to avoid any exposure of the fascicles.

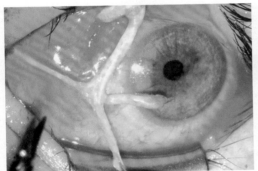 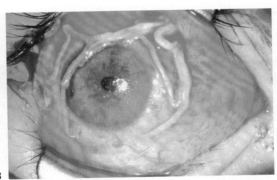

TECH FIG 3 • A. Once overlaying the cornea, the sural nerve graft is dissected into separate fascicles. **B.** Once divided into separate fascicles, these are distributed evenly around the cornea. In our experience, there are a variable number of fascicles in the sural nerve. We aim to have at least two fascicles, with a maximum of four when available. Each fascicle is then tunneled below the level of the conjunctiva through perilimbal incisions to surround the eye.

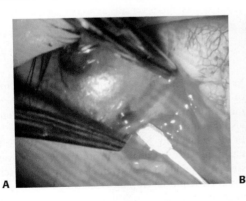 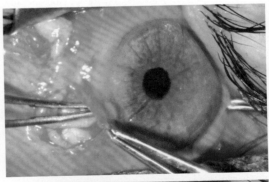 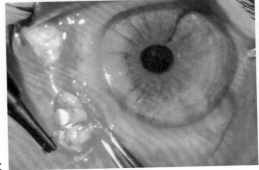

TECH FIG 4 • A. Through each perilimbal incision, an ophthalmic scalpel is used to make a pocket within the corneal stroma. **B.** Once the stromal pocket has been made, the fascicle is tunneled directly into the corneal stroma using forceps. In the image, the distal portion of the sural nerve graft can be seen protruding into the corneal stroma. Each fascicle is sutured into place proximal to the stromal pocket using 10-0 absorbable sutures. **C.** After the sural nerve fascicle has been tunneled into the corneal stroma and secured to the sclera with a 10-0 stitch, the perilimbal conjunctival incision is sutured closed.

TECHNIQUES

- A limbal incision and tunneling the nerve fascicles directly into the corneal stroma may significantly improve nerve regrowth as the limbus may act as a barrier to corneal nerve ingrowth.
- The affected eye is then closed with a temporary central tarsorrhaphy suture to protect the corneal surface after surgery, and this is left in place for 1 to 2 weeks.
- If a permanent lateral tarsorrhaphy has not been performed previously, it can be done at this step.

Nerve Coaptation

- As the final step, the distal portion of the sural nerve graft is coapted to the supratrochlear nerve in an end-to-end fashion with 10-0 nylon suture or fibrin glue (**TECH FIG 5**) or both glue and sutures, depending on surgeon preference.
- The supraorbital incisions are closed with a 6-0 subcuticular Monocryl stitch.

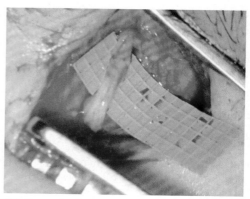

TECH FIG 5 • Once all conjunctival incisions have been closed, the distal portion of the sural nerve graft is coapted to the proximal stump of the transected supratrochlear nerve. We have also done side-to-end repair; however, we prefer this technique as we have found the donor site morbidity to be minimal and end-to-end repair recruits a greater number of donor sensory axons.

PEARLS AND PITFALLS

Preoperative considerations	▪ A thorough sensory examination is necessary prior to the operation to identify normal functioning donor nerves.

Acquired vs congenital cases	▪ Acquired cases usually have straightforward neuroanatomy.
	▪ Congenital cases often have aberrant anatomy.
	  ▪ These cases may have complete absence of any supratrochlear or supraorbital nerves despite intact glabellar sensation.
	  ▪ We have also used the ipsilateral infraorbital nerve to reconstruct corneal sensation.

Nerve harvest	▪ The tibial contribution to sural nerve is usually sufficient length. This can be harvested through a popliteal incision and a small counter incision in the midcalf.
Postoperative considerations	▪ Keep postoperative patients out of sports or vigorous activities for 6 weeks. ▪ Patients may experience pain once innervation occurs; this is actually a positive sign, but they should be warned in advance.

POSTOPERATIVE CARE

- Patients should be under the care of an ophthalmologist pre-, intra-, and postoperatively.
- The intraoperative tarsorrhaphy suture is left in place for 1 week.
- Patients are provided with postoperative topical medication:
  - Topical tobramycin and dexamethasone ointment until the tarsorrhaphy is removed
  - Topical moxifloxacin and prednisolone eyedrops
  - Preservative-free lubricating eyedrops
- Sensory and vision outcomes are monitored regularly by the ophthalmologist.

OUTCOMES

- To date, there are have been only two series published describing outcomes in patients with corneal neurotization by Terzis[22] and Borschel[23,24] and a case report by Samii.

- In Terzis' series, all 6 patients were followed for an average of 16.3 ± 2.42 years and demonstrated significant improvements in corneal sensibility with no further deterioration of visual acuity or overall corneal health.[22]
- In Borschel and Ali's series, using the described surgical technique for corneal neurotization, all patients demonstrated significant improvements in corneal sensation with some patients developing sensation indistinguishable from normal with Cochet-Bonnet esthesiometry; however, follow-up had not been carried out far enough to definitively determine vision outcomes.[23]

COMPLICATIONS

- Axon regrowth through the nerve graft and into the cornea may take several months with this sural nerve grafting technique.
- Using the contralateral supratrochlear nerve results in minimal sensory loss on the donor side.

- Inability to regain protective sensation after corneal neurotization may be caused by unrecognized insufficiency of the donor nerve.
- Loss of sensation on the lateral ankle and foot after sural nerve harvest is of minimal functional consequence.

REFERENCES

1. Bonini S, Rama P, Olzi D, Lambiase A. Neurotrophic keratitis. *Eye (Lond)*. 2003;17(8):989-995.
2. Rozsa AJ, Beuerman RW. Density and organization of free nerve endings in the corneal epithelium of the rabbit. *Pain*. 1982;14:105-120.
3. Müller LJ, Marfurt CF, Kruse F, Tervo TMT. Corneal nerves: structure, contents and function. *Exp Eye Res*. 2003;76(5):521-542.
4. de Castro F, Silos-Santiago I, de Armentia M, et al. Corneal innervation and sensitivity to noxious stimuli in trkA knockout mice. *Eur J Neurosci*. 1998;10:146-152.
5. De Felipe C, Gonzalez GG, Gallar J, Belmonte C. Quantification and immunocytochemical characteristics of trigeminal ganglion neurons projecting to the cornea: effect of corneal wounding. *Eur J Pain*. 1999;3:31-39.
6. LaVail JH, Johnson WE, Spencer LC. Immunohistochemical identification of trigeminal ganglion neurons that innervate the mouse cornea: relevance to intercellular spread of herpes simplex virus. *J Comp Neurol*. 1993;327:133-140.
7. Al-Aqaba MA, Fares U, Suleman H, et al. Architecture and distribution of human corneal nerves. *Br J Ophthalmol*. 2010;94(6):784-789.
8. Marfurt CF, Cox J, Deek S, Dvorscak L. Anatomy of the human corneal innervation. *Exp Eye Res*. 2010;90(4):478-492.
9. Lambley RG, Pereyra-Muñoz N, Parulekar M, et al. Structural and functional outcomes of anaesthetic cornea in children. *Br J Ophthalmol*. 2014:1-7.
10. Ramaesh K, Stokes J, Henry E, et al. Congenital corneal anesthesia. *Surv Ophthalmol*. 2007;52(1):50-60.
11. Rosenberg M. Congenital trigeminal anaesthesia. *Brain*. 1984;107:1073-1082.
12. Alper M. The anesthetic eye: an investigation of changes in the anterior ocular segment of the monkey caused by interrupting the trigeminal nerve at various levels along its course. *Trans Am Ophthalmol Soc*. 1975;73:313-365.
13. Beuerman R, Schimmelpfennig B. Sensory denervation of the rabbit cornea affects epithelial properties. *Exp Neurol*. 1980;69:196-201.
14. Cavanagh H, Colley A. The molecular basis of neurotrophic keratitis. *Acta Ophthalmol*. 1989;192:115-134.
15. Sigelman S, Friedenwald J. Mitotic and wound-healing activities of the corneal epithelium. *Arch Ophthalmol*. 1954;52:46-57.
16. Goins KM. New insights into the diagnosis and treatment of neurotrophic keratopathy. *Ocul Surf*. 2005;3(2):96-110.
17. Sacchetti M, Lambiase A. Diagnosis and management of neurotrophic keratitis. *Clin Ophthalmol*. 2014;8:571-579.
18. Chikama T, Fukuda K, Morishige N, Nishida T. Treatment of neurotrophic keratopathy with substance-p-derived peptide (FGLM) and insulin-like growth factor I. *Lancet*. 1998;351:1783-1788.
19. Brown SM, Lamberts DW, Reid TW, et al. Neurotrophic and anhidrotic keratopathy treated with substance P and insulinlike growth factor 1. *Arch Ophthalmol*. 1997;115:926-927.
20. Bonini S, Lambiase A, Rama P, et al. Tropical treatment with nerve growth factor for neurotrophic keratitis. *Ophthalmology*. 2000;107(7):1347-1352.
21. Lambiase A, Rama P, Bonini S, Caprioglio G, Aloe L. Topical treatment with nerve growth factor for corneal neurotrophic ulcers. *N Engl J Med*. 1998;338(17):1174-1180.
22. Terzis JK, Dryer MM, Bodner BI. Corneal neurotization: a novel solution to neurotrophic keratopathy. *Plast Reconstr Surg*. 2009;123(1):112-120.
23. Elbaz U, Bains R, Zuker RM, et al. Restoration of corneal sensation with regional nerve transfers and nerve grafts: a new approach to a difficult problem. *JAMA Ophthalmol*. 2014;132(11):1289-1295.
24. Bains R, Elbaz U, Zuker R, et al. Corneal neurotization from the supratrochlear nerve with sural nerve grafts: a minimally-invasive approach. *Plast Reconstr Surg*. 2015;135(2):397e-400e.

54
CHAPTER

Section XIII: Brachial Plexus (Obstetrical Injury)
Primary Treatment of Neonatal Brachial Plexus Palsy

Bryce R. Bell, Ji-Geng Yan, and Hani Matloub

DEFINITION

- Injury to the nerves supplying the upper extremity (C5-T1) during the birth process
- Epidemiology[1]
  - Incidence can vary greatly by institution.
  - The most recent nationwide study shows 1.51 per 1000 live births in the USA.
- Risk factors[1–3]
  - Shoulder dystocia
  - Macrosomia (greater than 4–4.5 kg)
  - Instrumented delivery
  - Prior delivery with brachial plexus injury
  - Prolonged labor resulting in hypotonia
  - Tachysystole during labor
  - Use of oxytocin
  - Studies have consistently shown that more than half of patients with neonatal brachial plexus palsy (NBPP) have no identifiable risk factor.

ANATOMY

- Normally, the brachial plexus has contributions from C5 to T1.
- Can have prefixed or postfixed cords with contributions from C4 (22%) and T2 (1%), respectively
- Roots combine to form upper (C5/C6), middle (C7), and lower trunks (C8/T1).
- Near the level of the clavicle, these trunks give off anterior and posterior divisions to form lateral, medial, and posterior cords, so named for their relation to the axillary artery. The lateral cord is formed from the confluence of the anterior divisions of the upper and middle trunks. The posterior cord is formed from the posterior divisions of all three trunks. Finally, the medial cord consists of only the anterior division of the lower trunk.
- Cords then divide into terminal branches (musculocutaneous, axillary, radial, median, and ulnar).
- Smaller branches originate from various levels in the brachial plexus and are important in localizing the level of injury by clinical examination (**FIG 1**).
- The sympathetic chain runs along the ventral aspect of the exiting roots and is often disrupted in root avulsions from the spinal cord. This accounts for the findings seen in Horner syndrome.

PATHOGENESIS

- Mechanism of injury
  - Most commonly a downward force on the shoulder causes deviation of the neck away from the involved extremity.

This typically involves at least the C5-C6 roots but can result in complete plexus injury.
- More rarely, injury can occur due to extreme cranial traction on the extremity with neck extension during breech delivery. These injuries often involve the lower roots.
- Traditionally, injury was thought to be caused by traction during delivery by the obstetrician, by either manual or instrumented delivery.
- However, given that more than half of children with brachial plexus injuries do not have an identifiable risk factor, some debate exists on the presence of an intrauterine mechanism of injury that is more difficult to identify. One study estimated uterine contractions exert up to 9 times greater force on the shoulder than that applied by the obstetrician.[4]
- In addition, Walsh et al. showed no significant decrease in incidence of NBPP despite structured training on management of shoulder dystocia and a rising cesarean section rate.[5]
- These injuries result in varying degrees of weakness in the ipsilateral extremity, ranging from subtle weakness to flaccid paralysis.
- Classifications of Seddon and Sunderland
  - Seddon divided nerve injuries into three categories: neurapraxia, axonotmesis, and neurotmesis.[6]

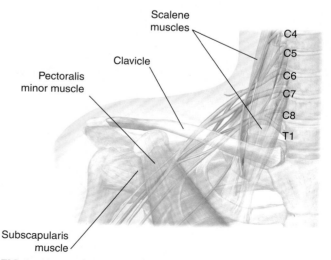

FIG 1 • The most common anatomy of the brachial plexus. The branching of the brachial plexus can be highly variable, and a thorough understanding of the most common variants is crucial prior to proceeding with brachial plexus exploration.

■ Neurapraxic injuries have a transient loss of conduction, but do not undergo wallerian degeneration. In axonotmesis, the nerve is still externally in continuity but undergoes wallerian degeneration due to axonal disruption. Neurotmesis indicates a complete division of a nerve.

■ Sunderland classified neurapraxia as type I and neurotmesis as type V. The axonotmesis category is divided into three separate categories, types II to IV, based on degree of internal injury short of complete division of the nerve.[7] MacKinnon and Dellon later added a type VI injury, indicating multiple degrees of injury in a single cross-sectional area of a nerve.[8] This has been termed a neuroma-in-continuity.

■ Wallerian degeneration occurs in axonotmetic and neurotmetic lesions due to axonal disruption. While there is some chance of recovery in axonotmetic lesions depending on the degree of internal injury, neurotmetic lesions will not recover without surgical repair or grafting.

■ Contractures
  ■ Denervation leads to a progressive joint contracture due to muscle paralysis. This joint contracture was generally believed to be caused by muscle imbalance and fibrosis of denervated muscle groups. However, animal studies have shown that muscle contracture precedes fibrosis, indicating a separate, yet to be determined mechanism.[9]
  ■ Two types of joint contractures are seen in NBPP patients. The first is due to overpowering of affected muscles by their antagonists, as is seen with the internal rotation contracture at the shoulder in Erb palsy. The second is due to muscle contracture and shortening, as seen in the glenohumeral abduction contracture caused by the paralyzed deltoid or the elbow flexion contracture caused by the brachialis in Erb palsy.
  ■ Global shoulder dysfunction and glenohumeral deformity develop as early as 3 months due to unbalanced forces on the shoulder and may require open or arthroscopic reduction and tendon transfers for treatment.
  ■ It has also been shown that each segment of the upper extremity exhibits decreased length and girth compared to the unaffected extremity.[10]

NATURAL HISTORY

■ In the past, full recovery had been reported to be as high as 95.7%.[11] However, more recent reports claim less optimistic spontaneous recovery rates in the 60% to 70% range.[12,13]

■ Upon closer analysis, it is clear that location and severity of injury, as well as the degree of spontaneous recovery by 3 to 6 months, can all dramatically change the prognosis for a given patient. Assessing these factors is essential to recommending a plan of care to the patient's parents.

■ In patients with only mild weakness and rapid recovery within weeks, complete neurologic recovery is highly likely without surgical intervention.

■ However, in patients with a flaccid upper extremity and Horner syndrome (indicating a complete brachial plexus injury with avulsion), acceptable recovery is extremely unlikely, and early surgical intervention at about 3 months is recommended. Even in the case where there is some degree of proximal muscle improvement, if the hand is still paralyzed at 3 months, one should proceed with surgical

intervention to reinnervate the hand, as these patients are unlikely to recover meaningful hand function on their own.

■ The remainder of neonatal brachial plexus patients fall between these two extremes, and the decision on the appropriate timing for intervention, if any, is still controversial.

PATIENT HISTORY AND PHYSICAL FINDINGS

■ History should include a detailed maternal gestational history as well as patient birth history. The physician should seek specific information on the course of delivery, shoulder dystocia, instrumented delivery, respiratory distress or signs of hypoxia, and Apgar scores. This information can be helpful in ruling out other causes of apparent limb weakness or paralysis (ie, cerebral palsy, infection, fracture of the involved limb).

■ Careful, systematic examination is crucial for making treatment decisions and comparisons over time. Given the importance of examination over time and the negative effects of delayed treatment, early referral to a multidisciplinary brachial plexus clinic is recommended. This will not only facilitate early surgical intervention when necessary but also ensure that patients receive prompt physical and occupational therapy to mitigate joint contracture formation while awaiting recovery.

■ Physical examination should be performed with the child naked from the waist up to assess the entire upper extremity as well as the neck, chest, back, scapula, and abdomen. In the infant, physical examination relies heavily on observance of limb posture, spontaneous motion, neonatal reflexes, and passive motion.

■ Certain postures have traditionally been associated with different levels of injury. The "waiter's tip" posture describes a patient with the shoulder internally rotated, elbow extended, and wrist flexed. This posture would be suggestive of an upper plexus injury. Inversely, a patient with a lower plexus injury may have near normal shoulder and elbow function with a flaccid hand. A totally flaccid extremity indicates a complete brachial plexus injury.

■ Horner syndrome describes a patient with ipsilateral ptosis, meiosis, and anhidrosis. This is indicative of a preganglionic avulsion from the spinal cord.

■ There are many assessment tools and classification systems that can help synthesize information from the physical examination and assist in treatment decision-making. The most commonly used scores include the modified Mallet scale, the Active Movement Scale, and the Toronto Test Score. All three of these scores have been assessed for inter- and intrarater reliability.

■ The modified Mallet scale is a widely used measure of global shoulder function and does not grade specific muscles. It requires that the patient is mature enough to follow directions.

■ The Active Movement Scale (AMS) is a detailed scoring of 15 different movements on a scale of 1 to 7. It was developed to quantify motor function in infants with NBPP and evaluate recovery over time. It can be used as early as 2 to 3 weeks of age by eliciting neonatal reflexes to assess specific joint movements.[15]

■ The Toronto Test Score was developed to help predict recovery in children with NBPP. It can be used in young children who are unable to follow directions and tests five specific motions: elbow flexion, elbow extension, wrist extension, thumb extension, and finger extension.[14]

IMAGING AND OTHER DIAGNOSTIC STUDIES

- Although the decision to proceed with primary nerve surgery for NBPP is a clinical one, further diagnostic testing can provide useful information in development of a surgical plan.
- Electrodiagnostic testing can be useful in determining preganglionic vs postganglionic lesions because avulsions will show normal sensory nerve action potential with no motor nerve conduction at the same level. However, these studies tend to overestimate the degree of recovery in NBPP and thus are not routinely used in surgical decision-making.
- Computed tomography (CT) myelography can also be useful in determining the presence of root avulsions preoperatively. One study showed 98% specificity, but only 37% sensitivity for CT myelography in diagnosing root avulsions if no rootlets are seen traversing the pseudomeningocele.[16]
- Another study compared CT myelography to MR myelography and found similar results for CT myelography to prior studies. However, MR myelography on a 3T magnet showed equivalent sensitivity and specificity without the need for lumbar puncture, intrathecal contrast injection, or ionizing radiation. Therefore, with improvements in technology, many now favor MR over CT myelography.[17]
- Other imaging modalities that some find useful are ultrasound to assess diaphragmatic motion and chest radiography to look for an elevated hemidiaphragm. Abnormal findings would indicate phrenic nerve injury. This is particularly important if one is considering using the phrenic or intercostal nerves for plexus reconstruction.

DIFFERENTIAL DIAGNOSIS

- Spinal cord injury
- Pseudoparalysis
  - Septic joint
  - Upper extremity fracture
- Cerebral palsy

NONOPERATIVE MANAGEMENT

- Patients should be referred early to an occupational therapist with experience in neonatal brachial plexus injuries. Ideally, this therapist will see the patient at the same time as the surgeon to facilitate communication.
- Therapy should focus stretching and range of motion of the entire upper extremity to prevent contractures and maladaptive motions. It is particularly important to stabilize the scapula during shoulder range of motion and stretching to make sure motion is truly glenohumeral and not scapulothoracic.

SURGICAL MANAGEMENT

- The decision to proceed with microsurgical repair or reconstruction of the brachial plexus is perhaps the most controversial topic in management of neonatal brachial plexus injuries.
- As discussed earlier, most surgeons agree that infants with a flaccid extremity, Horner syndrome, or other signs of a preganglionic avulsion warrant early exploration and microsurgical intervention.

- Gilbert and Tassin popularized the absence of biceps function at 3 months as an indication to proceed with microsurgery.[3] However, another study showed that when biceps function alone was used in decision-making, it would have incorrectly predicted recovery in 12.8% of cases.[14]
- The Hospital for Sick Children reports using AMS for initial evaluation of infants with NBPP. At 3 months, a conversion is made for scores of elbow flexion and elbow, wrist, thumb, and finger extension. The converted scores are then summed. If the score is above 3.5, then observation is continued and the patient re-evaluated every 3 months for continued improvement. If the patient fails to improve at each visit or fails the "cookie test" at 9 months, then microsurgery is scheduled.[18]
- After assessing the outcomes of patients managed by observation, microsurgery, and/or secondary orthopedic procedures (tendon transfer or external rotation osteotomy), Waters concluded that he would operate on infants with no return of biceps function by 5 months or a flail arm and Horner syndrome at 3 months.[19]
- We prefer to use the absence of any biceps function at 4 months as a trigger to proceed with surgery, re-evaluating monthly for continued improvement in those with some biceps function present at 4 months. Our center has performed surgery at up to a year for those that present late to our clinic for initial evaluation without biceps function. In these cases, we are likely to perform a bypass graft around the neuroma rather than neuroma resection and grafting, to avoid resecting any regenerated axons.

PREOPERATIVE PLANNING

- Once the clinical decision is made to proceed with surgery, develop a carefully considered operative plan that incorporates information from physical examination, imaging, and electrodiagnostic testing, if obtained.
- Review the results of the physical examination and imaging to estimate the number of roots involved and if they are ruptures or avulsions. The former are often amenable to neuroma resection and grafting, whereas the latter require neurotization from other levels or extraplexal nerves. If several levels are involved, prepare for transfer of nerves from outside the plexus to innervate critical targets for upper extremity function. This may require further workup with diaphragmatic ultrasound or chest radiographs to determine if the phrenic nerve or intercostal nerves are a suitable option for extraplexal neurotization.
- Consider what portion of the plexus is injured in a proximal to distal direction. Though most injuries are supraclavicular, more distal involvement may require a clavicular osteotomy and/or extension of the incision to expose the deltopectoral interval.
- In the case that the entire plexus is involved, the lower roots are usually avulsed, and options are limited for reinnervation. Although priority is usually given to elbow flexion and shoulder stability in adults, in NBPP, some advocate that priority should be given to grafting nerve roots supplying the hand because it is a shorter distance to regenerate than in adults, a greater capacity for healing, and more

neural plasticity in the brain. In addition, there are proven extraplexal nerve transfer options for shoulder and elbow function.

- Failure to plan for all potential scenarios and their solutions not only prolongs surgical time but may compromise the ultimate outcome for the patient if inappropriate decisions are made intraoperatively.
- The surgeon should request avoidance of muscle paralysis after induction of anesthesia to allow for assessment of signal transmission across neuromas via nerve stimulation.
- In some centers, pathology service is consulted to perform fresh frozen specimens for evaluation of neuromas to confirm resection to healthy axons before grafting.
- Neurology may be consulted for intraoperative evaluation of somatosensory evoked potentials (SSEPs). This can be extremely helpful when trying to distinguish between an intact root, an intraforaminal rupture, and an avulsion from the spinal cord. However, this requires special training on the part of the interpreting neurologist and is only available in a limited number of centers.

Positioning

- Some centers begin with the patient positioned in the prone position and perform bilateral sural nerve harvest prior to exploration. We prefer to begin in the supine position and perform the brachial plexus exploration prior to harvest, as this may avoid unnecessary nerve harvest if bilateral sural nerve grafts are not needed.
- For plexus exploration and reconstruction, the patient should be positioned supine with a small, transversely oriented roll placed at the level of the scapulae to extend the neck and to rotate to the contralateral side of the injury by improving access to the injured plexus.
- We also recommend placing the patient's head at the most proximal extent of the bed and the ipsilateral shoulder near the edge of the bed to improve positioning and access for the surgeon and assistants (**FIG 2**).
- It is crucial to assure that all bony prominences are well padded, as the procedure can last up to 12 hours. A Foley catheter with a temperature probe is also placed for urine output monitoring, fluid management, and avoidance of hypothermia.
- The patient should be prepped and draped from the level of the mandible proximally to just below the nipple on the ipsilateral chest and the ipsilateral extremity draped free (**FIG 3**).
- If considering use of the contralateral C7 nerve root, it will be necessary to prep and drape the contralateral chest and neck as well. In addition, both legs should have a tourniquet placed on the thigh and be prepped and draped for a possible sural nerve harvest.

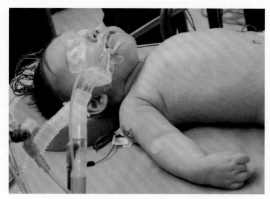

FIG 2 • The patient is positioned with the head at the most proximal extent of the bed and the ipsilateral shoulder near the edge of the bed to improve positioning and access for the surgeon and assistants. A transverse roll should be placed posteriorly at the level of the scapulae to allow neck extension and rotation away from the injured side.

Approach

- Although some surgeons use a straight incision paralleling the upper border of the clavicle for exposure, we prefer the use of an L-shaped incision.
- The proximal limb follows the posterior border of the sternocleidomastoid (SCM) muscle, and the transverse limb follows the superior border of the clavicle.
- We believe this improves access to the neural foramina to assess for proximal rupture vs avulsion from the spinal cord during initial exploration or end-to-side neurotization into the phrenic nerve, if necessary.

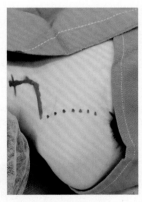

FIG 3 • The patient is prepped and draped from the level of the mandible proximally to just below the nipple on the ipsilateral chest, with the ipsilateral arm draped free. The incision is marked along the posterior border of the sternocleidomastoid (SCM) with the transverse limb following the superior border of the clavicle.

■ Exposure

- The expected incision should be marked out clearly and hashed for correct closure at the conclusion of the case (see **FIG 3**). Formerly, our center injected the line of the incision with epinephrine diluted 1 to 400 000 to minimize blood loss during initial dissection. However, we have found that with careful dissection using electrocautery, epinephrine infusion is not necessary and eliminates a potential source of error in appropriate dilution.
- Dissection is taken down through the platysma with meticulous care to coagulate superficial vessels, attempting to minimize blood loss during the case. The flap is raised in the plane just below the platysma and reflected superolaterally to expose the posterior triangle. This is tied back with suture for retraction throughout the case.
- At this point, it may be necessary to reflect the clavicular head of the SCM and ligate the nearby external jugular vein to improve exposure of the anterior and middle scalene muscles and the more proximal nerve roots. The clavicular head of the SCM should be tagged and repaired at the conclusion of the case.
- Moving laterally, the omohyoid is either divided at its tendinous portion or tagged and retracted. The omohyoid is a consistent marker for the level of the suprascapular notch.
- During this exposure, the branches of the cervical plexus extending across the clavicle to the upper chest will be encountered and divided. With careful dissection, these can be traced proximally to identify the C4 root and then excised and used as additional nerve graft.
- There will be a fat pad at the level deep to the omohyoid that should be released from the clavicle, tagged, and reflected superolaterally. This should be repaired back to the clavicle during closure.
- Additionally, the transverse cervical vessels will cross the surgical field and may need to be ligated and cut to facilitate access to the supraclavicular brachial plexus.
- After this, the upper and middle trunks are often visible exiting between the anterior and middle scalene muscles. The junction of the C5 and C6 roots is the most common

site for neuroma formation and is often visible now (**TECH FIG 1A**).
- Identify the phrenic nerve running in a cranial-to-caudal direction along the lateral border of the anterior scalene, and trace this proximally to its contribution from the C4 nerve root. Frequently the phrenic nerve gives off a contribution to the C5 nerve root. The identity of the phrenic nerve can be confirmed using a nerve stimulator and watching for contraction of the diaphragm. One should notify the anesthesia team to hold respiration during phrenic nerve stimulation to avoid confusion.
- This should give two markers confirming the levels of the brachial plexus. In many cases, the phrenic nerve is entrapped in scar tissue as it passes over the involved plexus, and care should be taken not to injure or excise it during dissection or neuroma resection.
- Often the anterior and middle scalene muscles are also included in the scar around the brachial plexus, and careful dissection is required to separate them and adequately expose the roots and the neural foramina (**TECH FIG 1B**).
- Once the levels have been appropriately identified, begin dissecting the C5 nerve root proximally to determine continuity all the way to the spinal cord. The branch to the long thoracic nerve should be identified during dissection of C5-C7 and protected initially. However, some or all of these branches may need to be sacrificed later during neuroma resection and grafting in the case of very proximal injuries.
- Carry out the same dissection proximally for C6-T1, inspecting closely for intraforaminal rupture or avulsion from the spinal cord. Again, the scalene muscles must be dissected free from the neuroma to allow enough retraction to inspect the more caudal C8 and T1 roots. In addition, caudal to C7, the subclavian vein and clavicle will need to be retracted to improve exposure. Take care to avoid violating the pleura just distal to T1.
- If there is uncertainty regarding whether or not a preganglionic avulsion exists, either a specimen can be sent for pathologic assessment to evaluate for involvement of the dorsal root ganglion or SSEPs can be evaluated if neurology service is available.

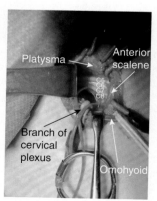

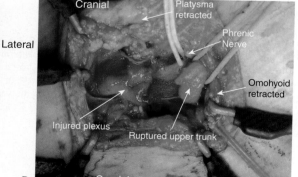

TECH FIG 1 • A. With the superficial dissection complete, the upper and middle trunks are often visible exiting between the anterior and middle scalene muscles. The junction of the C5 and C6 roots is the most common site for neuroma formation, and the neuroma is often visible now. **B.** In more severely scarred cases, accurate identification of individual roots and determining which levels are intact, ruptured, or avulsed is often difficult. A nerve stimulator and intraoperative electrodiagnostic testing can be helpful.

- Next, dissect from proximal to distal along the cranial border of the C5 root and upper trunk to locate the suprascapular nerve exiting posteriorly toward the suprascapular notch. It is classically described as branching from the upper trunk. However, recent cadaver studies have shown that it often branches at or after the split of the anterior and posterior divisions of the upper trunk (most often from the posterior division) and can even have contributions from both the anterior and posterior divisions of the upper trunk.[20]
- Continue laterally to identify the anterior division of the upper trunk and potentially the lateral pectoral nerve depending on its level of branching. This is traditionally described as branching from the lateral cord. However, it most often originates from the anterior division of the upper trunk rather than the lateral cord proper.[20]
- Next dissect from the C7 root distally to identify the middle trunk with its anterior and posterior divisions. Continue this dissection distally until nerves are free of neuroma.

- Carry out the same dissection of the lower trunk distally to its anterior and posterior divisions and, if necessary, to the medial cord. Identify its branches as you dissect distally. It will be necessary to carefully dissect and retract the clavicle and subclavian vein during this portion of the dissection.
- Once all components of the plexus are identified, a nerve stimulator should be used to determine which portions of the brachial plexus are transmitting sufficient signals distally. Catalogue this information clearly and carefully to avoid neglecting essential functions during reconstruction.
- If infraclavicular access is also needed, this incision can be joined laterally with a standard deltopectoral incision near the coracoid process.
- Once the conjoined tendon is identified, the tendon can be tagged, cut, and reflected to expose the lateral, posterior, and medial cords as well as their terminal branches. This will be repaired at the conclusion of the case.

■ Neuroma Resection With Nerve Grafting

- Although neurolysis alone of a neuroma-in-continuity was performed in the past, it is no longer recommended due to inferior outcomes when compared to neuroma resection and grafting.[21] Therefore, if it is determined that there is insufficient signal transmission across a neuroma, then resection and grafting should be performed.
- As mentioned in the prior section, careful dissection should be performed proximal and distal to the site of injury to ensure that there is a complete understanding of the injured structures. Do not presume a normal appearing nerve root proximal to a neuroma is not avulsed based solely on visual appearance. It is possible to have a two-level injury with avulsion from the spinal cord and a neuroma distally.
- Begin by sectioning the midportion of the neuroma and then at what appears to be normal nerve proximally and distally. Many centers will tag these specimens for orientation and send them for frozen section by the pathology department to determine whether the proximal and distal extent of the resection is free of fibrosis. Alternatively, perform an initial resection under loupe magnification, and then under the operating microscope, inspect the fascicular pattern to assess the adequacy of resection. Regardless, grafting to healthy stumps proximally and distally is important to assure fibrosis does not impair axon regeneration.
- Next, assess the length of nerve graft necessary to bridge each defect. This number will need to be multiplied by the number of cables necessary to match the size of the nerves being grafted. After a determination of the total

length of graft needed, sural nerve harvest can be performed on one or both legs. This can be done open or endoscopically depending on surgeon preference and training. These techniques are described elsewhere in this text.
- If avulsions make grafting impossible at some levels, existing roots should be preferentially grafted to the medial and then posterior cords to restore hand function. Extraplexal nerve transfers can be used to reliably restore shoulder and elbow function in these cases, as will be described below.
- Coaptation of the nerves can be carried out using 9-0 or 10-0 nylon suture or fibrin glue depending on surgeon preference (**TECH FIG 2**).

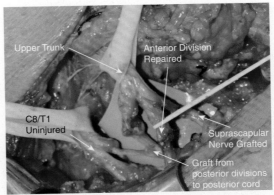

TECH FIG 2 • After confirming intact roots and adequate neuroma resection, use the available graft material to reinnervate as many priority targets as possible.

■ Accessory (CN XI) to Suprascapular Nerve Transfer

- If you cannot graft directly to the suprascapular nerve from the upper trunk or the C5/C6 root, either because of avulsion of the upper roots or the need to divert those roots to other targets, external rotation of the shoulder can be restored through transfer of CN XI.
- Trace the transverse cervical artery posteriorly to where it enters the trapezius muscle. Localize the accessory nerve using a nerve stimulator.
- Next, trace the accessory nerve distally, past its innervation of the upper and middle portions of the trapezius. Mobilize and then cut the nerve, making sure there is sufficient length to reach the stump of the suprascapular nerve. The stump of the suprascapular nerve should be prepared such that it is as close as possible to its origin while still resecting to healthy axons.
- Transpose the accessory nerve over to the suprascapular nerve stump, and coapt the two using either nylon suture or fibrin glue, depending on surgeon preference (**TECH FIG 3**).

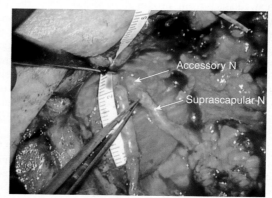

TECH FIG 3 • The spinal accessory nerve is followed caudally to the branch to lower trapezius, where it is transected and rotated laterally to innervate the suprascapular nerve.

■ Ulnar to Musculocutaneous Nerve Transfer

- If the lower trunk and medial cord are intact and the patient has demonstrated full ulnar nerve function preoperatively, a portion of the ulnar nerve can be used to reanimate the biceps muscle.
- Beginning at the inferior border of the pectoralis major tendon, make a longitudinal incision on the medial arm about 8 cm long. Dissect down to the biceps fascia, and separate it from coracobrachialis (**TECH FIG 4A**).
- Identify the motor branch to the biceps, which is about 13 cm distal to the acromion.[22] Dissect this as far proximally into the musculocutaneous nerve as possible, and then transect it for transfer to the ulnar nerve.

- Dissect posteriorly to locate the median and then ulnar nerves. If there is any confusion, a nerve stimulator can be used to differentiate the two.
- Using the microscope, make an epineurotomy in the ulnar nerve, and harvest two fascicles from the ulnar nerve. Use the nerve stimulator to confirm that they contain motor fibers, and section them distally enough that they can be transposed anteriorly to meet the biceps motor branch without tension.
- Coapt the ulnar nerve fascicles to the biceps motor branch under the microscope using either nylon suture or fibrin glue (**TECH FIG 4B**). Some surgeons will perform a similar transfer of median fascicles to the FCR flexor carpi radialis (FCR) to the motor branch to the brachialis in conjunction with this procedure for added elbow flexion strength.

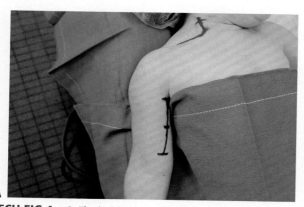
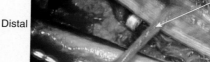

TECH FIG 4 • A. The incision is marked beginning at the inferior border of the pectoralis major tendon and extended distally along the medial border of the biceps tendon. **B.** After isolating the fascicles of the ulnar nerve to FCU as distally as possible, transect the motor branch to biceps as proximally as possible to assure there is no tension on the repair.

Intercostal to Musculocutaneous Nerve Transfer

- If the ulnar nerve is not an option for restoration of elbow flexion, two to three intercostal nerves can be transferred in a similar manner.
- If you have already made the incision in the deltopectoral groove to expose the infraclavicular plexus, then you can extend this inferomedially across the chest. If not, then make an anterior axillary incision and extend your incision inferomedially, perpendicular to the ribs down to the level just inferior to the nipple. Retract the pectoralis major tendon superiorly to expose the musculocutaneous nerve at its take off from the lateral cord. It should be sectioned here and mobilized for later coaptation with the cables from the intercostal nerves (**TECH FIG 5A**).
- Limit resection of the fat and the associated lymph nodes in the axillary fossa. However, dissect sufficiently to expose the involved structures and a more direct line for coaptation of the intercostal and musculocutaneous nerves.
- Dissect down to the ribs. It may be necessary to release portions of the origin of the pectoralis major and serratus

anterior muscles. These should be tagged for repair at the conclusion of the case.

- Expose the second, third, and fourth ribs subperiosteally. The intercostal nerves from roots T2 to T4 are inferior to their respective ribs after dissecting through the external and internal intercostal muscles.
- Carefully dissect the intercostal nerves anteriorly to the mammary line and posteriorly to the point where they will be transposed toward the musculocutaneous nerve.
- Cut the intercostal nerves about 1 cm medial to the mammary line, and carefully mobilize each nerve posteriorly such that there is sufficient length to reach the musculocutaneous nerve in the axilla.
- Coapt the intercostal nerves as a cable graft to the musculocutaneous nerve as far distal as possible without tension or kinking, to minimize the distance for regeneration. Coaptation can be performed with nylon suture or fibrin glue, per surgeon preference (**TECH FIG 5B**).
- Make sure that you there is no tension on the nerve coaptation site with the arm in 90 degrees of abduction and 90 degrees of external rotation.

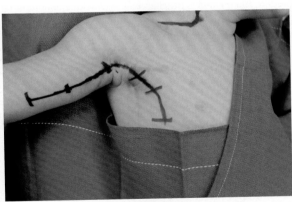 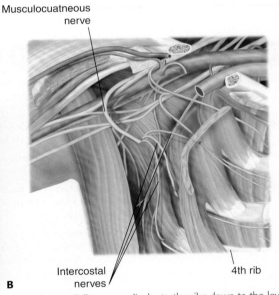

Musculocuatneous nerve

Intercostal nerves

4th rib

A   **B**

TECH FIG 5 • **A.** Mark out an anterior axillary incision, and extend your incision inferomedially, perpendicular to the ribs down to the level just inferior to the nipple. **B.** Cut the intercostal nerves about 1 cm medial to the mammary line, and carefully mobilize each nerve posteriorly such that there is sufficient length to reach the musculocutaneous nerve in the axilla. These will be transferred to the musculocutaneous nerve as a cable.

Radial to Axillary Nerve Transfer

- For this procedure, we prefer the patient to be flipped prone with the involved extremity prepped into the field and forearm either at the side or resting on the lower back. As mentioned before, paralysis should be avoided after induction of anesthesia to allow for use of the nerve stimulator.
- Make a J-shaped incision from the lateral border of the scapula, following the posterior border of the deltoid

and extending down the posterior aspect of the upper arm (**TECH FIG 6A**).
- Dissect down to the fascia overlying the triceps and deltoid, watching for the lateral cutaneous branch of the axillary nerve. This can be used to trace proximally to the axillary nerve as it passes through the quadrangular space.
- Transect the axillary nerve just proximal to the teres minor motor branch, and transpose the nerve distally.

- Find the radial nerve as it passes through the triangular space, and trace it as distally to locate the motor branch the medial head of the triceps muscle. Transect the nerve as distally as possible such that there is sufficient length for tension-free repair.
- Transpose the triceps nerve branch proximally. Remove the lateral cutaneous nerve from the axillary nerve.

- Under the microscope, coapt the triceps motor branch to the axillary stump using nylon suture or fibrin glue. 8-0 or 9-0 suture is appropriate. Intercalary grafts are usually not needed (**TECH FIG 6B**).
- Abduct and rotate the arm to make sure that there is no tension on the repair with shoulder motion.

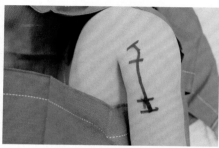
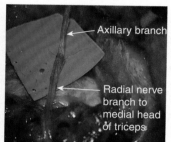

TECH FIG 6 • A. A J-shaped incision is marked from the lateral border of the scapula, following the posterior border of the deltoid and extending down the posterior aspect of the upper arm allowing exposure of the axillary nerve in the quadrangular space and the radial branch to the medial head of the triceps distally. **B,C.** The branch to the medial head of the triceps is transected as distally as possible and transposed proximally to meet the motor branch of the deltoid. A branch to the lateral or long head of the triceps could also be used if better for coaptation. No branch has been shown to be functionally superior to the others.

PEARLS AND PITFALLS

Preoperative planning	■ Develop a complete understanding of the injury prior to surgery, as well as a plan with multiple alternatives. This facilitates efficiency during a long procedure and minimizes the chance of overlooking important targets for reinnervation.
Exploration	■ It is crucial to fully explore each involved nerve root to its insertion in the spinal cord, even if it is involved in neuroma distally. Grafting from an avulsed nerve root assures complete failure of the surgery at that level.
Neuroma resection	■ Use available resources to confirm adequate neuroma resection as grafting to a fibrotic nerve ending will limit or completely block nerve regeneration.
Reconstruction	■ When there are limited intact nerve roots for grafting, preferentially graft to the lower trunk and medial cord as there are no proven extraplexal transfers for animating the hand but multiple options for extraplexal transfers for the shoulder and elbow.
Therapy	■ Appropriate therapy before and after surgery is at least as important as a technically excellent repair or reconstruction. Maintaining full passive motion of all involved joints gives the recovering neuromuscular units the best chance to succeed. A strong relationship with a trusted occupational therapist, experienced in brachial plexus injury, is crucial for success.

POSTOPERATIVE CARE

- Acute phase (0–4 weeks)
  - Place the patient in cervical collar and shoulder immobilization dressing for 3 weeks in order to protect repairs. We perform weekly dressing changes in our therapy clinic to monitor the incisions as well as for skin breakdown in the axilla and between the forearm and abdomen.
  - After 3 weeks of immobilization, begin gentle active and passive range-of-motion exercises for the neck, scapula, shoulder, elbow, and hand. We recommend two formal therapy visits per week initially.
- Subacute phase (4 weeks to 2 years)
  - Monitor active and passive range of motion and return of muscle function.

- Review and adjust home therapy program to emphasize the importance of consistency in performing exercises at home and to address any developing contractures early.

OUTCOMES

- Outcomes in brachial plexus surgery can be highly variable depending on the number of levels involved, the number of avulsion injuries, and the willingness or ability of the patient's family to participate in therapy.
- In patients undergoing nerve transfer or grafting, it may take 6 to 9 months to see any function in the involved muscle groups. Continued improvement can be seen for 2 to 4 years as patients continue to make gains in strength and coordination.

- It should be emphasized repeatedly to parents that therapy must continue at home until the child reaches skeletal maturity. Excellent early outcomes can be lost if therapy is neglected for any period of time, especially during a growth spurt.

COMPLICATIONS

- Injury to major vessels of the neck and upper extremity
- Failure to recover function after plexus reconstruction
- Pneumothorax
- Seroma formation
  - After axillary dissection during nerve transfers
  - With thoracic duct injury when exploring the left brachial plexus

REFERENCES

1. Foad SL, Mehlman CT, Ying J. The epidemiology of neonatal brachial plexus palsy in the United States. *J Bone Joint Surg Am.* 2008; 90(6):1258-1264.
2. Abzug JM, Kozin SH. Evaluation and management of brachial plexus birth palsy. *Orthop Clin North Am.* 2014;45(2):225-232.
3. Gilbert A, Brockman R, Carlioz H. Surgical treatment of brachial plexus birth palsy. *Clin Orthop Relat Res.* 1991;(264):39-47.
4. Gonik B, Walker A, Grimm M. Mathematic modeling of forces associated with shoulder dystocia: a comparison of endogenous and exogenous sources. *Am J Obstet Gynecol.* 2000;182(3):689-691.
5. Walsh JM, Kandamany N, Ni Shuibhne N, et al. Neonatal brachial plexus injury: comparison of incidence and antecedents between 2 decades. *Am J Obstet Gynecol.* 2011;204(4):324.e1-324.e6.
6. Seddon HJ. A classification of nerve injuries. *Br Med J.* 1942;2(4260): 237-239.
7. Sunderland S. A classification of peripheral nerve injuries producing loss of function. *Brain.* 1951;74(4):491-516.
8. Mackinnon SE. New directions in peripheral nerve surgery. *Ann Plast Surg.* 1989;22(3):257-273.
9. Nikolaou S, Liangjun H, Tuttle LJ, et al. Contribution of denervated muscle to contractures after neonatal brachial plexus injury: not just muscle fibrosis. *Muscle Nerve.* 2014;49(3):398-404.
10. Bae DS, Ferretti M, Waters PM. Upper extremity size differences in brachial plexus birth palsy. *Hand (N Y).* 2008;3(4):297-303.
11. Greenwald AG, Schute PC, Shiveley JL. Brachial plexus birth palsy: a 10-year report on the incidence and prognosis. *J Pediatr Orthop.* 1984;4(6):689-692.
12. Hoeksma AF, ter Steeg AM, Nelissen RGHH, et al. Neurological recovery in obstetric brachial plexus injuries: an historical cohort study. *Dev Med Child Neurol.* 2004;46(2):76-83.
13. Pondaag W, Malessy MJA, van Dijk JG, Thomeer RTWM. Natural history of obstetric brachial plexus palsy: a systematic review. *Dev Med Child Neurol.* 2004;46(2):138-144.
14. Michelow BJ, Clarke HM, Curtis CG, et al. The natural history of obstetrical brachial plexus palsy. *Plast Reconstr Surg.* 1994;93(4):675-680.
15. Curtis C, Stephens D, Clarke HM, Andrews D. The active movement scale: an evaluative tool for infants with obstetrical brachial plexus palsy. *J Hand Surg [Am].* 2002;27(3):470-478.
16. Chow BC, Blaser S, Clarke HM. Predictive value of computed tomographic myelography in obstetrical brachial plexus palsy. *Plast Reconstr Surg.* 2000;106(5):971-977.
17. Tse R, Nixon JN, Iyer RS, et al. The diagnostic value of CT myelography, MR myelography, and both in neonatal brachial plexus palsy. *AJNR Am J Neuroradiol.* 2014;35(7):1425-1432.
18. Clarke HM, Curtis CG. An approach to obstetrical brachial plexus injuries. *Hand Clin.* 1995;11(4):563-580.
19. Waters PM. Comparison of the natural history, the outcome of microsurgical repair, and the outcome of operative reconstruction in brachial plexus birth palsy. *J Bone Joint Surg Am.* 1999;81(5): 649-659.
20. Arad E, Li Z, Sitzman TJ, et al. Anatomic sites of origin of the suprascapular and lateral pectoral nerves within the brachial plexus. *Plast Reconstr Surg.* 2014;133(1):20e-27e.
21. Clarke HM, Al-Qattan MM, Curtis CG, Zuker RM. Obstetrical brachial plexus palsy: results following neurolysis of conducting neuromas-in-continuity. *Plast Reconstr Surg.* 1996;97(5):974-982.
22. Oberlin C, Beal D, Leechavengvongs S, et al. Nerve transfer to biceps muscle using a part of ulnar nerve for C5-C6 avulsion of the brachial plexus: anatomical study and report of four cases. *J Hand Surg [Am].* 1994;19(2):232-237.

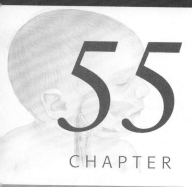

55

CHAPTER

Secondary Neonatal Brachial Plexus Palsy Reconstruction

Joshua M. Adkinson

DEFINITION

- Neonatal brachial plexus palsy (NBPP) results from injury to any brachial plexus nerve root (C5-T1) during a difficult delivery.[1,2]
- Persistent paralysis and progressive spasticity, contractures, joint instability, and bony deformities of the upper extremity may occur in children with incomplete recovery of nerve function.
- The type, severity, and manifestations of NBPP vary greatly between patients and surgical options for treatment must be individualized.

ANATOMY

- Most commonly, the C5C6 roots are involved (Erb palsy), leading to deficits of shoulder abduction and external rotation (supraspinatus, infraspinatus, and deltoid), elbow flexion (biceps brachii, brachialis), and forearm supination (supinator).
- C7 involvement causes paralysis of the subscapularis, teres major (TM), clavicular head of the pectoralis major (PM), brachioradialis (BR), extensor carpi radialis longus (ECRL) and brevis (ECRB), and possibly extensor carpi ulnaris and extensor digitorum communis (EDC). This leads to the classic "waiter tip" posture,[3] with deficits of wrist and finger extension.
- Rarely, the C8T1 roots alone are affected (Klumpke palsy), leading to weakness/paralysis in the wrist/finger flexors and hand intrinsic muscles.
- Complete plexus involvement (C5-T1) leads to a flail extremity.

PATHOGENESIS

- Between 50% and 92% of patients with NBPP experience complete recovery of function without primary nerve reconstruction.[1,4–8] In those with persistent deficits, the clinical findings will vary over time.
- Secondary deformities are impacted by the severity of the initial nerve injury, extent of muscle recovery, patient age at presentation, and previous treatments.
- In addition to paresis/paralysis of affected muscles, co-contracture of antagonistic muscles can occur in patients with partial recovery.[9] This may lead to contracture and/or joint deformity.
- The most common posture in children with NBPP is internal rotation of the shoulder, flexion of the elbow, supination of the forearm, and ulnar deviation of the wrist, with variable involvement of the fingers.[10] Many children also develop a limb-length discrepancy.

PATIENT HISTORY AND PHYSICAL FINDINGS

- The preoperative evaluation of children with secondary NBPP deformities includes a detailed history, an assessment of functional limitations, and measurements of active and passive range of motion.
- Grading function
  - No grading systems are universally recommended for assessment of elbow, forearm, wrist, and hand function in patients with NBPP.
- Physical Examination
  - Function is observed, active and passive ranges of motion are documented, and muscle strength is assessed with and without gravity.
- Elbow
  - Co-contracture of the elbow flexors and extensors are assessed. Dislocation of the radial head and proximal ulna are noted.
- Forearm
  - Long-standing supination or pronation deformities may lead to fixed contracture of the interosseous membrane (IOM). Continued growth can then lead to bowing of the radius and ulna, dorsal dislocation of the distal ulna, and/or posterior dislocation of the radial head.
- Wrist
  - Ulnar deviation is common because of paralysis of the ECRL and ECRB.
- Hand
  - Limited metacarpophalangeal (MCP) joint extension is common, as is thumb instability.[11]

IMAGING

- Anteroposterior and lateral radiographs of the elbow or wrist may be obtained to evaluate for joint subluxation/dislocation or articular deformities (**FIG 1**).

NONOPERATIVE MANAGEMENT

- All patients should undergo physical therapy, with the goal of muscle strengthening and full passive range of motion of the elbow, forearm, wrist, and fingers.
- Orthoses are used to maintain anatomic joint alignment and to prevent contracture.
- Botox injection into spastic musculature is effective for temporary (3–6 months) muscle weakening.

SURGICAL MANAGEMENT

- Surgical options include tendon transfers, arthrodeses, osteotomies, muscle/tendon releases, and functioning muscle transfers.
- Secondary reconstruction of the elbow, forearm, wrist, and hand is considered in children older than 4 years with

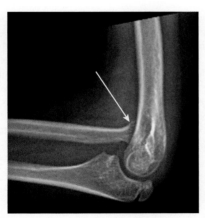

FIG 1 • Right radial head dislocation (*arrow*) in long-standing brachial plexus palsy.

incomplete recovery of upper extremity function after primary reconstruction or in those who present after the optimal window for nerve reconstruction.[10,12–15]

- Restoration of elbow flexion is the priority, followed by wrist extension, thumb/finger flexion, wrist flexion, thumb/finger extension, and intrinsic hand reconstruction.
- Elbow flexion contractures greater than 40 degrees are an indication for surgical release. Less significant contractures can be released, but this may cause clinically significant elbow flexion weakness.
- Weak elbow flexion (less than MRC grade 3) may be addressed via Steindler flexorplasty or transfer of the latissimus dorsi (LD), PM, or triceps.
- The surgical approach to the forearm depends upon the underlying deformity. Supination contractures are best treated by a biceps rerouting. If there is minimal passive range of motion, IOM release or pronation osteotomy of the radius is recommended.
- Pronation deformities are treated by pronator teres (PT) release or rerouting. One must ensure good passive supination prior to PT rerouting.
- Weak wrist extension can be managed by transfer of the flexor carpi ulnaris (FCU) to the ECRB or ECRL (to counterbalance an ulnar deviation force). Weak finger extension can be man-

aged with a combination of palmaris longus/flexor digitorum superficialis $(FDS)_{middle}$ or $FDS_{middle}FDS_{ring}$ transfer to the extensor pollicis longus (EPL) and EDC tendons, respectively.
- In patients with a total (pan-plexus) palsy, free functioning muscle transfers (eg, contralateral LD, gracilis, rectus femoris) are the procedure of choice.

Preoperative Planning

- Radiographs of the affected extremity should be reviewed, if relevant.

Positioning

- The patient is positioned supine on the operating room table with the affected extremity on a hand table. A well-padded tourniquet is placed high on the arm for procedures distal to and including the elbow.
- For pedicled LD muscle transfer, the patient is placed in the lateral decubitus position.
- The gracilis muscle harvest requires a frog leg position.

Approach

- Elbow approach: The muscles causing an elbow flexion contracture (brachialis, biceps brachii, and BR) are approached via an antecubital incision.
  - Procedures to restore elbow flexion require a technique-specific approach.
- Forearm approach: The biceps tendon is approached through an antecubital fossa incision. The entire length of the tendon and portion of the radius under which the tendon is rerouted must be visualized.
- Wrist/fingers approach: Procedures to restore wrist and finger function require a technique-specific approach. The FCU tendon may be approached through a single longitudinal incision or several stepcut incisions.
  - Free functioning muscle transfers to restore finger flexion require an extensile approach from the anterior upper arm across the acromion and lateral clavicle. This provides full visualization of the proposed site of origin of the transferred muscle as well the adjacent neurovascular structures to be protected and/or used for vascular anastomoses and nerve coaptation.

ELBOW RECONSTRUCTION

■ Elbow Release

- Landmarks: median nerve, radial nerve, lateral antebrachial cutaneous nerve (LABC), brachial artery, brachialis muscle, biceps brachii muscle, BR (**TECH FIG 1**)
- Depending on the severity of the contracture, a curvilinear or Z-plasty incision is made and the lacertus fibrosus is identified and divided (**TECH FIG 2A,B**).
- The median nerve/brachial artery is identified and retracted medially and the LABC is retracted laterally.

- If fractional lengthening is indicated, then two incisions 1 cm apart are made with electrocautery at the musculotendinous junction of the brachialis. The anterior half of the BR is elevated from the humerus while protecting the radial nerve. The medial half of the biceps tendon is incised distally and the lateral half proximally to provide lengthening. The release is reinforced with 3-0 braided suture, as needed.

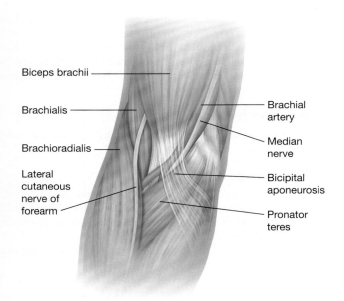

TECH FIG 1 • Structures crossing the elbow.

- If a full release is indicated, then the biceps tendon is Z-lengthened[16] (**TECH FIG 2C**), the brachialis is divided, and the BR is completely elevated from the humerus while protecting the radial nerve. The anterior elbow capsule is incised, if necessary. In long-standing contractures, foreshortened neurovascular structures will limit full passive elbow extension.
- The biceps tendon is reapproximated using 3-0 braided suture with the elbow in 30 degrees of flexion (**TECH FIG 2D**).
- The skin is closed in layers (**TECH FIG 2E**).

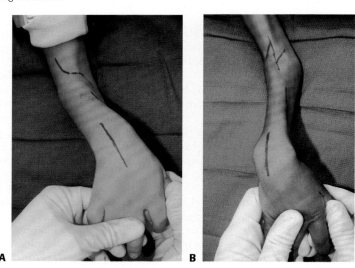

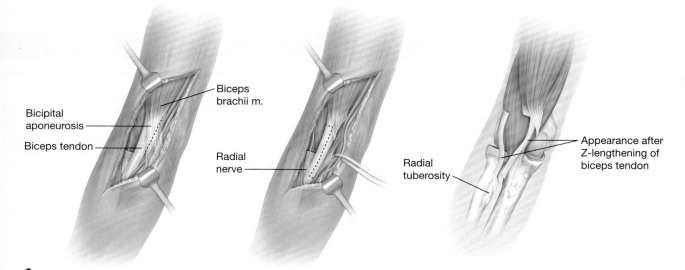

TECH FIG 2 • Approaches to elbow release. **A.** Curvilinear approach to the elbow. **B.** Z-plasty approach to the elbow. **C.** Steps in a biceps Z-lengthening.

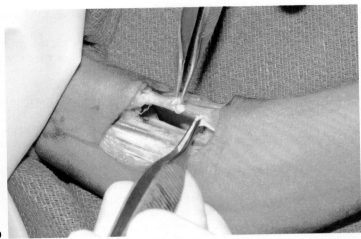
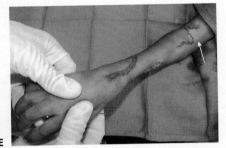

TECH FIG 2 (Continued) • **D.** Z-lengthened biceps tendon prior to reapproximation. **E.** Wound closure with a Z-plasty at the elbow (*arrow*).

■ Restoration of Elbow Flexion

Steindler Flexorplasty (TECH FIG 3)

- Landmarks: medial epicondyle, median nerve, ulnar nerve, brachial artery, humerus, biceps brachii muscle, brachialis muscle
- Fifteen-centimeter medial elbow curvilinear incision is made, and the skin flaps are elevated above the fascia while protecting the medial antebrachial cutaneous nerve.
- The ulnar nerve is retracted medially and the median nerve and brachial artery are retracted laterally.

- The flexor-pronator mass is freed from osseous attachments distally. Using an osteotome, the flexor-pronator origin at the medial epicondyle is elevated with a 2-cm segment of bone.
- The humerus is exposed deep to the brachialis. Approximately 5 to 7 cm proximal to the elbow joint, a bur is used to create a cortical window in the humerus.[17]
- With the elbow in 130 degrees of flexion, the medial epicondyle/flexor-pronator mass is secured to the humeral corticotomy using a 3.5-mm compression screw over a washer.

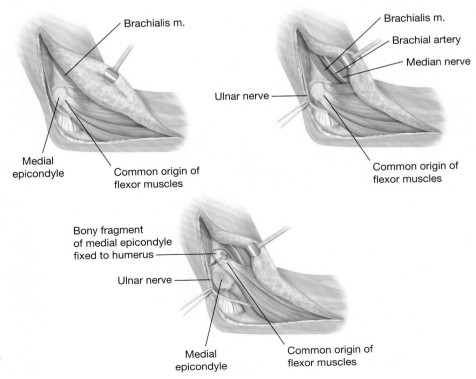

TECH FIG 3 • Steps in a Steindler flexorplasty.

- The ulnar nerve is transposed anteriorly to prevent tethering and the muscle is closed over the exposed osteotomy site using absorbable suture.
- The skin is closed in layers.

Latissimus dorsi Transfer (Pedicled) (TECH FIG 4)

- Landmarks: thoracodorsal neurovascular bundle, rhomboid muscle, teres major and minor muscles, acromion, clavicle, biceps brachii tendon
- Bipolar (moving the muscular origin and insertion) transfer is preferred because it increases the mechanical efficiency of the transfer and decreases the chance of vessel twisting/kinking.[18]
- Harvest—5-cm wide elliptically oriented skin paddle (8 cm distal to the axilla) is designed over the midaxis of the muscle and incised with superolateral and inferomedial extensions.
- The skin flaps are elevated off of the muscle and the arm is fully abducted and flexed.
- The muscle is marked at resting tension using 3-0 silk sutures placed at 5-cm intervals.

- The origin of the muscle is released and the muscle is elevated toward the axilla.
- The thoracodorsal neurovascular pedicle is identified on the deep surface of the muscle and dissected to its origin from the axillary artery. All adventitia is freed from the vessel to prevent tethering during transfer.
- The LD insertion is released from the bicipital groove of the humerus using electrocautery.
- Inset—a curvilinear longitudinal incision is made over the anterior upper arm with a transverse extension over the acromion and lateral clavicle.
- The skin flaps are elevated, and a deltopectoral window is created through which the muscle flap is passed, origin first. Confirmation of the neurovascular pedicle orientation is mandatory at this juncture.
- The insertion of the muscle is secured to the acromion and clavicle using two previously placed suture anchors.
- With the elbow in 100 degrees of flexion and full supination, the distal muscle is tubularized and secured to the distal biceps tendon with 2-0 braided suture or with suture anchors to the radial tuberosity.

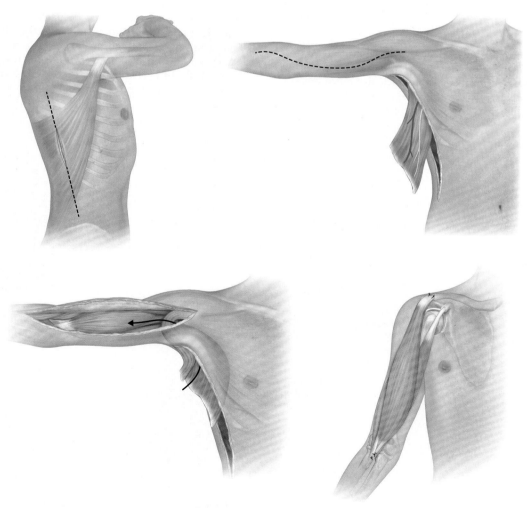

TECH FIG 4 • Steps in a latissimus dorsi transfer for elbow flexion.

- Two drains are placed in the donor site and all wounds are closed in layers.
- The skin paddle is used for postoperative muscle flap perfusion monitoring.

Free Functioning Gracilis Transfer

- Landmarks: thoracoacromial artery, acromion, clavicle, biceps brachii tendon, PM, intercostal muscles, adductor magnus, adductor longus
- Harvest—a longitudinal incision is made 2 cm posterior to the palpable adductor longus tendon on the medial upper thigh. The gracilis muscle is identified and freed from surrounding soft tissues.
- The obturator nerve is identified and dissected proximally toward the adductor hiatus where it is divided sharply.
- The medial circumflex femoral artery and vein are dissected to their origin on the deep femoral vessels between the adductor longus and magnus. Branches to the adductor longus must be carefully ligated and divided (**TECH FIG 5A**).
- The muscle is marked at resting tension using 3-0 silk sutures placed at 5-cm intervals.
- A 4-cm longitudinal incision is made overlying the medial proximal tibia. The sartorius fascia is divided and the distal gracilis tendon (the most superior structure of the pes anserinus) is identified and sharply release from the tibia.

- Inset—a curvilinear longitudinal incision is made over the anterior upper arm with a transverse extension 2 cm above the acromion and lateral clavicle. The distal biceps tendon is exposed while protecting the neurovascular structures.
- The thoracoacromial artery (or brachial artery) and cephalic vein are prepared and the spinal accessory nerve is dissected free from the deep surface of the anterior trapezius muscle, ensuring maximum length for transfer (**TECH FIG 5B,C**). The intercostal nerves are an alternative donor for motor reinnervation.[19]
- The medial circumflex vessels are ligated and the muscle is transferred to the arm.
- The muscle position is evaluated relative to the anticipated neurovascular repairs and the muscle is secured to the acromion and clavicle using two previously placed suture anchors.
- The vessel anastomoses and nerve coaptations are performed with 9-0 and 10-0 nylon suture, respectively.
- With the muscle at resting tension and the elbow flexed to 100 degrees, the gracilis tendon is woven into the distal biceps tendon with 2-0 braided suture or secured to the radial tuberosity with suture anchors.
- The wounds are closed in layers (**TECH FIG 5D**).
- An implantable venous Doppler is used to monitor perfusion in combination with clinical examination.
- The patient is placed on 81 mg of aspirin daily for 4 weeks.

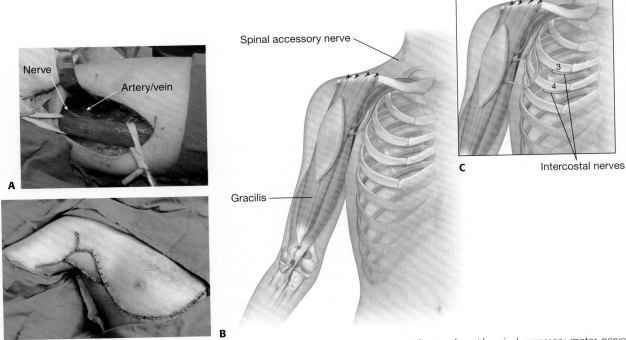

TECH FIG 5 • **A.** Free functioning gracilis muscle transfer harvest. **B.** Free functioning gracilis transfer with spinal accessory motor nerve. **C.** Free functioning gracilis transfer with intercostal motor nerves. **D.** Free functioning gracilis muscle transfer inset and closure.

FOREARM RECONSTRUCTION

■ Biceps Rerouting

- Landmarks: biceps muscle, brachialis muscle, BR muscle, lacertus fibrosus, brachial artery and branches, recurrent radial artery, median nerve, radial nerve, LABC
- A curvilinear incision is made over the antecubital fossa and the LABC is identified and protected.
- The radial nerve is identified between the brachialis and BR and protected. The brachial artery and median nerve are also identified and gently retracted for protection. The radial recurrent artery is ligated, if necessary.

- The lacertus fibrosus is divided and the biceps tendon is traced to the interval between the BR and PT such that the biceps insertion into the radius is visualized.
- The biceps tendon is then divided with a Z-lengthening technique.[20]
- The distal biceps tendon is rerouted dorsolaterally around the radial neck using a curved clamp. The rerouted tendon is then secured to the proximal biceps tendon in a side-to-side fashion using 3-0 braided with the elbow in 90 degrees of flexion and the forearm in full pronation (**TECH FIG 6**).

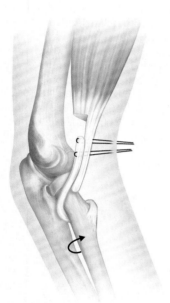 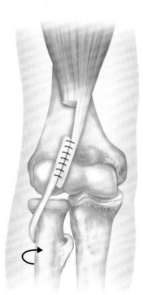

TECH FIG 6 • Biceps tendon rerouting.

■ PT Release/Rerouting

- Landmarks: BR, ECRL, ECRB, radius, radial artery, superficial radial nerve
- Six-centimeter skin incision at the volar radial aspect of the midforearm (**TECH FIG 7A**).
- The forearm fascia is divided and the BR and ECRL are retracted dorsally (**TECH FIG 7B**).
  - The superficial radial nerve lies under the BR and should be protected.
- The PT is detached from the insertion on the radius (the release is complete at this step). If rerouting is planned, then a 3-cm sleeve of the periosteum is taken with the PT to ensure adequate length for rerouting (**TECH FIG 7C**).

- The PT is mobilized proximally to allow for easy excursion.
- The IOM is released at the site of reinsertion and the PT is passed from volar to dorsal though a window in the IOM.
- The forearm is supinated and the PT is reinserted into the radius. In children, a 3-0 braided is woven into the PT tendon and passed through two transosseous drill holes to secure the PT to the radius (**TECH FIG 7D**). This is facilitated with the use of a Hewson suture passer.
  - In adults, a suture anchor may be used to secure the PT to the radius.
- The tourniquet is deflated, hemostasis is ensured, and the incision is closed in layers.

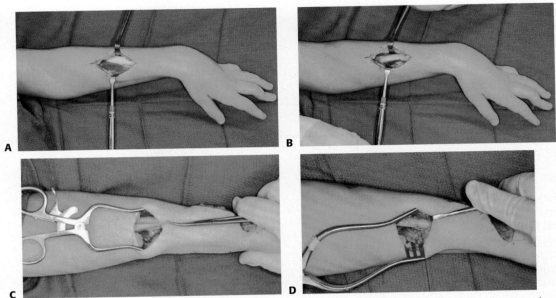

TECH FIG 7 • A. Approach for pronator teres exposure. **B.** Exposure of pronator teres insertion on the radius. **C.** Pronator teres elevation with a strip of the periosteum. **D.** Transosseous suture placement and docking of pronator teres onto dorsal radial shaft.

WRIST/FINGERS RECONSTRUCTION

■ FCU to ECRB Tendon Transfer for Wrist Extension

- Landmarks: FCU tendon, ulnar artery, ulnar nerve, ECRB tendon, ECRL tendon, EDC tendons
- A 10-cm incision made over the palpable FCU tendon extending proximally from the pisiform (**TECH FIG 8A**).

- The FCU is released from the pisiform, and the muscle/tendon unit is elevated while protecting the ulnar artery and nerve (**TECH FIG 8B**).
- A 6-cm incision is made over the distal dorsal forearm in line with the middle finger ray. The second extensor compartment is opened sharply, and the ECRB tendon is identified.

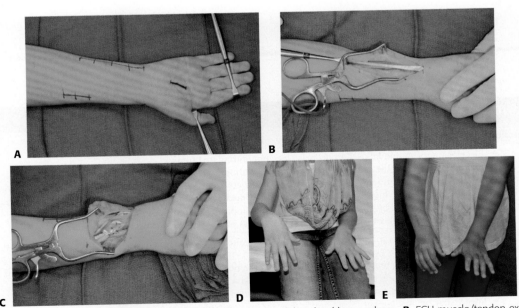

TECH FIG 8 • A. Markings for FCU to ECRB transfer, pronator rerouting, and thumb adductor release. **B.** FCU muscle/tendon exposure. Ulnar neurovascular bundle sits just deep to the tendon. **C.** The FCU to ECRB transfer was performed in combination with EPL rerouting. **D.** Preoperative right wrist extension. **E.** Postoperative right wrist extension.

TECHNIQUES

- A wide subcutaneous tunnel is created to directly connect the FCU muscle to the proposed intersection with the ECRB tendon.[11] In the setting of ulnar wrist deviation, the FCU is instead woven into the ECRL to achieve radial balance.
- With the wrist in 30 degrees of extension, the FCU tendon is interwoven into the ECRB tendon using an end-to-side Pulvertaft weave with 3-0 braided suture (**TECH FIG 8C**).
- Hemostasis is ensured, and the incisions are closed in layers.
- The preoperative and postoperative posture of the right wrist is shown in **TECH FIG 8D,E**.

■ Free Functioning Gracilis Transfer for Finger Flexion

- Landmarks: thoracoacromial artery, acromion, clavicle, intercostal muscles, adductor magnus, adductor longus, FPL, and FDP tendons
- See Restoration of Elbow Flexion technique, earlier, for harvest and proximal inset details. The muscle may also be directly attached to the humerus via suture anchors if additional distal length is necessary.
- A pulley is created at the elbow using either the PT or the FCU to optimize gracilis muscle excursion.[21]
- With the muscle tension set at resting length, the elbow at 90 degrees of flexion, and the MCP joints at 45 degrees of flexion, the gracilis tendon is woven obliquely through the FDP and FPL tendons in the distal third of the forearm and secured using 3-0 Ethibond suture. The FPL tendon junction with the FDP tendons is performed to ensure that the thumb does not flex prior to the digits (**TECH FIG 9**).
- Hemostasis is ensured and the incisions are closed in layers.
- An implantable venous Doppler is used to monitor perfusion in combination with clinical examination.
- The patient is placed on 81 mg of aspirin daily for 4 weeks.

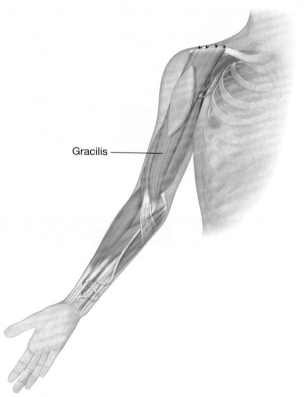

Gracilis

TECH FIG 9 • Free functioning gracilis muscle for finger flexion.

PEARLS AND PITFALLS

Elbow Reconstruction

Elbow release	■ Electrocautery should be used to decrease bleeding during myotomy. ■ Identify and protect the radial nerve during BR elevation. ■ In long-standing contractures, the neurovascular structures will shorten and prevent full passive extension. ■ Z-lengthening of the biceps tendon should be performed over as long a stretch of the tendon substance as possible. ■ Extreme care should be taken when handling the thin biceps tendon during repair. ■ Patients with weak flexion may have a functional loss of elbow flexion power after full release.
Steindler flexorplasty	■ Small nerve branches to the flexor-pronator muscles and the medial collateral ligament of the elbow must be protected. ■ Ensure good wrist extension power to counteract the possible development of a wrist flexion contracture. If active wrist extension is poor, simultaneous wrist arthrodesis can be performed. ■ Concomitant ulnar nerve transposition is recommended to prevent traction on the nerve after muscle transposition. ■ Ensure that the median nerve and brachial artery are free from compression or traction prior to securely fixing the transposed medial epicondyle/flexor-pronator mass.

PEARLS AND PITFALLS (Continued)

LD transfer	■ High brachial plexus lesions may preclude use of this transfer. ■ Inclusion of a skin island will simplify recipient site closure. ■ The muscle can be debulked to accommodate the upper arm soft tissue pocket. ■ The neurovascular structures should be assessed repeatedly during transfer in an effort to avoid kinking/twisting.
Free functioning gracilis transfer	■ Avoid nerve grafts, if at all possible. ■ If normal (unaffected by the NBPP), the LD transfer results in better elbow flexion strength than the free gracilis transfer. ■ Delay revision surgery for at least 1 year or after skeletal maturity.
Forearm Reconstruction	
Biceps rerouting	■ Overtensioning of the transfer may lead to an elbow flexion contracture. ■ The tendon may be fragile, and care should be taken to prevent fraying during handling. ■ It is essential to Z-lengthen the entirety of the tendon to ensure adequate length for rerouting. ■ The posterior interosseous nerve is at risk during rerouting because it lies directly on the radius. ■ A concomitant IOM release is recommended if there is no passive pronation. ■ A BR rerouting in the forearm is recommended in patients without adequate triceps function, because biceps rerouting will impart an unopposed flexion force across the elbow.
PT release/ rerouting	■ The superficial radial nerve and radial artery must be protected throughout the procedure. ■ The periosteal sleeve must be carefully elevated from the radius to provide adequate length for rerouting and reinsertion into the radius.
Wrist/Fingers Reconstruction	
FCU to ECRB tendon transfer	■ If passive flexion of the wrist to 20 degrees is not possible, the tension is too great and the muscle weave must be loosened. ■ Avoid lifting the tendons from the wound when performing the weave because this will result in a lax repair. ■ Ensure that the subcutaneous tunnel through which the tendon is passed is wide and straight. ■ Wrist arthrodesis is a better option in children with weak wrist flexors.
Free functioning gracilis transfer	■ Delay revision or adjunctive procedures for at least 1 year or after skeletal maturity. ■ In children with weak or absent wrist extension, wrist arthrodesis may be considered in the future to direct the full force of flexion to the finger flexors.

POSTOPERATIVE CARE

Elbow Reconstruction

■ Elbow release
  ■ No immobilization is necessary after a fractional lengthening of the elbow flexors. Immediate active and passive range of motion is initiated.
  ■ A full elbow release requires a long-arm orthosis for 4 weeks with initiation of active and passive range of motion. A nighttime extension orthosis is worn for 3 months.
■ Steindler flexorplasty
  ■ The elbow is immobilized in a long-arm orthosis for 6 weeks.
  ■ After 6 weeks, gentle elbow extension and flexion are initiated under guidance of a hand therapist.
  ■ Resistance exercises are introduced at 12 weeks.
■ LD transfer
  ■ The elbow is immobilized at 100 degrees of flexion in a sling for 6 to 8 weeks. At 4 weeks, the patient is instructed to begin muscle contraction exercises.
  ■ At 8 to 10 weeks, active elbow extension and flexion are initiated under guidance of a hand therapist; re-education of the transferred muscle is often necessary.
  ■ Resistance exercises are introduced at 12 weeks.
■ Free functioning gracilis transfer
  ■ The elbow is immobilized for 6 weeks in a position of 100 degrees of elbow flexion and the forearm in neutral.
  ■ Passive range of motion is initiated at 6 weeks, but passive flexion is restricted beyond 30 degrees for 12 weeks.

  ■ Re-education of the transferred muscle is necessary and EMG biofeedback is helpful.[22]
  ■ Contraction of the transferred muscle typically begins around 4-6 months postoperatively.

Forearm Reconstruction

■ Biceps rerouting
  ■ The arm is immobilized in a long-arm cast with the elbow in 30 degrees of flexion and maximal pronation.
  ■ At 4 weeks, passive range-of-motion exercises are initiated and the patient is transitioned to a long-arm orthosis.
  ■ At 6 weeks, active elbow extension and flexion are initiated under guidance of a hand therapist.
  ■ The orthosis is discontinued at 8 weeks and resistance exercises are introduced at 10 weeks.
■ PT release/rerouting
  ■ The forearm is placed in full supination using an above elbow orthosis for 6 weeks.
  ■ The patient is then allowed unrestricted motion under the supervision of a hand therapist.

Wrist/Fingers Reconstruction

■ FCU to ECRB tendon transfer
  ■ The wrist is immobilized in 30 degrees of extension for 4 weeks.
  ■ After 4 weeks, gentle range-of-motion exercises are begun and an orthosis is worn for an additional 4 weeks.

- Free functioning gracilis transfer
  - The arm is immobilized for 4 weeks with the elbow at 90 degrees of flexion, the wrist in neutral, and the fingers in at least 45 degrees of flexion at the MCP joints and interphalangeal joints.
  - At 4 weeks, a custom orthosis is created and a passive stretching program is initiated under the guidance of a hand therapist.
  - Upon spontaneous muscle contraction, the patient is directed to attempt active flexion of the fingers.
  - Therapy should continue for up to 1 year.
  - Re-education of the transferred muscle is necessary and EMG biofeedback is helpful.[22]
  - Contraction of the transferred muscle typically begins around 4-6 months postoperatively.

OUTCOMES

Elbow Reconstruction

- Elbow release: fractional lengthening will increase elbow extension by 40 to 60 degrees, with minimal loss of elbow flexion power.[23–25]
  - A full elbow release will increase elbow extension by 50 degrees but leads to a 19-degree loss of active flexion.[25] Many patients are able to accomplish tasks that were difficult before surgery.
- Steindler flexorplasty: Al-Qattan[26] reports that patients can expect 110 degrees of active elbow flexion against resistance, with a mean postoperative elbow flexion contracture of 35 degrees.
- LD transfer: Most patients will achieve M4 elbow flexion strength after transfer, with a mean arc of flexion of 90 to 140 degrees.[18,27]
- Free functioning gracilis transfer: El-Gammal et al. report an average arc of elbow flexion of 104 degrees. Elbow flexion power increased an average of 3.8 grades,[28] and 79% of patients achieve at least M4 elbow strength.[29] Average passive elbow range of motion significantly decreased from 147 to 117 degrees.[28]

Forearm Reconstruction

- Biceps rerouting: Rühmann and Hierner reported an average increase in pronation of 87 degrees (range 70 to 100 degrees). Active pronation to neutral was achieved in 91% of patients and 46% were able to pronate 30 degrees or more.[30] Results are less favorable in those with limited preoperative passive supination[31] or active pronation.
- PT release/rerouting: PT release results in approximately 50 degrees of decreased forearm pronation.[32] PT rerouting results in an improvement of active supination between 45 and 90 degrees.[23,33] Over time, there may be attenuation at the insertion site, leading to loss of supination.[34]

Wrist/Fingers Reconstruction

- FCU to ECRB tendon transfer: Transfer results in an average gain in wrist extension of approximately 47 degrees.[35] Al-Qattan[14] reported that average wrist extension muscle strength increased from 0 to 4 on a modified MRC system for motor grading. All patients, regardless of gains in wrist extension, discontinued use of a wrist orthosis.[35]

- Free functioning gracilis transfer: Terzis and Kostopoulos reported a postoperative mean MRC grade of 3.17 and 4.00 when innervated by the intercostal or spinal accessory nerve, respectively.[36] In a series by Chim et al.,[21] the youngest patients in their series (ages 6 and 8) developed elbow joint flexion contractures. Many patients require secondary procedures to optimize finger flexion and hand function.

COMPLICATIONS

Elbow Reconstruction

- Elbow release: neurovascular injury, weakening of elbow flexion, recurrent contracture
- Steindler flexorplasty: neurovascular injury, nonunion of fusion site, elbow flexion contracture, wrist flexion contracture
- LD transfer: hematoma/seroma, muscle nonfunction or ischemic failure, loss of muscle tension, clavicle fracture, elbow flexion contracture, compartment syndrome
- Free functioning gracilis transfer: neurovascular injury, muscle nonfunction or ischemic failure, clavicle fracture, elbow flexion contracture

Forearm Reconstruction

- Biceps rerouting: neurovascular injury, persistent supination or pronation contracture, tendon rupture
- PT release/rerouting: neurovascular injury, persistent pronation or supination contracture, attenuation of the reinsertion site

Wrist/Fingers Reconstruction

- FCU to ECRB tendon transfer: neurovascular injury, attenuation of the transfer, limited finger release resulting from weak finger extensors or tight finger flexors.
- Free functioning gracilis transfer: neurovascular injury, muscle nonfunction or ischemic failure, adhesions, bowstringing across the elbow, elbow flexion contracture

REFERENCES

1. Hoeksma AF, ter Steeg AM, Nelissen RG, et al. Neurological recovery in obstetric brachial plexus injuries: an historical cohort study. *Dev Med Child Neurol.* 2004;46(2):76-83.
2. Waters PM. Obstetric brachial plexus injuries: evaluation and management. *J Am Acad Orthop Surg.* 1997;5(4):205-214.
3. Terzis JK, Kokkalis ZT. Pediatric brachial plexus reconstruction. *Plast Reconstr Surg.* 2009;124(6 suppl):e370-e385.
4. Gordon M, Rich H, Deutschberger J, Green M. The immediate and long-term outcome of obstetric birth trauma. I. Brachial plexus paralysis. *Am J Obstet Gynecol.* 1973;117(1):51-56
5. Greenwald AG, Schute PC, Shiveley JL. Brachial plexus birth palsy: a 10-year report on the incidence and prognosis. *J Pediatr Orthop.* 1984;4(6):689-692.
6. Bager B. Perinatally acquired brachial plexus palsy: a persisting challenge. *Acta Paediatr.* 1997;86(11):1214-1219.
7. Lagerkvist AL, Johansson U, Johansson A, et al. Obstetric brachial plexus palsy: a prospective, population-based study of incidence, recovery, and residual impairment at 18 months of age. *Dev Med Child Neurol.* 2010;52(6):529-534.
8. Michelow BJ, Clarke HM, Curtis CG, et al. The natural history of obstetrical brachial plexus palsy. *Plast Reconstr Surg.* 1994;93(4):675-680.
9. Chuang DC, Hattori Y, Ma And HS, et al. The reconstructive strategy for improving elbow function in late obstetric brachial plexus palsy. *Plast Reconstr Surg.* 2002;109(1):116-126.
10. Zancolli EA, Zancolli ER Jr. Palliative surgical procedures in sequelae of obstetric palsy. *Hand Clin.* 1988;4(4):643-669.

11. Chuang DC, Ma HS, Borud LJ, et al. Surgical strategy for improving forearm and hand function in late obstetric brachial plexus palsy. *Plast Reconstr Surg.* 2002;109(6):1934-1946.

12. Soucacos PN, Vekris MD, Zoubos AB, et al. Secondary reanimation procedures in late obstetrical brachial plexus palsy patients. *Microsurgery.* 2006;26(4):343-351.

13. Duclos L, Gilbert A. Restoration of wrist extension by tendon transfer in cases of obstetrical brachial plexus palsy. *Ann Chir Main Memb Super.* 1999;18(1):7-12.

14. Al-Qattan MM. Tendon transfer to reconstruct wrist extension in children with obstetric brachial plexus palsy. *J Hand Surg Br.* 2003;28(2):153-157.

15. Bertelli JA. Brachialis muscle transfer to the forearm muscles in obstetric brachial plexus palsy. *J Hand Surg Br.* 2006;31(3):261-265.

16. Price AE, Grossman JA. A management approach for secondary shoulder and forearm deformities following obstetrical brachial plexus injury. *Hand Clin.* 1995;11(4):607-617.

17. Mayer R, Green W. Experiences with the Steindler flexorplasty at the elbow. *J Bone Joint Surg Am.* 1954;36-A(4):775-789.

18. Chaudhry S, Hopyan S. Bipolar latissimus transfer for restoration of elbow flexion. *J Orthop.* 2013;10(3):133-138.

19. Terzis JK, Kostopoulos VK. Free muscle transfer in posttraumatic plexopathies part II: the elbow. *Hand (N Y).* 2010;5(2):160-170.

20. Zancolli EA. Paralytic supination contracture of the forearm. *J Bone Joint Surg Am.* 1967;49(7):1275-1284.

21. Chim H, Kircher MF, Spinner RJ, et al. Free functioning gracilis transfer for traumatic brachial plexus injuries in children. *J Hand Surg [Am].* 2014;39(10):1959-1966.

22. Manktelow RT. Functioning microsurgical muscle transfer. *Hand Clin.* 1988;4(2):289-296.

23. Mital MA. Lengthening of the elbow flexors in cerebral palsy. *J Bone Joint Surg Am.* 1979;61(4):515-522.

24. Mital MA, Sakellarides HT. Surgery of the upper extremity in the retarded individual with spastic cerebral palsy. *Orthop Clin North Am.* 1981;12(1):127-141.

25. Carlson MG, Hearns KA, Inkellis E, et al. Early results of surgical intervention for elbow deformity in cerebral palsy based on degree of contracture. *J Hand Surg [Am].* 2012;37(8):1665-1671.

26. Al-Qattan MM. Elbow flexion reconstruction by Steindler flexorplasty in obstetric brachial plexus palsy. *J Hand Surg Br.* 2005;30(4):424-427.

27. Cambon-Binder A, Belkheyar Z, Durand S, et al. Elbow flexion restoration using pedicled latissimus dorsi transfer in seven cases. *Chir Main.* 2012;31(6):324-330.

28. El-Gammal TA, El-Sayed A, Kotb MM, et al. Free functioning gracilis transplantation for reconstruction of elbow and hand functions in late obstetric brachial plexus palsy. *Microsurgery.* 2015;35(5):350-355.

29. Barrie KA, Steinmann SP, Shin AY, et al. Gracilis free muscle transfer for restoration of function after complete brachial plexus avulsion. *Neurosurg Focus.* 2004;16(5):E8.

30. Rühmann O, Hierner R. Z-plasty and rerouting of the biceps tendon with interosseous membrane release to restore pronation in paralytic supination posture and contracture of the forearm. *Oper Orthop Traumatol.* 2009;21(2):157-169.

31. Gellman H, Kan D, Waters RL, et al. Rerouting of the biceps brachii for paralytic supination contracture of the forearm in tetraplegia due to trauma. *J Bone Joint Surg Am.* 1994;76(3):398-402.

32. Strecker WB, Emanuel JP, Dailey L, et al. Comparison of pronator tenotomy and pronator rerouting in children with spastic cerebral palsy. *J Hand Surg [Am].* 1988;13(4):540-543.

33. Bunata RE. Pronator teres rerouting in children with cerebral palsy. *J Hand Surg [Am].* 2006;31(3):474-482.

34. Sakellarides HT, Mital MA, Lenzi WD. Treatment of pronation contractures of the forearm in cerebral palsy by changing the insertion of the pronator radii teres. *J Bone Joint Surg Am.* 1981;63(4):645-652.

35. van Alphen NA, van Doorn-Loogman MH, Maas H, et al. Restoring wrist extension in obstetric palsy of the brachial plexus by transferring wrist flexors to wrist extensors. *J Pediatr Rehabil Med.* 2013;6(1):53-57.

36. Terzis JK, Kostopoulos VK. Free muscle transfer in posttraumatic plexopathies: part III. The hand. *Plast Reconstr Surg.* 2009;124(4):1225-1236.

56
CHAPTER

Section XIV: Lower Extremity

Rotationplasty of the Lower Extremity

Samer Attar, Robert J. Steffner, and Terrance Peabody

DEFINITION

- Rotationplasty of the lower extremity is a reliable and durable reconstructive option in the setting of bone loss in the lower extremity due to tumor, infection, or trauma.
- With resection of the bone around the knee joint, the rotated tibia is attached to the remaining femur.
- With appropriate preoperative education and proper patient selection, it is a functional alternative to an above-knee amputation or endoprosthetic reconstruction—especially in the skeletally immature patient.

ANATOMY

- The distal limb is rotated 180 degrees. This technique permits the rotated ankle joint to function as a knee joint for prosthetic fitting (**FIG 1**).
- The stump can fit into a modified below-knee prosthesis that is end-bearing, as opposed to ischial-bearing prostheses for above-knee amputations.

PATIENT HISTORY AND PHYSICAL FINDINGS

- Historically, rotationplasty has been described in the management of femoral bone loss from tuberculosis, proximal femoral focal deficiency, and sarcomas.[1,2]
- Indications for rotationplasty
  - Congenital bone loss or deficiency
  - Sarcomas of the lower extremity
  - Trauma
  - Failed arthroplasty
  - Skeletally immature patient or active adult patient
- Contraindications
  - Pre-existing nerve damage or ankle stiffness
  - Sciatic nerve involvement in tumor requiring its resection
- Physical examination
  - The soft tissues proximal and distal to the area of tumor must be intact and free of disease.
  - The ankle joint must be inspected for any contractures or limitations to motion.
  - The dorsalis pedis and posterior tibialis pulses must be inspected for flow.
  - Ankle extension, ankle flexion, and extensor hallucis longus motor strength must be documented.
  - A sensate foot with 5/5 motor strength and full ankle range of motion is ideal.

IMAGING

- Limb lengths of both lower extremities are obtained.

- Bone age should be approximated as the nonoperative limb will continue to grow.
- In malignant bone tumors about the knee undergoing resection, the distal femoral and proximal tibial growth plates are usually removed.
- When the patient reaches skeletal maturity, the rotated tibiotalar joint of the operative limb should be located at the center of rotation of the knee of the nonoperative limb.
- The projection of growth of the nonoperative limb must be taken into consideration at the time of surgery. Therefore, in a skeletally immature individual, the operative leg must be longer than the nonoperative femur.
- In the setting of sarcoma, magnetic resonance imaging determines where to resect the femur with an adequate margin, whether the joint is contaminated, and whether vascular structures are contaminated.
  - If there is joint invasion, an extra-articular resection should be performed.
  - If tumor infiltrates or encases vessels, vascular resection with anastomosis should be considered.
  - The tibial and peroneal nerves should be intact and free of disease as they will be required to power ankle motion.

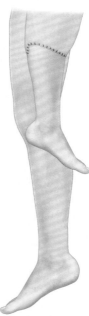

FIG 1 • Limb after rotationplasty, allowing the rotated ankle joint to function as a knee joint for prosthetic fitting.

SURGICAL MANAGEMENT

- Operative intervention must focus on the creation of appropriate flaps, wide resection of bone and soft tissue margins, and stable fixation of the remaining femur to the rotated tibia.

Preoperative Planning

- Extensive discussions with the patient and family are essential prior to performing a rotationplasty. The options of an amputation vs internal prosthesis must be reviewed in addition to explaining their respective risks/benefits.
- Imaging is reviewed to determine levels of resection of the femur and tibia in order to:
  - Achieve a sound oncologic margin
  - Account for a projected center of rotation of the rotated tibiotalar joint to be at the same level of the nonoperative knee when the patient reaches skeletal maturity

Positioning

- The patient is placed supine on a radiolucent table.
- The entire lower extremity from the pelvis to the foot must be prepped and draped.
- This setup provides vascular access and enables internal fixation to the level of the hip joint if needed.

- Intraoperative fluoroscopy is recommended in order to aid placement of hardware.

Approach

- The skin incision must be planned to accommodate the disproportion between thigh and calf circumference.
- Circumferential incisions are commonly made at acute angles to each other to account for this thigh/calf discrepancy (**FIG 2**).
- A longitudinal incision is then drawn to connect the proximal and distal circumferential flaps. This line is placed ideally to expose a plane for tumor resection and neurovascular dissection.[3-6]

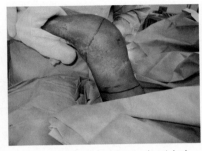

FIG 2 • Intraoperative outline of incision in the right lower extremity of a pediatric patient with a distal femur osteosarcoma.

■ Incision

- Skin and subcutaneous tissues are incised and raised as flaps along the circumferential thigh and calf tissues and the longitudinal line connecting them (**TECH FIG 1A,B**).

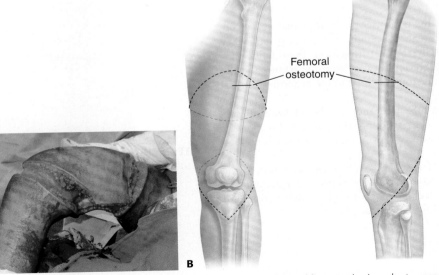

TECH FIG 1 • **A.** Incision with thick skin flaps. Note the circumferential incisions placed at oblique angles in order to accommodate the difference in thigh and calf diameter during rotation and closure of the wounds. **B.** The rhomboid incision should have an anterior axis that is about 5 to 10 cm longer than the intended length of the bone resection. The bone resection itself should be located at the proximal and middle thirds of the more proximal incision.

TECHNIQUES

■ Nerves

- The peroneal nerve is identified deep to the biceps tendon coursing laterally around the proximal fibula. It is dissected free of the surrounding soft tissue and followed proximally into the posterior thigh until its bifurcation with the tibial nerve (**TECH FIG 2A**).

- The tibial nerve is traced distally through the popliteal space and distal to the proposed osteotomy site. It is also dissected proximally until the sciatic nerve is identified and traced above the level of the proposed femoral osteotomy.
- Alternatively, the sciatic nerve may be identified proximally and traced distally through its bifurcation into the tibial and peroneal nerves (**TECH FIG 2B**).

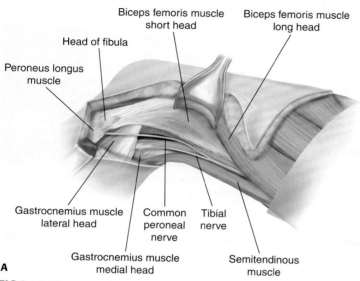

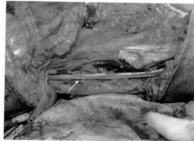

TECH FIG 2 • **A.** The peroneal nerve is dissected more proximally to the location where it joins the tibial nerve at the bifurcation. The tibial nerve can then be dissected distally into the popliteal space. **B.** Sciatic nerve (*arrow*) dissected from surrounding soft tissues.

■ Vessels

- Transection of the pes anserinus and medial gastrocnemius tendons reveals the popliteal artery and vein. They are traced distally to the trifurcation. Proximally, they are delivered posteriorly away from the femur, and the dissection should stop proximal to the proposed femoral osteotomy site.[7]
- The vessels must be free and untethered from all surrounding soft tissues from proximal to distal to prevent kinking and tension when the tibiotalar joint is rotated (**TECH FIG 3**).
- In the setting of vascular involvement with tumor, the vessels can be resected and the remnants anastomosed. However, this technique possesses a higher risk and higher potential for complications.

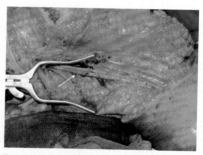

TECH FIG 3 • Femoral vessels (*arrow*) dissected from surrounding soft tissues.

■ Osteotomies

- Once the neurovascular structures are dissected and freed, attention should be turned to the femoral and tibial osteotomies.
- Steinmann pins can aid in rotation of the limb (**TECH FIG 4A**).
  - Proximal to the level of bone resection, a pin can be placed anterior to posterior with the patella directed straight anteriorly.
  - Distal to the tibial resection, a second pin is placed in the medial tibia perpendicular to the femoral pin.
- The surrounding soft tissues are then incised down to the proposed osteotomy sites.
  - Distally, the patellar tendon, the cruciate and collateral ligaments, the knee menisci, and the posterior knee capsule are incised and released at the level of the tibial insertion.
  - Proximally, the quadriceps, hamstring, and adductor musculature are incised down to the level of the femoral osteotomy site.

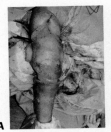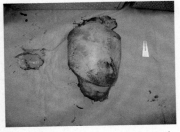

A **B**

TECH FIG 4 • A. Steinman pin placed anterior to posterior in the proximal femur and medial to lateral in the distal tibia. **B.** Intercalary specimen with resected proximal tibia.

- Attention must always be paid to maintaining tumor margin and protecting neurovascular structures during these steps.
- The femur and tibia can then be osteotomized with an oscillating saw, and the specimen is passed off the field (**TECH FIG 4B**).

■ Marrow Margin

- A femoral bone marrow margin should be sent to pathology for a frozen section. It should be confirmed that this margin is negative prior to proceeding with reconstruction.
  - During this wait time, the wound can be irrigated. The continuity of the vessels and nerves should be examined and should be tension-free (**TECH FIG 5**).

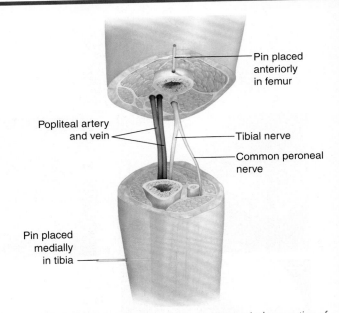

Pin placed anteriorly in femur

Popliteal artery and vein

Tibial nerve

Common peroneal nerve

Pin placed medially in tibia

TECH FIG 5 • Depiction of the limb after extra-articular resection of the distal femur before rotation of the limb.

■ Rotation/Reconstruction

- Reconstruction involves external rotation of the tibia by 180 degrees. If a medial tibial pin was placed, it should be perpendicular to the femoral pin from the lateral direction once rotation is complete (**TECH FIG 6A–C**).
- The vessels and nerves should coil in a relaxed fashion with no excessive tension. Any kinking or tension of neurovascular structures suggests adherent soft tissues that should be released (**TECH FIG 6D–F**).
- The lateral aspect of the femur and medial aspect of the tibia are then exposed to permit compression plating

fixation of the femoral-tibial junction. Fixation of six to eight cortices on either side of the junction is ideal if the remaining bone allows. Alternative methods of fixation are intramedullary rods or external fixators.
- Intraoperative fluoroscopy aids final images documenting limb alignment and positioning of hardware (**TECH FIG 6G,H**).
- Flow to the foot must be documented prior to closure by palpation and/or Doppler ultrasound of the dorsalis pedis and posterior tibialis pulses.

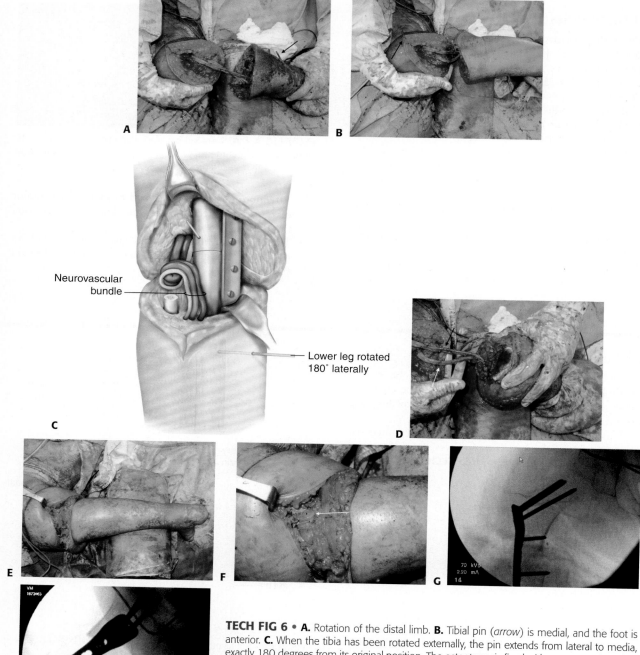

TECH FIG 6 • A. Rotation of the distal limb. **B.** Tibial pin (*arrow*) is medial, and the foot is anterior. **C.** When the tibia has been rotated externally, the pin extends from lateral to media, exactly 180 degrees from its original position. The osteotomy is fixed with a compression plate and screws. The vessels coil medially. **D.** The neurovascular structures should be relaxed and tension-free. Continuity of the sciatic nerve (*white arrow*) and femoral vessels (*black arrow*). **E.** View of the lower extremity after rotation. **F.** Close-up view of the coiled vessels and nerves (*arrow*). **G.** Intraoperative fluoroscopic radiographs of compression plate fixation between the remaining proximal femur and rotated distal tibia. **H.** AP view. Lateral view.

■ Closure

- Drains are placed per surgeon discretion.
- A layered closure is then performed. The quadriceps fascia is usually sutured to the gastrocnemius musculature and deep fascia of the calf. The hamstring fascia is sutured to the pretibial fascia (**TECH FIG 7**).
- A bulky dressing is ideal to maximize padding and minimize swelling. The internal fixation should be rigid, so no cast is usually needed.

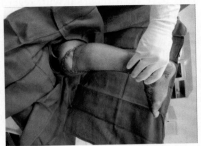

TECH FIG 7 • Extremity after closure and before dressing applied.

TECHNIQUES

PEARLS AND PITFALLS

Indications	■ Indicated in skeletally immature or active individuals. Preoperative education of the patient and family with literature, photos, and communication with patients who have undergone rotationplasty is beneficial.
Preoperative planning	■ Plan the length of the operative limb so that at skeletal maturity, the rotated tibiotalar joint of the operative limb should be located at the center of rotation of the knee of the nonoperative limb.
Approach	■ Angle circumferential incisions to account for discrepancies in thigh and calf circumference.
Technique	■ Vessels and nerves should be coiled in a relaxed fashion with no tension. ■ Use landmarks or pins to approximate rotation of the tibiotalar joint to 180 degrees. ■ Confirm vascular flow after rotation and fixation.

POSTOPERATIVE CARE

- The status of the limb must be followed closely with frequent neurovascular and compartment checks.
- Mobilization out of bed with assistive devices is encouraged as soon as possible Active motion of the hip and ankle should be promoted as well.
- If there is a nerve palsy, an ankle-foot orthosis may be placed, and the foot and ankle should be passively ranged to prevent a contracture until motor function returns.
- Adequate wound healing usually occurs in 2 to 6 weeks. At that point, provisional prosthetic fitting may begin. However, no weight bearing through the prosthesis should be allowed until clinical and radiographic healing is evident at the femoral-tibial junction (**FIG 3**).
- Once healing has occurred, activities as tolerated are allowed with a prosthesis.

OUTCOMES

- Rotationplasty provides local recurrence rates comparable to other forms of wide resection such as limb salvage and amputation.
- Gait velocity and the energy cost for mobility are improved compared to a transfemoral amputation.
- Rotationplasty permits participation in recreational and sports activities due to an end-bearing prosthesis, whereas endoprosthetic reconstruction has limitations due to concerns over prosthetic wear and loosening.
- Psychosocial problems due to the cosmetic appearance of a rotated limb are not usually reported.
- Psychosocial issues can be avoided through preoperative education of the patient and family with literature, photographs, and interactions with patients who have had rotationplasties.

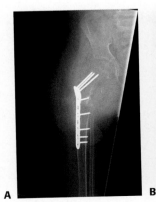
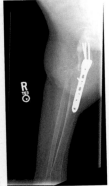

FIG 3 • Radiographs of the hip at 6 months postop. **A.** AP view. **B.** Lateral view.

- No adverse events have been reported with regard to the ability to pursue an education or career or develop and maintain relationships.
- There are no phantom pains or neuromas reported due to nerve continuity unlike in amputations.
- Rotationplasty is a reliable, predictable, and durable reconstructive option in the active or skeletally immature patient with a malignant bone tumor about the knee. Functionally, it can be equivalent or better than a transfemoral amputation, and it has comparable oncologic outcomes.[8-16]

COMPLICATIONS

- Ischemia and vascular compromise can occur—especially in the setting of vascular resection with anastomosis.
- Transient or permanent nerve palsy can lead to soft tissue contractures or a delay in rehabilitation with a prosthesis.
- Delayed or incomplete wound healing may require debridement with soft tissue coverage.
- Infection.
- Fracture nonunion.
- Hardware failure.
- Compartment syndrome.
- Rotational malalignment.

REFERENCES

1. Van Nes CP. Rotation-plasty for congenital defects of the femur. *J Bone Joint Surg Br.* 1950;32(1 suppl):12-16.
2. Salzer M, Knahr K, Kotz R, Kristen H. Treatment of osteosarcomata of the distal femur by rotation-plasty. *Arch Orthop Trauma Surg.* 1981;99(2 suppl):131-136.
3. Gebhart MJ, McCormack RR Jr, Healey JH, et al. Modification of the skin incision for the Van Nes limb rotationplasty. *Clin Orthop Relat Res.* 1987;216:179-182.
4. Ossendorf C, Exner GU, Fuchs B. A new incision technique to reduce tibiofemoral mismatch in rotationplasty. *Clin Orthop Relat Res.* 2010;468(5 suppl):1264-1268.
5. Fuchs B, Sim FH. Rotationplasty about the knee: surgical technique and anatomical considerations. *Clin Anat.* 2004;17(4 suppl):345-353.
6. Anderson M, Green WT, Messner MB. Growth and predictions of growth in the lower extremities. *J Bone Joint Surg Am.* 1963;45:1-14.
7. Mahoney CR, Hartman CW, Simon PJ, et al. Vascular management in rotationplasty. *Clin Orthop Relat Res.* 2008;466(5 suppl):1210-1216.
8. Agarwal M, Puri A, Anchan C, et al. Rotationplasty for bone tumors: is there still a role? *Clin Orthop Relat Res* 2007;459:76-81.
9. Sawamura C, Hornicek FJ, Gebhardt MC. Complications and risk factors for failure of rotationplasty: review of 25 patients. *Clin Orthop Relat Res.* 2008;466(6 suppl):1302-1308.
10. Gottsauner-Wolf F, Kotz R, Knahr K, et al. Rotationplasty for limb salvage in the treatment of malignant tumors at the knee: a follow-up study of seventy patients. *J Bone Joint Surg Am.* 1991;73(9 suppl):1365-1375.
11. Fuchs B, Kotajarvi BR, Kaufman KR, Sim FH. Functional outcome of patients with rotationplasty about the knee. *Clin Orthop Relat Res.* 2003;415:52-58.
12. Rödl RW, Pohlmann U, Gosheger G, et al. Rotationplasty: quality of life after 10 years in 22 patients. *Acta Orthop Scand.* 2002;73(1 suppl):85-88.
13. Hillmann A, Rosenbaum D, Gosheger G, et al. Rotationplasty type B IIIa according to Winkelmann: electromyography and gait analysis. *Clin Orthop Relat Res* 2001;384:224-231.
14. Hopyan S, Tan JW, Graham HK, Torode IP. Function and upright time following limb salvage, amputation, and rotationplasty for pediatric sarcoma of bone. *J Pediatr Orthop.* 2006;26(3 suppl):405-408.
15. McClenaghan BA, Krajbich JI, Pirone AM, et al. Comparative assessment of gait after limb-salvage procedures. *J Bone Joint Surg Am.* 1989;71(8 suppl):1178-1182.
16. Hillmann A, Rosenbaum D, Schroter J, et al. Electromyographic and gait analysis of forty-three patients after rotationplasty. *J Bone Joint Surg Am.* 2000;82(2 suppl):187-196.

Poland Syndrome

57

CHAPTER

Patrick J. Buchanan and Paul S. Cederna

DEFINITION

- Poland syndrome is a developmental defect characterized by varying degrees of unilateral pectoralis major aplasia, thoracic skeletal defects, breast hypoplasia or aplasia, and ipsilateral syndactyly.[1,2]
- A congenital unilateral absence of the sternocostal head of the pectoralis major muscle is pathognomonic for this congenital anomaly.

ANATOMY

- There are two predominant variations of Poland syndrome: simple form (mild) and complex form (severe).
- The simple form is the most common and is characterized by the absence of the sternocostal head of the pectoralis major muscle and effacement of the ipsilateral axillary fold.
    - The clavicular head of the pectoralis major muscle remains as a thin triangular muscle bundle that attaches the humerus to the inferomedial third of the clavicle.
    - The ipsilateral breast is hypoplastic or aplastic.
    - The ipsilateral nipple-areolar complex is typically smaller in diameter and displaced laterally and superiorly toward the axilla (**FIG 1**).
- The complex form is characterized by the absence of the sternocostal head of the pectoralis major muscle, ipsilateral rib and/or sternal hypoplasia or absence, and other ipsilateral muscular abnormalities (**FIG 2**).
    - The clavicular head of the pectoralis major muscle may be diminutive.
    - The ipsilateral latissimus dorsi, trapezius, pectoralis minor, serratus anterior, external oblique, and/or rectus abdominis muscles may be abnormal.
        - The pectoralis minor muscle is commonly hypertrophic.
        - Absence of the serratus anterior muscle results in a winged scapula.
        - Insertion of the ipsilateral rectus abdominis muscle is displaced cranially.
    - The sternum is foreshortened and bifid with a pectus excavatum appearance.
    - The ipsilateral scapula is small and cranially displaced, causing an internal shoulder rotation when compared to the contralateral side.
    - The ipsilateral anterior second through fifth ribs are thin, short, and devoid of their superolateral cartilage.

PATHOGENESIS

- To date, no definitive cause of Poland syndrome has been elucidated.
- However, there are theories identifying developmental and familial causes.
    - Developmentally, in the 6th week of gestation, there is an interruption of the subclavicular arterial branches causing maldevelopment of the tissues supplied by these vascular pedicles
    - Currently, geneticists believe Poland syndrome is rarely inherited; however, there is documentation of a 1% inheritance pattern from affected individuals.

NATURAL HISTORY

- The true incidence and etiology of Poland syndrome still remains unknown; however, it tends to occur more on the right side, 2 to 3:1, is more common in males, 2:1, and is estimated to occur 1 in 20 000 to 30 000 live births.[3]
- The most common presentation is that of a patient with a unilateral absence of the sternocostal head of the pectoralis major muscle with hypoplastic or absent breast parenchyma.[1]

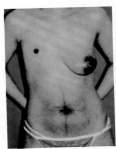

FIG 1 • Simple form of Poland syndrome depicting an ipsilateral breast anomaly with a smaller and superolaterally displaced nipple-areolar complex.

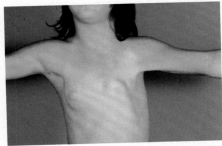

FIG 2 • Complex form of Poland syndrome showing ipsilateral axillary webbing, ipsilateral rib and sternal hypoplasia, ipsilateral trapezius, serratus anterior, rectus abdominis, and external oblique muscle abnormalities.

- The vast majority of patients with Poland syndrome present with concerns about the shape and appearance of their chest or abnormal breast development.[1]

PATIENT HISTORY AND PHYSICAL FINDINGS

- The surgeon must be acutely aware of the social impact of Poland syndrome on the patient and their parents.
- Patients with the simple form of Poland syndrome may be aware of their abnormality earlier than their family, as it can remain unannounced until early adolescence, as muscle and breast development occur.
  - Early in childhood, parents may notice a slight chest asymmetry.
  - Adolescent children with Poland syndrome spend an inordinate amount of time trying to conceal their asymmetry from their parents and others.
- The severe form, on the contrary, is readily known during infancy by the parents, as the chest wall is grossly asymmetric.
- In all patients, there will be a noticeable soft tissue deficiency of the affected side of the chest due to volume loss from the partial or complete absence of the pectoralis musculature.
  - The noticeable asymmetry often leads to adverse psychosocial sequelae.
  - Patients often report an adverse impact on their social functioning, emotional well-being, and psychological health.

IMAGING

- Diagnostic imaging is available but usually not necessary in cases other than the most severe variants.
  - Ultrasonography will show an absence of a portion of the pectoralis major muscle and asymmetry of the rib cage.[4]
  - Mammography is typically not used as an imaging modality for Poland syndrome; however, absence of the pectoralis major muscle can be incidentally discovered on the mediolateral oblique view of a hypoplastic breast.[4]
  - A CT scan can be used for presurgical planning to confirm the presence of the latissimus dorsi muscle and to better define the structural chest wall deformity.[5]
  - MRI may be useful to better define the patient's anatomy as it offers a multiplanar view without the ionizing radiation of a CT scan.[5]
  - Both color-coded duplex sonography and contrast-enhanced magnetic resonance angiography allow for the evaluation of selected arteries and vessels.[5]

DIFFERENTIAL DIAGNOSIS

- Unilateral accentuated thelarche
- Unilateral amazia
- Unilateral amastia

NONOPERATIVE MANAGEMENT

- Because reconstruction is rarely ever performed to restore a severe functional deficit, providing reassurance to the patient and their family is an important aspect of care that should not be overlooked by the surgeon.
- Removable external breast prostheses help correct the appearance of a female patient's chest and breast in clothing.

SURGICAL MANAGEMENT

- The reconstructive options for patients presenting with chest wall deformities from Poland syndrome depend on several key factors, including anatomical severity, gender, patient preferences, and associated anomalies.
- The timing and number of reconstructive stages is also of paramount importance.
  - A tissue expander can be placed early to gradually expand the affected side to decrease the amount of noticeable asymmetry as the contralateral breast developmentally matures.
  - Fat grafting can be initiated early to camouflage the asymmetry until the definitive reconstructive procedures are performed.
- Tissue expander-based reconstruction is ideal for the female patient with a hypoplastic and fibrotic breast or a patient with an aplastic breast.
- The latissimus dorsi muscle transfer can be used with any of the reconstructive approaches.
  - It is the best method to reconstruct the anterior axillary fold.
  - It can be performed on any patients, male or female, with a robust latissimus dorsi muscle.
  - The surgeon should discuss with the patients that harvesting of the latissimus dorsi muscle can create asymmetry in their back.
- Customized chest wall implants may be adjunctively needed in women and are often the treatment of choice in men.[6]
  - Author preference is for a custom silicone chest wall prosthesis.
  - The advantages of the customized chest wall implant reside in its ease of fabrication and insertion.
    - There is a relatively low morbidity for this technique compared to flap reconstruction.[6]
  - Disadvantages include implant migration, contour irregularities, patient reported discomfort, and potentially palpable or visible edges.[6]
- The endoscopic approach is typically performed in two stages when using a tissue expander and latissimus dorsi muscle transfer

Preoperative Planning

- Documenting the presence or absence of the serratus anterior and latissimus dorsi muscles is necessary, because this may affect desired reconstruction.
- The degree of pectoralis major muscle hypoplasia is also critical to determining the most appropriate reconstructive option for the patient.
- The sternal notch-to-acromion, acromion-to-olecranon, and olecranon-to-ulnar styloid distances are measured and compared to the contralateral side, in cases of notable skeletal abnormality.
- In women, the size of the breast and position of the nipple complex are assessed, particularly in regard to the contralateral, normal side.
- In the occasional male who seeks muscular strength improvement due to absence of the pectoralis musculature, objective testing of strength of the upper extremity via comparison to the contralateral side is needed.[1]
  - Male patients often lift weights in an attempt to increase the bulk of their affected chest.

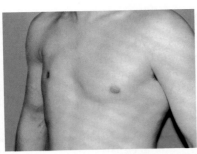

FIG 3 • Male patient with Poland syndrome showing hypertrophy of the ipsilateral pectoralis minor and clavicular head of the pectoralis major muscles.

- Weight lifting typically causes the pectoralis minor and the clavicular head of the pectoralis major muscle to become more hypertrophic (**FIG 3**).

Positioning

- The traditional latissimus dorsi muscle transfer harvest is performed by positioning the patient in a semilateral decubitus position with the ipsilateral arm elevated on an arm sling.

- **TECH FIG 1A** shows the intraoperative positioning for muscle harvest.
  - **TECH FIG 1B** depicts the large incisional scar that can be expected from this traditional approach.
- Alternatively, the latissimus dorsi muscle harvest and implant placement can be performed via a single axillary incision with the patient's ipsilateral arm extended cranially.

Approach

- Reconstructive options include the use of tissue expansion with implants, latissimus dorsi muscle transfers, customized chest wall implants, fat grafting, and rarely, free tissue transfers.[1,7–10]
  - Frequently, contralateral procedures are performed after definitive reconstruction of the affected side to achieve better symmetry.
  - Symmetry procedures include, but are not limited to, contralateral breast reduction, mastopexy, repositioning of the nipple-areolar complex (NAC), and reducing the size of the NAC.
- Both implant-based and latissimus dorsi muscle transfer reconstructions can be performed with an endoscopic approach to minimize scarring.[7]

■ Tissue Expansion with Implants

- The fibrotic breast tissue requires radial scoring prior to tissue expander placement to allow for adequate expansion.[11]
- The degree of muscle coverage of the expander is dependent on the extent of pectoralis major muscle absence.
  - Partial superior coverage will be achievable in some patients.

- Subglandular or subcutaneous placement is necessary when the pectoralis major muscle is notably hypoplastic or fully absent.
- Expansion is performed as necessary, followed by permanent implant placement, similar to breast reconstruction.
  - This technique can be performed in stages separated by many years.
  - The tissue expander can be placed early to allow for gradual expansion as the contralateral breast grows, prior to permanent implant placement.

■ Latissimus Dorsi Muscle Transfer

- Most often, a skin paddle is not required and, as such, a single incision can be used.
  - A dorsal incision above the lateral border of the latissimus dorsi muscle, approximately 6 to 10 cm long, is one option to gain access to the muscle[12,13] (see **TECH FIG 1A,B**).

- An endoscope can also be used to gain access to the muscle with a single, 5- to 6-cm incision placed within the axilla[7] (**TECH FIG 1C**).
- The skin/soft tissue is elevated off of the fascia overlying the latissimus muscle to expose the borders of the entire muscle. The muscle is divided distally and the fascial and muscular attachments to the chest wall

TECHNIQUES

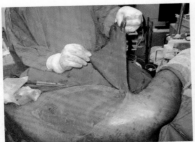

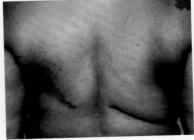

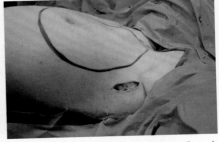

TECH FIG 1 • **A.** Traditional open approach to latissimus dorsi muscle harvest with the patient positioned in a lateral decubitus with the ipsilateral arm extended at 90 degrees on an operative armrest. **B.** Surgical scar created after a traditional, open harvest of the latissimus dorsi muscle for Poland syndrome reconstruction. **C.** Endoscopic approach with the patient in a supine position and the ipsilateral arm extended at 90 degrees allowing for a 5- to 6-cm incision placed within the apex of the axilla.

are divided, elevating the muscle toward the axilla[12,13] (see **TECH FIG 1**).
- The ipsilateral chest skin is undermined through the axillary incision or through a periareolar approach.
- The chest and previous axillary dissection planes are then joined.
- The mobilized latissimus dorsi muscle is then transferred.

- Release the insertion of the latissimus dorsi muscle and suture it anteriorly near the bicipital groove, on the humerus, to recreate the anterior axillary fold.
- The origin, lumbosacral fascia, is affixed to the lateral border of the sternum.
- Care must be taken to preserve the innervation to minimize the amount of muscle atrophy over time.

■ Customized Chest Wall Implants

- The entire operation, with implantation, can be performed through a single 4-cm incision.
- A malleable custom silicone chest wall prosthesis is positioned using endoscopic techniques (**TECH FIG 2**).

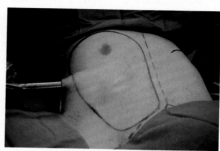

TECH FIG 2 • Customized chest wall implant insertion using the endoscopic approach with a single 4-cm incision.

■ Endoscopic Approach

- First stage[7]:
  - The patient is positioned supine, and a 5- to 6-cm incision is placed in the apex of the axilla (see **TECH FIG 1C**).
  - The dissection is performed in the subcutaneous plane to expose the border of the clavicular head of the pectoralis major muscle.
  - A 10-mm, 30-degree endoscope is attached to an endoretractor and placed within the dissected pocket to extend it medially to the sternum and inferiorly to the proposed inframammary fold.
  - Once this pocket is developed, a tissue expander is then placed.
- Second stage occurs once the tissue expander is expanded to its desired volume and the patient has reached his or her full developmental maturity.[7]
  - Performed in the lateral decubitus position.
  - The same 5- to 6-cm incision is used for the harvest of the latissimus dorsi muscle.
  - The 10-mm, 30-degree endoscope is inserted to complete the superficial and deep dissection of the latissimus dorsi muscle as previously described (**TECH FIG 3**).
  - With the thoracodorsal neurovascular pedicle directly visualized, the origin and insertion of the muscle are divided.
  - The patient is then repositioned supine, and the anterior dissection is performed to regain access to the tissue expander.
  - The tissue expander is removed and the latissimus dorsi muscle is transferred into the anterior pocket and sutured into place.
    - The lumbosacral fascia is affixed to the sternum and along the new position of the inframammary fold.
    - The former lateral border of the latissimus dorsi muscle is secured to the inferior border of the clavicular head of the pectoralis major muscle.

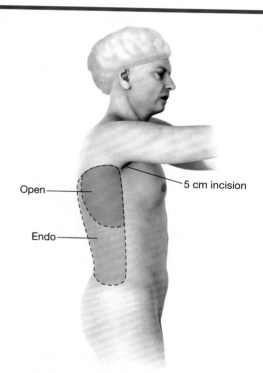

Open

5 cm incision

Endo

TECH FIG 3 • Two-stage endoscopic approach using a 5-cm axillary incision. The initial dissection is performed under direct, open, visualization. The subsequent dissection is performed under endoscopic visualization for muscle harvest.

  - The insertion of the latissimus dorsi muscle is attached anteriorly to the bicipital groove of the humerus.
- A breast implant can then be positioned deep to the latissimus dorsi muscle.

PEARLS AND PITFALLS

Hemostasis	■ Maintain adequate hemostasis to avoid hematomas that may subsequently become infected causing removal of implants.
Latissimus dorsi muscle transfer	■ Avoid dissecting under the teres major at the inferior angle of the scapula. ■ Maintain visualization of the thoracodorsal pedicle during the endoscopic harvest of the latissimus dorsi muscle to avoid injury to the pedicle. ■ Perform dissection of the vascular pedicle under direct visualization in the axilla to permit safe mobilization of the latissimus dorsi muscle.
Tissue expander and implant	■ Score the deep surface of the breast parenchyma to allow complete expansion of the breast.
Customized chest implants	■ Paying special attention to "feathering" of the implant's border during design and fabrication of the implant can hide visible, palpable edges (**FIG 4**). ■ Fat grafting during implantation can also help reduce visible and palpable edges. ■ Fat grafting can also be done secondarily to correct visible and palpable edges noted postimplantation.
Secondary procedures	■ Often contralateral mammoplasty is needed to maintain symmetry. ■ Nipple-areolar complex reconstruction is occasionally needed. ■ Translocation of the nipple-areolar complex to create symmetry with the contralateral side may be indicated.

POSTOPERATIVE CARE

■ Following Poland syndrome reconstruction, standard incisional postoperative care is required.

■ For patients who require an implant-based reconstruction, postoperative protocols apply.

  ■ Perioperative oral antibiotics are commonly given.

  ■ Closed-suction drains, when placed, are not removed until the output from each drain is less than 30 cc for 2 consecutive days.

OUTCOMES

■ The goals for reconstruction of the female patient are to achieve breast symmetry, recreate the anterior axillary fold, and provide adequate infraclavicular fullness.

  ■ These goals are successfully achieved with any of the aforementioned reconstructive options.

  ■ To optimize breast symmetry, female patients most often request a contralateral mastopexy and/or reduction.

  ■ Seyfer et al.[14] performed 57 operations on 29 women and incurred no revision operations when they performed the latissimus dorsi transfer in conjunction with breast implant. Most complications seen were due to the breast implant itself. Capsular contractures were revised using open capsulotomies.[14]

■ The general goal for reconstruction of the male patient is to achieve symmetric chest wall contour (**FIG 4**).

  ■ As in their female counterpart, the latissimus dorsi transfer had better overall outcomes.[3]

  ■ When performed as an isolated procedure, the latissimus dorsi muscle transfer is prone to undercorrect the deformity; however, fat grafting can be used as an adjunctive procedure to improve symmetry over time.

■ The reconstructive results for Poland syndrome tend to be long-lasting, accompanied by high patient satisfaction.[3]

COMPLICATIONS

■ Complications of Poland syndrome reconstruction include seroma, hematoma, infection, scar, delayed wound healing, and pain/paresthesias.

  ■ Seroma formation was most often seen after the removal of the closed-suction drains in the latissimus dorsi transfer donor site.[14]

  ■ However, as in the Seyfer et al.[14] study, these seromas are typically small and treated conservatively until they resolve on their own.

■ Long-term complications can occur with implant-based reconstruction and are manifested predominantly by capsular contracture and implant rupture.[3,14]

  ■ Progressive asymmetries can also become apparent over time due to discordant amount of breast tissue and differences in the skin envelope.

  ■ Implant infection and malposition may also occur.

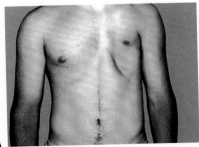 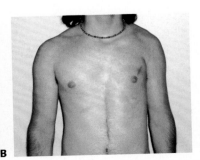

A   **B**

FIG 4 • Left Poland Syndrome. **A.** Preoperative. **B.** Four years postoperative using a customized chest wall implant reconstruction with a "feathering" technique to camouflage the edges of the implant.

REFERENCES

1. Buchanan P, Leyngold M, Mast BA. Bipolar latissimus dorsi transfer for restoration of pectoralis major function in Poland syndrome. *Ann Plast Surg.* 2016;77(1):85-89.
2. Ram AN, Chung KC. Poland's syndrome: current thoughts in the setting of a controversy. *Plast Reconstr Surg.* 2009;123(3):949-953.
3. Seyfer AE, Icochea R, Graeber GM. Poland's anomaly. Natural history and long-term results of chest wall reconstruction in 33 patients. *Ann Surg.* 1988;208(6):776-782.
4. Hurwitz DJ, Stofman G, Curtin H. Three-dimensional imaging of Poland's syndrome. *Plast Reconstr Surg.* 1994;94(5):719-723.
5. Wright AR, et al. MR and CT in the assessment of Poland syndrome. *J Comput Assist Tomogr.* 1992;16(3):442-447.
6. Gatti JE. Poland's deformity reconstructions with a customized, extrasoft silicone prosthesis. *Ann Plast Surg.* 1997;39(2):122-130.
7. Borschel GH, Izenberg PH, Cederna PS. Endoscopically assisted reconstruction of male and female Poland syndrome. *Plast Reconstr Surg.* 2002;109(5):1536-1543.
8. Fokin AA, Robicsek F. Poland's syndrome revisited. *Ann Thorac Surg.* 2002;74(6):2218-2225.
9. Haller JA Jr, et al. Early reconstruction of Poland's syndrome using autologous rib grafts combined with a latissimus muscle flap. *J Pediatr Surg.* 1984;19(4):423-429.
10. Longaker MT, et al. Reconstruction of breast asymmetry in Poland's chest-wall deformity using microvascular free flaps. *Plast Reconstr Surg.* 1997;99(2):429-436.
11. Borschel GH, Costantino DA, Cederna PS. Individualized implant-based reconstruction of Poland syndrome breast and soft tissue deformities. *Ann Plast Surg.* 2007;59(5):507-514.
12. Santi P, et al. Anterior transposition of the latissimus dorsi muscle through minimal incisions. *Scand J Plast Reconstr Surg.* 1986;20(1):89-92.
13. Santi P, Berrino P, Galli A. Poland's syndrome: correction of thoracic anomaly through minimal incisions. *Plast Reconstr Surg.* 1985;76(4):639-641.
14. Seyfer AE, Fox JP, Hamilton CG. Poland syndrome: evaluation and treatment of the chest wall in 63 patients. *Plast Reconstr Surg.* 2010;126(3):902-911.

Gynecomastia

Dennis C. Hammond and Eric Yu Kit Li

DEFINITION

- Gynecomastia involves the abnormal proliferation of glandular breast tissue in men, resulting in breast enlargement.[1,2]
- It is distinguished from pseudogynecomastia or lipomastia, which is characterized by fatty deposition without glandular development.

ANATOMY

- In healthy patients, the male breast resembles that of a prepubescent female.
- Fat is the predominant tissue and lobules are absent, in contrast to ductal and lobular development in females (**FIG 1**).
- The ideal male breast is also flat, to accentuate the contour of the underlying pectoralis major muscle.
- The arterial supply, venous drainage, lymphatic drainage, and sensory supply mimic those of the female breast.
- Although there is general consensus on the ideal size, shape, and location of the nipple-areolar complex (NAC) in women, this subject has been less extensively studied in men.
  - Various authors have published equations to calculate the ideal NAC on the male torso, often as a function of measurements such as patient height and chest circumference.[3-8]

- Some general themes exist among the various formulas, in that the ideal male NAC is
  - Slightly oval (horizontal greater than vertical)
  - Smaller (with diameter lesser than 3 cm)
  - Positioned around the 4th or 5th intercostal space
- Recent studies have characterized the shape of gynecomastia specimens as having a head, body, and tail[9,10] (**FIG 2**).
  - The head is semicircular in shape and extends toward the midline.
  - The body is located directly underneath the NAC and intimately attached to it.
  - The tail tapers off and extends toward the axilla.
  - Awareness of this shape may help guide intraoperative dissection.

PATHOGENESIS

- Gynecomastia occurs due to a hormonal imbalance between the level or action of estrogens and androgens.[1,2]
  - Estrogens stimulate breast development, whereas androgens inhibit it.
- Causes of this imbalance may be idiopathic, physiologic, pharmacologic, or pathologic.[11]

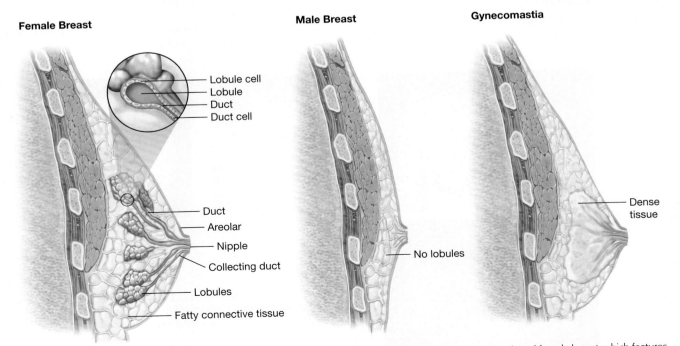

Female Breast

Lobule cell
Lobule
Duct
Duct cell

Duct
Areolar
Nipple
Collecting duct
Lobules
Fatty connective tissue

Male Breast

No lobules

Gynecomastia

Dense tissue

FIG 1 • In the normal male breast, fat is the predominant tissue and lobules are absent. This is in contrast to the developed female breast, which features lobules and ducts.

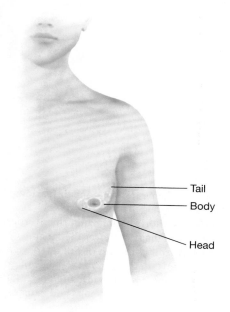

Tail
Body
Head

FIG 2 • A typical gynecomastia specimen with head, body, and tail sections.

■ Obesity is also strongly associated with gynecomastia, due to increased levels of circulating estrogens from peripheral aromatization of androgens in adipose tissue.[1]

■ Histopathologically, early-stage gynecomastia is characterized by ductal proliferation with loose stromal tissue (florid type).[12]

■ Over time, generally over the course of a year, the stromal tissue undergoes fibrosis (fibrotic type).[12]
  ■ Gynecomastia that has undergone fibrosis is unlikely to be responsive to medical treatment.

NATURAL HISTORY[1,2]

■ Physiologic gynecomastia (**FIG 3A–C**)
  ■ Often seen in newborns, adolescents, and older men

  ■ Adolescent gynecomastia:
    • May begin as early as age 12
    • Can occur in up to 65% of adolescent boys[13]
    • Breast enlargement typically lasts 6 to 12 months.
    • Ninety percent of cases spontaneously resolve without treatment.[14]
    • Generally, presents as a subareolar, firm, concentric, fibrous mass with surrounding fibrofatty tissue that is proportional to the body habitus of the patient
  ■ Senescent gynecomastia (**FIG 3D**):
    • Can occur in up to 65% of men over 65 years of age[15]
    • Generally presents as diffuse fibrofatty tissue that gradually enlarges over time
■ Pathologic gynecomastia
  ■ Can occur at any age, related to a tumor or medical condition (eg, liver or kidney disease)
  ■ There may be a history of rapid eccentric growth, nipple discharge, skin changes, or constitutional symptoms.[12]
■ Pharmacologic gynecomastia
  ■ Can occur at any age, related to a drug exposure.
  ■ Generally presents as a subareolar, firm, concentric, mass.
  ■ If the mass is not fibrotic, stopping the offending medication may resolve the condition.
  ■ If the mass is fibrotic, stopping the offending medication may halt progression of gynecomastia, but it is unlikely to reduce the breast enlargement already present.

PATIENT HISTORY AND PHYSICAL FINDINGS

■ Patients with the suspected diagnosis should be evaluated for both signs and symptoms related to the abnormal breast growth.
■ A detailed history should inquire about:
  ■ The onset and velocity of breast growth
  ■ The onset of puberty and ongoing pubertal development (if applicable)
  ■ Any tendency for spontaneous resolution of the breast hypertrophy
  ■ Associated symptoms, including pain, tenderness, weight loss, night sweats, and general malaise

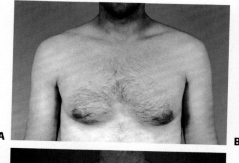
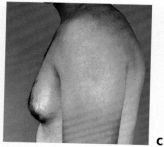
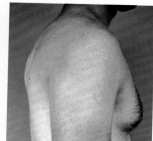
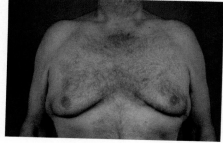

FIG 3 • **A–C.** Frontal and lateral views of a 24-year-old man who presented with bilateral physiologic gynecomastia. Both sides were characterized by a subareolar fibrous mass and surrounding fibrofatty tissues. **D.** Frontal view of a 52-year-old man who presented with bilateral senescent gynecomastia with skin excess and NAC ptosis. Both sides were characterized by diffuse fibrofatty tissues.

- Any social, vocational, or avocational dysfunction due to the breast enlargement
- The effect of the breasts on the patient's psychological well-being and self-esteem
- Any personal or family history of breast cancer or disorders
- Medication history, especially recreational and off-the-counter drugs (eg, marijuana and exogenous steroids)
- Symptoms suggestive of underlying thyroid, liver, or kidney disease
- A detailed physical should examine
  - The patient's height, weight, and body mass index
  - For the development of secondary sexual characteristics (if applicable)
  - For the presence of a subareolar mass and its area of involvement
  - For the presence of fibrofatty tissue and its area of involvement
  - For other masses, irregularities, or deformities involving the breasts or chest wall
  - Overall breast aesthetics, including the shape, size, and symmetry of the breasts and NACs, the degree of ptosis, excess skin, and the position and symmetry of the inframammary folds (IMFs)
  - Standard breast measurements to highlight asymmetries, including the sternal notch to nipple, midclavicular to nipple, nipple to midline, and nipple to IMF distances
  - The patient's neck, abdomen, and testicles for any masses or irregularities

IMAGING

- Imaging is not typically required if the history and physical examination are consistent with physiologic gynecomastia.
- In suspected cases of pathologic gynecomastia, appropriate imaging (mammogram, ultrasound, etc.) should be carried out based on the identified or suspected abnormalities.

DIFFERENTIAL DIAGNOSIS

- Idiopathic gynecomastia
- Physiologic gynecomastia
- Pseudogynecomastia or lipomastia
- Benign breast tumors (eg, fibroadenoma, giant fibroadenoma, phyllodes tumor, lipoma, or cysts)
- Malignant breast tumors (eg, ductal or lobular carcinoma, lymphoma, or metastases)

NONOPERATIVE MANAGEMENT

- Patient reassurance is the foremost treatment in adolescent gynecomastia.
  - About 90% of adolescent cases spontaneously resolve, so no treatment may be needed at all.[14]
  - Treatment is indicated when gynecomastia has persisted for more than 2 years, or if there are overriding functional, medical, or psychosocial concerns that warrant earlier intervention.[16]
- In gynecomastia related to reversible etiologies, the offending medication should be stopped or the underlying condition treated as soon as possible.
- Weight loss through dietary restriction and exercise are important first-line treatments in any gynecomastia related to obesity.

- Pharmacologic therapies, including danazol, tamoxifen, and anastrozole, may be effective in preventing or treating early-stage gynecomastia but are less effective once breast tissues undergo fibrosis.[2]
  - Of these medications, tamoxifen is most widely used, but there are no clear guidelines on the ideal dose or duration.
  - All medications also have unfavorable side effects that must be considered.
- If pathologic gynecomastia is suspected, patients should be urgently referred to the appropriate specialist(s).

SURGICAL MANAGEMENT

- Surgical treatment is indicated when gynecomastia is persistent or causes functional or aesthetic concerns.
- Options include liposuction, excision of the subareolar fibrous tissue, or a combination of the two.
- In patients with significant breast enlargement with skin excess and ptosis, mastopexy may be incorporated as well.
- Although weight loss should be the first-line strategy in any obese patient with gynecomastia, it is still reasonable to proceed with surgery in obese patients since normalizing the chest wall contour may allow the patient to lead a more active lifestyle.[16]
- Whether resected gynecomastia tissues should be routinely sent for histopathological examination is debatable.
  - The likely risk of finding occult malignancy in gynecomastia specimens is less than 0.01%.[12,17]
  - Of note, the College of American Pathologists does not specifically require the use of cancer protocols for gynecomastia, nor do they offer any formal guidelines for the examination of gynecomastia tissue.

Preoperative Planning

- The patient is seen preoperatively 1 to 3 days before surgery to achieve several objectives:
  - To review the procedure in detail, and revisit goals and expectations of surgery with the patient
  - To complete all perioperative paperwork, including orders, prescriptions, and instruction sheets
  - To mark the patient in an unrushed, quiet, and controlled environment
  - To obtain preoperative photographs of the marked patient
- For all procedures, the patient is marked in a standing position with arms at the sides.
  - Preoperative markings are done with a variety of colored markers.
- A laser leveler can be used to confirm the horizontal plane across the chest.
- Preoperative photographs serve several functions:
  - They document the surgical plan electronically.
  - They can be brought to the operating room to guide intraoperative decision-making.
  - They can be compared to postoperative photographs to critically appraise surgical technique and final results.
  - They can be used to educate patients in the preoperative and postoperative settings.
- Photographs, at the minimum, should capture three standard views of the breasts including the front and each side.
  - Supplemental views, including ¾s, hands over head, and with breasts lifted by the patient, can also be taken.
  - Patients should be framed from the top of the shoulders to midway between the breast and umbilicus, with the width extending just outside the arms.

Positioning

- The patient is positioned supine on an operating room table that is capable of sitting up 90 degrees.
  - This positioning will allow the patient to be placed upright intraoperatively and the chest to be evaluated in the sitting position, which may guide intraoperative decision-making.
- The patient's head is positioned at the top of the table, supported by a foam headrest.
- The patient's arms are placed on arm boards and secured to allow safe upright positioning of the patient.
  - Arm boards are placed at the shoulder level.
  - Foam pads are placed between the arm and arm boards.
  - The arm is then secured to both with a soft towel followed by a gentle circumferential wrap of gauze, which runs from the axilla to the hand to provide a uniform layer of support.
- The patient's knees are elevated with a pillow to relieve pressure on the back while the patient is upright, and the patient's heels are supported with foam pads.
- A heated air-warming device is placed on the lower body.
- The area from the top of the shoulders to midway between the inferior pole of the breast and umbilicus is prepped and draped to allow full visualization of the shoulders, chest, and breasts during surgery.

Approach

- All surgical techniques can be performed under local anesthesia, intravenous sedation, or general anesthesia.

- Development of a surgical plan is based on the need to address two issues.[16]
  - How to best remove the excess volume
  - When and how to best remove the excess skin
- Volume reduction techniques:
  - Direct glandular excision is performed when gynecomastia presents as an isolated subareolar fibrous mass.
  - Liposuction is performed when gynecomastia presents largely as a diffuse accumulation of fibrofatty tissue.
  - When both a subareolar fibrous mass and diffuse fibrofatty tissue are present, both direct excision and liposuction techniques are used to effectively recontour the chest wall.
- Skin reduction techniques:
  - In general, most patients do not require skin envelope excision after volume reduction, because the propensity of the chest wall skin to retract is significant, especially in younger patients.
  - Only in cases of significant skin excess or laxity is a skin-reducing procedure required.
  - Small localized areas of skin excess can be directly treated with skin excision.
  - Small reductions in the skin envelope or ptotic NACs can be treated with periareolar mastopexies.
  - Large reductions in the skin envelope or extremely ptotic NACs can be treated with circumvertical mastopexies.

TECHNIQUES

■ Direct Excision

- Landmarks:
  - The patient is marked in a standing position with arms at the sides.
  - The subareolar mass underneath the NAC is palpated and outlined with a surgical marker.
  - The planned incision on the inferior areolar border is marked.
- The planned incision on the inferior areolar border is first infiltrated with local anesthetic.
- Local anesthetic is also injected deep to the NAC and in the subcutaneous tissues overlying the fibrous mass.
  - In this fashion, the plane between the subcutaneous and glandular tissues is intentionally hydrodissected to facilitate later dissection with cautery.
- Using a no. 15 blade, the periareolar incision is made through the deep dermis.
- A Senn retractor is then placed on the dermal edge, upward traction is applied, and the plane between the deep dermis and glandular tissue is carefully dissected with monopolar cautery (**TECH FIG 1A**).
- The dissection is performed both medial and lateral to the area underneath the nipple first (where a true plane exists) and then joined in the middle transecting the ducts (where no true plane exists).
  - Care is taken to ensure that the NAC maintains a uniform thickness of 5 to 10 mm.

- Once beyond the boundaries of the NAC, the dissection is continued with monopolar cautery in the plane between the subcutaneous and glandular tissues, peripherally in all directions.
  - It is important to stay in this plane to preserve the overlying subcutaneous fat and maintain an even contour to the breast skin flaps.
- Once the fibrous mass is freed to its peripheral margins, it is elevated from the pectoralis major fascia.
  - Extra care is taken to avoid violating the fascia.
  - If possible, leave a bed of fat above the fascia to avoid a "saucer" contour deformity deep to the NAC.

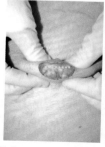 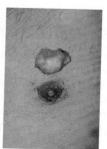

A **B**

TECH FIG 1 • A. The plane between the dermis and glandular tissues. **B.** The completed inferior areolar closure. The gynecomastia specimen is shown above.

- After the fibrous tissue is removed, the chest wall is carefully palpated and inspected for any remaining contour irregularities.
  - Further scissor dissection or cautery excision can be done at this point to feather the peripheral contours and excise any remaining glandular tissue.
- The dissected space is irrigated with normal saline and hemostasis checked.

- The wound layers are closed with 4-0 Monocryl (Ethicon Inc., Somerville, NJ, USA) or equivalent absorbable monofilament dermal interrupted suture, followed by a 3-0 Stratafix (Ethicon Inc., Somerville, NJ, USA) or equivalent absorbable barbed subcuticular suture (**TECH FIG 1B**).
- Dermabond (Ethicon Inc., Somerville, NJ, USA) is lastly applied to the skin incision.

■ Liposuction

- Landmarks:
  - The patient is marked in a standing position with arms at the sides.
  - The fibrofatty issues surrounding the breast are palpated and outlined for liposuction (**TECH FIG 2A**).
  - The planned access incisions for liposuction are marked at the lower border of the NAC and/or along the lateral aspect of the IMF.
  - The planned incisions are infiltrated with local anesthetic.
  - Wetting solution is next infiltrated deep to the NAC and in the surrounding areas of fibrofatty tissue.
    - Typical wetting solution consists of 40 to 60 mL of 1% lidocaine with 1 amp of Epi added to 1 L of NS.
    - Fluid is added to each breast until the tissue consistency is firm.

- After allowing time for the wetting solution to take effect, standard liposuction is performed (**TECH FIG 2B**).
  - A 3- to 4-mm cannula is used by the author.
  - Care is taken to feather the boundaries of the marked areas.
  - In bilateral cases, the access incision on the opposite NAC can be used and the cannula passed across the midline to liposuction the subareolar area (**TECH FIG 2C**).
  - Underneath the NAC, external pinching compression with the opposite hand is used to drive the dense subareolar fat into the cannula.
- In breasts with a well-defined IMF, the cannula can be used to discontinuously undermine it and soften it.
- All wounds are closed with dermal 4-0 Monocryl (Ethicon Inc., Somerville, NJ, USA) or equivalent absorbable monofilament dermal interrupted suture, and Dermabond (Ethicon Inc., Somerville, NJ, USA) is applied to the skin.

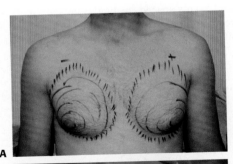
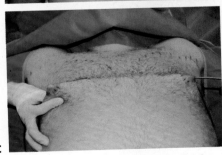
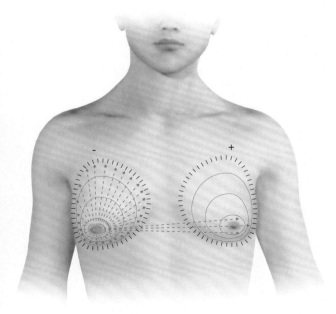

TECH FIG 2 • A. Preoperative markings of the fibrofatty tissue surrounding the breast and the planned area of liposuction. **B.** The path of the liposuction cannula to reach all areas of the breast. In bilateral cases, the NAC access incision can be used to pass the cannula across the midline to liposuction the opposite subareolar area. **C.** The liposuction cannula is shown passing through the NAC access incision and across the midline to reach the opposite subareolar area.

■ Combination Technique

- Landmarks:
  - The patient is marked in a standing position with arms at the sides.
  - The subareolar mass underneath the NAC is palpated and outlined with a surgical marker.
  - The fibrofatty issues surrounding the breast are palpated and outlined for liposuction.
  - The planned incisions on the inferior areolar border and/or the lateral aspect of the IMF are marked.
- The planned incisions on the inferior areolar border and lateral IMF are first infiltrated with local anesthetic.

- Local anesthetic is also injected deep to the NAC and in the subcutaneous tissue overlying the fibrous mass.
- Wetting solution is then infiltrated into the surrounding areas of the fibrofatty tissue until the breast is firm.
- After allowing time for the wetting solution to take effect, liposuction is then performed using a 3- to 4-mm cannula, as described above.
- Once no further liposuction can be performed, the mass effect of the remaining fibrous portion is assessed.
- If there remains a persistent and protuberant fibrous mass, the inferior areolar border is incised and the glandular tissue excised via direct excision, based on the technique as described above.

■ Periareolar Skin Reduction

- Landmarks:
  - The patient is marked in a standing position with arms at the sides.
  - The midsternal line, IMF, and lateral breast contour are marked.
  - The top of the periareolar incision is drawn, and symmetry on both sides is confirmed with a laser leveler.
    - The author typically positions the new NAC 2 to 3 cm above the existing IMF.
  - A circular pattern is next drawn around the NAC (**TECH FIG 3A**).
  - Under maximum stretch, the NAC is outlined with a nipple marker with a maximum diameter of 3 cm.
- Local anesthetic is injected in the deep dermis of the periareolar pattern.
- Wetting solution is also infiltrated deep to the NAC and in the surrounding areas of fibrofatty tissue.
- Liposuction and/or direct excision is first carried out, as described above.
- The breast is accessed through an incision on the caudal portion of the periareolar pattern.

- The NAC is incised to the deep dermis, and the previously marked periareolar pattern preliminarily stapled.
- The patient is then placed upright to visualize the resultant breast shape, and the staple line is adjusted as needed to create the desired chest contour and NAC elevation.
- After the staple line is deemed satisfactory, the patient is returned supine.
- The staple line is marked with a surgical marker, and the staples are removed.
- The intervening skin within the periareolar pattern is then de-epithelialized.
- Typically, the periareolar dermis is minimally incised or not incised at all to maintain the subdermal plexus that supplies the NAC.
- The dermis may be incised, however, in staged scenarios in which the NAC has secondarily revascularized via its wound base.
- The periareolar defect is lastly closed using a periareolar purse-string technique.[18]
  - Eight evenly spaced cardinal points are marked on the areola and periareolar incision.
- A 2-0 Cytoplast (Surgiform Technologies Ltd., Columbia, SC, USA) or equivalent polytetrafluoroethylene (PTFE) suture on a straight needle is selected.

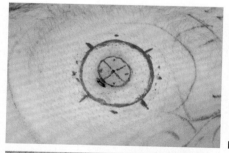
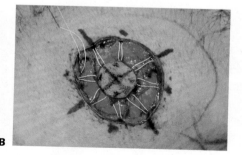
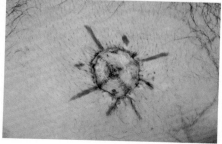

TECH FIG 3 • A. A circular pattern is drawn around the NAC to outline the periareolar pattern. **B.** Appearance of the periareolar pattern after weaving of the purse-string suture. **C.** The completed periareolar closure.

- The suture is then passed, from deep to superficial, starting on the medial dermal shelf of the periareolar incision, through the corresponding cardinal point on the dermis of the areola, inserted back into the outer dermal shelf, and then passed through the periareolar dermis to the next cardinal point.
- This weaving is continued until the suture has weaved completely around the periareolar defect, culminating in the appearance of a wagon wheel (**TECH FIG 3B**).

- The free suture ends are then tightened to cinch the periareolar incision down to match the diameter of the areola, followed by placement of 8 to 10 square knots to secure the suture.
- The knot complex is placed underneath the medial dermal shelf, and the periareolar closure is completed with 3-0 Stratafix or equivalent absorbable barbed suture (Ethicon Inc., Somerville, NJ, USA) (**TECH FIG 3C**).

■ Circumvertical Skin Reduction

- Landmarks:
  - The patient is marked in a standing position with arms at the sides.
  - The midsternal line, IMF, and lateral breast contour are marked.
  - The top of the periareolar incision is drawn, and symmetry on both sides is confirmed with a laser leveler.
    - The author typically positions the new NAC 2 to 3 cm above the existing IMF.
  - A circular pattern is next drawn around the NAC, followed by a vertical pattern below the NAC extending in a curvilinear fashion toward the IMF (**TECH FIG 4**).
  - Under maximum stretch, the NAC is outlined with a nipple marker with a maximum diameter of 3 cm.
- Local anesthetic is injected in the deep dermis of the periareolar pattern.
- Wetting solution is also infiltrated deep to the NAC and in the surrounding areas of fibrofatty tissue.
- Liposuction and/or direct excision is first carried out, as described above.
  - The breast is accessed through an incision on the caudal portion of the periareolar pattern.
- The NAC is incised to the deep dermis, and the previously marked circumvertical pattern preliminarily stapled.

- The patient is then placed upright to visualize the resultant breast shape, and the staple line is adjusted as needed to create the desired chest contour and NAC elevation.
- After the staple line is deemed satisfactory, the patient is returned supine.
- The staple line is marked with a surgical marker, and the staples are removed.
- The intervening skin within the periareolar pattern is de-epithelialized, while the intervening skin within the vertical pattern may be de-epithelialized or removed altogether.
  - Typically, the periareolar dermis is minimally incised or not incised at all to maintain the subdermal plexus that supplies the NAC, but the dermis of the vertical pattern may be incised to gain further access to the breast and/or facilitate flap advancement and closure.[16]
- The vertical pattern is closed with 4-0 Monocryl (Ethicon Inc., Somerville, NJ, USA) or equivalent interrupted deep dermal sutures followed by subcuticular closure with 3-0 Stratafix (Ethicon Inc., Somerville, NJ, USA) or equivalent absorbable barbed suture.
- The periareolar defect is closed using the periareolar purse-string technique,[18] as described earlier.

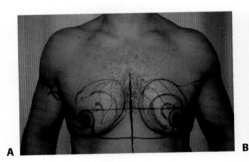
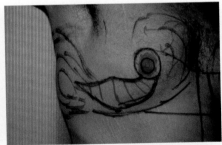
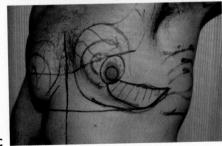

TECH FIG 4 • A-C. Preoperative markings of the planned circumvertical pattern skin reduction.

PEARLS AND PITFALLS

Landmarks	■ The top of the NAC is typically positioned 2 to 3 cm above the IMF by the authors. Although other techniques can be used to calculate the ideal position of the NAC,[3–8] it is ultimately the surgeon's artistic judgment that should prevail. To this end, sitting the patient up intraoperatively and tailor-tacking the periareolar or circumvertical patterns will preview the desired result and NAC position before irreversible incisions are made.
Technique	■ Patients with hairy chests are advised to shave preoperatively. This will save time the day of surgery and also allow easier identification of the inferior areolar border for incision placement.
	■ If there is any doubt whether skin resection is required after volume reduction techniques, stage the mastopexy. Even when skin retraction is insufficient and a second-stage procedure is required, the amount of skin reduction required is usually less than originally thought, and it may be possible to reduce the amount of cutaneous scarring.[16]
	■ In cases of delayed skin envelope reduction, no additional internal dissection is required. As well, the dermal edges of the periareolar and circumvertical patterns can be safely incised at this point to facilitate tension-free closure since the NAC will have adequate secondary revascularization from its wound base.[16]
	■ A common area for persistent skin excess and fatty accumulation, particularly in obese patients, is under the arm along the lateral chest wall. The extra skin in this area can be directly excised to achieve the appropriate chest contour (**FIG 4**).
	■ In breasts with significant fibrofatty tissue, liposuctioning the breast tissue via various access incisions can be of mechanical advantage and help achieve a more uniform reduction in breast volume. In bilateral cases, it is helpful to use the contralateral breast incisions to liposuction the ipsilateral subareolar area (see **TECH FIG 2C**).
	■ When elevating the fibrous mass off the chest wall, avoid violating the pectoralis major fascia to minimize postoperative pain, bleeding, and scar tethering deep to the NAC. If possible, leave a thin layer of fat above the fascia to maintain a natural gliding plane and to avoid a "saucer" concave deformity involving the NAC.
	■ In patients presenting for revision gynecomastia surgery, use small liposuction cannulas to carefully control the amount of liposuction performed and avoid contour irregularities. Particularly in patients who have had only liposuction performed as the primary procedure, it is wise to perform direct excision in revision surgery to eliminate any residual breast bud and avoid further patient dissatisfaction.
Postoperative care	■ It may be difficult to find compression dressings designed specifically for men. In our practice, we recommend that patients purchase a sports compression shirt that is a size smaller than the patient's normal size. If the shirt is too uncomfortable for the patient for prolonged use, the arms and bottom portion of the shirt may be trimmed so that the compression is isolated to the chest.

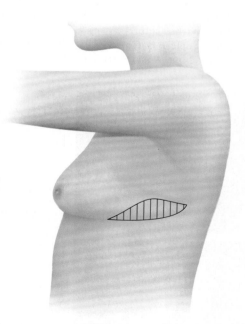

FIG 4 • A common area for persistent skin excess and fatty accumulation is the lateral chest wall.

POSTOPERATIVE CARE

■ All incisions are covered with Dermabond; no additional external dressings are required.

■ Patients are typically discharged the same day after surgery.

■ Drains are usually unnecessary but, if placed, are typically removed at the first follow-up visit.

■ Routine follow-up visits are scheduled at 1 week, 6 weeks, 6 months, and yearly thereafter.

■ A sports compression shirt is worn for the first 2 weeks.

■ Patient may resume full activities generally 4 to 6 weeks after surgery.

OUTCOMES

■ Gynecomastia surgery is generally well tolerated with patient satisfaction rates over 90%[19–21] (**FIG 5**).

■ Most patients benefit from improved emotional comfort, functional capacity, and social acceptance.[22,23]

■ Overall surgical complication rates vary from 5% to 30%, depending on the technique used.[11,20,23–26].

■ Recurrence is possible in incomplete resections or if the offending medication(s) is continued after surgery.

■ Recurrence is also more likely in patients with glandular vs fibrofatty gynecomastia.[21]

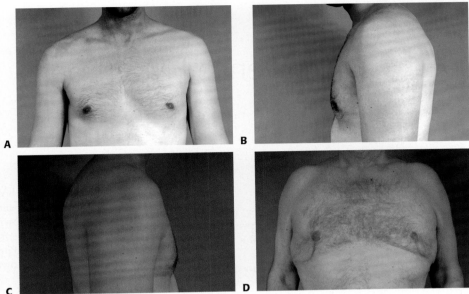

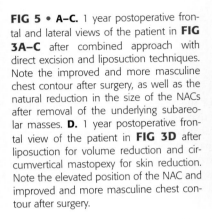

FIG 5 • A–C. 1 year postoperative frontal and lateral views of the patient in **FIG 3A–C** after combined approach with direct excision and liposuction techniques. Note the improved and more masculine chest contour after surgery, as well as the natural reduction in the size of the NACs after removal of the underlying subareolar masses. **D.** 1 year postoperative frontal view of the patient in **FIG 3D** after liposuction for volume reduction and circumvertical mastopexy for skin reduction. Note the elevated position of the NAC and improved and more masculine chest contour after surgery.

COMPLICATIONS

- Early
  - Hematoma
  - Seroma
  - Infection
  - Delayed wound healing or wound dehiscence
  - NAC necrosis
- Late
  - Adverse scarring
  - Shape change
  - Loss of nipple-areolar complex function (sensation or lactation)
  - Fat necrosis
  - "Saucer" contour deformity to the NAC

REFERENCES

1. Thiruchelvam P, Walker JN, Rose K, et al. Gynaecomastia. *BMJ.* 2016;354:i4833.
2. Narula HS, Carlson HE. Gynaecomastia: pathophysiology, diagnosis and treatment. *Nat Rev Endocrinol.* 2014;10(11):684-698.
3. Atiyeh BS, Dibo SA, El Chafic AH. Vertical and horizontal coordinates of the nipple-areola complex position in males. *Ann Plast Surg.* 2009;63(5):499-502.
4. Murphy TP, Ehrlichman RJ, Seckel BR. Nipple placement in simple mastectomy with free nipple grafting for severe gynecomastia. *Plast Reconstr Surg.* 1994;94(6):818-823.
5. Kasai S, Shimizu Y, Nagasao T, et al. An anatomic study of nipple position and areola size in Asian men. *Aesthet Surg J.* 2015;35(2):NP20-NP27.
6. Shulman O, Badani E, Wolf Y, Hauben DJ. Appropriate location of the nipple-areola complex in males. *Plast Reconstr Surg.* 2001;108(2):348-351.
7. Beckenstein MS, Windle BH, Stroup RT Jr. Anatomical parameters for nipple position and areolar diameter in males. *Ann Plast Surg.* 1996;36(1):33-36.
8. Beer GM, Budi S, Seifert B, et al. Configuration and localization of the nipple-areola complex in men. *Plast Reconstr Surg.* 2001;108(7):1947-1952.
9. Blau M, Hazani R, Hekmat D. Anatomy of the gynecomastia tissue and its clinical significance. *Plast Reconstr Surg Glob Open.* 2016;4(8):e854.
10. Blau M, Hazani R. Correction of gynecomastia in body builders and patients with good physique. *Plast Reconstr Surg.* 2015;135(2):425-432.
11. Bailey SH, Guenther D, Constantine F, Rohrich RJ. Gynecomastia management: an evolution and refinement in technique at UT Southwestern Medical Center. *Plast Reconstr Surg Glob Open.* 2016;4(6):e734.
12. Senger JL, Chandran G, Kanthan R. Is routine pathological evaluation of tissue from gynecomastia necessary? A 15-year retrospective pathological and literature review. *Plast Surg (Oakv).* 2014;22(2):112-116.
13. Nydick M, Bustos J, Dale JH Jr, Rawson RW. Gynecomastia in adolescent boys. *JAMA.* 1961;178:449-454.
14. Akgul S, Kanbur N, Derman O. Pubertal gynecomastia: what about the remaining 10%? *J Pediatr Endocrinol Metab.* 2014;27(9-10):1027-1028.
15. Niewoehner CB, Nuttal FQ. Gynecomastia in a hospitalized male population. *Am J Med.* 1984;77(4):633-638.
16. Hammond DC. Surgical correction of gynecomastia. *Plast Reconstr Surg.* 2009;124(1 Suppl):61e-68e.
17. Koshy JC, Goldberg JS, Wolfswinkel EM, et al. Breast cancer incidence in adolescent males undergoing subcutaneous mastectomy for gynecomastia: is pathologic examination justified? A retrospective and literature review. *Plast Reconstr Surg.* 2011;127(1):1-7.
18. Hammond DC, Khuthaila DK, Kim J. The interlocking Gore-Tex suture for control of areolar diameter and shape. *Plast Reconstr Surg.* 2007;119(3):804-809.
19. Colombo-Benkmann M, Buse B, Stern J, Herfarth C. Indications for and results of surgical therapy for male gynecomastia. *Am J Surg.* 1999;178(1):60-63.
20. Li CC, Fu JP, Chang SC, et al. Surgical treatment of gynecomastia: complications and outcomes. *Ann Plast Surg.* 2012;69(5):510-515.
21. Fricke A, Lehner GM, Stark GB, Penna V. Long-term follow-up of recurrence and patient satisfaction after surgical treatment of gynecomastia. *Aesthetic Plast Surg.* 2017;41:491-498.
22. Davanço RA, Sabino Neto M, Garcia EB, et al. Quality of life in the surgical treatment of gynecomastia. *Aesthetic Plast Surg.* 2009;33(4):514-517.
23. Kasielska A, Antoszewski B. Surgical management of gynecomastia: an outcome analysis. *Ann Plast Surg.* 2013;71(5):471-475.
24. Fagerlund A, Lewin R, Rufolo G, et al. Gynecomastia: a systematic review. *J Plast Surg Hand Surg.* 2015;49(6):311-318.
25. Hammond DC, Arnold JF, Simon AM, Capraro PA. Combined use of ultrasonic liposuction with the pull-through technique for the treatment of gynecomastia. *Plast Reconstr Surg.* 2003;112(3):891-895.
26. Zavlin D, Jubbal KT, Friedman JD, Echo A. Complications and outcomes after gynecomastia surgery: analysis of 204 pediatric and 1583 adult cases from a national multi-center database. *Aesthetic Plast Surg.* 2017;41:761-767.

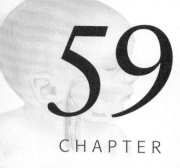

59

CHAPTER

Juvenile Hypertrophy

Dennis C. Hammond and Eric Yu Kit Li

DEFINITION

- Juvenile or virginal breast hypertrophy is a rare condition characterized by atypical and pronounced breast growth during puberty in the absence of a discrete mass or nodularity.[1,2]
- The term gigantomastia may be used to describe extreme cases.[1]

ANATOMY

- At thelarche, the breast develops into glandular tissue composed of lobules and ducts and supporting stromal tissue.
- Breast development continues until the age of 18 to 20, at which point growth is complete.
- The arterial supply of the breast is derived from numerous sources, including perforators from the internal thoracic, external thoracic, thoracoacromial, and anterior and posterior branches of intercostal arteries.
  - The internal thoracic artery is the dominant source.
  - The blood supply to the nipple-areolar complex (NAC), in particular, is augmented by a rich vascular arcade that travels in a distinct fascial septum known as *Wuringer septum*[3] (**FIG 1A**).
    - The arcade takes origin from the thoracoacromial, external thoracic, and intercostal arteries.
    - The septum arises approximately at the level of the 5th rib, dividing the breast into a superior two-thirds and inferior one-third, and courses from the pectoralis major fascia to the NAC (**FIG 1B,C**).
    - Preservation of the septum and its vascular arcade is key to maintaining a robust NAC during pedicle dissection in breast surgery.
- The venous drainage of the breast parallels the arterial supply.
- The lymphatic drainage of the breast is generally to the axillary and internal mammary lymph nodes.
- A variety of sensory nerves innervate the breast, including the anterior and lateral branches of the 2nd through 6th intercostal nerves and supraclavicular nerves.
  - The NAC is predominantly innervated by the lateral branch of the 4th intercostal nerve.
- The breast is enveloped by the Scarpa fascia, which forms anterior and posterior lamellae.
- Cooper ligaments are intraparenchymal fibers, which span both lamellae and confer structural support to the breast.
- The inframammary fold (IMF) is the foundation of the breast and is the point of convergence of the Scarpa fascia of the abdomen inferiorly with the anterior and posterior lamellae of the breast superiorly.[4]

- The fat layer above the Scarpa fascia is thicker, denser, and more compact than the fat layer below it.
- Avoidance of downward deforming pressures on the subscarpal fatty layer/space, whether by an implant or parenchyma, is key to preventing "bottoming out" of the breast and undesired lowering of the IMF.

PATHOGENESIS

- The exact cause of juvenile hypertrophy is unknown.[1,2]
- Theories include either increased end-organ sensitivity to normal levels of gonadal hormones or increased levels of gonadal hormones, although previous studies have identified normal hormone levels in juveniles diagnosed with this disease.

NATURAL HISTORY

- Juvenile hypertrophy is characterized by rapid and atypical breast growth during puberty.
- Initial growth over the first 6 months may be extreme, followed by a longer period of slower growth.
- Disease onset can be anytime during puberty, but in most cases, it is shortly after thelarche (ages 9 to 13).
- Involvement can be either unilateral, which is more common, or bilateral.

PATIENT HISTORY AND PHYSICAL FINDINGS

- Juveniles with the suspected diagnosis should be evaluated for both signs and symptoms related to rapid breast growth.
- A detailed history should inquire about:
  - The onset and velocity of breast growth
  - The onset of puberty and ongoing pubertal development
  - Associated symptoms, including headaches; neck, shoulder, or back pain; shoulder grooving from brassiere straps; and skin irritation or intertrigo along the IMF
  - Any social, vocational, or avocational dysfunction due to the hypertrophied breasts
  - The effect of the breasts on the patient's psychological well-being and self-esteem
  - Any personal or family history of breast cancer or disorders
- A detailed physical should examine
  - The patient's height, weight, and body mass index
  - For signs related to hypertrophied breasts, including skin striae or hyperemia, peau d'orange skin, dilated subcutaneous veins, or, in severe cases, tissue necrosis involving the breast
  - For specific masses, irregularities, or deformities involving the breasts or chest wall

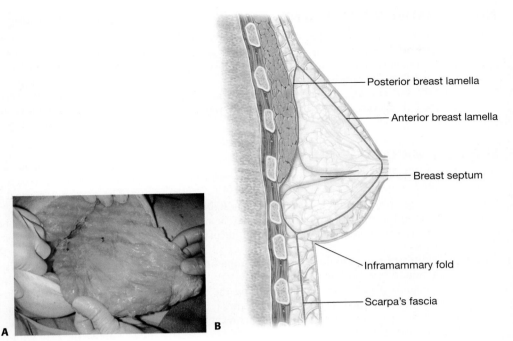

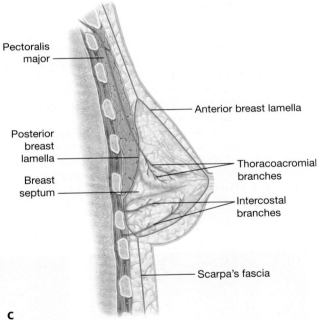

FIG 1 • **A.** Intraoperative appearance of the Wuringer septum, which is seen as a distinct white fascial layer during pedicle dissection. **B.** The Wuringer septum is a horizontally oriented fascial condensation that spans from the pectoralis major fascia, at the level of the 5th rib, to the nipple-areolar complex. The septum contains a rich vascular arcade, which receives contributions from thoracoacromial, external thoracic, and intercostal arteries. The septum divides the breast into a superior 2/3rd and inferior 1/3rd. **C.** The IMF is the point of convergence of the Scarpa fascia of the abdomen inferiorly with the anterior and posterior lamellae of the breast superiorly. Wuringer septum is illustrated in the middle of the breast.

- Overall breast aesthetics, including the shape and size of the breasts and NACs, the degree of ptosis, and the position and symmetry of the IMFs
- Standard breast measurements to highlight asymmetries, including the sternal notch to nipple, midclavicular to nipple, nipple to midline, and nipple to IMF distances

IMAGING

- Mammography tends to be of limited value because of the density of the breast tissues in juvenile hypertrophy.
- Ultrasonography or magnetic resonance imaging may be useful in select situations, especially if masses or irregularities

are identified on examination and the diagnosis is in question.
- Ultimately, diagnosis of juvenile hypertrophy is often clinical and based on history and examination.[2]

DIFFERENTIAL DIAGNOSIS[5]

- Physiologic breast hypertrophy (including normal growth or pregnancy-related growth)
- Benign breast tumors (eg, fibroadenoma, giant fibroadenoma, phyllodes tumor, or cysts)
- Malignant breast tumors (eg, ductal or lobular carcinoma, lymphoma, or metastases)

NONOPERATIVE MANAGEMENT

- Pharmacologic therapies, including tamoxifen, dydrogesterone, danazol, and bromocriptine, have been used as both primary treatment options or in combination with surgery, in either a neoadjuvant or adjuvant fashion.[6]
  - The safety and efficacy of these therapies are not well established, however, due to the scarcity of reported cases.

SURGICAL MANAGEMENT

- Surgical treatment of juvenile hypertrophy is reduction mammoplasty.
- Surgery is ideally performed once breast size has stabilized for 6 to 12 months, but earlier intervention may be necessary if there are overriding functional, medical, or psychosocial concerns.[2,7]
- All resected breast tissues should be sent for histopathological examination to rule out breast pathologies.
- Reduction mammoplasties are completed using the short scar periareolar inferior pedicle (SPAIR) technique.[8,9]
- The SPAIR technique is advantageous over other techniques for numerous reasons:
- It is versatile and can be used for breast reductions of varying size.
- Most plastic surgeons have been trained and are comfortable using the inferior pedicle.
- The circumvertical skin resection pattern minimizes scar burden, creates a more rounded breast shape, and improves breast projection while avoiding wound healing difficulties at the T junction or vertical segments associated with other breast reduction techniques.
- Lessening the scar burden is a significant priority in young female patients.
- The breast can be actively shaped with various intraoperative maneuvers to achieve the final desired contour.
- The IMF is preserved, thus minimizing the risk of long-term "bottoming out" of the breast.

Preoperative Planning

- The patient should be seen preoperatively 1 to 3 days before surgery to achieve several objectives:
  - To review the procedure in detail and revisit goals and expectations of surgery with the patient
  - To complete all perioperative paperwork, including orders, prescriptions, and instruction sheets
  - To mark the patient in an unrushed, quiet, and controlled environment
  - To obtain preoperative photographs of the marked patient
- Preoperative markings can be done with a variety of colored markers, each representing a specific surgical step.
  - The patient is marked in a standing position with arms at the sides.
    - A laser leveler can be used to confirm the horizontal plane across the chest.
  - The midsternal line, IMF, lateral breast contour, and breast meridian are first marked (**FIG 2A**).
    - The IMF is drawn across the chest so that it can be visualized with the breasts at rest (**FIG 2B**).
  - The periareolar pattern is outlined next:
    - The top point is the intersection of a line 2 to 4 cm above the IMF with the breast meridian (**FIG 2C**).
    - The bottom points are the top points of a rectangle, which is drawn 8 cm wide, centered on the breast meridian and arising from the IMF, with a height of 8 to 10 cm (**FIG 2D**).
    - The lateral and medial points are identified by lifting the breast up and outward and up and inward with just enough tension to create a rounded contour and transposing the breast meridian onto the breast (**FIG 2E,F**).
    - The above points are then joined together to create an elongated oval, which outlines the periareolar pattern (**FIG 2G**).
  - The superior aspect of the inferior pedicle is outlined last within the periareolar pattern:
    - The top points of the rectangle are joined with a curved line skirting the areola by 2 cm (**FIG 2H**).
    - The final design of the inferior pedicle thus comprises the area encompassed by the rectangle and the curved line.

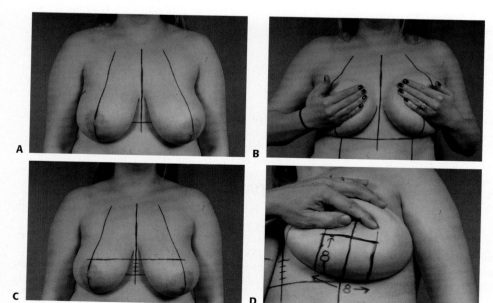

FIG 2 • A. The midsternal line, IMF, lateral breast contour, and breast meridian are marked. **B.** The IMF is drawn across the chest. **C.** The top point is the intersection of a line 2 to 4 cm above the IMF with the breast meridian. **D.** The bottom points are the top points of an 8- × 8- to 8- × 10-cm rectangle, centered on the breast meridian, arising from the IMF.

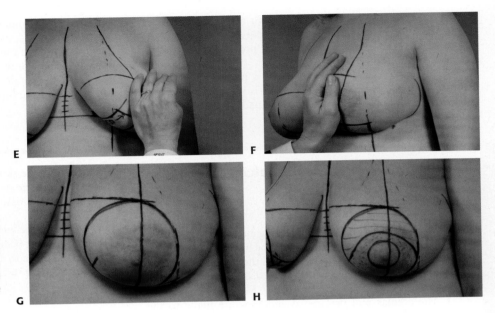

FIG 2 (Continued) • **E,F.** The lateral and medial points are identified by manipulating the breast and transposing the breast meridian. **G.** The periareolar pattern is outlined. **H.** The top points of the rectangle are joined with a curved line skirting the areola by 2 cm.

- Preoperative photographs serve several functions:
  - They document the surgical plan electronically.
  - They can be brought to the operating room to guide intraoperative decision-making.
  - They can be compared to postoperative photographs to critically appraise surgical technique and final results.
  - They can be used to educate patients at both the pre- and postoperative settings.
- Photographs, at the minimum, should capture three standard views of the breasts including the front and each side.
  - Supplemental views, including ¾s, hands over head, and with breasts lifted by the patient, can also be taken.
  - Patients should be framed from the top of the shoulders to midway between the breast and umbilicus, with the width extending just outside the arms.

Positioning

- The SPAIR technique is performed under general anesthesia.
- The patient is positioned supine, on an operating room table that is capable of sitting up 90 degrees.
  - This will allow the patient to be placed upright intraoperatively and the breasts to be evaluated in the sitting position, which may guide intraoperative decision-making.
- The patient's head is positioned at the top of the table, supported by a foam headrest (**FIG 3A**).
- The patient's arms are placed on arm boards and secured to allow safe upright positioning of the patient.
  - Arm boards are placed at the shoulder level.
  - Foam pads are placed between the arm and arm boards (**FIG 3B**).

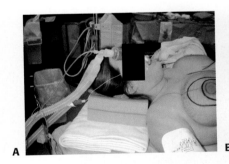
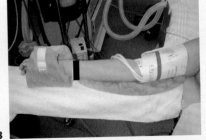
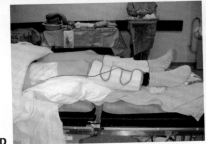
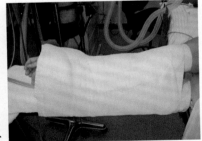
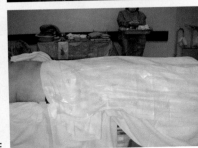

FIG 3 • A. The patient's head is positioned at the top of the table, supported by a foam headrest. **B.** Foam pads are placed between the arm and arm boards. **C.** The arm is secured with a soft towel followed by a gentle circumferential wrap of gauze. **D.** The patient's knees are elevated with a pillow, and the patient's heels are supported with foam pads. **E.** A heated air-warming device is placed on the lower body.

- The arm is then secured to both with a soft towel followed by a gentle circumferential wrap of gauze, which runs from the axilla to the hand to provide a uniform layer of support (**FIG 3C**).
- The patient's knees are elevated with a pillow to relieve pressure on the back while the patient is upright, and the patient's heels are supported with foam pads (**FIG 3D**).

- A heated air-warming device is placed on the lower body (**FIG 3E**).
- The area from the top of the shoulders to midway between the inferior pole of the breast and umbilicus is prepped and draped to allow full visualization of the shoulders, chest, and breasts during surgery.

■ Short Scar Periareolar Inferior Pedicle (SPAIR) Technique[8,9]

Incisions

- With the breast under stretch using a tourniquet, a 40- to 52-mm areolar mark is made on the breast (**TECH FIG 1A**).
- Local anesthetic is injected into all the planned incisional areas and in the dermis of the area encompassed by the inferior pedicle.
- The areolar and periareolar incisions are made to the deep dermis, and the periareolar area de-epithelialized, except in the planned crescentric resection area above the NAC (**TECH FIG 1B**).
- The periareolar area is incised through the dermis leaving a 5-mm dermal cuff from the skin edge (**TECH FIG 1C**).
  - This dermal edge will be used ultimately for placement of the periareolar purse-string suture.

Flap Creation

- Breast flaps are then developed medially, superiorly, and laterally from the periareolar incision (**TECH FIG 2A,B**).
  - The medial and superior breast flaps are dissected thicker, aiming for 4 to 6 cm thickness (**TECH FIG 2C,D**).
  - The lateral breast flap is dissected thinner, along the plane of the outer lamina (**TECH FIG 2E**).
  - At the base of the superior breast flap dissection, the cephalic aspect of the breast septum is identified and preserved, while medially and laterally the septum is incised/released (**TECH FIG 2F**).

- The curved line skirting the areola is incised. and dissection proceeds to the pectoralis fascia to define the segment of breast tissue to be removed and free the inferior pedicle.
  - The final specimen resembles a horseshoe, with the lateral segment being larger (**TECH FIG 2G**).
  - Care is taken to avoid inadvertent undermining of the pedicle and preserve the septum.

Shaping

- Various maneuvers are now used to further shape the breast as needed.
- If the upper pole is concave, the leading edge of the superior breast flap can be advanced superiorly and fixated to the pectoralis fascia using 3-0 PDS (Ethicon Inc., Somerville, NJ, USA) or equivalent absorbable interrupted sutures to autoaugment the upper pole (**TECH FIG 3A,B**).
- If the medial pole is deficient, the medial breast flap can be imbricated upon itself on its deep surface using 3-0 PDS (Ethicon Inc., Somerville, NJ, USA) or equivalent absorbable interrupted sutures to create a more rounded contour (**TECH FIG 3C,D**).
- If either contour is excessive, the breast flaps can be further debulked as needed.
- To centralize the pedicle, the superior aspect of the inferior pedicle is sutured to the pectoralis fascia (**TECH FIG 3E,F**).

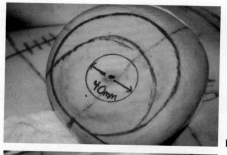
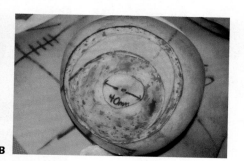
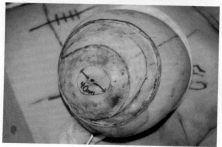

TECH FIG 1 • A. A 40- to 52-mm areolar mark is made on the breast. **B.** The areolar and periareolar incisions are made to the deep dermis, and the periareolar area de-epithelialized. **C.** The periareolar area is incised through the dermis, leaving a 5-mm dermal cuff.

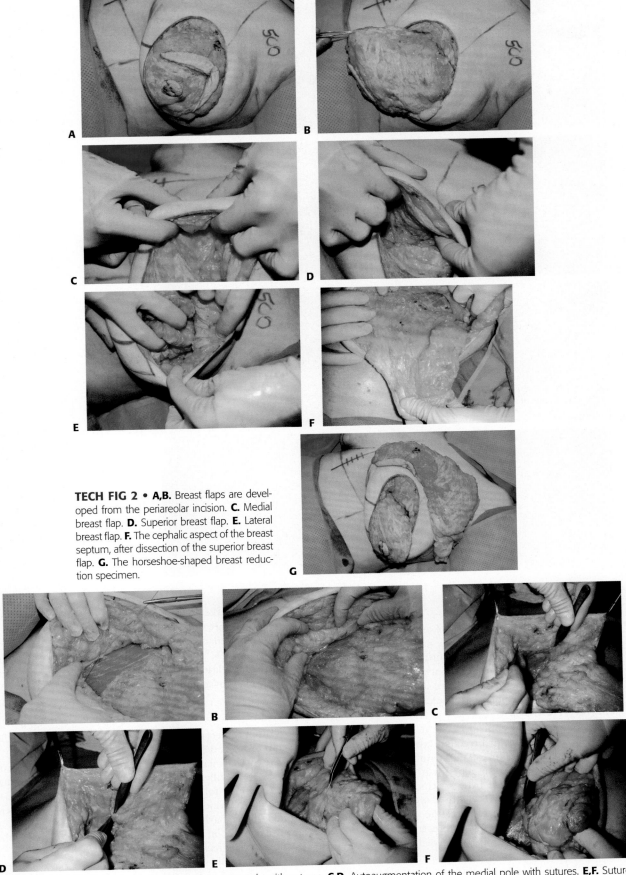

TECH FIG 2 • A,B. Breast flaps are developed from the periareolar incision. **C.** Medial breast flap. **D.** Superior breast flap. **E.** Lateral breast flap. **F.** The cephalic aspect of the breast septum, after dissection of the superior breast flap. **G.** The horseshoe-shaped breast reduction specimen.

TECH FIG 3 • A,B. Autoaugmentation of the upper pole with sutures. **C,D.** Autoaugmentation of the medial pole with sutures. **E,F.** Suture suspension of the inferior pedicle to the pectoralis fascia.

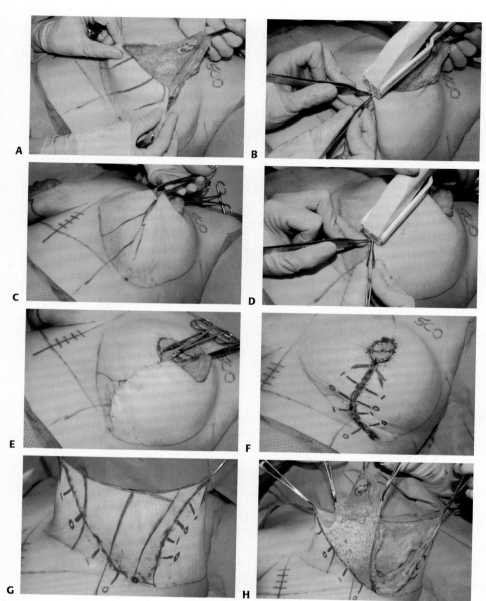

TECH FIG 4 • A,B. Two lateral buckle points are identified, which are the starting points of the inferior pole skin plication. **C–E.** The inferior pole skin is progressively stapled from superior to inferior, curving inferolaterally toward the IMF. **F,G.** The plication line is marked with a surgical marker. **H.** The outlined resection area is de-epithelialized, and the redundant medial and lateral wedges of tissue are removed.

Skin Plication

- The vertical pattern to manage the excessive skin enveloped is next created.
- A hemostat is applied to the superior pedicle and cephalic traction applied in line with the breast meridian to reveal two lateral buckle points, which are stapled together and represent the starting point of the inferior pole skin plication (**TECH FIG 4A,B**).
- With two hemostats applied to the dermal edge of the buckle points and upward traction (away from patient) in line with the breast meridian, the inferior pole skin is progressively stapled from superior to inferior, curving inferolaterally toward the IMF to achieve a smooth and contoured breast shape (**TECH FIG 4C–E**).
- After preliminary staple closure, the patient is placed upright to visualize the resultant breast shape and make adjustments to the staple line as needed.
- After the staple line is deemed satisfactory, the patient is returned supine, the plication line is marked with a

surgical marker with hash marks to guide closure, and the staples are remove (**TECH FIG 4F,G**).
- The outlined resection area, which typically resembles a "slanted V," is de-epithelialized, and the redundant medial and lateral wedges of tissue adjacent to the pedicle are removed en bloc (**TECH FIG 4H**).

Closure

- A drain is placed as desired, coursing around the pedicle, and brought out through the lateral breast.
- The vertical incision is closed with 4-0 Monocryl (Ethicon Inc., Somerville, NJ) or equivalent interrupted deep dermal sutures followed by subcuticular closure with 3-0 Stratafix (Ethicon Inc., Somerville, NJ) or equivalent absorbable barbed suture.
- The periareolar defect is closed last using the periareolar purse-string technique.[10]
  - Eight evenly spaced cardinal points are marked on the areola and periareolar incision (**TECH FIG 5A**).

- A 2-0 Cytoplast (Surgiform Technologies Ltd., Columbia, SC) or equivalent PTFE suture on a straight needle is selected.
- The suture is then passed, from deep to superficial, starting on the medial dermal shelf of the periareolar incision, through the corresponding cardinal point on the dermis of the areola, inserted back into the outer dermal shelf, and then passed through the periareolar dermis to the next cardinal point.
- This weaving is continued until the suture has weaved completely around the periareolar defect, culminating in the appearance of a wagon wheel (**TECH FIG 5B**).
- The free suture ends are then tightened to cinch the periareolar incision down to match the diameter of the areola (**TECH FIG 5C**), followed by placement of 8 to 10 square knots to secure the suture.
- The knot complex is placed underneath the medial dermal shelf, and the periareolar closure is completed with 3-0 Stratafix or equivalent absorbable barbed suture (Ethicon Inc., Somerville, NJ, USA) (**TECH FIG 5D**).

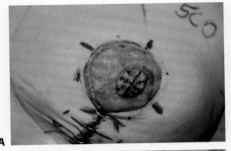
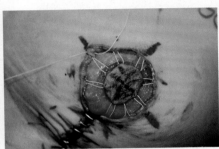
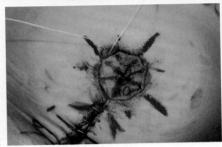
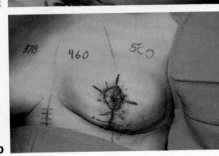

TECH FIG 5 • **A.** Eight evenly spaced cardinal points are marked on the areola and periareolar incision. **B.** Intraoperative appearance of the periareolar pattern after weaving of the purse-string suture. **C.** The periareolar incision is cinched down to match the size of the areola. **D.** Completed periareolar closure.

PEARLS AND PITFALLS

Landmarks	■ Place the top of the periareolar pattern 4 cm above the IMF for smaller reductions and 2 cm above the IMF for larger reductions because the vertical skin resection is more significant in larger breasts, which tends to create a more pronounced lifting effect. ■ Draw the rectangle below the periareolar pattern with a height of 8 cm for smaller breasts and 10 cm for larger breasts to preserve more breast skin for redraping in larger reductions. ■ Push the breasts medially after all markings are completed to confirm symmetry (**FIG 4A**). ■ To ensure that there is sufficient skin medially to allow tension-free redraping of the breast, the distance from the midsternal line to the medial mark of the periareolar pattern should be at least 12 cm (**FIG 4B**).
Technique	■ Periareolar patterns greater than 20 cm and reductions greater than 1000 g tend to be more difficult; they require more tedious dissection and greater operator skill and culminate in more pleating and scalloping around the periareolar closure. ■ The thickness of the superior and medial breasts flaps can be directly controlled by adjusting the path of dissection toward the chest wall; bevel inward for lesser thickness and vice versa. ■ With upward traction of the two hemostats applied to the dermal edge of the buckle points, and gentle inward pressure on the inferior pedicle along the breast meridian, the inferior breast tissues will imbricate and reveal a curvilinear path toward the IMF, which guides preliminary staple closure of the breast. ■ Instead of being resected, the medial wedge of tissue adjacent to the pedicle may be de-epithelialized and preserved for more medial fullness to the reduced breast. ■ If the nipple to IMF distance of the inferior pedicle is long, plication sutures can be placed on the dermis of the pedicle to shorten the distance and improve the lower pole contour of the pedicle (**FIG 5A,B**). ■ If the resultant periareolar defect after closure of the vertical segment is not circular, it can be resected again and de-epithelialized to create a circular defect that matches the areola; this will better approximate the wound edges using the periareolar purse-string technique (**FIG 5C**).
Postoperative care	■ If there is any concern about the vascularity of the NAC, especially in cases in which the inferior pedicle is long, a support bra should not be worn postoperatively to avoid compression on the pedicle, and patients should be specifically educated about this to avoid unnecessary anxiety about not wearing a bra.

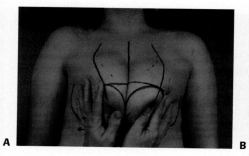
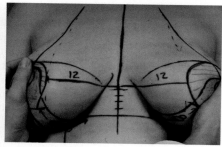

FIG 4 • **A.** The breasts are pushed medially to check that the markings are symmetrical. **B.** The minimum distance from the midsternal line to the medial periareolar pattern is 12 cm.

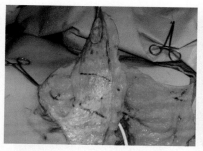
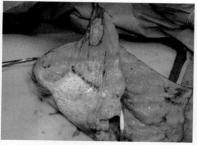
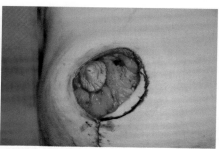

FIG 5 • **A,B.** Suture plication of the inferior pedicle to improve its contour. **C.** Planned re-resection of the periareolar pattern to create a more circular defect.

POSTOPERATIVE CARE

- All incisions are covered with Steri-Strips and Tegaderm dressings, and a support bra is worn.
- Patients are typically discharged the same day after surgery.
- Dressings remain in place for 7 to 10 days and are removed at the time of the first follow-up visit.
- Drains, if placed, are removed when their daily output is less than 30 mL.
- Routine follow-up visits are scheduled at 1 week, 6 weeks, 6 months, and yearly thereafter.
- Paper tape is applied to the healing wounds for the first 6 weeks and is changed as needed.
- A support bra is worn for the first 6 weeks.
- Patient may resume full activities, except vigorous running and weight lifting, generally 2 weeks after surgery.

OUTCOMES

- Reduction mammoplasty is generally well tolerated by adolescents from a physical and psychological perspective.[7]
- Approximately 60% of women are able to breastfeed after breast reduction.[11]
- Approximately 2% of women lose sensation to the nipple-areolar complex after breast reduction.[11]
- Recurrent hypertrophy is possible, especially if the reduction mammoplasty is performed during breast growth.

COMPLICATIONS

- Early
  - Hematoma
  - Seroma
  - Infection
  - Delayed wound healing or wound dehiscence
  - Nipple-areolar complex necrosis
- Late
  - Adverse scarring
  - Shape change
  - Loss of nipple-areolar complex function (sensation or lactation)
  - Fat necrosis

REFERENCES

1. Wolfswinkel EM, Lemaine V, Weathers WM, et al. Hyperplastic breast anomalies in the female adolescent breast. *Semin Plast Surg.* 2013;27(1):49-55.
2. Hoppe IC, Patel PP, Singer-Granick CJ, Granick MS. Virginal mammary hypertrophy: a meta-analysis and treatment algorithm. *Plast Reconstr Surg.* 2011;127(6):2224-2231.
3. Würinger E, Mader N, Posch E, Holle J. Nerve and vessel supplying ligamentous suspension of the mammary gland. *Plast Reconstr Surg.* 1998;101(6):1486-1493.
4. Muntan CD, Sundine MJ, Rink RD, Acland RD. Inframammary fold: a histologic reappraisal. *Plast Reconstr Surg.* 2000;105(2):549-556.
5. Chang DS, McGrath MH. Management of benign tumors of the adolescent breast. *Plast Reconstr Surg.* 2007;120(1):13e-19e.
6. Pruthi S, Jones KN. Nonsurgical management of fibroadenoma and virginal breast hypertrophy. *Semin Plast Surg.* 2013;27(1):62-66.
7. Xue AS, Wolfswinkel EM, Weathers WM, et al. Breast reduction in adolescents: indication, timing, and a review of the literature. *J Pediatr Adolesc Gynecol.* 2013;26(4):228-233.
8. Hammond DC. The short scar periareolar inferior pedicle reduction (SPAIR) mammaplasty. *Semin Plast Surg.* 2004;18(3):231-243.
9. Hammond DC. Short scar periareolar inferior pedicle reduction (SPAIR) mammaplasty. *Plast Reconstr Surg.* 1999;103(3):890-901.
10. Hammond DC, Khuthaila DK, Kim J. The interlocking Gore-Tex suture for control of areolar diameter and shape. *Plast Reconstr Surg.* 2007;119(3):804-809.
11. Cruz, NI, Korchin L. Lactational performance after breast reduction with different pedicles. *Plast Reconstr Surg.* 2007;120(1):35-40.

Pectus Excavatum and Pectus Carinatum

Jamie C. Harris and Fizan Abdullah

DEFINITION

- Pectus excavatum is the most common chest wall deformity that involves a concave deflection of the sternum posteriorly, with a wide range of severity from slight depression to almost reaching the level of the vertebrae. This abnormality can be present at birth but more frequently becomes apparent during puberty when rapid growth occurs.
- It occurs more frequently in males than females (3:1 ratio).
- Indications for repair include symptomatic relief, improved appearance, or to alleviate psychosocial anxiety due to the defect.
- Pectus carinatum is a congenital chest wall anomaly sometimes referred to as "pigeon chest," less common than excavatum, which is associated with a convex deformity of the sternum, leading to protrusion of the chest wall.
- Two general types are described: chondrogladiolar, which is symmetric protrusion of the body of the sternum and cartilage, and chondromanubrial, which is protrusion of the manubrium sternum with inward depression of the inferior portion. This generally presents during adolescence and has a male predominance.[1]

DIFFERENTIAL DIAGNOSIS

- Pectus carinatum vs excavatum
- Poland syndrome: absence of pectoris major and minor muscles, missing ribs, and chest wall depression
- Scoliosis: abnormal curvature of the spine that can make the chest wall appear deformed

PATIENT HISTORY AND PHYSICAL FINDINGS

- As with any patient, the first approach is a thorough history. The time course of presentation is important to identify, as it can vary from infancy to adolescence.
  - The progression of the deformity is important to note. For example, during puberty the deformity can rapidly become much more prominent.
  - Symptoms associated with pectus excavatum (PE) are rare but can include dyspnea or exercise intolerance. However, the majority of patients will not report symptoms.
  - Often, the presenting complaint is poor appearance due to the enlarging deformity at puberty.
  - Clear documentation of dyspnea, exercise intolerance, or worsening dyspnea is important to facilitate insurance coverage.
  - Family history regarding chest wall deformities should be obtained; there is a 25% rate of positive family history.

- Cardiopulmonary sequela has long been investigated; however, definitive results are still lacking. It has been shown that patients have normal spirometry preoperatively but can report subjective improvement in breathing postoperatively.
- On physical exam, symmetry of the chest should be examined. Often, asymmetry can occur, most frequently favoring the right side. Calipers can be used to determine the depth and width of the deformity; however, computed tomography (CT) scan has become a more standardized way to categorize defects.
- Chest wall inspection includes observing chest wall symmetry or asymmetry, as well as the type of deformity present.
- Auscultation can reveal displaced cardiac sounds. Additionally, a systolic ejection murmur can sometime be appreciated due to the proximity of the chest wall to the pulmonary artery. Mitral regurgitation can also be present.
- Examination of the rest of the body, looking for stigmata of Marfan syndrome including long digits or history of bruising. If present, a full evaluation for Marfan syndrome should be done.

IMAGING AND OTHER DIAGNOSIS STUDIES

- Computed tomography of the chest has now become important for diagnosing severity of the PE. The Haller index is calculated from the axial images using the ratio of the transverse diameter from the inner ribs to the length of the greatest point on defect between the posterior sternum and anterior vertebrae. A ratio greater than 3.2 is considered a severe defect.[2]
- Plain chest radiograph, posteroanterior (PA) and lateral views, has been described to calculate the Haller index as well and in some studies has been found to be equivalent for predicting severity.[3] However, most patients will generally still have CT scan for evaluation.
- Pulmonary function tests in patients with pectus excavatum have been shown to have 10% to 20% less of the expected lung volume on spirometry. Additionally, the forced expiratory volume has been shown to be less than 80% of the predicted value for patients of similar age without pectus abnormalities.[4]
- Echocardiogram for cardiac evaluation is very important in this group of patients. There is a higher prevalence of cardiac abnormalities including right ventricular compression, mitral valve prolapse and arrhythmias. An echocardiogram is important to evaluate if cardiac structure is abnormal to allow for proper operative planning if identified.[4]

SURGICAL MANAGEMENT

Preoperative Planning

Pectus Excavatum

- In general, it is preferred to time repair during the pubertal growth phase, usually from ages 10 to 15.[5] This is because the rapid growth phase can worsen pectus and therefore cause a previously repaired defect to recur. However, for children with severe exercise intolerance, earlier repair can be considered.
- Indications for operative correction include Haller index greater than 3.2, progression of severity of disease, pulmonary function tests (PFTs) demonstrating obstructive or restrictive lung patterns, or cardiac abnormalities such as displacement, arrhythmias, or murmurs.[6]
- There are two different types of repair: open (or Ravitch procedure) and the minimally invasive procedure (Nuss). There are a few important considerations to make when deciding which approach is appropriate. In patients with severe asymmetry, the open approach is often favored. Additionally, in patients presenting with a failed Nuss procedure, the open procedure should be considered for the second repair. However, overall, the Nuss procedure tends to be the procedure of choice for consideration in lower postoperative pain as well as improved appearance from its minimally invasive nature.

- If pursuing noninvasive repair with a Nuss bar, it is crucial to determine if the patient has allergies to metal, or a family history of metal allergy. If a family history is present, subsequent skin testing for metal allergy is necessary before proceeding. If an allergy is present, a titanium bar should be used instead of the standard stainless steel.
- The bar length for the Nuss procedure should be 2.5 cm shorter than the distance from the right to left midaxillary line.[7]
- General anesthesia should be achieved prior to beginning the operation, and a secure airway must be obtained at the beginning of the case.

Pectus Carinatum

- In general, most children with pectus carinatum will not require surgery. For children that are younger and have not yet completed puberty, orthotic bracing regimens are attempted to mold the chest into the correct position. Up to 75% of patients will achieve significant or complete correction of the pectus carinatum deformity using bracing alone.[8]
- The most common reason for incomplete or failed correction is patient noncompliance with bracing regimen. Noncompliance often results from failure to wear the brace often enough or in time periods long enough to correct the deformity.
- If the defect fails to improve, surgical correction can then be pursued.

■ Nuss Procedure: Minimally Invasive Approach for Pectus Excavatum

Positioning and Incision

- Patient is supine with arms extended.
- The operating surgeon is on the right and assistant surgeon on the left.
- The initial incisions should be at the transverse midaxillary line at the level of the deepest depression of the sternum, 4 cm in length on each side.

Endoscopic Bar Placement

- Once the incisions are made, carry the right-sided incision down to the pleura, entering under direct vision.
- A 5-mm thoracoscope is inserted in two rib spaces caudal to the right-sided incision to allow for direct vision of passage of the introducer.
- Deep subcutaneous tunnels are made on both the left and right sides, staying superficial to the muscle layer.
- Next, the introducer is inserted on the right, at the level just lateral to the beginning of the indentation. The introducer is passed through the intercostal muscles.
- Under direct visualization, the introducer is passed just posterior to the sternum, using extreme caution to avoid injury to the heart (**TECH FIG 1A**).
- Upon crossing the midline, the introducer is then passed through the left-sided intercostal muscles just lateral to the edge of the depression and taken out the skin incision.

- Next, umbilical tape is tied to the introducer on the left side of the chest, pulled through the tract, and removed on the right side.
- The preformed bar is then attached to the umbilical tape, and it is then pulled through the track, with the apex of the bar angled away from the sternum (**TECH FIG 1B**).
- The bar is then rotated 180 degrees, such that the convex portion of the bar is against the sternum (**TECH FIG 1C**).
- This is secured in place using bar stabilizers on both sides. Either wire of heavy PDS suture is passed around the stabilizers and the rib to avoid bar displacement.
- For patients that have severe deformity, a second bar can be used. This is placed in the same manner, slightly inferior to the original bar.

Closure

- A 16-French red rubber catheter is placed in the tract of the camera port. A positive end expiratory pressure of 5 mm Hg is given, and a Valsalva is done by anesthesia to evacuate any residual air within the thoracic cavity. Alternatively, Valsalva without a red rubber catheter can also be used to evacuate residual air.
- The lateral incisions are then closed in layers using an absorbable suture
- The skin is closed with a running subcuticular suture
- Rarely, a chest tube is required for this procedure.

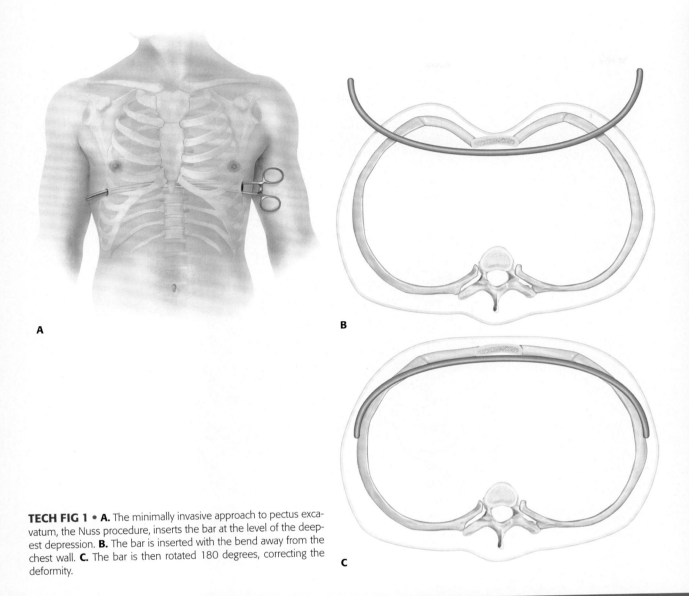

TECH FIG 1 • A. The minimally invasive approach to pectus excavatum, the Nuss procedure, inserts the bar at the level of the deepest depression. **B.** The bar is inserted with the bend away from the chest wall. **C.** The bar is then rotated 180 degrees, correcting the deformity.

■ Open Ravitch Procedure for Pectus Excavatum

Positioning and Incisions

- The patient should be in the supine position with their arms out to the side on the operating room table.
- Both the chest and abdomen should be prepped and draped into the sterile field.
- The operating surgeon will be positioned on the patient's right, the assisting surgeon on the patient's left, and the anesthesiologist at the head of the bed.
- Two incisions can be used depending on the cosmetic outcomes. A sternal incision or transverse incision at the fourth intercostal space is used in males.
- In females, better cosmetic outcomes can be achieved using a transverse incision instead of a sternal incision. Care should be taken to make this incision within the projected inframammary crease to prevent injury to the breast bud (**TECH FIG 2**).

Exposure and Resection of the Abnormal Ribs

- Continue the incision creating skin flaps that are centered at the sternum. The skin flap should extend cephalad to the angle of Louis, the manubriosternal junction, and caudally to the xiphoid, allowing for adequate visualization of sternum and costal cartilage.
- Next, the pectoralis major muscle flaps should be elevated; passing an empty knife anterior to the costal cartilage insures the correct plane. This is continued cephalad until the highest abnormal cartilage is seen.
- Next, the rectus abdominis is mobilized off of the inferior border of the sternum.
- The perichondrium is excised anteriorly to expose the bony rib up to the sternum, exposing the cartilage at its insertion site on the sternum
- Using a Haight elevator to protect the mediastinum, the deformed cartilage is cut from the sternum using a knife. The deformed cartilage is then removed and cut at the costal cartilage junction, leaving a 5-mm margin.

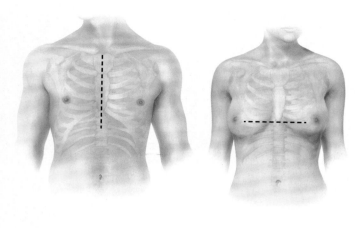

TECH FIG 2 • Open repair, Ravitch procedure, is used for both pectus excavatum and carinatum. Incision is made either midline for males or inframammary in females.

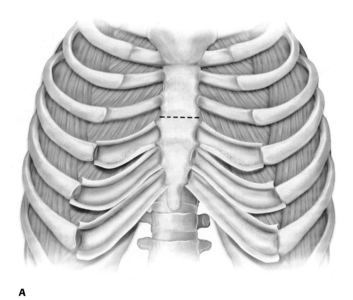

A

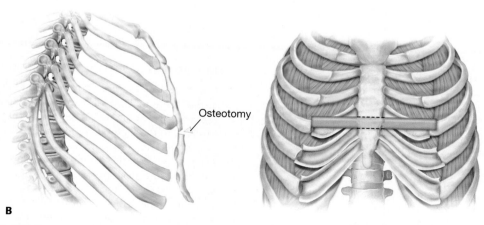

Osteotomy

B

TECH FIG 3 • A. Skin flaps are made, and the periosteum is cleared from both sides of the sternum. The deformed cartilage is cut from the sternum using a knife and removed. **B.** The sternum is then either flattened with a wedge osteotomy (for carinatum) or elevated with a transverse osteotomy (for excavatum).

- This is continued until all deformed cartilage has been resected. Then, a sternal wedge osteotomy is made just cranial to the final resected cartilage (**TECH FIG 3**).

Sternal Closure

- At the level of the osteotomy, the sternum is fractured and lifted into a flat orientation.

- Although not necessary in all cases, a sternal bar can be inserted posterior to the sternum at this point. This is secured to the adjacent ribs for greater stabilization.
- If a bar is not used, heavy silk suture is used to close the sternal ostomy, fixing the sternum at the corrected position.
- Perichondrial sheaths are then reappoximated if necessary.

Closure

- A Hemovac drain is inserted through the inferior skin flap and placed along the sternal edge of the cut cartilage.

- The pectoralis muscle is then closed in the midline and secured to the sternum.
- The rectus muscles are then closed in the midline using an absorbable suture and reattached to the sternum.
- Layered closure of the subcutaneous tissues is done, and the skin is closed using a subcuticular stitch.

■ Open Ravitch Procedure for Pectus Carinatum

- The initial steps of the carinatum repair mirror that of the Ravitch procedure for pectus excavatum.
- The difference in technique from excavatum begins when the sternal osteotomy is made. Unlike in pectus excavatum in which a wedge osteotomy is made, a transverse linear osteotomy is made for correction

of pectus carinatum at the point where the superficial deflection begins.
- The xiphoid process is detached from the sternum to allow for better sternal mobilization. The sternum is then flattened posteriorly to create a flat surface. The xiphoid process is then reattached once the sternum is in correct position.[9]
- Closure is the same as for Ravitch procedure for pectus excavatum.

PEARLS AND PITFALLS

Pectus excavatum	■ Most patients with symmetric pectus excavatum are well suited for a Nuss procedure. ■ Most patients who require redo surgery for pectus excavatum may benefit from a Ravitch procedure or a combined Ravitch and Nuss procedure.
Pectus carinatum	■ Nonoperative treatment is the mainstay of treatment for carinatum; however, asymmetric lesions tend to require surgery more often. For symmetric deformities, bracing is first-line treatment. ■ In some hands, the combination of postoperative antibiotics with sterile operative techniques has resulted in almost no wound infections in patients with pectus carinatum[10]

POSTOPERATIVE CARE

Pectus Excavatum

- Chest radiograph should be performed in the recovery room. This should confirm appropriate placement of the bar and also evaluate for pneumothoraces. It is not uncommon to have very small bilateral pneumothoraces that can be monitored; these usually do not require tube thoracostomy.
- Pain can be significant in the postoperative period for both procedures. Additionally, for some patients, pain can continue during the entire time the Nuss bar is in place. This pain can be managed generally with physical therapy and medications. Rarely, the bar is removed for severe pain.
- For the initial 6 weeks postoperatively, patients must refrain from any sports.
- Patients are forbidden from participating in any heavy contact sports, such as wrestling, football, and hockey for the entire duration that the Nuss bar is in place. Aerobic activities, such as running or soccer, are allowed after the initial 6 weeks.
- The Nuss bar must remain in place for at least 2 years. Timing of removal is based upon patient growth; for older patients in their rapid growth phase, removal is usually

closer to 2 years. For younger patients who have not yet reached puberty, the bar can remain in place for up to 4 years.

Pectus Carinatum

- Postoperative pain is initially managed with intravenous analgesia and then transitioned to oral pain medication.
- Generally, patients are discharged within 2 to 3 days postoperatively.
- Intravenous antibiotics can be considered for 48 hours postoperatively, and oral antibiotics are continued for another 4 days.

OUTCOMES

- No difference in length of stay between open and Nuss procedures has been demonstrated. Procedure length was slightly increased with open operation.
- The Nuss procedure is associated with higher rates of reoperation, pneumothorax, and hemothorax.[11]
- Postoperative seroma formation is the most common complication in the open procedure. Due to this, a drain is left in the potential space within the skin flaps.

- Patient satisfaction scores have not been found to differ significantly between Nuss and open procedures, with 93.3% and 92% reported overall improved cosmetic outcomes, respectively. Symptomatic relief was also reported by both groups of patients.[12]
- Overall recurrence rates vary among studies but have been quoted between 2% and 10% in both open and Nuss procedures.[13]

COMPLICATIONS

Pectus Excavatum

- Cardiac perforation: this is an exceedingly rare intraoperative complication; however, if it does occur, it has an extremely high rate of mortality. Immediate sternotomy with cardiac repair should be done. This complication is more often associated with the Nuss procedure.
- Pneumothorax: in general, asymptomatic pneumothorax can be observed. Rarely, this may be symptomatic and require insertion of a chest tube.
- Bar dislodgement in the Nuss procedure can occur in up to 5% of patients; this can happen through the immediate or late postoperative period. If early, it can lead to immediate recurrence, and reoperation is required.
- Allergic reaction to the metal bar, ranging from rash to anaphylaxis.
- Prolonged pain, requiring bar removal in some cases.
- Recurrence has been documented after bar removal.

Pectus Carinatum

- Fortunately, complications are rare following repair of pectus carinatum.[10]
- Pneumothorax has been quoted at rate of 2% after repair[10,14] but were less than 10% of total lung volume.
- Wound infection is a risk with any surgery and occurs at a very low rate.
- Recurrence/continued exercise intolerance: almost all patients report an improvement in exercise tolerance 3 to 4 months post procedure, and only 2.8% did not report an excellent result.

REFERENCES

1. Desmarais TJ, Keller MS. Pectus carinatum. *Curr Opin Pediatr.* 2013;25(3):375-381.
2. Haller JA Jr, Kramer SS, Lietman SA. Use of CT scans in selection of patients for pectus excavatum surgery: a preliminary report. *J Pediatr Surg.* 1987;22(10):904-906.
3. Khanna G, Jaju A, Don S, Keys T, Hildebolt CF. Comparison of Haller index values calculated with chest radiographs versus CT for pectus excavatum evaluation. *Pediatr Radiol.* 2010;40(11):1763-1767.
4. Nuss D, Kelly RE Jr. Indications and technique of Nuss procedure for pectus excavatum. *Thorac Surg Clin.* 2010;20(4):583-597.
5. Sacco-Casamassima MG, Goldstein SD, Gause CD, et al. Minimally invasive repair of pectus excavatum: analyzing contemporary practice in 50 ACS NSQIP-pediatric institutions. *Pediatr Surg Int.* 2015;31(5):493-499.
6. Frantz FW. Indications and guidelines for pectus excavatum repair. *Curr Opin Pediatr.* 2011;23(4):486-491.
7. Kelly RE, Goretsky MJ, Obermeyer R, et al. Twenty-one years of experience with minimally invasive repair of pectus excavatum by the Nuss procedure in 1215 patients. *Ann Surg.* 2010;252(6):1072-1081.
8. Banever GT, Konefal SH, Gettens K, Moriarty KP. Nonoperative correction of pectus carinatum with orthotic bracing. *J Laparoendosc Adv Surg Tech A.* 2006;16(2):164-167.
9. Robicsek F, Watts LT, Fokin AA. Surgical repair of pectus excavatum and carinatum. *Semin Thorac Cardiovasc Surg.* 2009;21(1):64-75.
10. Fonkalsrud EW. Surgical correction of pectus carinatum: lessons learned from 260 patients. *J Pediatr Surg.* 2008;43(7):1235-1243.
11. Nasr A, Fecteau A, Wales PW. Comparison of the Nuss and the Ravitch procedure for pectus excavatum repair: a meta-analysis. *J Pediatr Surg.* 2010;45(5):880-886.
12. Jo WM, Choi YH, Sohn YS, et al. Surgical treatment for pectus excavatum. *J Korean Med Sci.* 2003;18(3):360-364.
13. Antonoff MB, Erickson AE, Hess DJ, et al. When patients choose: comparison of Nuss, Ravitch, and Leonard procedures for primary repair of pectus excavatum. *J Pediatr Surg.* 2009;44(6):1113-1118.
14. Fonkalsrud EW, DeUgarte D, Choi E. Repair of pectus excavatum and carinatum deformities in 116 adults. *Ann Surg.* 2002;236(3):304-312.

Section XVI: Thorax and Back

Myelomeningocele: Postnatal Repair

Gregory G. Heuer and Jesse A. Taylor

61

CHAPTER

DEFINITION

- Myelomeningocele (MMC) is a congenital malformation of the spinal cord in the family of neural tube defects and spina bifida.[1]
- MMC develops from a failure of neurulation of the spinal cord during the fourth week of gestation. The exposure of the spinal cord results in dysfunction of neural tissue as a result of the malformation itself and damage to the exposed neural tissue.
- MMCs occur in roughly 1 in 1000 live births and lead to significant morbidity including bowel and bladder dysfunction, gait disturbances, and even paralysis. Importantly, lack of sensation caudal to the MMC may result in significant decubital wound issues.

ANATOMY

- The MMC results from failure of neurulation, which results in an "open book" of distinct elements that are normally closed over the spinal cord[2] (**FIG 1**).
  - The placode, the exposed flat spinal cord tissue, is present in the center, with nerve roots running ventrally and exiting through the spine foramen. Atrophic nerve roots can often be seen exiting the placode and running to the skin and soft tissue. These are nonfunctional elements.
  - The zona epitheliosa surrounds the placode and contains cerebrospinal fluid (CSF). This is part of the sac or "bubble" seen on imaging studies.
  - The dura of the meninges is open and reflected and covers the fascia and muscle.
  - The skin is located laterally to the lesion. Some of this tissue is extremely thin and atrophic. The quality of the skin needs to be taken into account, as it impacts surgical closure.

- Elements of the posterior vertebral body—the spinous process and lamina—are absent, and the spinal column is open dorsally. The open spinal column can be seen laterally as the bifida bone elements.
- In some cases, a sac is not present, and the placode is flat and in the spinal elements. This condition is known as myeloschisis and is managed in the same way as a MMC.

PATHOGENESIS

- During neurulation, normally the neural tube undergoes an ordered process of formation and closure. During this process, the neural folds meet and fuse, followed by closure of the layers around the spinal cord—including the dura, bone, muscle, and skin.[1]
- MMC results from a failure of the neural tube to close at the caudal end, resulting in the exposure of the spinal cord—the placode—to the external environment.
- Most cases are idiopathic, though risk factors include genetic susceptibility and environmental risks such as toxins or medication exposure.
- Risk factors include genetic susceptibility and environmental risks such as toxins or medication exposure. In most cases, there is not an identifiable cause and is thus idiopathic.
- In some populations, the use of high-dose folic acid supplementation prior to conception can reduce the risk of neural tube defects, as folate is a known cofactor in many of the folding processes involved in neurulation.

NATURAL HISTORY

- MMC leads to irreversible loss of nerve function at the level of the exposed spinal cord.
- This loss of function occurs from[3]:
  - Abnormal development of the spinal cord
  - Direct damage to the exposed spinal cord from trauma and toxic injury

PATIENT HISTORY AND PHYSICAL FINDINGS

- Patients with MMC are typically identified prior to birth.
- Ultrasound examination is performed for three reasons:
  - To define the MMC defect and its spinal level
  - To look at associated abnormalities of the central nervous system
  - To analyze the fetus for other structural abnormalities
- Patients with known MMC lesions are typically delivered via cesarean section.
- Newborn MMC patients are cared for in a systematic fashion (http://www.chop.edu/clinical-pathway/myelomeningocele-myeloschisis-neonatal-clinical-pathway).

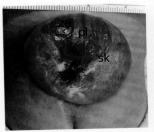 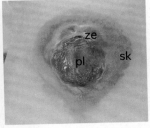

A **B**

FIG 1 • Appearance of an MMC defect. The neural placode (*pl*) is seen at the center. This is surrounded by the zona epitheliosa (*ze*) and the skin (*sk*). The myofascial layer can often be seen through the translucent portion of the arachnoid surrounding the ze.

- General neonatal care must be the first priority, assuring that the newborn is stable and healthy and avoiding the temptation to focus solely on the MMC lesion.
- In the presence of a MMC, the patient is generally positioned prone to avoid undue pressure on the exposed spinal elements. A sterile gauze is placed on the MMC lesion, and this is kept moist with a constant drip of sterile saline from a bag suspended above the patient.
- The patient is placed on antibiotics (ampicillin and amoxicillin) as prophylaxis against bacterial seeding of the spinal elements.
- Consults are obtained including the physical therapy, neurosurgery, orthopedics, plastic surgery, urology, and spina bifida team.
- An ultrasound of the head is obtained to establish a baseline of the ventricular system.
- A physical exam is performed on the infant.
    - The infant is examined for signs of hydrocephalus such as a full fontanelle, large head circumference, or splayed sutures.
        - In most instances, newborn MMC patients do not show clinical signs of hydrocephalus until after the MMC closure is performed.
        - The anatomy of the MMC defect is similar (see **FIG 1**) even if the overall appearance of the lesion may be grossly variable (**FIG 2**).
    - The size of the MMC lesion is noted as well as the quality of the skin. These factors are important to anticipate the need for specialized closure techniques such as rotational flaps, allograft patches, or skin grafts.
    - A neurologic exam is performed to assess the clinical level of function. The clinical exam is very difficult to interrupt in a newborn and should be done by a trained clinician

and followed over time for any changes. Movement secondary to direct stimulation that is not clinically significant can be present below the level of the lesion and should not be confused with volitional movement.[4]
    - The infant should be examined for orthopedic deformities, such as talipes or hip contractures. These are important to note prior to the MMC closure as they may affect patient positioning both before and after surgery.
- Surgical closure of the MMC is typically performed within the first 48 hours after birth.
    - However, this can be delayed if the patient is not clinically stable as long as the positioning, wound care, and prophylactic antibiotics are administered. The risks of delaying surgery must be carefully weighed against the risks of infection and further neurological deterioration. If the surgery is delayed for weeks to months, the granulation tissue that develops can increase the technical difficulty of the closure.
- MMC closure is performed in a stepwise fashion to close the layers over the spinal cord that should be present.

SURGICAL MANAGEMENT

- The overall goal of the surgical closure is to obtain a multi-layer closure of all three layers of the back—dura, muscle, skin—that is watertight.

Positioning

- The infant is placed prone with the abdomen suspended to promote venous return and reduce bleeding during surgery (**FIG 3**).
- The back is widely prepped on the table with Betadine. The back must be prepped in a wide fashion to allow for skin rotational procedures.

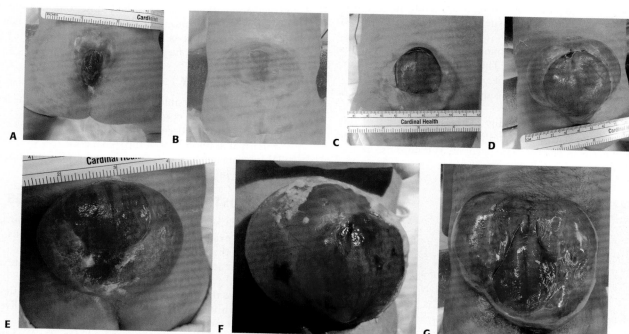

FIG 2 • Various MMC lesions. Note the variability in the size and appearance of the lesions.

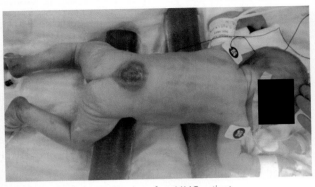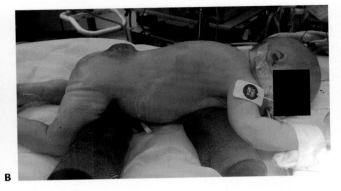

FIG 3 • Intraoperative positioning of an MMC patient.

■ Release of the Placode

- The tissue just lateral to the placode is sharply incised, releasing the placode to float ventrally into the spinal column (**TECH FIG 1A**).

- It is often necessary to make this incision further from the placode and the residual tissue should be dissected from the placode.
- The placode can be rolled back into a tubular structure by placing sutures in the pial layer. This is often accomplished with 6-0 Prolene interrupted sutures (**TECH FIG 1B**).

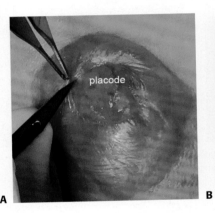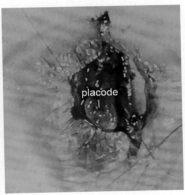

TECH FIG 1 • **A.** Dissection of the placode from the surrounding tissue. **B.** The released placode is brought into a tubular shape with fine sutures.

■ Skin Release and Mobilization

- The skin is then released from the underlying fascia and muscle (**TECH FIG 2**).
- The skin is undermined widely, resulting in greater exposure of the underlying fascia and freeing up soft tissues that can be more easily rotated over the fascia during the skin closure.
- Care needs to be taken to stay in the proper plane and avoid tearing the skin and soft tissues during this undermining process.
- The edges of the skin are then trimmed back to the tissue that will support dermal and skin sutures.

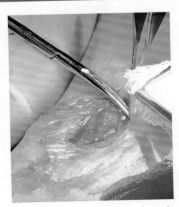

TECH FIG 2 • The skin is extensively undermined.

■ Dura, Myofascial, and Skin Closure

- The next step is closure of the lateral tissue over the placode. The goal of the closure is a watertight closure over the placode.
- The skin is held with a retractor, exposing the lateral dura and fascia.
- An incision is made in the lateral tissue. This tissue is normally the dura that is present over the top of the muscle and fascia.
  - This is carefully mobilized over the underlying tissue and rotated over the placode (**TECH FIG 3A**).
  - The dura may be thin or absent in the sacral portion of the MMC.
- The next layer is the myofascial layer (**TECH FIG 3B**).
  - An incision is made in the fascial layer. This needs to be several centimeters away from the opening to allow it to be rotated over the dural closure without tension.

Mobilization of the layer can be assisted by releasing this layer from the opening spina bifida elements.
- This layer is rotated to the midline and closed (**TECH FIG 3C**).
- After closure of the myofascial flaps, the skin is further undermined. Additionally, extension of the superior and inferior skin edges can increase the mobilization of the skin flap.
- The skin flaps are then rotated to the midline and closed in two layers (**TECH FIG 3D**).

Additional Maneuvers

- If the skin cannot be mobilized, additional maneuvers are sometimes needed.
- This can include placing an AlloDerm patch (LifeCell, Branchburg, NJ) (**TECH FIG 4**), relaxing incisions in the posterior axillary line, or Z-plasty extensions.

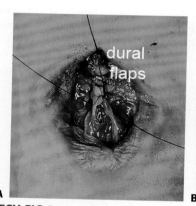 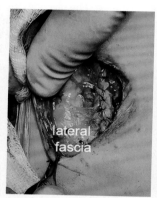 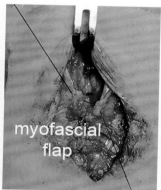 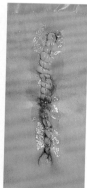

TECH FIG 3 • **A.** The dural flaps are rotated over the placode and closed in the midline. **B.** Exposure of the lateral myofascia. **C.** Rotation and closure of the myofascial flaps. **D.** Appearance of the skin after closure.

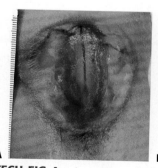 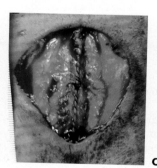 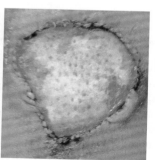

TECH FIG 4 • Appearance of a large MMC preoperatively **(A)**, which resulted in a skin wound **(B)** that required an AlloDerm patch **(C)**.

PEARLS AND PITFALLS

Closure	■ A multilayer watertight closure is essential to prevent wound breakdown and protect the placode from further damage or infection. ■ If fluid collections form that are consistent with pseudomeningoceles, this needs to be treated, normally with CSF diversion. ■ It is important to be aware of the vascular supply to skin flaps to prevent necrosis of the skin when performing Z-plasty or relaxing incisions.
Intraoperative care	■ The patient needs to be positioned to take pressure off the abdomen and other pressure points; this will promote venous return, reduce bleeding, and prevent pressure sores. ■ The patient should be prepped and draped widely to allow multiple options for skin closure.

POSTOPERATIVE CARE

■ The patient is cared for in the neonatal ICU. Close observation for bladder dysfunction, pressure points, and orthopedic issues is paramount.

■ Special attention should be paid to the examination of the wound. Wound care is very important as the wound is in the lumbosacral area and is prone to contamination with stool or urine. A drape separating the anal region from the MMC closure should be placed to divert stool, but local wound care must be maximal to prevent infection.

■ The child needs to be monitored for the development of hydrocephalus. In patients with a full fontanelle, enlarging pseudomeningoceles, or other clinical signs of hydrocephalus, they should be treated with CSF diversion, either with a ventriculoperitoneal shunt or an external ventricular catheter.

REFERENCES

1. Copp AJ, Adzick NS, Chitty LS, et al. Spina bifida. *Nat Rev Dis Primers.* 2015;1:15007.
2. Heuer GG, Adzick NS, Sutton LN. Fetal myelomeningocele closure: technical considerations. *Fetal Diagn Ther.* 2015;37(3):166-171.
3. Walsh DS, Adzick NS, Sutton LN, Johnson MP. The rationale for in utero repair of myelomeningocele. *Fetal Diagn Ther.* 2001;16:312-322.
4. Rintoul NE, Sutton LN, Hubbard AM. A new look at myelomeningoceles: functional level, vertebral level, shunting, and the implications for fetal intervention. *Pediatrics.* 2002;109:409-413.

62

CHAPTER

Myelomeningocele, Prenatal (Fetal) Repair

Gregory G. Heuer and N. Scott Adzick

DEFINITION

- Myelomeningocele (MMC) is a congenital malformation of the spinal cord in the family of neural tube defects and spina bifida as described in the previous chapter (Myelomeningocele, Postnatal Closure).
- Prenatal surgery was first attempted in the 1990s. A randomized controlled trial, the Management of Myelomeningocele Study (MOMS), demonstrated that closure during the prenatal period could be performed relatively safely and can result in significant benefit to the child.[1]

ANATOMY

- The MMC results from failure of neurulation resulting in an "open book" of distinct elements that are normally closed over the spinal cord (**FIG 1**) as described in the Myelomeningocele, Postnatal Closure chapter.

PATHOGENESIS

- During neurulation, normally the neural tube undergoes an ordered process of formation and closure as described in the Myelomeningocele, Postnatal Closure chapter.

NATURAL HISTORY

- MMC leads to irreversible loss of nerve function at the level of the exposed spinal cord as described in the previous chapter (Myelomeningocele, Postnatal Closure).
- In addition, a fetus with MMC will progressively develop two associated conditions as the result of the continued cerebrospinal fluid (CSF) leak, a Chiari malformation with hindbrain herniation and hydrocephalus.[2]

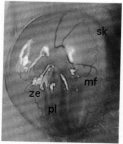

FIG 1 • Appearance of an exposed MMC defect during a fetal repair. The neural placode (*pl*) is seen at the center. This is surrounded by the zona epitheliosa (*ze*) and the skin (*sk*). The myofascial layer (*mf*) covered by dura can be seen through the translucent arachnoid.

PRENATAL EVALUATION

- Expectant mothers receive extensive prenatal testing to determine if they are candidates for prenatal surgery. The inclusion and exclusion criteria in the MOMS trial are still used by most fetal therapy centers (Table 1).[3]
- Ultrasound (US) examination is performed for three reasons: to define the MMC defect and its spinal level, look at associated CNS abnormalities, and evaluate the fetus for other structural abnormalities.
- With regard to the MMC defect and CNS-associated conditions, US is used specifically:
  - To define the level of bone and skin opening
  - To analyze the posterior fossa, specifically to look for the presence of hindbrain herniation (must be present as it confirms an open neural tube defect)
  - To determine the size of the lateral ventricles and degree of ventriculomegaly
  - To look for any associated abnormalities such as a spinal cord syrinx, a split cord malformation, or a significant kyphosis that may affect the eligibility of the patient for fetal MMC repair.
- Patients also receive a fetal magnetic resonance imaging (MRI) scan. These scans provide a more detailed anatomic evaluation of the MMC defect and associated abnormalities, particularly the presence of hindbrain herniation.
- In addition to imaging, the fetus undergoes an analysis for genetic or chromosomal abnormalities. Also, amniotic fluid analysis is performed to confirm an open neural tube defect.
- A detailed medical history for the mother is obtained, specifically looking for significant maternal health issues and risk factors associated with premature delivery.

SURGICAL MANAGEMENT

- The overall goal of the surgical repair is to obtain a multilayer closure that is watertight. To provide the greatest possible benefit to the fetus, the closure needs to protect the neural structures from direct trauma, prevent the leakage of CSF, and prevent the exposure of the neural structures to amniotic fluid. Additionally, the closure needs to be done in a manner that is safe for the fetus and the mother, as extreme premature birth can erase all potential gains of the surgical procedure. There are some modifications of the general technique outlined below, but the principles above should not be compromised.

Preoperative Planning[3]

- A preoperative US is obtained to confirm the location of the fetus and the placenta.

Table 1 MOMS Trial Inclusion and Exclusion Criteria

Inclusion	Singleton pregnancy
	Lesion level T1-S1
	Evidence of hindbrain herniation
	Gestational age of 19.0–25.9 weeks
	Normal karyotype
	U.S. residency
	Maternal age of 18 years or older
Exclusion	Fetal anomaly unrelated to myelomeningocele
	Severe kyphosis greater than or equal to 30 degrees
	Multiple gestation
	Previous spontaneous preterm birth less than 37 weeks
	Short cervix less than 20 mm
	Placental abruption or abnormal placentation (placenta previa)
	Obesity defined as BMI > 35
	Maternal medical condition that would place an additional risk to maternal health/surgical risk or the pregnancy (insulin-dependent diabetes, poorly controlled hypertension)
	Documented history of incompetent cervix or planned/current cerclage
	Maternal-fetal Rh isoimmunization, Kell sensitization, or a history of neonatal alloimmune thrombocytopenia
	Maternal HIV, hepatitis B or hepatitis C positivity
	Uterine anomaly such as multiple fibroids or müllerian duct abnormality; previous hysterotomy in the active segment of the uterus
	Patient does not have a support person
	Inability to comply with the travel and follow-up requirements
	Patient does not meet other psychosocial criteria to handle the implications of the trial
	Participation in another study that influences maternal and fetal morbidity and mortality or participation in this trial in a previous pregnancy

- The mothers receive an epidural catheter for delivery for intraoperative and postoperative pain control.
- Antibiotics and indomethacin are given.

Positioning and Anesthetic Concerns[3]

- The mother is placed supine on the operating room table with a bump placed under the right side to avoid inferior vena cava compression by the gravid uterus and compromise of venous return.
- The surgery is performed under deep general anesthesia, with the goal to achieve maximum uterine relaxation. In addition to maternal anesthetic, the fetus receives a direct dose of intramuscular anesthesia (vecuronium and fentanyl).

- The cardiac function of the fetus is continually monitored by fetal echocardiography. If a decrease in cardiac function is seen, the anesthetic to the mother is adjusted or the fetus is examined for signs of umbilical cord or placental compression.[4]
- An arterial line is placed in the mother.

Approach

- The uterus is approached via a low transverse maternal laparotomy. Of note, the uterus is opened in the upper muscular portion and not the lower segment used for typical cesarean sections (**TECH FIG 1A**).
- The site of the placenta is mapped out on the surface of the uterus. If the placenta is anterior, the uterus is rotated out of the abdomen to gain access to the fundus and posterior uterine wall. The goal is to open the uterus at least 6 cm away from the placental edge. In addition to the placenta, the location of the fetus is noted so that the hysterotomy is made directly over the MMC defect to minimize the need for manipulation of the fetus. In some cases, the fetus is moved prior to opening the uterus to aid in this exposure.
- The uterus is opened under continuous sonographic visualization.
  - Two monofilament traction sutures are placed through the full thickness of the uterus.
  - A Bovie cautery is then used between the sutures and the uterus opened.
  - An atraumatic clamp is placed through this opening to compress the uterine tissue and to facilitate the firing of a specialized uterine stapling device that is only partially inserted. This device places a row of absorbable polyglycolic acid staples across the uterine wall and fetal membranes. This device cuts the uterine wall at the same time it places the staples, holding the layers together in a normal anatomic position and occluding crossing blood vessels. This is then repeated in the opposite direction to create the 6-cm hysterotomy.
  - An infusion of body temperature lactated Ringers with a level I infusion device is used to maintain the uterine volume and keep the fetus warm and buoyant.
  - The fetus is then held in the hysterotomy incision so that the back and MMC defect are in the opening.
- After the MMC repair the uterus and then the maternal laparotomy are closed in a layered fashion.
  - Full-thickness stay suture is placed first, followed by a running full-thickness layer that incorporates the absorbable staples. During this closure the uterus is filled with the lactated Ringers solution to reconstitute the amniotic fluid volume, and intra-amniotic antibiotics are added.
  - The running layer suture is tied followed by tying of the individual stay sutures.
  - The uterine closure is then covered with an omental patch to help seal it and provide blood supply.
  - The laparotomy wound and skin are then closed.

■ Fetal MMC repair is performed in the same manner as postnatal repair. There are three important differences to the prenatal repair compared to the postnatal repair.[5]
  ■ First, one advantage of fetal MMC closure is the chance to maintain spinal function, and therefore, even greater care is needed in the fetal patient to minimize any trauma to the placode and neural tissue.

■ Second, the fetal tissue is more delicate than in a newborn, and therefore it may tear with even minor manipulation.
■ Lastly, maneuvers, such as pulling the skin tightly, that may be tolerated in a newborn may lead to cardiac depression in the fetus and are therefore avoided.

■ Release of the Placode

■ The tissue just lateral to the placode is sharply incised, releasing the placode to float ventrally into the spinal column (**TECH FIG 1B**).

■ It is often necessary to make this incision further from the placode than desired to avoid damaging the spinal cord or exiting nerve roots. In these cases, the residual tissue should be dissected from the placode to reduce the risk of subsequent inclusion cyst formation.

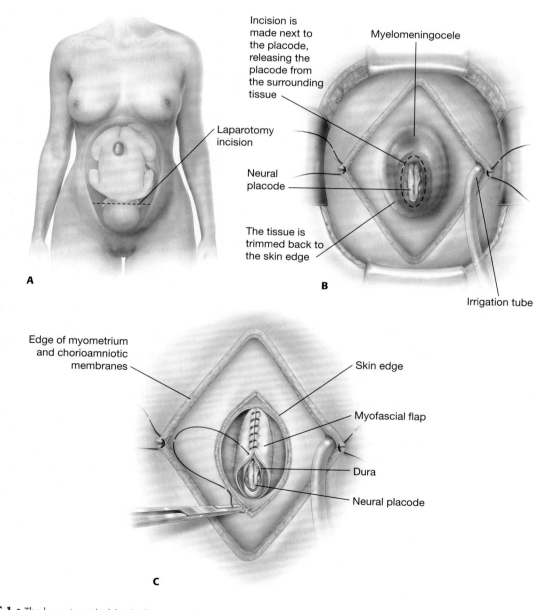

TECH FIG 1 • The laparotomy incision is shown in **A**. The incision in the uterus is performed in the upper segment. **B.** The exposed MMC defect. The fetus is positioned to allow access to the MMC defect and monitor the fetal cardiac function. **C.** The exposed MMC defect is then repaired.

■ Skin Release and Mobilization

- The skin is then released from the underlying fascia and muscle.
- The skin is undermined using scissors in an elliptical fashion for several centimeters.

- Undermining of the skin allows the skin to be mobilized, resulting in greater exposure of the underlying fascia and skin that can be more easily rotated over the fascia during the skin closure.
- Care needs to be taken to stay in the proper plane and avoid tearing the skin during this undermining process.

■ Dura and Myofascial Closure

- The next step is closure of the lateral tissue over the placode.
- The goal of the closure is a watertight closure over the placode.
  - The skin is held with a retractor, exposing the lateral dura and fascia. The skin opening can be extended superiorly and inferiorly to aid in the exposure of the fascia.
  - An incision is made in the lateral tissue and this tissue is then rotated over the released placode. Some authors close only the dural layer, but we prefer a thick myofascial flap with the dural layer on the mesial surface to ensure watertight closure and direct contact between the delicate dural layer and the neural placode.
  - The myofascial flaps are then closed with a running suture such as a 4-0 polydioxanone (PDS). When this thick layer is closed in the midline, care is taken to approximate the dural surfaces and to protect the placode. This protection can be assisted with placement of a freer retractor over the placode during the suturing (**TECH FIG 1C**).

Skin Closure

- After closure of the myofascial flaps, the skin is further undermined.
- The skin flaps are then rotated to the midline; an assessment is then made if flaps can be rotated to the midline without tearing the tissue significantly or leading to tension-related cardiac depression.
- A running monofilament, such as 4-0 PDS, is placed. The suture should be placed loosely; once the suture has been placed across the opening, the suture is pulled tight after each stitch in a stepwise fashion until the skin edges meet. This "lacing" technique allows the tension to be spread across the incision and reduces tearing. Additionally, to reduce the chance for tearing the suture through the skin, the suture should be placed away from the skin edge and in the thicker portion of the skin flaps.
- If the skin cannot be closed, a graft is then sized to the opening. This graft is normally constructed with AlloDerm (LifeCell, Branchburg, NJ) and is elliptical in shape. It is sutured with two running monofilament sutures.
- Other groups have described the use of relaxing incisions in the flank to aid in mobilization. However, these are generally not used because they are at risk to fail from devascularization after skin mobilization.

PEARLS AND PITFALLS

Selection	■ A detailed study of the mother and fetus is necessary for proper patient selection, confirming the presence of an open neural tube defect and no other associated fetal or maternal abnormalities that will prevent a good outcome.
Closure	■ A multilayer watertight closure is essential for maximal benefit to the fetus. ■ The goal of the surgery is to release the neural tissue and then rotate and close the layers over the placode, consisting of the dura, muscle, and skin.
Intraoperative Care	■ A dedicated fetal team is essential for a good outcome. This team should include fetal surgery, experienced anesthesia, obstetrics, and fetal cardiology.
Outcome	■ Fetal MMC repair can result in significant benefits for motor function, reversal of hindbrain herniation, and reduction in hydrocephalus.

POSTOPERATIVE CARE

- Postoperative care is focused on maintaining the pregnancy.
- During the operative procedure, the mother is given a bolus of magnesium sulfate and started on an infusion. This reduces uterine contractions and the risk for premature delivery. This infusion is continued for the first 18 to 24 hours.
- The mother is started on oral nifedipine after the magnesium sulfate infusion.
- The mother is given indomethacin prior to surgery, and this is continued for 48 hours postoperatively.
- The mother is observed as an inpatient for an average of 4 days and then is discharged to modified bed rest. The mother is followed closely for signs of premature labor or amniotic fluid leakage.
- Delivery is performed via an elective cesarean section prior to the development of labor and contractions, as this could lead to uterine rupture. The goal is to deliver at 37 weeks, but often the delivery is performed earlier than this time.

REFERENCES

1. Adzick NS, Thom EA, Spong CY; for the MOMS Investigators. A randomized trial of prenatal versus postnatal repair of myelomeningocele. *N Engl J Med.* 2011;364:993-1004.
2. Sutton LN, Adzick NS, Bilaniuk LT, et al. Improvement in hindbrain herniation demonstrated by serial fetal magnetic resonance imaging following fetal surgery for myelomeningocele. *JAMA.*1999;282: 1826-1831.
3. Danzer E, Adzick NS. Fetal surgery for myelomeningocele: patient selection, perioperative management and outcomes. *Fetal Diagn Ther.* 2011;30:163-173.
4. Rychik J, Cohen D, Tran KM, et al. The role of echocardiography in the intraoperative management of the fetus undergoing myelomeningocele repair. *Fetal Diagn Ther.* 2015;37:172-178.
5. Heuer GG, Adzick NS, Sutton LN. Fetal myelomeningocele closure: technical considerations. *Fetal Diagn Ther.* 2015;37:166-171.

Sacrococcygeal Teratoma

Nicholas J. Ahn and William H. Peranteau

DEFINITION

- Usually benign extragonadal germ cell tumor that develops prenatally, involving the coccyx with various degrees of pelvic and intra-abdominal involvement.
- It is the most common congenital neoplasm found in fetuses and neonates.
- Between 11% and 35% of the tumors may contain malignant elements such as yolk sac tumor or embryonal carcinoma.[1]
- Large or solid tumors may lead to poor clinical outcomes due to high-output cardiac failure, hydrops fetalis, tumor rupture, or internal hemorrhage.[2]
- Surgical resection is the mainstay of treatment but has associated morbidities such as problems with micturition, defecation, or cosmetic dissatisfaction up to 40% to 50%.[3] Large tumors with significant pelvic/intra-abdominal involvement have the most significant risk for urologic and anorectal complications.[4]

ANATOMY

- All sacrococcygeal teratomas (SCTs) involve the coccyx but are classified into four categories according to the location and extent of the tumor—the Altman Classification Scheme.[5]
  - Type I: primarily external with a small presacral component
  - Type II: external with intrapelvic extension
  - Type III: primarily pelvic and intra-abdominal with external component
  - Type IV: completely intrapelvic with no external component

PATHOGENESIS

- SCTs are thought to originate from the primitive knot (also known as Hensen node), where the three germ cell layers start to form.
- SCTs may be cystic, solid, or a mix of both. Solid tumors tend to be more vascular and are associated with an increased risk of high-output cardiac failure, hydrops fetalis, tumor rupture, hemorrhage, and fetal demise.

PATIENT HISTORY AND PHYSICAL FINDINGS

- The majority of the lesions are now diagnosed by the time of birth as early as 18 to 19 weeks of gestation due to advancement in antenatal imaging.
- Type I to III lesions that are not diagnosed prenatally are identified at birth by an obvious protruding mass originating from the sacral region.
- A rectal exam must be performed to assess the degree of intrapelvic extension of the tumor, especially for tumors that were diagnosed postnatally.

- Rarely, some type IV lesions can go undiagnosed until the child is up to 4 years of age and present with compressive symptoms of the bladder or rectum, such as urinary retention, obstruction, or constipation.

IMAGING

- Most SCTs are diagnosed prenatally at the time of approximately 20-week gestation fetal anatomy ultrasound. If diagnosed, the mother and fetuses should be referred to a high-volume multidisciplinary fetal diagnosis and treatment center where a high-resolution fetal ultrasound will be performed to assess the anatomical extension of the tumor and the characteristics of the mass (solid, cystic, vascularity) (FIG 1A).
- Ultrafast fetal MRI is used as an adjunct to ultrasonography to better assess the SCT, including the pelvic or abdominal extension of the tumor and its involvement with surrounding structures such as the colon, urinary tract, vagina, hip, and especially the spine (FIG 1B).
- After birth, hemodynamically stable infants may undergo a CT scan or MRI to assess the extent of the tumor for preoperative planning (FIG 2).

DIFFERENTIAL DIAGNOSIS

- Meningocele
- Lymphangioma
- Enteric duplication cyst
- Dermoid cyst
- Retrorectal hamartoma
- Meconium pseudocyst
- Tail remnant
- Lipoma

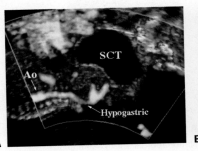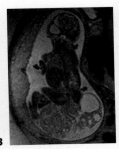

FIG 1 • Prenatal SCT imaging. **A.** High-resolution fetal ultrasound demonstrating a predominantly cystic type I SCT with blood supply originating from the hypogastric vessel. **B.** Ultrafast fetal MRI demonstrating a large type I SCT that has solid and cystic components.

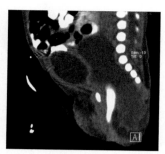

FIG 2 • Postnatal SCT imaging. Postnatal CT scan demonstrating a predominantly type II SCT.

SURGICAL MANAGEMENT

Preoperative Planning

■ Fetuses with external tumors that are larger than 5 cm, predominantly solid, or have a significant vascular supply should be delivered by cesarean delivery to decrease the risk of catastrophic bleeding or tumor rupture.

■ If the patient is stable, the tumor can be resected within the first week of life.

■ CBC, type and screen, and cross-match must be performed in anticipation of surgery.

■ Alpha-fetoprotein (AFP) and β-HCG levels should be obtained prior to surgery.

■ CT scan or MRI of the abdomen and pelvis with contrast should be performed as discussed above in stable patients.

Positioning

■ Most type I and type II lesions can be resected with the patient in prone jackknife position and completely resected from the posterior approach (**FIG 3**).

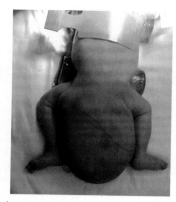

FIG 3 • Positioning. Prone position of newborn with large type I SCT.

■ Lesions with significant intra-abdominal components often require an anterior (laparotomy) as well as posterior approach for complete resection and thus should be positioned supine for the anterior approach initially.

■ Towel rolls or gel pads should be used to support the patient's shoulder and pelvis from underneath when in the prone position.

■ If uncertain regarding possible laparotomy, the patient should be sterilely prepped from the chest to the toes to allow for free intraoperative repositioning without repreparation and draping.

Approach

■ Most type I and II lesions can be completely resected from the posterior approach.

■ Lesions with large intra-abdominal components (some type III and type IV) require a combined anterior approach via a laparotomy and a posterior approach.

■ Posterior Approach (TECH FIG 1)

■ Landmarks: gluteal crease, sacrococcygeal junction, anal orifice

■ A Foley catheter is placed prior to placing the patient in the prone jackknife position.

■ The incision is made over the external component of the tumor in an orientation that allows for the development of large skin flaps. This often involves a transverse incision in an inverted V shape that starts at the sacrococcygeal junction.

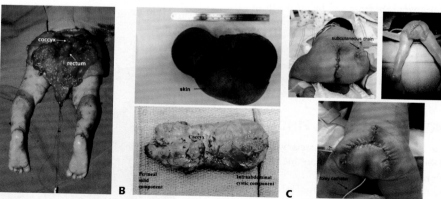

TECH FIG 1 • Posterior approach for postnatal SCT resection. **A.** Most type I and II SCTs can be approached from the posterior approach. Care must be taken to identify the anus/rectum to avoid injuring it. The coccyx is identified and resected with the specimen. The surgeon must also try to save the attenuated muscle fibers to reconstruct the pelvic floor following tumor resection. **B.** Resected specimen. Ideally the tumor and coccyx are resected as a single specimen. Often thin, extra skin is resected with the tumor specimen as there is frequently redundant skin available for appropriate skin closure. **C.** Skin closure following SCT resection.

- The incision is carried down to the tumor capsule, which, in many cases, is very superficial.
- Being cognizant to stay on the tumor capsule to preserve attenuated muscle fibers that will later be used to reconstruct the pelvic floor, the tumor is circumferentially dissected out as skin/muscle flaps are raised.
- Identify and always be cognizant of the position of the anus and rectum, which are often displaced and closely opposed by the SCT. Placement of a Hegar dilator or large red rubber catheter in the anal opening helps the surgeon identify and avoid injury to the anus/rectum.
  - For tumors with a large intrapelvic component, similar attention should be paid to the ureters.
- Dissection of the tumor along its posterior superior border will lead the surgeon to the coccyx, which must be identified and resected.
  - The sacrococcygeal junction is identified and circumferentially dissected out.
  - Care is taken to stay on the anterior surface of the sacrococcygeal junction during dissection to avoid

injury to the vascular supply to the tumor that usually originates from the middle sacral artery or branches from the hypogastric.
  - With an instrument on the anterior surface of the coccyx to protect underlying vessels, the sacrococcygeal junction is transected with a Bovie.
- Ligate the vascular supply to the tumor after the coccyx is transected at the sacrococcygeal joint.
- The tumor and coccyx are ideally resected as a single specimen (**TECH FIG 1B**).
- The muscles of the pelvic floor and anorectal sphincter are reconstructed.
- Excess skin is removed to allow for the best appearance.
- The skin is often closed in a "Mercedes" sign but can be closed in a vertical incision (often following complete resection after an initial debulking, see below) if more cosmetically appropriate (**TECH FIG 1C**).
  - If large skin flaps are raised, the skin is closed over a small drain.

■ Anterior Approach

- Tumors with large intra-abdominal/intrapelvic components often require a laparotomy via an anterior approach in combination with the above posterior approach.
- The anterior approach is done initially with the goal of identifying and controlling the vascular supply to the tumor prior to significant dissection of the tumor.
- Large intra-abdominal/intrapelvic tumors may be closely associated with the colon, intestinal mesentery, and the ureters all of which should be identified and preserved.

- The laparotomy is performed via a transverse incision between the umbilicus and pubic symphysis or, in cases with a very large intra-abdominal component, may be approached via a midline incision.
- After controlling the vascular supply to the tumor and dissecting out the intra-abdominal component of the tumor, the patient is flipped to the prone position and the remainder of the tumor and coccyx resected.

■ Special Considerations—Debulking
(TECH FIG 2)

- Large, predominantly solid lesions often have increased tumor vascularity and may be associated with high-output cardiac failure prenatally or immediately after birth. Fetuses with these lesions require close prenatal follow-up with assessment by high-resolution ultrasound often twice a week to monitor combined cardiac output and for signs of hydrops fetalis.
- If the SCT has a significant solid external component and there are signs of hydrops or early heart failure, the fetuses may be a candidate for debulking of the external component of the SCT. Depending on the gestational age of the fetus, this may occur as a cesarean delivery with immediate debulking after birth or open fetal surgery.[2,6]
- The techniques of open fetal surgery are beyond the scope of this chapter.
- Surgical debulking includes the following:
  - A posterior approach to the tumor
  - The anus is identified and a Hegar dilator or red rubber catheter placed to assess the tract of the rectum.

- The skin at the base of the external component of the SCT is scored with a Bovie.
- A tourniquet consisting of an umbilical tie, and a cut large red rubber catheter is placed at the base of the SCT where the skin had been scored.
- The tourniquet is tightened, and a harmonic scalpel is used to transect the tumor above the level of (distal to) the tourniquet.
- The tourniquet is slowly released, and hemostasis is obtained by oversewing bleeding vessels with a 5-0 Prolene.
- The skin is reapproximated and sutured over the cut edge of the tumor.
- The infant is then resuscitated and cared for in the neonatal intensive care unit.
- All patients undergoing surgical debulking will require a second operation to complete the resection of the tumor, including the coccyx, once the infant is stable and well recovered (usually greater than 6 weeks after debulking).

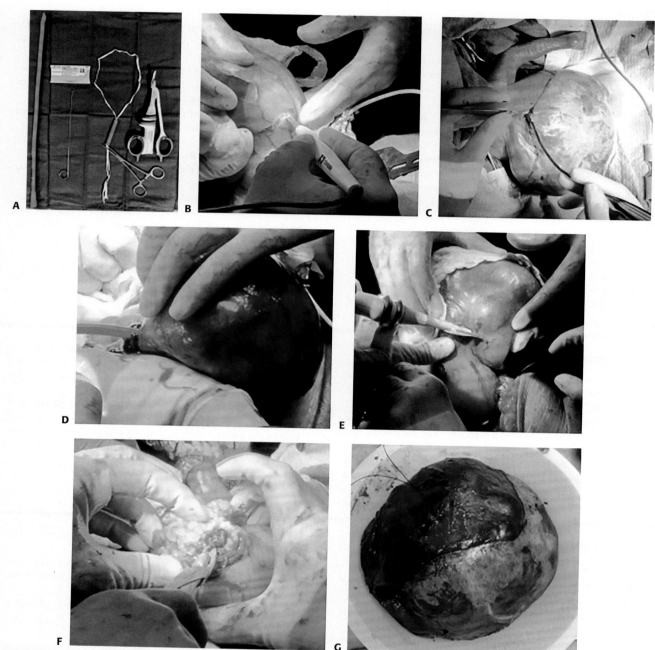

TECH FIG 2 • SCT debulking. Large type I SCTs that threaten hemodynamic stability may require debulking prior to or immediately after birth. Some of the main instruments required for debulking **(A)**. The skin of the tumor is scored with a Bovie near the base of the SCT **(B,C)**. A tourniquet constructed from an umbilical tie, and a cut large red rubber catheter is placed around the base where the skin was scored **(D)**. A harmonic scalpel is used to transect the tumor above the tourniquet **(E,F)**. The tourniquet is released and bleeding vessels oversewn. Note, unlike formal resection of an SCT, debulking does not remove the coccyx or intrapelvic/intra-abdominal tumor components **(G)**. These components will be resected after recovery and stabilization from debulking.

PEARLS AND PITFALLS

Positioning and prep	▪ If uncertain of need for laparotomy, prep the patient from lower chest to toes to allow for repositioning during the case without the need for new prep and drapes.
Technique	▪ A Hegar dilator can be used to identify the rectum and avoid damage.
Complete resection	▪ The coccyx must be resected to lower the risk of recurrence.

POSTOPERATIVE CARE

▪ Immediate postoperative care
  ▪ The patient should be positioned to avoid pressure on the wound as much as possible.
  ▪ The wound should be monitored for bleeding, dehiscence, or infection.
  ▪ If the tumor had a significant intrapelvic extension, urinary retention may occur, requiring a Foley catheter or intermittent catheterization.
▪ Follow-up
  ▪ Final pathology should be followed up to rule out malignancy.
    • Benign lesions may be managed with surgical resection and observation alone.
    • If malignant elements are noted on histology, a consultation with oncology may be needed.
  ▪ All patients should be followed long term with rectal examinations and AFP levels every 3 to 6 months until the age of 3.
    • The AFP level should return to normal by 9 months.
    • If still elevated after 9 months or a mass is palpated on rectal exam, an MRI or CT scan must be performed in suspicion of a recurrence.
▪ Recurrence
  ▪ Tumor spillage, incomplete resection, and malignant or immature histology are risk factors for recurrence.
  ▪ If recurrence is noted, a full metastatic workup including a CT chest, abdomen, pelvis, and laboratory studies are required.
  ▪ Management of recurrence requires re-excision with or without chemotherapy.

OUTCOMES

▪ The survival rate is greater than 90% if SCT is diagnosed on routine prenatal ultrasound.
▪ If the indication for the ultrasound examination was due to another complication of pregnancy, the mortality rate increases to 60%.

▪ If hydrops or placentomegaly is present, the mortality almost reaches 100%[2,7] if no intervention performed.
▪ Recurrence after resection occurs in about 10% to 15% of all patients with SCT, as early as 1 month to as far out as 59 months post-op (median 10–16 months).
▪ Survival rate is decreased with recurrence: 90% without recurrence and 65% with recurrence.

COMPLICATIONS

▪ Prevalence of anorectal morbidities including severe constipation and fecal incontinence ranges from 6% to 60% of the patients.
▪ Urologic bladder, vesicoureteral reflux, and urinary incontinence can manifest in 5% to 45% of the patients.
▪ Large intrapelvic extension of the tumor is associated with these morbidities.[4]

REFERENCES

1. Egler RA, Gosiengfiao Y, Russell H, et al. Is surgical resection and observation sufficient for stage I and II sacrococcygeal germ cell tumors? A case series and review. *Pediatr Blood Cancer.* 2016;64(5 suppl).
2. Hedrick HL, Flake AW, Crombleholme TM, et al. Sacrococcygeal teratoma: prenatal assessment, fetal intervention, and outcome. *J Pediatr Surg.* 2004;39:430-438.
3. Kremer ME, Derikx JP, Peeters A, et al. Sexual function after treatment for sacrococcygeal teratoma during childhood. *J Pediatr Surg.* 2016;51(4 suppl):534-540.
4. Partridge EA, Canning D, Long C, et al. Urologic and anorectal complications of sacrococcygeal teratomas: prenatal and postnatal predictors. *J Pediatr Surg.* 2014;49:139-142.
5. Altman RP, Randolph JG, Lilly JR. Sacrococcygeal teratoma: American Academy of Pediatrics Surgical Section Survey-1973. *J Pediatr Surg.* 1974;9(3 suppl):389-398.
6. Roybal JL, Moldenhauer JS, Khalek N, et al. Early delivery as an alternative management strategy for selected high-risk fetal sacrococcygeal teratomas. *J Pediatr Surg.* 2011;46:1325-1332.
7. Makin EC, Hyett J, Ade-Ajayi N, et al. Outcome of antenatally diagnosed sacrococcygeal teratomas: single-center experience (1993-2004). *J Pediatr Surg.* 2006;41:383-393.

Section XVII: Abdomen

CHAPTER 64

Prune Belly

Jamie C. Harris and Fizan Abdullah

DEFINITION[1,2]

- Prune belly is an extremely rare disease, occurring in 1/35 000 live births. The majority of patients are male (**FIG 1**).
- It is characterized by three components: abdominal wall flaccidity, bilateral undescended testes, and urologic anomalies.
  - Abdominal wall laxity is associated with increased rates of respiratory infections, due to a poor cough mechanism, as well as increased incidence of lordosis.
  - Urinary tract anomalies lead to increased rates of infectious complications as well as ureteral obstruction; 81% of patients have megaureter.
    - Urinary tract abnormalities can include renal dysplasia and ureteral enlargement.
  - Additionally, both testes are intra-abdominal in the majority of patients.
- Overall outcome of the children is variable, with some not surviving past the neonatal period due to complications to some with minimal disease complications.

DIFFERENTIAL DIAGNOSIS

- Prune bellylike variant: abdominal flaccidity. However, unlike in prune belly, the rectus muscles are not involved.

Patient History and Physical Findings[3]

- Prenatal history is often unremarkable. However, oligohydramnios may be present.
- Physical examination
  - A wrinkled abdomen with more laxity noted in the medial and inferior regions. This is a distinctive feature of prune belly. There will be redundant skin over the abdomen.

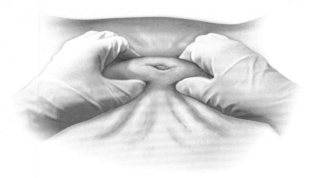

FIG 1 • This demonstrates the laxity in the abdominal wall of prune belly.

- As the children age, the abdomen will look more protuberant and less wrinkled.
- If portions of the urinary system are massively dilated, these can sometimes be palpated on abdominal exam.[4]
- Scrotal exam will reveal bilateral absence of testes in the majority of cases.
- Cardiac anomalies can be associated with prune belly; a cardiopulmonary exam should be included to listen for murmurs.
- Close monitoring of urine output is important to identify any obstructive uropathy that may be present. If present, nephrostomy tubes can be considered for urinary decompression.

IMAGING AND OTHER DIAGNOSTIC STUDIES

- Prenatal ultrasound
  - Hydroureteronephrosis, bladder distension, oligohydramnios, and cryptorchidism can be seen on prenatal ultrasound.[5]
- Postnatal urinary tract evaluation
  - Serum creatinine measurements
    - This will identify any worsening renal function.
    - Baseline measurements should be obtained at birth and trended to determine changes in function, creatinine greater than 0.7 mg/dL has a higher rate of developing renal failure.[6]
  - Kidney Ureter Bladder radiograph (KUB):
    - Evaluation of the bowel for dilatation can be done using a KUB. Bowel will extend over the lateral edge of the abdominal wall, which is diagnostic of prune belly.
    - Due to the lack of abdominal wall structure, intestinal malrotation can occur due to poor fixation to the abdominal wall.[4]
  - Renal and bladder ultrasound[4]:
    - An ultrasound will demonstrate atresia or absent kidney, hydronephrosis, megaureter, tortuous ureters, or megabladder.[7]
  - Voiding cystourethrogram (VCUG):
    - This is used for evaluation of the urethra. It can evaluate for vesicoureteral reflux. If identified, prophylactic antibiotics are indicated.
- Evaluation for associated anomalies:
  - Echocardiogram: should be considered if murmur is appreciated on physical exam.
  - Chest radiograph: if signs of respiratory distress are present, a chest radiograph can identify pneumothorax or pulmonary hypoplasia.

SURGICAL MANAGEMENT[3,8]

Preoperative Planning

- Respiratory status should be optimized prior to abdominal reconstruction.
- Urinalysis without evidence of infection should be done prior to surgery.
- Nasogastric tube placed prior to operation to decompress intestinal contents.

Positioning

- The patient is placed in the supine position.
- The abdomen is prepped with antiseptic.

Approach

- Two main open exposures have been described for umbilical preservation, described by Ehrlich and Monfort.
- The Ehrlich approach[8]:

- A midline vertical incision is made from xiphoid to pubis; an inferior transverse incision is made at the lower end of the incision. The umbilicus is left on a vascular pedicle.
- The midline incision is carried down to the peritoneum.
  - If a urologic repair is to be performed in the same operation, this will now take place.
- The Monfort approach[9] (**FIG 2**):
- An elliptical incision is used to remove redundant abdominal wall skin from xiphoid to pubis.
- The umbilicus is preserved from the full-thickness skin excision with a second incision to preserve its original location.
- The skin and subcutaneous tissue is dissected away from the underlying fascia, exposing the lateral abdominal wall.

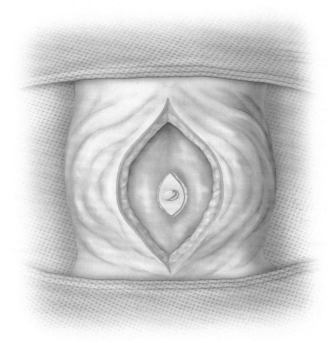

FIG 2 • The area of laxity where the skin will approximate is identified and excised.

■ Ehrlich Approach

- Skin flaps are created from the midline incision laterally until the level of the midaxillary line, separating the abdominal musculature from the skin and subcutaneous tissue.[8]

- Fascial advancement is then done bilaterally until the two sides are aligned in the midline.
- If umbilical sparing abdominoplasty is being done, the side with the umbilicus should be anterior.
- Horizontal mattress sutures are used to align the fascia.
- At this time, excess skin is excised bilaterally.

■ Monfort Approach

- Access to the abdomen is created using two fascial incisions to the epigastric arteries.[9] If urological correction is to be done concurrently, these incisions expose the genitourinary system (**TECH FIG 1A**).

- Once the intra-abdominal portion is completed, the lateral fascia is closed by overlapping the central remaining fascia to decrease abdominal wall laxity bilaterally (**TECH FIG 1B**).

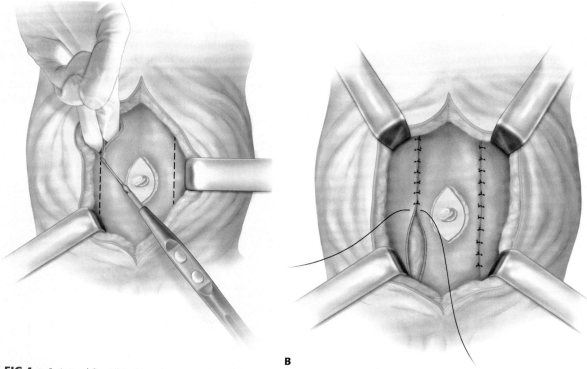

A   **B**

TECH FIG 1 • A. Lateral fascial incisions are made in the Monfort repair, which provides access to the abdominal cavity if urologic corrections are needed. **B.** The lateral fascia is closed by overlapping the central remaining fascia to decrease abdominal wall laxity bilaterally.

■ Closure

- The skin and subcutaneous tissues are closed in two layers (**TECH FIG 2**).
- A drain is placed in the subcutaneous tissue and maintained to suction to prevent formation of seromas.
- The nasogastric tube is removed prior to extubation.

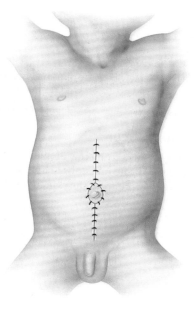

TECH FIG 2 • The skin is finally reapproximated in the midline, and closed in two layers.

PEARLS AND PITFALLS

Intraoperative monitoring	■ It is important to monitor airway pressures during abdominal wall reconstruction to identify abdominal compartment syndrome.
Laparoscopy	■ Laparoscopic abdominoplasty has been described and has been proposed to result in decreased rates of intra-abdominal adhesion formation. The fascia at the level of the anterior rectus muscle is plicated intra-abdominally, and then tacked to the medial fascial wall to reduce laxity.[10]

POSTOPERATIVE CARE

■ Pain control, initially with intravenous analgesia.

■ Subcutaneous drains are maintained to suction until drain output decreases, thereby minimizing the risk of seroma formation.

■ An abdominal binder should be worn for 8 to 10 weeks postoperatively.

■ Close monitoring of respiratory status is needed, as patients can develop respiratory distress in the postoperative period and may require intubation.

COMPLICATIONS[3]

■ Continued abdominal wall laxity.

■ Necrosis of skin flaps; close attention to blood supply of the flaps should be done to maintain adequate perfusion.

■ Long-term complications can be related to urological complications.

■ Overall mortality of prune belly is about 20% and is usually related to renal complications.

REFERENCES

1. Denes FT, Arap MA, Giron AM, et al. Comprehensive surgical treatment of prune belly syndrome: 17 years' experience with 32 patients. *Urology.* 2004;64(4):789-793.

2. Routh JC, Huang L, Retik AB, Nelson CP. Contemporary epidemiology and characterization of newborn males with prune belly syndrome. *Urology.* 2010;76(1):44-48.

3. Lesavoy MA, Chang EI, Suliman A, et al. Long-term follow-up of total abdominal wall reconstruction for prune belly syndrome. *Plast Reconstr Surg.* 2012;129(1):104e-109e.

4. Jennings RW. Prune belly syndrome. *Semin Pediatr Surg.* 2000;9(3):115-120.

5. Papantoniou N, Papoutsis D, Daskalakis G, et al. Prenatal diagnosis of prune-belly syndrome at 13 weeks of gestation: case report and review of literature. *J Matern Fetal Neonatal Med.* 2010;23(10):1263-1267.

6. Noh PH, Cooper CS, Winkler AC, et al. Prognostic factors for long-term renal function in boys with the prune-belly syndrome. *J Urol.* 1999;162(4):1399-1401.

7. Zugor V, Schott GE, Labanaris AP. The Prune Belly syndrome: urological aspects and long-term outcomes of a rare disease. *Pediatr Rep.* 2012;4(2):e20.

8. Ehrlich RM, Lesavoy MA. Umbilicus preservation with total abdominal wall reconstruction in prune-belly syndrome. *Urology.* 1993;41(3):231-232.

9. Monfort G, Guys JM, Bocciardi A, et al. A novel technique for reconstruction of the abdominal wall in the prune belly syndrome. *J Urol.* 1991;146(2 (Pt 2)):639-640.

10. Levine E, Taub PJ, Franco I. Laparoscopic-assisted abdominal wall reconstruction in prune-belly syndrome. *Ann Plast Surg.* 2007;58(2):162-165.

65

CHAPTER

Gastroschisis and Omphalocele

Jamie C. Harris and Fizan Abdullah

DEFINITION

Gastroschisis

- Gastroschisis is the most common congenital abdominal wall defect in the newborn period. This results from failure of the intestines to return back into the abdomen during development around week 10 of gestation.
- The abdominal wall defect is usually less than 4 cm in diameter and is more commonly located to the right of midline.

Omphalocele

- Omphalocele is the second most common abdominal wall defect, 1/5000 live births.
- This is characterized by a large defect, greater than 4 cm, and is covered by a membrane of peritoneum.
- This can contain intestines, as well as liver, spleen, and gonads. Unlike gastroschisis, omphalocele has a high rate of associated anomalies, including chromosomal abnormalities and cardiac defects.

DIFFERENTIAL DIAGNOSIS

- Ruptured omphalocele can be distinguished from gastroschisis based on the size of the defect (greater than 4 cm), as well as contents other than intestines in the defect.
- An umbilical cord hernia will be smaller than omphalocele, and does not contain abdominal organs.
- Pentalogy of Cantrell is a rare constellation of ectopia cordis, omphalocele, sternal cleft, anterior diaphragmatic hernia, and intracardiac defect.
- In ectopia cordis, the defect is located at the midline of the sternum and contains the heart.

Patient History and Physical Findings

- Prenatal history
  - Often, abdominal wall defects are diagnosed on prenatal screening. Maternal serum and amniotic fluid demonstrates elevated alpha fetoprotein (AFP).
  - Amniotic fluid demonstrates elevated acetylcholinesterase.
  - There is a higher specificity of elevated AFP for gastroschisis compared to omphalocele.
- Postnatal history and physical (**FIG 1**)
  - For both defects, birth history as well as patient stabilization from a cardiopulmonary standpoint should be completed first.
  - Initial inspection should be done to determine:
    - The presence of a covering membrane (indicating omphalocele) (**FIG 1A**).
    - The viability of the intestines, evidence of necrosis, atresias, or perforation.

- Contents in the defect, including liver, gonads, and other intra-abdominal organs.
  - If these are seen without a covering membrane, ruptured omphalocele should be considered.
- Full cardiopulmonary exam should be done to determine if there are audible murmurs appreciated, which suggest an underlying cardiac defect.
- Examination of the rest of the body to examine for any associated anomalies should be done.
  - Omphalocele is associated with multiple different syndromes including Beckwith-Wiedemann (omphalocele, macroglossia, and gigantism), and trisomy 13, 18, and 21.[1]

IMAGING AND OTHER DIAGNOSTIC STUDIES

- Prenatal ultrasound
  - Gastroschisis
    - Prenatal ultrasound will demonstrate intestines within the amniotic fluid, outside of the abdomen.
    - This is most commonly seen around 20 weeks of gestation.[2]
    - Anomalies, most commonly intestinal atresias, can also be identified on prenatal ultrasound. Bowel dilatation greater than 14 mm is predictive of atresias.[1]
  - Omphalocele
    - Intestinal contents will be seen outside of the abdomen.
    - The sac can be visualized on ultrasound, helping distinguish from gastroschisis.
    - Additionally, liver can be visualized in the defect.
    - This is seen around 18 weeks of gestation.
    - Evaluations of other associated anomalies, including cardiac, can be done on prenatal ultrasound as well.
- Postnatal echocardiogram
  - The rate of cardiac anomalies in omphalocele is higher (14%–47%) than in gastroschisis (3%–33%).[3]
  - Common cardiac anomalies that are seen are ventricular septal defect, atrial septal defect, and tricuspid atresia. A complete cardiac evaluation for omphalocele should be done in the perinatal period.

SURGICAL MANAGEMENT

Preoperative Planning

- Gastroschisis
  - There are two management strategies for gastroschisis:
    - Delayed closure with silo placement, allowing for reduction of the abdominal contents over the following days
    - Immediate reduction with closure at birth

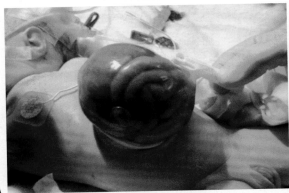 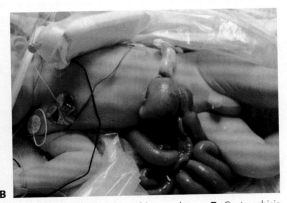

FIG 1 • A. Omphalocele presents with a membrane covering and the umbilicus originating from this membrane. **B.** Gastroschisis presents with a defect in the abdominal wall without a membrane covering the extruded intestines.

- Many studies monitor intra-abdominal pressures for signs of abdominal compartment syndrome to guide decisions on immediate vs delayed closure.[3,4]
- When the diagnosis is known prenatally, delivery should be done at a hospital in which pediatric surgeons can be present.
- The current guidelines have shown no difference in outcomes between vaginal delivery and cesarean section for gastroschisis. Delivery modality should be at the discretion of the obstetrician. Additionally, older gestational age is associated with less complications, where 37 weeks is considered term.[5]
- Immediately after birth, the intestines should be covered with sterile moist towels to minimize fluid losses. Intravenous access should be started to replace losses.
- Assessment of the viability of the bowel should be done.
  - If any atresias are noted, this should be documented. These are generally repaired 4 to 6 weeks after birth to allow the intestinal inflammation gastroschisis to decrease.
  - Atretic segments of intestine, if not compromised, are reduced into the abdomen.
- If necrotic or perforated intestines are encountered, termed complex gastroschisis, these are resected and enterostomies are created.
- An orogastric tube should be placed at birth to aid in bowel decompression to facilitate reduction into the abdominal cavity.
- Omphalocele
  - When the diagnosis is known prenatally, delivery should be done at a hospital in which pediatric surgeons can be present.

- Surgical repair is dependent upon the size of the omphalocele. For giant omphaloceles with loss of abdominal domain, primary closure is generally not attempted. These are often complex and require a level of creativity to close. Closure methods that are used include promoting sac granulation by treating with topical agents such as diluted betadine, xeroform, or bacitracin to allow the peritoneal sac to become firmer and more durable.
  - Skin flaps and grafts, such as Gore-Tex mesh, can be used to cover the sac, and negative pressure wound VAC used to promote granulation.
- If the omphalocele is not a giant omphalocele, primary closure of the small omphalocele can be done.

Positioning

- Gastroschisis
  - The patient is positioned in the supine position, with the arms at the patient's side.
  - The abdomen should be prepped and draped into the operative field.
  - The surgeon is positioned on the right of the patient, while the assistant is on the left.
  - Omphalocele
    - The patient is positioned in the supine position, with the arms at their sides.
    - Antiseptic prep is used and should include the entire abdomen up to the chest.
    - Reduction of the sac contents into the abdomen is performed at this point.

■ Repair of Gastroschisis

Immediate Reduction

- If primary closure is feasible at the time of birth, the umbilical cord can be used to elevate the abdominal cavity to reduce the intestines within the cavity.
- Once the intestines are returned to the abdominal cavity, closure of the defect can be managed in a similar fashion with both methods.

Delayed Closure With Silo Placement

- The infant is placed supine[6] (**TECH FIG 1**).
- The silo bag can either be spring loaded, which is placed below the fascia, or sutured to the fascia.
- The intestines are maintained in the silo.
- It is important to maintain upward traction on the silo to maintain bowel orientation and minimize any twisting or kinking of the mesentery to minimize the risk of ischemia.
- Once secured, serial reduction of the intestine within the silo is done, and complete reduction is usually accomplished within 2 to 3 days of life.
- Often, the silo can be placed with light sedation to minimize the need for general anesthesia in an infant.

Closure

- Sutured closure of the defect is done after the intestines are reduced to the abdomen.
  - The fascia is then closed using either a purse-string or interrupted suture closure.
  - The skin is closed using a running subcuticular stitch.
- Alternatively, sutureless closure has been demonstrated to be a viable option for closure[7,8] (**TECH FIG 2**).
  - The umbilical cord remnant is cut to fit over the fascial defect.
  - The remnant is then secured in place using Tegaderm or adhesive tape to reinforce the defect.
  - Tegaderm or tape is maintained for 3 days postoperatively and is then removed.
  - The defect closes circumferentially around the umbilical cord.

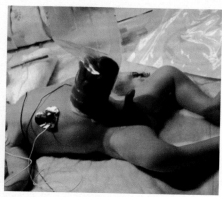

TECH FIG 1 • Initial management of gastroschisis involves placing a spring-loaded silo below the fascia and the intestines are suspended. This is serially reduced over the next few days until the abdominal contents are completely reduced and closure can be completed.

Primary Closure of Omphalocele

- The sac is incised circumferentially at the level of the skin.
- Any remaining herniated intestinal contents are completely reduced into the abdomen, monitoring airway pressures as they are reduced.
- After reduction, the sac is excised and the fascia is closed primarily.
- The fascia can be closed with either interrupted fascial sutures or running fascial closure.
- If the defect is large, primary fascial closure is not feasible and temporary closures or mesh closures can be considered.[9]
- Once the fascia is closed, the subcutaneous tissue is closed in layers.
- A running subcuticular suture is used to close the skin.
- Generally, drains are not used following skin closure.

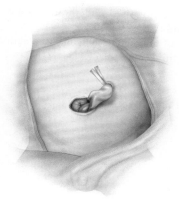
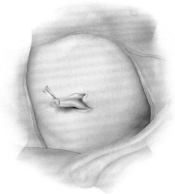
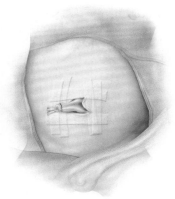

A **B** **C**

TECH FIG 2 • Sutureless closure. **A.** The intestines are reduced completely into the abdominal cavity. **B.** The umbilical cord remnant is then placed over the defect and **(C)** secured in place with Tegaderm.

PEARLS AND PITFALLS

Gastroschisis	▪ 5%–8% of gastroschisis patients have intestinal atresia; therefore, careful running of the bowel should be done whenever feasible. ▪ Gastroschisis defects placed in a silo bag can typically be reduced over 24–72 hours.
Omphalocele	▪ For patients with omphalocele, maintaining the membrane and not allowing it to rupture is paramount, as the membrane? provides significantly more tissue to adequately cover the defect. ▪ Surgical options for closure and/or temporary surgical silo are used only if it is not possible to preserve the peritoneal sac in omphalocele, or if the sac ruptures.

POSTOPERATIVE CARE

▪ Gastroschisis
  ▪ During intestinal reduction, observation for signs of abdominal compartment syndrome including elevated airway or bladder pressures, as well as decreasing urine output should be monitored.
  ▪ Return of bowel function is very slow in gastroschisis, and postoperative parenteral nutrition is necessary to support the infant until oral intake can be instated.
  ▪ If atresias are present, resection and primary anastomosis can be completed once intestinal inflammation has decreased. This usually takes place 4 to 6 days after birth.
▪ Omphalocele
  ▪ Airway pressures as well as bladder pressures should be monitored for signs of abdominal compartment syndrome.
  ▪ If granulation of the sac is the initial method of closure, close inspection of defects within the sac should be done regularly.
  ▪ Management of associated anomalies should continue to be done, as these are what cause the largest morbidity in this group.

COMPLICATIONS

▪ Most often, complications associated with gastroschisis have to do with prematurity rather than the surgical repair.[2]
▪ Similarly, complications associated with omphalocele are most often related to the associated anomalies.

▪ Gastroschisis has a high rate of necrotizing enterocolitis (NEC), and the surgeon should be cognizant of this if bloody stools or abdominal distention occur in the perioperative period.
▪ Overall survival rates in gastroschisis are 90%; overall survival rates in omphalocele are 70% to 95%.

REFERENCES

1. Lakshminarayanan B, Lakhoo K. Abdominal wall defects. *Early Hum Dev.* 2014;90:917-920.
2. Mortellaro VE, St Peter SD, Fike FB, et al. Review of the evidence on the closure of abdominal wall defects. *Pediatr Surg Int.* 2011;27:391-397.
3. Gamba P, Midrio P. Abdominal wall defects: prenatal diagnosis, newborn management, and long-term outcomes. *Semin Pediatr Surg.* 2014;23:283-290.
4. Boutros J, Regier M, Skarsgard ED, et al. Is timing everything? The influence of gestational age, birth weight, route, and intent of delivery on outcome in gastroschisis. *J Pediatr Surg.* 2009;44:912-917.
5. Pastor AC, Phillips JD, Fenton SJ, et al. Routine use of a SILASTIC spring-loaded silo for infants with gastroschisis: a multicenter randomized controlled trial. *J Pediatr Surg.* 2008;43:1807-1812.
6. Kidd JN Jr, Jackson RJ, Smith SD, et al. Evolution of staged versus primary closure of gastroschisis. *Ann Surg.* 2003;237:759-764.
7. Sandler A, Lawrence J, Meehan J, et al. A "plastic" sutureless abdominal wall closure in gastroschisis. *J Pediatr Surg.* 2004;39:738-741.
8. Emami CN, Youssef F, Baird RJ, et al. A risk-stratified comparison of fascial versus flap closure techniques on the early outcomes of infants with gastroschisis. *J Pediatr Surg.* 2015;50:102-106.
9. Marven S, Owen A. Contemporary postnatal surgical management strategies for congenital abdominal wall defects. *Semin Pediatr Surg.* 2008;17:222-235.

66 CHAPTER

Management of the Open Abdomen

Alexander F. Mericli and Charles E. Butler

DEFINITION

- The phrase "open abdomen" is used to describe a defect in the abdominal wall that exposes the viscera.
- There are several challenging clinical scenarios that can necessitate leaving the abdominal cavity opened or that can result in an open abdomen (**FIG 1**):
  - Damage control laparotomy after trauma
  - Excessive visceral edema as seen in severe abdominal sepsis
  - Following a decompressive laparotomy for management of abdominal compartment syndrome
  - Strategies involving a planned relaparotomy (second look for intestinal ischemia)
  - Staged abdominal wall reconstruction after fascial dehiscence and evisceration
- The central tenant of open abdomen management is the construction of a temporary abdominal closure until definitive abdominal wall reconstruction can be performed.
- When one is confronted with a clinical situation that requires an open abdomen or results in an opened abdomen, there is a number of reasons why it may be prudent to stage the abdominal reconstruction with a temporary abdominal closure:
  - Decreases tension on the musculofascial abdominal wall and prevents abdominal compartment syndrome
  - Reduces risk of evisceration
  - Facilitates regaining access to the abdominal cavity
  - Reduces lateral retraction of the skin, subcutaneous tissue, muscle and fascia
  - Ideally, it facilitates a delayed primary abdominal wall closure.

ANATOMY

- The abdominal wall is a layered structure consisting of muscle and fascia.

- The paired rectus abdominis muscles comprise the central portion, ensheathed in the fascia of the anterior and posterior rectus sheaths.
- The rectus muscles are flanked on either side by the oblique family of muscles: the external oblique, followed by the internal oblique, followed by the transversus abdominis.
- Above the arcuate line (approximately at the level of the anterior superior iliac spine), the anterior rectus sheath is made up by contributions from the external oblique aponeurosis and internal oblique; the posterior rectus sheath is made up by the internal oblique, transversus, and transversalis fascia.
- Below the arcuate line, there is no posterior sheath, only transversalis fascia is below the rectus muscle (**FIG 2**).

PATHOGENESIS

- The scientific rationale for the creation and maintenance of an open abdomen is centered on the phenomenon of intestinal edema and decreasing the impact of the inflammatory cascade.
- The intestine is a highly vascularized structure with a rich network of arteries, veins, capillaries, and lymphatic vessels. In pathologic states, such as after an abdominal trauma, after abdominal surgery, or in abdominal sepsis, a decrease in clearance of fluid from the extracellular space can result in swelling of the intestinal wall several times the normal diameter, potentially interfering with perfusion of the bowel.
- Multiple inflammatory cells are present within the bowel wall and peritoneal membrane.
- In the postsurgical abdomen, the trauma abdomen, and in abdominal sepsis, there is a profound local inflammatory response, which quickly progresses to systemic inflammatory response syndrome (SIRS), which can easily contribute to multiple organ dysfunction syndrome (MODS).

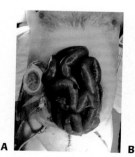 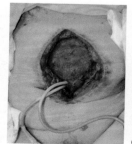 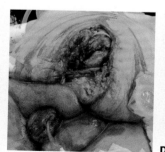 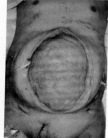

FIG 1 • Various clinical scenarios commonly managed using the technique of temporary open abdomen. From left to right: open abdomen after postsurgical evisceration; multiple enterocutaneous fistulae; open abdomen associated with abdominal sepsis; open abdomen after damage control laparotomy.
© Charles E. Butler, MD.

Above Arcuate Line

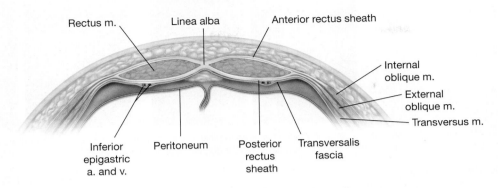

Rectus m. — Linea alba — Anterior rectus sheath — Internal oblique m. — External oblique m. — Transversus m. — Inferior epigastric a. and v. — Peritoneum — Posterior rectus sheath — Transversalis fascia

Below Arcuate Line

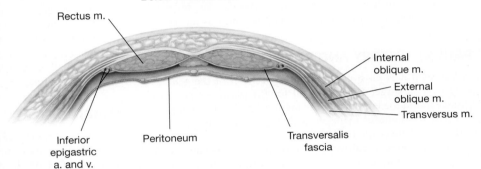

Rectus m. — Internal oblique m. — External oblique m. — Transversus m. — Inferior epigastric a. and v. — Peritoneum — Transversalis fascia

FIG 2 • Cross-sectional anatomy of the abdominal wall superior and inferior to the arcuate line.

- Premature closure of the abdomen can exacerbate the inflammatory response and accelerate these syndromes as well as contribute to abdominal compartment syndrome.[1]
- Utilizing the open abdomen technique is associated with survival rates up to 80% after abdominal trauma, severe intra-abdominal sepsis, and acute evisceration.[2–5]

Abdominal Compartment Syndrome

- Abdominal compartment syndrome is a syndrome of uncontrolled intra-abdominal hypertension. Any factor that raises intra-abdominal pressure can contribute to abdominal compartment syndrome, including free blood and clots, bowel edema, vascular congestion, excessive crystalloid resuscitation, intraperitoneal packing, and nonsurgical bleeding, acidosis, hypothermia, and postoperative ileus.
- Normal intra-abdominal pressure is 0 to 5 mm Hg and can easily be quantified by measuring bladder pressure.
- Abdominal compartment syndrome is defined as a sustained bladder pressure of 20 mmHg or greater with dysfunction of 1 or more organ systems (ie, heart, lungs, kidneys, neurologic, etc.) OR a sustained bladder pressure of greater than 25 mmHg without organ dysfunction.
- Once diagnosed, emergent abdominal decompression is indicated. Typically, organ function returns to normal after decompression, but a mortality rate of 50% has been recorded, secondary to ongoing MODS.[6]

NATURAL HISTORY

- There are numerous physiologic changes that accompany an open abdomen. These changes are not insignificant and can contribute to substantial morbidity; however, the potential for morbidity of an intentional open abdomen is outweighed by the possible complications that could ensue, should the abdomen be closed prematurely.
- Fluid balance
  - A significant amount of peritoneal fluid is lost through an open abdomen, typically 1 L/h for a 70 kg person.
  - If a closed suction system is used as part of the temporary abdominal closure, such as negative pressure therapy, then this fluid loss can be quantified and therefore accurately replaced.
- Maintenance of normothermia
  - The large cutaneous defect oftentimes present with an open abdomen impairs the body's thermoregulatory system.
  - The loss of peritoneal fluid exacerbates heat loss through convection.
  - Frequent temperature monitoring, forced air warming blankets, and a warmed room are all techniques that can be employed to counteract this effect.
- Protein loss
  - Peritoneal fluid is protein rich, with 2 g protein/L.[7] This must be replaced through diet or enteral feeds in order to maintain nitrogen balance.
- Fistula
  - With the open abdomen, the bowel is at risk for injury. Patients with a fresh bowel anastomosis are at greatest risk.[8]
  - Whenever possible, the viscera should be covered by the omentum for an additional layer of protection.

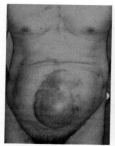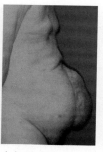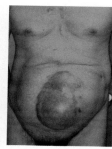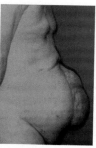

FIG 3 • Anterior and lateral views of a patient with abdominal loss of domain. The rectus and oblique muscles have retracted laterally overtime. The exposed viscera is skin grafted in anticipation of delayed abdominal wall reconstruction. © Charles E. Butler, MD.

- Loss of domain
  - The creation of an open abdomen places the patient at risk for losing abdominal domain as the musculofascial abdominal wall retracts laterally over time (**FIG 3**).
  - Methods of temporary abdominal closure are designed to prevent this situation by keeping the fascia as medial as possible.

PATIENT HISTORY AND PHYSICAL FINDINGS

- Although it is most commonly the decision of the general or trauma surgeon, it is helpful for the plastic surgeon to understand the factors that are involved in deciding whether a patient should be managed with an open abdomen.
- Trauma/damage control
  - Preoperative predictors: penetrating torso trauma with hypotension, need for resuscitative thoracotomy, blunt abdominal trauma with intraperitoneal hemorrhage, and hypotension
  - Intraoperative predictors: development of a coagulopathy, intraoperative exsanguination requiring greater than 10 units of packed red blood cells, pH less than 7.2, base deficit greater than −6 in patients older than 55 years or greater than −15 in patients younger than 55 years, temperature less than 34°C, and/or estimated blood loss greater than 4 L.[2]
- Abdominal compartment syndrome
  - Patients with sustained intra-abdominal pressure greater than 20 mm Hg with onset of new organ dysfunction
  - Patients with acutely increased intra-abdominal pressures greater than 25 mm Hg without acute organ dysfunction should be considered for prophylactic decompression.
  - Patients at high risk for development of abdominal compartment syndrome: those requiring greater than 15 L crystalloid or 10 units of packed red blood cells, patients with increased peak inspiratory pressures greater than 40 mm Hg upon fascial closure.[2]
- Planned relaparotomy
  - Management of intestinal ischemia potentially requiring repeat bowel resections

- Severe abdominal sepsis necessitating repeated debridements, such as in pancreatic necrosis or intra-abdominal abscesses
- Acute postoperative evisceration
  - Fascial dehiscence in the acute or subacute postoperative period can result in evisceration. Given that this often occurs during the inflammatory stage of wound healing, visceral edema and friable, inflamed abdominal wall soft tissue may preclude immediate fascial reapproximation.

IMAGING

- Computed tomographic imaging of the abdomen and pelvis are imperative for surgical planning and preoperative evaluation. **FIG 4** demonstrates images from a patient with an open abdomen and associated lateral musculofascial retraction (loss of domain) (left) as well as a patient with an incisional ventral hernia after laparotomy (right).

SURGICAL MANAGEMENT

- A variety of surgical techniques for temporary abdominal closure are available, ranging from a skin-only closure to the more sophisticated ABThera System (KCI, San Antonio, TX).
- The ideal temporary closure contains the viscera, minimizes skin maceration and damage to the underlying bowel or fascia, and facilitates durable fascial reapproximation. Although there are advantages and disadvantages to each technique (Table 1), the method of temporary abdominal closure is largely dependent upon surgeon preference.

Preoperative Planning

- Preoperatively, a full history should be obtained and physical exam should be performed.
- A basic laboratory panel should be obtained and preoperative CT scan should be performed.

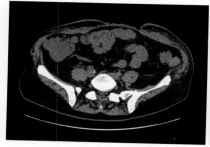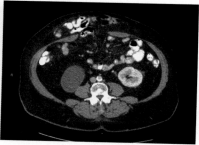

FIG 4 • Computed tomography images from a patient with an open abdomen and associated lateral musculofascial retraction (loss of domain) (left) as well as a patient with an incisional ventral hernia after laparotomy (right).

Table 1 Temporary Abdominal Closure Techniques

	Materials/Technique	Advantages	Disadvantages
Skin-only closure	Suture; staples	Inexpensive; fast; minimizes fluid and heat loss	100% hernia rate; high risk of evisceration; risk of abdominal compartment syndrome
Silo technique	"Bogota" bag; 3 L IV bag; suture; drains; bag secured to edges of fascia to contain viscera within "silo"	Inexpensive; visualization of intra-abdominal contents; minimizes fluid and heat loss	Risk of evisceration; loss of domain; poor fluid management
Absorbable synthetic mesh	Polyglactin 910 mesh, suture; mesh placed as bridge between fascial edges	Absorbable, can apply skin graft once granulation tissue forms over mesh	100% ventral hernia rate; risk of enterocutaneous fistula and evisceration
Bioprosthetic mesh	Acellular dermal matrix; mesh placed as bridge between fascial edges	Incorporates; low risk of infection or extrusion in contaminated settings; can be skin grafted once granulation tissue forms	Expensive; extremely high ventral hernia rate at 5 years if used in bridging format
Nonabsorbable synthetic mesh	Polypropylene; polytetrafluoroethylene patch; patch anchored to fascia laterally and serial plication of the patch at the midline progressively medializes the fascial edges	Extends the life span of the temporary abdominal closure; inexpensive; limits loss of domain	Fascial trauma; adhesions; enterocutaneous fistula formation; compartment syndrome possible if plication too aggressive
Patch	Wittmann patch (Starsurgical, Inc., Burlington, WI); two pieces of mesh approximated to lateral fascial edges, two pieces latch onto each other similar to Velcro; mesh is sequentially tightened	Limits loss of domain; high rate of primary fascial approximation; allows for extended open abdomen	Requires multiple fascial manipulations; requires special equipment; adhesions can occur to undersurface of mesh
Vacuum pack closure	Nonadherent sheet placed over bowel, followed by surgical towels, drains, and iodoform-impregnated occlusive dressing; wall suction	Inexpensive; ability to monitor fluid losses; temperature control	Poor control of domain; theoretical potential for massive exsanguination. Enterocutaneous fistula formation
Commercial negative pressure system	V.A.C. Therapy (KCI, San Antonio, TX)	Plastic-encased sponge designed to be placed in contact with the viscera; prevents adhesions; fluid management; temperature control; minimizes visceral edema; high rate of success with primary fascial reapproximation if used in conjunction with fascial retention sutures	Theoretical potential for massive exsanguination. Enterocutaneous fistula formation; expensive

■ Fascial Closure Techniques

- Fascial closure techniques use an interposition graft material sutured to the abdominal fascia to bridge the laparotomy defect.
- These techniques can utilize *absorbable synthetic* materials such as polyglactin 910 mesh, *bioprosthetic mesh* such as Strattice (Acelity, Inc.), Surgimend (TEI biosciences, Inc.), or *nonabsorbable synthetic* materials such as the Wittmann Patch (Starsurgical, Inc.), expanded polytetrafluoroethylene, or polypropylene mesh.
- Initially, the mesh material should be loose in order to allow for visceral edema.
- As the edema resolves, the mesh is either serially excised, plicated, or advanced (Wittmann patch) to facilitate fascial approximation during reexploration.
- Typically, the patient is taken to the operating room every 48 hours for repeated washouts, reexplorations, and mesh tightening until the fascia can be reapproximated primarily.

- These techniques provide a mechanism to limit or reverse the loss of domain that occurs with an open abdomen. Therefore, fascial closure techniques should be considered when the open abdomen is likely to be prolonged greater than 1 week.
- Fascial closure techniques do require suturing to the abdominal fascia, which may increase the risk of fascial injury.

Fascial Approximation Anticipated During Present Hospital Admission

- Fascial closure technique if the possibility of fascial approximation is anticipated during hospital admission: Wittmann Patch (Starsurgical, Inc.)
  - Intraperitoneal drains are placed.
  - Patch sutured to fascial edges on either side of laparotomy.
  - Material has hooks and eyes similar to Velcro, which facilitates repeated openings and reclosures (**TECH FIG 1**).

TECHNIQUES

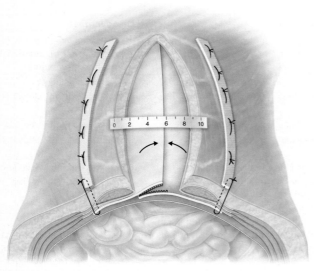

TECH FIG 1 • Artistic rendition of the Wittmann patch for management of the temporary open abdomen in situations where fascial approximation is anticipated during present hospital admission. Note the hooks and loops on the opposing pieces of mesh allowing sequential fascial medialization.

- The rate of primary closure for this method is 78% to 100%.[9]
- The rate of fistula is 2%.[9]

Delayed Fascial Approximation Anticipated

- Fascial closure technique if fascial approximation is likely not possible during initial hospital admission: bridged polyglactin 910 mesh or bridged bioprosthetic mesh
  - Intraperitoneal drains are placed.
  - Mesh is fixed to the fascial using polydioxanone sutures, bridging the fascial defect (**TECH FIG 2A**).
  - The mesh is covered with a moist dressing and changed twice daily.
  - The mesh is evaluated for redundancy on a daily basis; if redundancy is present, the pleating is plicated in the midline at the bedside with running absorbable suture.
  - If the fascial edges are able to be approximated to within 2 to 4 cm of each other before the formation of granulation tissue overlying the mesh, then the patient is returned to the OR for delayed primary fascial reapproximation.

- If granulation tissue forms over the mesh before fascial reapproximation is possible, then a skin graft is applied and delayed reconstruction is planned for 6 to 12 months following the injury (**TECH FIG 2B–D**).
- In this scenario, bioprosthetic mesh may have several advantages over polyglactin 910, including a greater tensile strength and structural support of the abdominal wall comparatively. The disadvantages include expense and difficulty to plicate at the bedside. Therefore, if a biologic is used, it should be inset with sufficient tension. Similarly, it too can be skin grafted once granulation tissue has formed.

Negative Pressure Wound Therapy for Temporary Abdominal Closure

- Negative pressure stimulates cell division, angiogenesis, and cell proliferation.[10,11]
  - Negative pressure for temporary abdominal closure was first described by Barker and colleagues.[12] They described a system in which a fenestrated plastic draped was placed in contact with the viscera, followed by surgical towels and drains; this middle layer was then covered by a bioocclusive adhesive sheet (Ioban). The drains were then connected to the wall suction at −150 mm Hg. Using this system, the authors achieved a primary fascial reapproximation rate of 55.4%. Fistula rate was 4.5%. The authors describe that within 7 to 10 days, the bowel would adhere to the abdominal wall, preventing primary reapproximation. Therefore, if definitive abdominal wall closure could not be achieved within 7 to 10, then the bowel should be skin grafted and definitive closure planned for 6 to 12 months.
- There are now several commercially available options for negative pressure management of the open abdomen. The most studied and popular system is the VAC System by KCI, Inc. (San Antonio, TX).
- The VAC System consists of an inner plastic-encased sponge designed to be in direct contact with the viscera. The plastic interface protects the bowel, prevents adhesion formation, and is perforated to allow drainage of peritoneal fluid.
- Next, a macroporous polyurethane sponge is then applied over the inner layer and is in direct contact with the overlying fascia and subcutaneous tissues.
- Fascial retention sutures can then be placed, if desired, to further medialize the fascial edges.

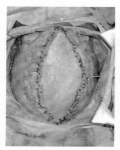
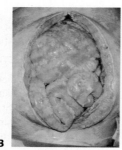
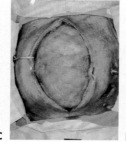
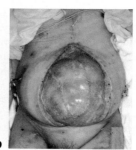

TECH FIG 2 • **A.** Abdominal wall closure with bilateral component separation and bridged bioprosthetic mesh. **B–D.** Series of photographs demonstrating temporary abdominal closure with a split-thickness skin graft. From left to right: Due to visceral edema, fascial approximation is not possible. A bridging mesh is placed and granulation tissue forms over the mesh. Skin grafts are placed over the mesh and granulation tissue. © Charles E. Butler, MD.

- The entire construct is then covered with an occlusive dressing and the machine is set to −125 mm Hg (**TECH FIG 3**).
- The patient is returned to the operative room every 2 to 3 days for irrigation, debridement, negative pressure dressing change, and further fascial medialization.
  - Primary fascial closure rates using this system average 67%[9] but can achieve 100% with the adjunctive use of fascial retention sutures.[13]
  - Fistula rate is 2.9%.

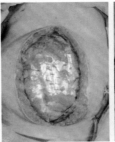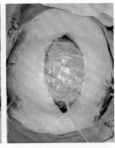

TECH FIG 3 • Negative pressure therapy for management of the open abdomen. A sterile fenestrated plastic drape is placed over the exposed viscera, followed by a macroporous sponge, and covered with an occlusive plastic dressing. © Charles E. Butler, MD.

PEARLS AND PITFALLS

Physiologic rationale for temporary abdominal closure?	■ Premature closure of the abdomen can exacerbate the inflammatory response and accelerate SIRS and MODS as well as contribute to abdominal compartment syndrome ■ Utilizing the open abdomen technique is associated with survival rates up to 80% after abdominal trauma, severe intra-abdominal sepsis, and acute evisceration
When to consider temporary abdominal closure?	■ Laparotomy for intra-abdominal trauma ■ Abdominal compartment syndrome ■ Abdominal sepsis ■ Planned relaparotomy ■ Acute evisceration
What are the two main methods of temporary abdominal closure?	■ Progressive fascial closure techniques ■ Negative pressure wound therapy
Postoperative care	■ Intensive fluid management due to insensible losses associated with open abdomen ■ Nutrition and protein intake ■ Return to the operating room every other day for repeat debridement, dressing change, and integral fascial advancement

POSTOPERATIVE CARE

- Because of the physiologic derangement that is associated with the clinical conditions necessitating an open abdomen, these patients often require intensive care.
- Postoperatively, the focus should be on resuscitation, fluid and electrolyte management, and nutrition. There is a multitude of information available on these topics, a review of which is outside the scope of this chapter.
- Time interval for repeated debridements
  - Regardless of the technique of temporary abdominal closure, the patient is typically returned to the operating room every 2 or 3 days.
  - There are no data to support a specific interval, and every clinical situation is different.
  - A shorter interval between episodes of general anesthesia may be physiologically challenging for the patient, whereas a longer period will allow for the formation of intestinal adhesions, increasing the risk for enteral injury.

- Nutrition
  - Assuming there are no contraindications (enteral anastomosis, ileus), enteral nutrition can and should continue during the period of open abdomen and temporary abdominal closure.
  - Because of the necessary repeated trips to the operating room, it can be difficult to meet nutritional requirements; therefore, a combination of both enteral and parenteral nutrition is prudent.
- Neuromuscular blockade
  - A short course of neuromuscular blockade may decrease fascial edge retraction and be a useful adjunct to negative pressure devices.
  - In one study, 192 open abdomen patients were divided into two groups: one receiving a continuous infusion of a neuromuscular blocker for greater than 24 hours and one receiving standard care.
  - The patients receiving the neuromuscular blockade were more likely to achieve primary fascial closure by

7 days (93% vs 83% $P < .024$) and had no increase in pneumonia.[14]

- Antibiotics
  - There is no evidence for prophylactic administration of antibiotics in patients with open abdomens other than the typical perioperative prophylactic antibiotic dosing.
  - Antibiotic use and duration should be determined by the treatment appropriate for the primary abdominal pathology (ie, abdominal sepsis, abscess, etc.).
- Sedation and analgesia
  - There are no studies regarding optimal pain control or sedation in patients with an open abdomen.
  - Epidural anesthesia has been shown to reduce intra-abdominal pressure and pain control in patients with open abdomen due to abdominal compartment syndrome.[15]

OUTCOMES

- Once the indication for open abdomen has resolved, a delayed primary abdominal wall reconstruction should be performed as soon as possible.
- Delayed primary closure of the abdominal wall is most possible if performed within 8 days of initial open abdomen.[16,17] A recent study of the damage control population demonstrated that delayed primary abdominal closure is only possible in 65% of patients.[9]
- If negative pressure temporary closure is combined with fascial retention sutures, a 100% primary repair rate can be achieved.[13]
- In situations where delayed primary abdominal closure cannot be obtained, a bridged biologic or synthetic absorbable mesh repair is performed, followed by skin grafting over the mesh once granulation tissue has formed. This controlled ventral hernia is then repaired 6 to 12 months later.[18]
- In certain clinical scenarios, the iatrogenic creation of a ventral hernia with skin graft coverage is not in the patient's best interest. For instance, in the oncologic population, a durable soft tissue reconstruction must be established expeditiously so that the patient can proceed with adjuvant radiation and chemotherapy.
- In these situations, adjunctive abdominal wall reconstruction techniques can oftentimes be employed to achieve primary fascial reapproximation in the acute setting.
- These techniques are covered in other chapters and include component separation, the use of inlay mesh, and various autologous flaps.

COMPLICATIONS

- The open abdomen leads to fluid and electrolyte derangements that must be actively monitored and corrected. The prolonged open abdomen, bowel fistulization, and loss of abdominal domain can complicate management. The main goal of temporary abdominal closure is fluid management and minimizing the loss of domain.
- Methods of temporary abdominal closure are associated with a bowel fistulization rate of 2% to 4.5%. Factors that increase the likelihood of fistula are abdominal sepsis, bowel anastomosis, and negative pressure therapy in direct continuity with a new bowel anastomosis.
- If using a "fascial closure technique," primary fascial approximation should be achieved within 7 to 12 days; otherwise, the

formation of intestinal adhesions may necessitate a delayed closure approach at a later date.

- If using a modern negative pressure technique, such as the ABThera System, primary fascial approximation can be achieved over a longer period of time, up to 30 days.
- Temporary abdominal closure techniques result in primary fascial approximation in 65% to 100% of patients. In the 35% of patients where primary fascial approximation is not possible, then either a delayed closure approach is taken (skin grafting followed by abdominal closure at a later date after the resolution of inflammation), an adjunctive abdominal reconstruction technique is utilized (component separation, flap), or some combination of both.

REFERENCES

1. Malbrain ML, Deeren D, De Potter TJ. Intra-abdominal hypertension in the critically ill: it is time to pay attention. *Curr Opin Crit Care.* 2005;11:156-171.
2. Regner JL, Kobayashi L, Coimbra R. Surgical strategies for management of the open abdomen. *World J Surg.* 2012;36:497-510.
3. Rotondo MF, Schwab CW, McGonigal MD, et al. "Damage control": an approach for improved survival in exsanguinating penetrating abdominal injury. *J Trauma.* 1993;35:375-382.
4. Ivatury RR, Nallanthambi M, Rao PM, et al. Open management of the septic abdomen: therapeutic and prognostic considerations based on the APACHE II. *Crit Care Med.* 1989;17:511-517.
5. Garcia-Sabrido JL, Tallado JM, Christou NV, et al. Treatment of severe intra-abdominal sepsis and/or necrotic foci by and "open-abdomen" approach: zipper and zipper-mesh techniques. *Arch Surg.* 1988;123:152-156.
6. Balough Z, McKinley BA, Holcomb JB, et al. Both primary and secondary abdominal compartment syndrome can be predicted early and are harbingers of multiple organ failure. *J Trauma.* 2003;54:848-859.
7. Cheatham ML, Safcsak K, Brzezinski SJ, Lube MW. Nitrogen balance, protein loss, and the open abdomen. *Crit Care Med.* 2007;35:127-131.
8. Ramsay PT, Mejia VA. Management of enteroatmospheric fistulae in the open abdomen. *Am Surg.* 2010;76:637-639.
9. Boele van Hensbroek P, Wind J, Dijkgraaf MG, et al. Temporary closure of the open abdomen: a systematic review on delayed primary fascial closure in patients with an open abdomen. *World J Surg.* 2009;33:199-207.
10. Ingber D. In search of cellular control: signal transduction in context. *J Cell Biochem Suppl.* 1998;30-31:232-237.
11. Chen SZ, Li J, Li XY, Xu LS. Effects of vacuum-assisted closure on wound microcirculation: an experimental study. *Asian J Surg.* 2005;28(3):211-217.
12. Barker DE, Kaufman HJ, Smith LA, et al. Vacuum pack technique of temporary abdominal closure: a 7-year experience with 112 patients. *J Trauma.* 2000;48:201-207.
13. Cothren CC, Moore EE, Johnson JL, et al. One hundred percent fascial approximation with sequential abdominal closure of the open abdomen. *Am J Surg.* 2006;192:238-242.
14. Abouassaly CT, Dutton WD, Zaydfudim V, et al. Postoperative neuromuscular blocker use is associated with higher primary fascial closure rates after damage control laparotomy. *J Trauma.* 2010;69:557-561.
15. Hakobyan RV, Mkhoyan GG. Epidural analgesia decreases intraabdominal pressure in postoperative patients with primary intra-abdominal hypertension. *Acta Clin Belg.* 2008;63:86-92.
16. Miller PR, Thompson JT, Faler BJ, et al. Late fascial closure in lieu of ventral hernia: the next step in open abdomen management. *J Trauma.* 2002;53:843-849.
17. Miller PR, Meredith JW, Johnson JC, Chang MC. Prospective evaluation of vacuum-assisted fascial closure after open abdomen: planned ventral hernia rate is substantially reduced. *Ann Surg.* 2004;239:608-614.
18. Bee TK, Croce MA, Magnotti LJ, et al. Temporary abdominal closure techniques: a prospective randomized trial comparing polyglactin 910 mesh and vacuum-assisted closure. *J Trauma.* 2008;65:337-342.

Umbilicoplasty

Sergey Y. Turin, Chad A. Purnell, and Gregory A. Dumanian

DEFINITION

- Reconstruction of the umbilicus is an essential part of restoring the natural aesthetic of the abdomen.
- It is the focal point of the anterior abdominal wall, helps define the middle abdominal sulcus and if absent or malformed, will draw attention to the abdomen.[1]
- We present two simple techniques for creation of a neoumbilicus.
  - One is to be used for patients with vertical midline incisions.
  - The other is for patients undergoing abdominoplasty when the umbilical stalk cannot be maintained.
- Umbilicoplasty for a scarred umbilicus after a standard abdominoplasty will also be discussed.

ANATOMY

- The umbilicus is generally described as a depressed circular indentation approximately 1.5 to 2 cm in diameter positioned in the midline of the abdomen at the level of the superior iliac crests[2] (**FIG 1A**).
- The vertical position has also been variably described as 30% to 47% of the way up between the symphysis pubis and the xiphoid.[3,4]

- The aesthetic ideal of the female umbilicus has been described as T or vertical in shape with a superior hood or shelf.[1] Protrusion, transverse orientation, or excessive size are rated as less attractive. There is a linear depression running from the xiphoid to the umbilicus, and this compares to the smooth contour of skin without a depression from the umbilicus to the symphysis pubis. Surrounding the umbilicus is a zone of decreased fat approximately 3 cm in diameter total, and this fat thickens to its maximum dimension for the ventral abdomen over the anterior rectus fascia.

PATIENT HISTORY AND PHYSICAL FINDINGS

- Past surgical history, including prior transection of the umbilical stalk at the time of an umbilical hernia repair, must be obtained. Prior laparoscopy umbilical portal sites can be the cause of incisional hernias and scar formation around the umbilicus.
- A reversed sit-up maneuver should be done for evaluation of rectus diastasis.
- Significant abdominal hirsutism should be appreciated preoperatively and is a relative contraindication to umbilicoplasty, as hair-bearing skin is placed deep against the abdominal wall and could create an iatrogenic pilonidal cyst.

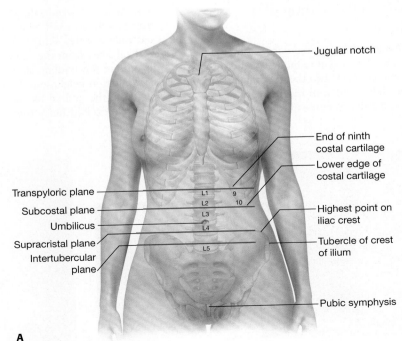

Jugular notch

End of ninth costal cartilage

Lower edge of costal cartilage

Transpyloric plane

Subcostal plane

Umbilicus

Supracristal plane

Intertubercular plane

Highest point on iliac crest

Tubercle of crest of ilium

Pubic symphysis

L1 9
L2 10
L3
L4
L5

A

FIG 1 • A. Location of umbilicus.

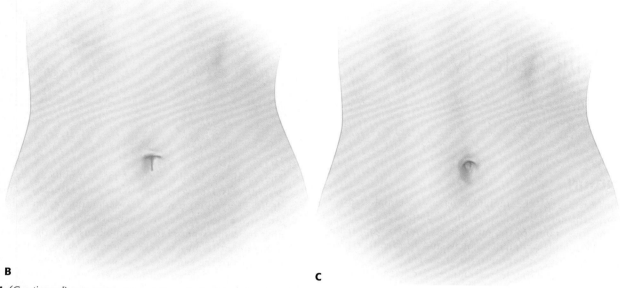

B

C

FIG 1 (Continued) • **B.** T-shaped umbilicus. **C.** Aesthetic abdominal contour with supraumbilical depression.

SURGICAL MANAGEMENT

Preoperative Planning

- The decision-making process for umbilicoplasty begins in the operating room after repair of the rectus muscles in the midline. The critical issue is whether or not the umbilical stalk remains vascularized and attached to the abdominal wall. For midline laparotomies, there is typically skin excess, and we find it easier to discard a marginal umbilical stalk and simply reconstruct it with pumpkin-teeth flaps.

- Patients undergoing an abdominoplasty where the stalk will not remain viable will need to be counseled that the reconstructed umbilicus with local flaps is not as aesthetic as the umbilical stalk that they currently have.

Positioning

- The patient is positioned in the usual supine position. The entire abdomen from xiphoid to pubis should be prepped to allow accurate determination of the midline and landmarks for appropriate umbilicus positioning.

■ Umbilicoplasty in the Setting of a Midline Incision

- Once the abdominal wall is reapproximated in the midline, we assess the amount of skin redundancy and if the umbilical stalk is still connected to the abdominal wall. In the majority of abdominal wall reconstructions, the skin is redundant and requires removal to decrease dead

space and improve healing. The markings for what we term "pumpkin-teeth" flaps are made at the time of this vertically oriented skin excision (**TECH FIG 1A–C**).

- Vertical lines from the xiphoid to the pubis are drawn to outline the midline skin to be excised. Rectangular flaps 2 cm in height and 2 cm wide are drawn and preserved in the desired location of the neoumbilicus. The flaps are excised fairly thinly, with minimal dermal fat

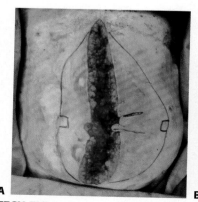

A

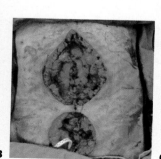

B

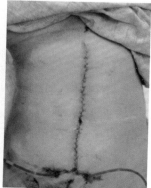

C

TECH FIG 1 • Markings for "pumpkin-teeth" flaps as final step in abdominal wall reconstruction.

remaining attached. After incising these pumpkin teeth, the full-thickness vertical incision for the length of the abdominal skin closure is then completed.

- We also perform a small amount of excision lipectomy just superior to the site of the neoumbilicus to allow for a depression in that area—this provides an aesthetically pleasing contour to the umbilicus.
- As the closure progresses, two 3-way sutures between the edges of the flaps and the final planned position of the neoumbilicus on the abdominal wall are placed and then tied using a 3-0 polydioxanone suture. The remaining dermal sutures are then placed in standard fashion, "folding in" these pumpkin-teeth skin flaps as the neoumbilicus (**TECH FIG 2**).

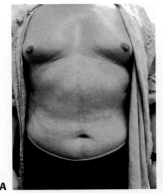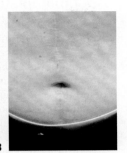

TECH FIG 2 • Postoperative result for "pumpkin-teeth" flaps.

De Novo Umbilicoplasty Without a Midline Incision

- For situations when the native umbilicus is removed and there is no vertical midline incision but still some laxity in the transverse plane, we present a variation on the technique described above (**TECH FIG 3A**).
- Two laterally based rectangular flaps are incised, and the fat deep to this entire area for a diameter of 3 cm is excised. These rectangular flaps are then sewn down to the abdominal wall with 3-0 polydioxanone sutures.
- For closure of the donor site, again A is brought to A prime, and B is brought to B prime. This creates excessive tissue above and below the neoumbilicus, which is handled as two separate W-plasties. The hashed triangles are excised, and point C and C prime are sewn down to the abdominal wall to create a circular depression (**TECH FIG 3B–E**).

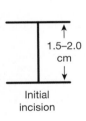

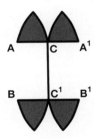
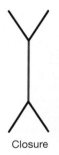
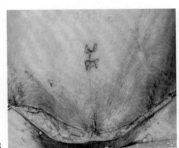
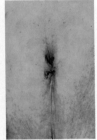
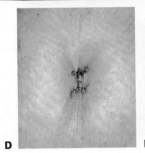
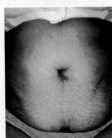

TECH FIG 3 • A. Umbilicoplasty design showing the initial H-shaped incision; excision of the redundant triangles of skin (shaded in); final closure design. **B.** Skin incised and approximated in midline, excess skin excised as W-plasties. **C.** Skin flaps tacked down to abdominal wall. **D.** Result at the end of the surgical procedure. **E.** Postoperative result.

T E C H N I Q U E S

■ Umbilical Stenosis After Abdominoplasty

- The goal of this umbilicoplasty is to bring the abdominal skin down to healthy umbilical stalk remnants (**TECH FIG 4**).
- In the office, the pinhole umbilicus opening is probed to ensure that a viable umbilicus stalk exists deep. The area around the scarred pinhole umbilicus opening is injected with 10 cc of xylocaine with epinephrine.
- The circular umbilical scar is excised.
- A 3-cm ring of fat is excised, especially superiorly, both to assist in local closure as well as to better identify the viable umbilicus stalk.
- The stalk is freed of scar tethering it to the abdominal wall and is mobilized superficially. The inferior aspect

of stalk is opened in the Heineke Mikulicz fashion to enlarge the circular suture line.
- The closure is performed in one layer with 5-0 polypropylene sutures to the abdominal skin.

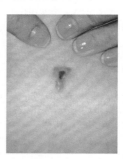

TECH FIG 4 • Umbilical stenosis after full abdominoplasty.

PEARLS AND PITFALLS

Patient selection	■ Umbilicoplasty is not to be performed in hirsute skin, as this will bring hair-bearing skin deeply and create an iatrogenic pilonidal sinus.
Technical considerations	■ These procedures require a transverse excess of skin. If the skin is tight transversely, the umbilicoplasty will be pulled open. ■ Umbilicoplasties tend to drain for 1–2 weeks after creation. ■ Optimal appearance will include a depression of fat in the midline from the umbilicus to the xiphoid (see **FIG 1C**).
Scarred umbilicus	■ Treatment of a scarred umbilicus after abdominoplasty will require pressure on the circular scar with a marble or equivalent daily to stretch and maintain patency of the stalk.
Stenosis of the neoumbilicus	■ This may occur after insetting the umbilicus in an abdominoplasty or with a de novo umbilicus. Stenting is the first-line management options and can be accomplished with daily use of a Vaseline-impregnated gauze bolster or even a firm noise-reducing ear plug for the 1–2 months following reconstruction.[5]
Umbilicus malposition in sagittal or coronal planes	■ This occurs especially when skin is extremely redundant as in cases of massive weight loss. Preoperative placement of staples 10 cm from the midline aids in having the final skin closure in the midline.

POSTOPERATIVE CARE

- We encourage the patients to gently wash these closures with soap and water twice daily and to cover them with a dry gauze for cleanliness.

OUTCOMES

- Creation of a neoumbilicus at the time of a midline hernia repair is reliable and significantly improves appearance. Pumpkin-teeth flaps tack the skin down to the abdominal wall as an ultimate "quilting" suture to help limit seroma formation. The only complications have been excessive hair growth in males, and one female patient where the umbilicus lost its depth due to a lack of transverse skin laxity.

COMPLICATIONS

- Drainage has on occasion lasted for several weeks after umbilicoplasty. Although difficult to quantify, on occasion, there has been restenosis of the scarred umbilicus after umbilicoplasty.

REFERENCES

1. Craig SB, Faller MS, Puckett CL. In search of the ideal female umbilicus. *Plast Reconstr Surg.* 2000;105:389.
2. Dini G, Ferreira L. A simple technique for umbilicus dilatation. *Plast Reconstr Surg.* 2006;117:336-337.
3. Dubou R, Ousterhout D. Placement of the umbilicus in an abdominoplasty. *Plast Reconstr Surg.* 1978;61:291.
4. Gallo J. Vertical relocation of the umbilical scar in abdominoplasty of Bozola and Psillakis Group IV cases—standardization of procedures. *Br Rev Plast Surg.* 2014;29:1.
5. Parnia R, Ghorbani L, Sepehrvand N, et al. Determining anatomical position of the umbilicus in Iranian girls, and providing quantitative indices and formula to determine neo-umbilicus during abdominoplasty. *Indian J Plast Surg.* 2012;45(1):94-96.

Hypospadias Repair

Christopher D. Morrison and Earl Y. Cheng

DEFINITION

- Hypospadias is defined as a ventrally located meatus proximal to its expected orthotopic location.
- Hypospadias is often associated with chordee, an abnormal ventral curvature of the penis.
- The prevalence of hypospadias is estimated at 1 per 200 to 300 live births, and the prevalence appears to be increasing.[1,2]

ANATOMY

- The hypospadiac meatus can be located anywhere along the course of the urethra:
  - Posterior/proximal: perineal, scrotal, penoscrotal
  - Middle: along the shaft of the penis
  - Distal/anterior: subcoronal, glandular
- In general, a more proximal hypospadiac meatus is associated with a more significant degree of chordee.
- The glans can vary in size, and the urethral plate can range from grooved to completely flat.
- In most cases, the prepuce does not extend ventrally, resulting in a noncircumferential dorsal hooded foreskin.
- The skin overlying the ventral aspect of the urethra can be dysplastic or insufficient, leading to ventral tethering of the penis.
- The corpus spongiosum diverges laterally or is completely atretic, which can result in a urethra that is only covered by a very thin layer of ventral skin.

PATHOGENESIS

- Hypospadias results from the incomplete development of the penis and urethra between 8 and 14 weeks gestation.
- Tubularization of the urethra is thought to be androgen mediated, and disruption of this process results in a hypospadiac meatus.[3]
- Both genetic and environmental factors have been associated with hypospadias.[4]
  - Hypospadias is heritable and can be associated with several syndromes (less than 10% of cases).
  - Over 20 genes have been implicated in the pathogenesis of hypospadias.
  - Environmental factors such as maternal medication/ drug use, maternal age, maternal obesity, and placental insufficiency have been associated with hypospadias and may account for the rising prevalence of hypospadias.

PATIENT HISTORY AND PHYSICAL FINDINGS

- Hypospadias is typically recognized at the time of birth during newborn examination.
- Newborn circumcision (if desired) is contraindicated in the setting of hypospadias because the foreskin may be needed for surgical repair of the hypospadias.
- History
  - A complete prenatal and family history should be performed to identify possible contributing factors.
  - If possible, ask the parents about the direction and strength of the patient's urinary stream, as well as the curvature of the penis with erections. A downward deflected urinary stream or significant curvature of the penis may affect the patient's urinary and sexual function later in life.
- Exam
  - Penile exam:
    - Location and appearance of the meatus
    - Quality and depth of urethral plate
    - Size and configuration of the glans
    - Degree of chordee
    - Integrity of the ventral skin
    - Amount of dorsal hooded foreskin available
  - A careful scrotal and inguinal exam should be performed to look for other abnormalities such as cryptorchidism, hydrocele, or hernia.[5]
  - If a patient also has undescended testicles (unilateral or bilateral), it is important to consider the possibility of a disorder of sex development (DSD).
    - If undiagnosed, a DSD condition such as congenital adrenal hyperplasia (CAH) can be life threatening.
    - These patients should undergo an endocrine workup and karyotype.
    - Approximately 20% to 30% of patients with hypospadias and cryptorchidism will have a karyotype abnormality.[3]
    - The most common DSD seen in patients with hypospadias and cryptorchidism is mixed gonadal dysgenesis.

IMAGING

- Proximal hypospadias can be associated with renal anomalies. However, routine imaging is not performed in most cases of hypospadias. If the patient has a severe proximal hypospadias, one could consider obtaining a renal ultrasound.

NONOPERATIVE MANAGEMENT

- For patients with distal/anterior hypospadias in which the urinary stream is relatively straight and there is no significant chordee, surgical correction is generally considered optional and is usually performed more for appearance and psychosocial reasons rather than for correction of a functional need.
- There is controversy among some urologists as to whether correction of distal hypospadias confers long-term benefits for patients.
  - A 1995 study of 500 men found great variability in the meatal location. Thirteen percent of these men had anterior hypospadias with no functional compromise, and two-thirds of these patients were unaware of their hypospadiac condition.[5]
  - In contrast, a 2014 study examined the self-reported outcomes for patients who had uncorrected hypospadias and found that these patients were more likely to have worse voiding symptoms, more penile curvature making sexual intercourse difficult, and worse satisfaction with the appearance of their penis.[6]

SURGICAL MANAGEMENT

- Multiple different surgical techniques have been described for distal hypospadias, including the MAGPI and the Mathieu repair. However, the tubularized incised plate (TIP) urethroplasty, as described by Snodgrass, is the technique that is now most commonly performed by hypospadias surgeons. It is suitable for patients with a sufficiently healthy and wide (greater than 7 mm) urethral plate and less than 30-degree chordee.
- Midshaft hypospadias is often approached similarly to distal hypospadias; however, it tends to be associated with more significant chordee.
  - If there is less than 30-degree chordee and the urethral plate is sufficiently healthy and wide, a TIP urethroplasty can be performed.
  - If there is less than 30-degree chordee but the urethral plate is too narrow, hypospadias repair can be performed using a transverse preputial island flap or an inner preputial inlay graft.
- Proximal hypospadias repair presents a greater challenge for several reasons:
  - There is a longer length of urethra that must be tubularized.
  - The urethral plate may be narrow, fibrotic, or even nonexistent.
  - There tends to be a more significant degree of chordee.

Preoperative Planning

- If diagnosed at the time of birth, most urologists will delay treatment until the child is 6 months of age to decrease potential anesthetic risks.

- Ideally, the surgery should be performed prior to the child being old enough to remember the surgery.
  - Many advocate hypospadias repair between 6 and 12 months of life.[7]
- Historically, hormonal stimulation with testosterone, dihydrotestosterone, or human chorionic gonadotropin was given preoperatively to increase penile length, glans circumference, and vascularity as this was thought to aid in surgical correction.
  - However, there is now concern that hormonal stimulation may affect normal wound healing and may lead to an increased risk of postoperative complications.[8]
  - Nevertheless, hormone stimulation is still felt to be beneficial in more severe cases of hypospadias.

Positioning

- After the induction of general anesthesia, if possible, a caudal anesthetic block is recommended for perioperative pain control.
- The patient is positioned supine for the surgery.

Approach

- The operative approach varies based on the following:
  - Location of the hypospadiac meatus
  - Severity of chordee
  - Characteristics (width, depth, and health) of urethral plate
  - Quality of penile shaft and dorsal hood skin
  - Surgeon preference/experience
- The main components of a hypospadias repair consist of the following:
  - Evaluation and correction of chordee
  - Urethroplasty
  - Glanuloplasty
  - Skin coverage
- Hypospadias repair is typically performed with the use of 2.5 times surgical loupes or with an operating microscope.
- Hypospadias repair can be either a one- or two-staged repair. The decision to perform a one- or two-stage repair depends primarily on the degree of chordee and the health of the urethral plate.
  - If the chordee can be corrected with dorsal plication and the urethral plate is healthy and wide, a TIP urethroplasty should be performed.
  - If the chordee can be corrected with dorsal plication but the urethral plate is NOT healthy and wide, the surgeon can perform either a one-staged preputial onlay island flap urethroplasty or a two-staged inner preputial inlay graft with subsequent tubularization.
  - If division of the urethral plate is required for correction of chordee, this should be performed during the initial stage. The urethroplasty should be performed in a second stage at least 6 months later.
- An algorithm for intraoperative decision-making during hypospadias repair is presented in **FIG 1**.

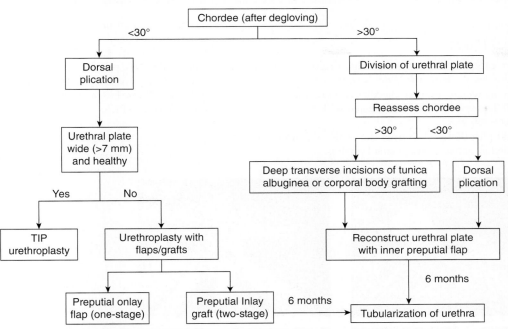

FIG 1 • Algorithm for hypospadias repair.

■ # Tubularized Incised Plate Urethroplasty for Distal Hypospadias Repair

■ ## Examination Under Anesthesia

- Prior to beginning the surgery, examine the anatomy.
- Visually inspect the meatus.

- Calibrate the meatus with bougies and examine the ventral penile skin overlying the urethra.
- If the urethra and overlying skin is too thin, it may be necessary to perform a cutback procedure to healthier tissue and perform a more proximal hypospadias repair.
- Examine the urethral plate for width, depth, and overall health.

■ # Initial Approach (TECH FIG 1)

- Place a 4-0 Ethibond suture longitudinally at the tip of the glans for retraction purposes.
- Make a reverse chevron incision on the dorsum of the penis to preserve the mucosal collar flaps.
- Working laterally to medially, carefully elevate the ventral skin off of the urethra. (Avoid incising into the urethra. If necessary, it is better to buttonhole the overlying skin than to incise into the native urethra.)

- Deglove the penis down to the penopubic and penoscrotal junction.
- Induce an artificial erection and evaluate degree of chordee by constricting the corpora cavernosa at the base of the penis with a tourniquet device (ie, rubber band, dental roll, and hemostat) and injecting saline through a small-gauge butterfly needle into the corpora cavernosa.

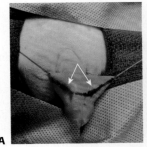
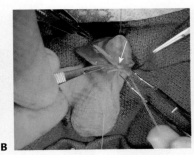
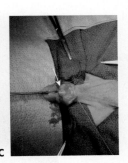

TECH FIG 1 • Initial incisions. **A.** Reverse chevron incision to preserve mucosal collars (*arrows*). **B.** Elevation of skin off of urethra behind hypospadiac meatus (*arrow*). **C.** Example of thin ventral urethra (*arrow*) that will require cut back.

TECHNIQUES

■ Correction of Chordee With Dorsal Plication

- In most cases of distal hypospadias, degloving of the penis alone will adequately straighten the penis.
- In cases in which residual chordee remains that is less than 30 degrees, this can be corrected with dorsal plication (**TECH FIG 2**).
  - Dorsal plication will shorten the penis and should be avoided in patients with a small phallus.

- Make an incision in Buck fascia at the 12 o'clock position over the dorsal vasculature.
- Place a 3-0 or 4-0 Ethibond suture (Ethicon Inc., Somerville, NJ) parallel to the shaft, ensuring not to injure the neurovascular bundles laterally.
- Imbricate Buck fascia over the plication suture using interrupted 6-0 PDS.

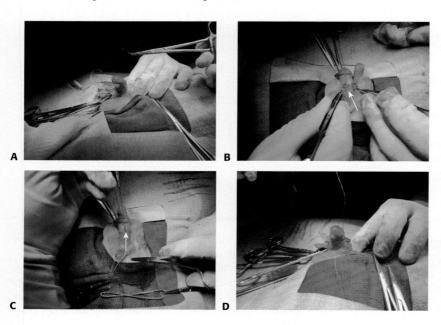

TECH FIG 2 • Dorsal plication. **A.** Artificial erection to assess chordee (less than 30 degrees). **B.** Dorsal incision at 12 o'clock (*arrow*; between neurovascular bundles). **C.** Plication suture (*arrow*) with 3-0 Ethibond suture. **D.** Corrected chordee following dorsal plication.

■ TIP Urethroplasty (TECH FIG 3)

- Elevate the spongiosum and create glans wings.
  - Often, the corpora spongiosum can be identified diverging lateral to the urethral plate.
  - If easily identified, elevate the divergent spongiosal tissue off the corporal bodies.
  - The corpus spongiosum can be used as an additional layer of closure over the urethral repair.
  - To create glans wings, incise along the lateral borders of the urethral plate to the top of the glans.
  - Dissect down to the corporal bodies.
  - Ensure that the glans wings are sufficiently wide to allow midline approximation without tension.

- Incise the urethral plate and tubularize the urethra (**TECH FIG 3B,C**).
  - Make a longitudinal incision at the base to deepen the groove.
  - Place a urethral stent (size varies based on urethral diameter, usually 6–8 French).
  - Close the urethra in two layers with a 7-0 PDS suture in a running subcuticular fashion with careful attention to turn in the epithelial edges.
  - Take care to not make the neomeatus too tight.
  - If the divergent spongiosal tissue was identified and easily mobilized, reapproximate over the urethral repair using interrupted 7-0 Vicryl sutures.

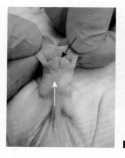
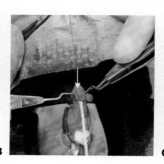
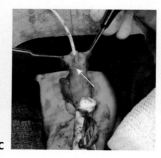

TECH FIG 3 • Distal hypospadias repair with TIP urethroplasty. **A.** Preoperative examination reveals coronal hypospadiac meatus (*white arrow*) and blind urethral dimple (*black arrow*). **B.** Incision of urethral plate (*arrow*). **C.** Urethroplasty repair (*arrow*).

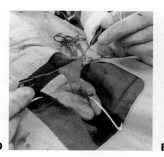
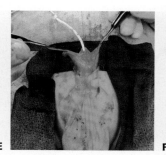
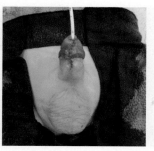

TECH FIG 3 (Continued) • **D.** Harvesting of dartos flap. **E.** Overlying urethral repair with dartos flap. **F.** Hypospadias closure.

- The dartos flap is used as an additional layer of coverage over the urethral repair and can be harvested from either the ventral or dorsal penis, but typically, the dorsal dartos is more supple and better vascularized (**TECH FIG 3D,E**).
  - Rotate the dartos flap over the urethral repair and suture in place using 7-0 Vicryl sutures.
- Close the glans in two layers. Use 6-0 PDS (Ethicon, Somerville, NJ) to close the deep layer and 7-0 Vicryl (Ethicon, Somervill, NJ) to close the superficial layers.

- For skin closure, transpose the mucosal collar flaps ventrally, excise the redundant tissue, and suture together with 7-0 Vicryl (**TECH FIG 3F**).
  - If there is inadequate ventral skin for closure, mobilize flaps from the excessive dorsal preputial skin, transpose the flaps ventrally, and suture in place with 7-0 Vicryl.
- Secure the stent to the glans with two 6-0 Vicryl sutures.

Midshaft Hypospadias Repair

Transverse Preputial Island Flap (TPIF)

- Performed in a single-stage repair.
- The urethral plate is preserved as the posterior urethral wall and a TPIF is used to make up the anterior wall of the neourethra.

- Harvest a strip of skin from the inner preputial skin along its native blood supply.
- Rotate the flap ventrally and position over the urethral plate to form the anterior urethral wall.
- Suture the skin flap to the lateral edges of the urethral plate using a running 7-0 Vicryl suture.
- Complete hypospadias repair as previously discussed (glanuloplasty, skin coverage, etc.).

Inner Preputial Inlay Graft (TECH FIG 4)

- An inner preputial graft is used to augment the urethral plate by placement of the graft into the defect that results following incision of the urethral plate.
- Measure the dimensions of the existing urethral plate to assess the length and width of an inlay graft needed for tubularization.
- Harvest an inner preputial graft of appropriate size.
- Defat the graft.
- Apply the tourniquet to reduce bleeding.
- Make a deep incision within the native urethral plate from the hypospadiac meatus to the tip of the penis.
- Elevate the urethral plate off the underlying corporal bodies.
- Place the inner preputial graft along the vascular bed and quilt it with 7-0 Vicryl sutures.
- Mature the graft to the surrounding urethral plate tissue with interrupted 7-0 Vicryl sutures.

- Fenestrate the graft with a micro knife to prevent hematoma formation beneath the graft.
- Following placement of the graft, one can perform a single-stage repair in which the lateral aspect of the urethral plate on each side of the graft is tubularized. Alternatively, one can perform a two-stage repair in which tubularization is delayed for 6 months later to allow maturation and neovascularization of the graft prior to creation of the neourethra. At our institution, we generally favor a two-stage approach in this setting.
- Rotate the mucosal collar flaps ventrally alongside the urethral plate and suture with 7-0 Vicryl sutures.
- The graft is allowed to heal for 6 months and then is tubularized during the second stage.
- If there is greater than 30-degree chordee such that dorsal plication is insufficient to correct the curvature, the hypospadias repair should be approached similarly to that of a proximal hypospadias.

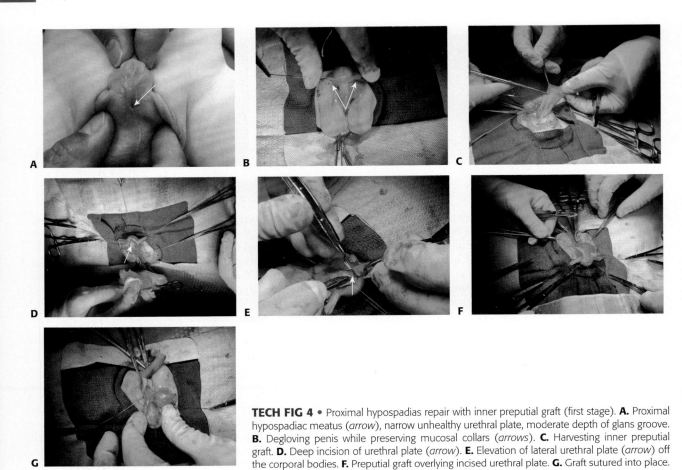

TECH FIG 4 • Proximal hypospadias repair with inner preputial graft (first stage). **A.** Proximal hypospadiac meatus (*arrow*), narrow unhealthy urethral plate, moderate depth of glans groove. **B.** Degloving penis while preserving mucosal collars (*arrows*). **C.** Harvesting inner preputial graft. **D.** Deep incision of urethral plate (*arrow*). **E.** Elevation of lateral urethral plate (*arrow*) off the corporal bodies. **F.** Preputial graft overlying incised urethral plate. **G.** Graft sutured into place.

◼ Proximal Hypospadias Repair

- Both one- and two-stage repairs for proximal hypospadias have been described.
- In most cases, there is significant (greater than 30 degrees) chordee that cannot be corrected with dorsal plication. Consequently, a two-stage repair is most often needed for proximal hypospadias repair.
- One-stage repair is reserved for the rare cases in which there is minimal chordee that can be corrected with dorsal plication.

- If the urethral plate is healthy and sufficiently wide (greater than 7 mm), a TIP urethroplasty can be performed.
- If the urethral plate is healthy but too narrow to tubularize, a one-stage repair can be performed with a transverse preputial island flap or an inner preputial inlay flap, as described for midshaft hypospadias repair.
- Two-stage repair **is** recommended for patient with significant chordee and/or an unhealthy urethral plate.
  - The goal of the first stage is to correct the chordee and/or augment the urethral plate for tubularization at the second stage.

◼ Stage 1: Correction of Chordee

- If there is greater than 30-degree chordee, dorsal plication is usually insufficient and the following techniques should be used to correct the curvature.

Division of Urethral Plate

- Make a transverse incision in the urethral plate at the level of the maximal curvature.
- Elevate the urethra off the corporal bodies.
- Excise dysgenetic tissue away from the corporal bodies.
- Repeat artificial erection. If chordee is now less than 30 degrees, proceed with dorsal plication.

Deep Transverse Incisions of Tunica Albuginea (DTITA)

- If significant chordee still remains that is more than 30 degree despite division of the urethral plate, the next step is to make multiple nearly full-thickness incisions in the tunica albuginea at the level of the maximal curvature.
- No full-thickness incisions into the erectile tissue should be made and thus should not affect future erectile function.
- For severe chordee, DTITA is often insufficient and corporal body grafting is necessary.

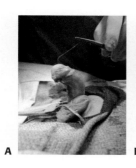
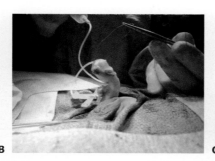
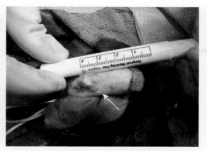
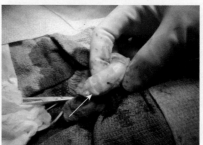

TECH FIG 5 • Division of urethral plate with corporal body grafting. **A.** Significant chordee after degloving. **B.** Chordee persists despite division of urethral plate. **C.** Corporal body incision (*arrow*) with subsequent defect. **D.** SIS grafting (*arrow*) of corporal body defect.

Corporal Body Grafting (TECH FIG 5)

- Make a full-thickness ventral incision through the tunica albuginea at the area of greatest curvature and extend to the lateral borders of the neurovascular bundles.
- Elevate the corporal wall off of the underlying erectile tissue to create a diamond-shaped defect.
- Graft the defect with either a dermal graft (harvested from the inguinal area) or small intestine submucosal (SIS) (off-the-shelf xenograft material).
- Suture the graft in place with a running 6-0 PDS.

Bridging of Urethral Plate Defect

- Following division of the urethral plate and correction of chordee, it is necessary to bridge the gap between the proximal and distal native urethral plates.
- Traditionally, this is performed utilizing Byars flaps. However, at our institution, we favor an inner preputial skin flap.
- Byars flaps (**TECH FIG 6**)
  - Make a midline dorsal incision in the preputial skin.
  - Rotate each preputial skin flap (Byars flap) ventrally along with their respective dartos vascular pedicles.

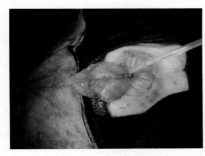

TECH FIG 6 • Byars flaps using ventrally rotated preputial flaps.

- Bring the flaps together in the midline and interpose the combined Byars flaps between the proximal and distal urethral plate. If the urethral plate in the glans is flat and insufficient, the plate can be incised and the Byars flaps can be placed into the defect with extension of the flaps out to the tip of glans.
- Suture the flaps in place utilizing 7-0 interrupted Vicryl sutures.
- At the time of the second stage, the Byars flaps are tubularized to form the urethra.
- Because of the nature of the preputial skin used for Byars flaps, the resultant tubularized urethra can be more prone to be hypermobile or difficult to catheterize. Furthermore, in our experience, the patient is more prone to urethral diverticula formation. Thus, we have favored use of an inner preputial skin flap for bridging of the urethral defect.
- Inner preputial skin flap (**TECH FIG 7**)
  - Harvest an appropriate-sized flap from the dorsal inner preputial skin while preserving the blood supply from the dartos fascia.
  - Defat the distal one-third of the flap while maintaining the blood supply to the proximal two-thirds.
  - Incise the glans urethral plate.
  - Inlay the defatted distal one-third of the flap into the incised distal urethra.
  - The proximal two-thirds of the flap is positioned along the shaft of the penis.
  - The flap is quilted to the tunica albuginea utilizing interrupted 7-0 Vicryl sutures.
  - Fenestrate the flap to reduce subcutaneous hematoma formation.
  - The urethra is tubularized at the time of the second-stage repair.

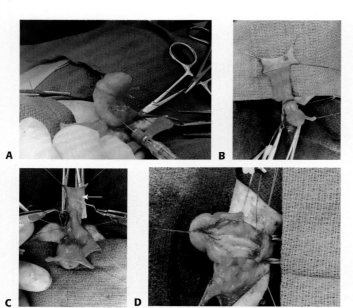

TECH FIG 7 • Division of urethral plate with preputial inlay flap. **A.** This curvature of more than 30 degrees required division of the urethral plate. **B.** Harvested preputial inlay flap. **C.** Defatted distal third of preputial flap (*arrow*). **D.** Preputial inlay flap quilted to tunica albuginea.

■ Stage 2: Tubularization of the Urethra and Glanuloplasty

Tubularization

- Deglove the penis.
- Induce artificial erection and ensure that any previous significant chordee has been corrected.
- Make parallel incisions along the inlay graft and residual urethral plate from the level of the hypospadiac meatus to the distal aspect of the glans.
- Tubularize the urethral plate over a 6 or 8 French stent and close in two layers, with interrupted 7-0 PDS for the first layer and a running subcuticular 7-0 PDS for the second layer.
- If available, harvest a vascularized dartos flap from the dorsum and transpose over the repair with interrupted 7-0 PDS.

Tunica Vaginalis Flap

- If a vascularized dartos flap is insufficient, harvest a tunica vaginalis flap.
- Make a transverse scrotal incision over either the left or right scrotum.

- Create a subdartos pouch.
- Deliver the testicle.
- Harvest a rectangular tunica vaginalis flap large enough to completely cover the length of the repair, ensuring not to disrupt its proximal blood supply along the cord structures.
- Create a tunnel between the scrotal incision and the penoscrotal junction.
- Deliver the tunica vaginalis flap and cover the entire repair.
- Suture the tunica vaginalis flap in place with interrupted 7-0 Vicryl sutures.
- Place the testicle into the developed subdartos pouch, and pexy it in place with interrupted 4-0 chromic sutures at the 3 o'clock and 9 o'clock positions.

Completion

- Perform glanuloplasty.
- Close in two layers. Use 7-0 PDS to close the deep layer and 7-0 Vicryl to close the superficial layers.
- Mobilize and transpose the mucosal collar flaps ventrally and suture with 7-0 Vicryl sutures.
- Mobilize skin flaps as necessary for skin closure.
- Place a catheter into the bladder for drainage purposes.

■ Buccal Mucosa Graft for Redo Hypospadias Repair

- Unfortunately, not all primary hypospadias repairs are successful. As a result, some patients may require a redo hypospadias repair.
- In instances of a redo hypospadias repair, the urethral plate is often no longer healthy and requires excision.
- In addition, inner preputial skin is typically not available for redo hypospadias repairs.

- As a result, a hypospadias repair using a buccal mucosa graft is required.
- Harvest a buccal mucosa graft from either cheek or the upper/lower lip.
- Mark out the edges of the desired graft.
- Infiltrate the edges of the graft with 1% lidocaine with epinephrine.
- Harvest the graft using scissors while preserving the underlying fatty tissue (avoid dissecting too deep as this will risk injuring the underlying muscles/nerves).

- Control bleeding from the graft site using bipolar cautery.
- Defat the graft.
- Excise the scarred urethra and surrounding scar tissue to create a healthy vascular bed along the surface of the corporal bodies. Make the buccal graft as wide as possible.
- Tack down the buccal mucosal graft to the location of the urethral plate with 7-0 Vicryl sutures in a quilted fashion.

- Fenestrate the graft with a micro knife to prevent hematoma formation beneath the graft.
- Allow at least 6 months for the buccal graft to mature.
- In a second stage, the buccal mucosa graft is tubularized and the hypospadias repair is completed (**TECH FIG 8**).

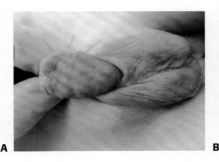 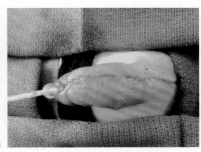

TECH FIG 8 • Second stage of proximal hypospadias repair with buccal mucosa. **A.** Healed first-stage repair with buccal mucosa. **B.** Tubularization and closure of buccal mucosa urethral plate.

PEARLS AND PITFALLS

Indications	▪ Proximal and middle hypospadias should be repaired to improve urinary and sexual function. ▪ Distal hypospadias typically will not impact overall function but correction can be performed to improve the appearance.
Approach	▪ The approach for each hypospadias repair should be dictated by the intraoperative assessment of the chordee and the urethral plate. ▪ Counsel the patient and/or parents preoperatively regarding the possibility of needing a staged repair.
Technique	▪ Know the limitations of the tissue available for repair. Attempting to do too much in a single stage may result in failure of the repair and increased morbidity for the patient. ▪ Use all available tissue to cover the urethral repair to reduce the risk of urethrocutaneous fistula.
Complications	▪ If a urethrocutaneous fistula or urethral diverticulum forms, the distal urethra and meatus must be interrogated. If a stricture or meatal stenosis is present, correction of the fistula or diverticulum without addressing the distal obstruction will inevitably lead to recurrence.

POSTOPERATIVE CARE

- **Dressing**
  - At the conclusion of the surgery, a slightly compressive dressing is typically placed around the penis to reduce swelling and promote hemostasis.
  - At our institution, we place a benzoin-soaked Owen gauze around the incisions followed by Coban gauze secured with plastic tape.
  - Care should be taken to ensure that the dressing is not too tight as this can decrease blood flow to the glans.
  - The dressing is removed by a physician or nurse 4 to 5 days postoperatively.
  - After removal of the dressing, a topical antibiotic ointment should be applied to the incisions routinely for 1 to 2 weeks as the incisions continue to heal.
- **Urinary diversion**
  - As mentioned previously, a urethral stent is sutured in place at the end of the surgery.
  - Urinary diversion with a urethral stent allows for proper urethral healing and prevents postoperative urinary retention.

- Some physicians utilize suprapubic tubes for urinary diversion as these may limit bladder spasms. In patients with a history of severe bladder spasms, a suprapubic tube should be considered as strong bladder spasms can expel the urethral catheter.
  - The urethral stent is typically removed 1 to 2 weeks postoperatively.
- **Postoperative antibiotics**
  - Historically, postoperative antibiotics were routinely prescribed while the urethral stent was in place.[9] However, it is currently unclear whether postoperative antibiotics confer a benefit.
  - While awaiting more conclusive studies, we routinely prescribe postoperative antibiotics (ie, Bactrim, Keflex) while the urethral stent is in place.
- **Postoperative evaluation**
  - Take a thorough history of the patient's urinary stream (direction, force, urethral bulging during urination, leakage of urine from along the repair, etc.).
  - Carefully examine the repair and look for evidence of urethrocutaneous fistula (early signs consist of erythema or inflammation along the urethra proximal to the meatus).

- Examine the meatus for evidence of meatal stenosis.
- If concern for meatal stenosis or urethral stricture, uroflowmetry can help gauge the strength of the stream.

OUTCOMES

- A successful hypospadias repair should meet the following primary goals:
  - Patent urethra with a good functional urinary stream
  - Intact sexual function (ie, erections, ejaculation)
  - Good appearance
  - Patient satisfaction
- Success of a hypospadias repair is directly correlated with the severity of the hypospadias. Patients with a history of a proximal hypospadias and/or significant chordee requiring a multistaged repair with multiple grafts are more likely to have diminished function or worse appearance.
- Patients with a history of more proximal hypospadias are more likely to have a shorter phallus, more voiding dysfunction, and lower maximum urinary flow compared to matched controls.[10] Patients are also more likely to report erectile dysfunction and decreased sexual quality of life as adults.[11]
- However, a study of patient-reported outcomes found that patients with a history of a successful hypospadias repair were more satisfied with the appearance of their phallus and fewer voiding symptoms than compared to patients who had uncorrected hypospadias.[12]

COMPLICATIONS

- Complication rates following hypospadias repair are also directly related to the severity of the hypospadias and the complexity of the repair.[13]
- In expert hands, distal hypospadias using the TIP urethroplasty can be performed with few complications.[14] Most series quote a less than 10% incidence of complications for distal hypospadias repair.
- Short-term complications
  - Glans dehiscence is the most common acute postoperative complication seen following urethroplasty repair and is typically due to closure of the glans under too much tension or by too much ventral pressure from the urethral stent. If the patient has a functional urinary flow and direction, the decision to correct the glans dehiscence typically depends on the patient's or parents' concern for appearance.
  - Hematoma formation and infection are other potential short-term complications.
- Long-term complications
  - Urethrocutaneous fistula formation is the most commonly seen long-term complication and typically presents within 1 year of repair.[15]
    - Rates of urethrocutaneous fistula formation with proximal hypospadias repairs have been reported as high as 30% to 50%.[16,17]
    - The patient or parents typically notices urine leaking from a site proximal to the meatus.
    - Often, there is an associated area of inflammation or wound breakdown.
    - A fistula is unlikely to close on its own with conservative management and reoperation is typically necessary.

- In general, it is recommended to wait 6 to 12 months prior to reoperation to allow inflammation and edema to resolve.
- Options for repair include primary closure vs redo urethroplasty.
- For primary closure, the fistula tract is excised and the urethra is closed with multiple layers of well-vascularized tissue. For primary closures, it is essential to calibrate the distal urethra to ensure no obstruction that will increase risk of recurrence.
- Meatal stenosis
  - The rates of meatal stenosis range from 0% to 17%.[18]
  - Obstruction created by meatal stenosis will increase the risk of urethrocutaneous fistula and urethral diverticula formation.
  - At follow-up appointments, it is important to query the patient and/or his family regarding urine stream and to closely examine the meatus.
  - If evidence of meatal stenosis, a simple meatotomy performed in the operating room is typically sufficient.
- Recurrent chordee
  - If the patient develops recurrent significant ventral curvature of the penis, the patient may require reoperation if there is concern that it will affect urinary or sexual function in the future.
  - For minor recurrent chordee (less than 30 degrees), dorsal plication is usually sufficient.
  - For significant chordee (≥30 degrees), repeat hypospadias repair may be necessary (although this is uncommon).
- Urethral diverticulum
  - Patients with a urethral diverticulum typically describe a bulging of the ventral aspect of the penis during urination. At completion of urination, compression of the bulge will cause the expulsion of more urine.
  - Urethral diverticula typically warrant correct. At the time of repair, excision of the excess urethra is typically sufficient. However, it is crucial to evaluate the distal urethra as there is likely an obstruction, which contributed to the initial diverticulum formation.
- Urethral stricture
  - Patients who present with urethral strictures often complain of a long, slow stream or having to strain to empty their bladder.
  - Diagnosis is typically performed by cystourethroscopy.
  - For mild, thin strictures, endoscopic management with direct visual incision of the urethra (DVIU) can be attempted; however, in many instances, the stricture will recur.
  - For denser strictures or strictures that have failed endoscopic management, reoperation is indicated.

REFERENCES

1. Canon S, Mosley B, Chipollini J, et al. Epidemiological assessment of hypospadias by degree of severity. *J Urol.* 2012;188(6):2362-2366.
2. Paulozzi LJ, Erickson JD, Jackson RJ. Hypospadias trends in two US surveillance systems. *Pediatrics.* 1997;100(5):831-834.
3. Cox MJ, Coplen DE, Austin PF. The incidence of disorders of sexual differentiation and chromosomal abnormalities of cryptorchidism and hypospadias stratified by meatal location. *J Urol.* 2008;180(6):2649-2652.

4. Shih EM, Graham JM. Review of genetic and environmental factors leading to hypospadias. *Eur J Med Genet.* 2014;57(8):453-463.

5. Fichtner J, Filipas D, Mottrie AM, et al. Analysis of meatal location in 500 men: wide variation questions need for meatal advancement in all pediatric anterior hypospadias cases. *J Urol.* 1995;154(2 Pt 2): 833-834.

6. Schlomer B, Breyer B, Copp H, et al. Do adult men with untreated hypospadias have adverse outcomes? A pilot study using a social media advertised survey. *J Pediatr Urol.* 2014;10(4):672-679.

7. Timing of elective surgery on the genitalia of male children with particular reference to the risks, benefits, and psychological effects of surgery and anesthesia. American Academy of Pediatrics. *Pediatrics.* 1996;97(4):590-594.

8. Wright I, Cole E, Farrokhyar F, et al. Effect of preoperative hormonal stimulation on postoperative complication rates after proximal hypospadias repair: a systematic review. *J Urol.* 2013;190(2): 652-659.

9. Hsieh MH, Wildenfels P, Gonzales ET. Surgical antibiotic practices among pediatric urologists in the United States. *J Pediatr Urol.* 2011;7(2):192-197.

10. Örtqvist L, Fossum M, Andersson M, et al. Long-term followup of men born with hypospadias: urological and cosmetic results. *J Urol.* 2015;193(3):975-981.

11. Chertin B, Natsheh A, Ben-zion I, et al. Objective and subjective sexual outcomes in adult patients after hypospadias repair performed in childhood. *J Urol.* 2013;190(4 suppl):1556-1560.

12. Keays MA, Starke N, Lee SC, et al. Patient reported outcomes in preoperative and postoperative patients with hypospadias. *J Urol.* 2016;195(4 Pt 2):1215-1220.

13. Arlen AM, Kirsch AJ, Leong T, et al. Further analysis of the Glans-Urethral Meatus-Shaft (GMS) hypospadias score: correlation with postoperative complications. *J Pediatr Urol.* 2015;11(2):71.e1-71.e5.

14. Cheng EY, Vemulapalli SN, Kropp BP, et al. Snodgrass hypospadias repair with vascularized dartos flap: the perfect repair for virgin cases of hypospadias? *J Urol.* 2002;168(4 Pt 2):1723-1726.

15. Snodgrass W, Villanueva C, Bush NC. Duration of follow-up to diagnose hypospadias urethroplasty complications. *J Pediatr Urol.* 2014;10(2):208-211.

16. Snodgrass W, Yucel S. Tubularized incised plate for mid shaft and proximal hypospadias repair. *J Urol.* 2007;177(2):698-702.

17. Mcnamara ER, Schaeffer AJ, Logvinenko T, et al. Management of proximal hypospadias with 2-stage repair: 20-year experience. *J Urol.* 2015;194(4):1080-1085.

18. Wilkinson DJ, Farrelly P, Kenny SE. Outcomes in distal hypospadias: a systematic review of the Mathieu and tubularized incised plate repairs. *J Pediatr Urol.* 2012;8(3):307-312.

69 CHAPTER

Vaginal and Vulvar Reconstruction

Elizabeth B. Yerkes and Julia Corcoran

DEFINITION

- Neovaginal creation or augmentation of the vaginal canal may be requested in several congenital conditions and in acquired vaginal stenosis. This chapter will address vaginal and vulvar reconstruction in emerging and young adults. It does not include vaginoplasty or labioplasty techniques that may be applied in reconstruction of urogenital sinus in cases of ambiguous genitalia, intersex states, and differences of sex development.
  - Vaginal agenesis or congenital vaginal atresia (Mayer-Rokitansky-Küster-Hauser syndrome)
  - Vaginal agenesis or insufficiency in the setting of complete androgen insensitivity and intersex/differences of sex development
  - Classic bladder exstrophy or cloacal exstrophy
  - Vaginal stenosis after early childhood surgery (congenital adrenal hyperplasia, intersex/differences of sex development, or persistent cloaca)
  - Secondary changes after pelvic malignancy or graft versus host disease (GVHD)
- Vulvar reconstruction in the form of monsplasty and labioplasty may be requested to align the laterally displaced or offset mons tissue and pubic hair and to reconfigure and stabilize the labia minora after pubertal development in congenital conditions such as exstrophy-epispadias and its covered variants.
- Reduction labioplasty may be requested to address physically bothersome bulk of the labia minora.

ANATOMY

- The paired Müllerian (paramesonephric) bodies fuse in the midline and contact the urogenital sinus. The sinovaginal bulb is induced and the vaginal plate is formed.
- Müllerian development occurs within first 10 weeks of gestation.
- The labia minora are formed from the urogenital folds and the labia majora and mons from the labioscrotal folds (**FIG 1**).

PATHOGENESIS

- Absent or incomplete development of the Müllerian bodies results in absence or atresia of the female genital tract.
  - Ovaries have a different embryologic development and are spared.
- Failure of the fusion of the Müllerian bodies results in duplication of the vagina or unilateral obstruction or atresia.
- Anomalous descent of the urorectal septum in dividing the cloaca, as in anorectal malformations, may interfere with fusion of the Müllerian bodies.

- Renal development and a portion of skeletal development occur at a similar time to Müllerian development, so anomalies may coexist.
- Pelvic diastasis associated with abdominal wall defects such as bladder exstrophy and cloacal exstrophy also results in nonfusion of the labial and mons tissues. Bifid clitoris also occurs in these conditions.
- Thickening of the labia minora with puberty results in extensive variation in size and shape. Sufficient hypertrophy may occur that some clothing and physical activity are physically bothersome.
  - Hygiene and tissue health may be a concern in young women with limited mobility or ability for self-care.

NATURAL HISTORY

- Vaginal agenesis or atresia does not resolve over time, but maturation of the vulvar tissues and proximal vaginal segment, if present, may facilitate the reconstruction.
- If a uterus and proximal vagina are present, judiciously allowing the vagina to distend with menstrual products may bring it closer to perineum or expand to create more tissue for pull-through reconstruction.
  - Local tissue flaps or nongenital grafts can be used to bridge the distance to the perineum.
  - Surgical benefits of this natural resource must be balanced against pain and the potential for retrograde menstrual flow and peritoneal irritation and deposits that could compromise future fertility.

PATIENT HISTORY AND PHYSICAL FINDINGS

- Patient age and autonomy as well as family values and motivations will impact discussions about goals and surgical options.
  - General discussions may have already involved the parent due to the professional relationship from infancy.
  - Once ready to discuss interventions, private discussions with the patient are essential but the parent must also be included for surgical discussions in minors.
- Patient readiness and goals for long-term results must be ascertained.
- Readiness to undertake daily vaginal dilations for indefinite period.
  - Goal may be simply unobstructed menstrual flow or use of tampon.
  - Understanding of need for progressive dilations, and potential additional procedures, thereafter for functional canal
- Readiness or anticipated timeline for intimate sexual contact.

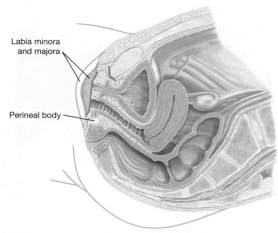

FIG 1 • Sagittal view of pelvic anatomy depicting relationship of urethra, vagina, and rectum in typical development.

Labia minora and majora

Perineal body

- Maturity level to be able to discuss with partner
- Desire for heterosexual penetrative intercourse vs nonpenetrative sexual activities
- Anticipated life events (graduation, prom, marriage) that could be complicated by surgical recovery or complications
- Conflicts between family values/guarantor values and patient's desire for surgery
- Anatomical and patient factors that may inform management
  - Quality of distal UG sinus/vaginal pouch and vulvar skin
    - Presence of functional uterus and proximal vaginal segment
    - Degree of estrogenization and maturation of tissues
  - Location of hair bearing tissues
  - Prior pelvic or genital surgery
  - Prior abdominal, urinary, or rectal surgical procedures
  - Prior chemotherapy or regional radiation therapy in setting of pelvic malignancy
  - Inflammatory bowel disease
  - Dermatologic conditions
  - Continence status for urine and stool
- Patient factors that may impact perioperative care and success
  - Resilience
  - Willingness to ask for and accept support in the perioperative period
  - Compliance
  - Lack of privacy to complete required care (college dorm)
- Timing relative to next expected menstrual period
- History of hypercoagulable state or bleeding diathesis
  - Increased surgical risk in terms of bleeding after deep dissection or from graft donor site
  - Increased risk of perioperative thromboembolic complications after pelvic surgery and prolonged bed rest
- Gastrointestinal or dermatologic conditions
- Continence status for urine and stool

IMAGING

- Imaging is not specifically required for surgical planning, although pelvic ultrasound or MRI is often obtained in the course of establishing certain diagnoses and individual anatomy.

NONOPERATIVE MANAGEMENT

- Daily serial dilation program can achieve a functional vaginal canal in properly selected and motivated candidates.
  - Preferred initial therapy in vaginal agenesis, CAIS, and other intersex/differences of sex development with a vaginal pit or pouch to guide positioning of dilator.
  - May be used to progressively dilate vaginal stenosis.
  - Tissue health and surgical scarring may limit success.
- Assess maturity and commitment to goals of program
  - Program is voluntary and timing should be dictated by patient.
- Ongoing office support is important to verify technique and to enhance success.
- Daily or twice daily dilation for 10 to 20 minutes
  - Goal is to achieve and maintain vaginal depth while increasing caliber.
  - Dilations may cease when consistently sexually active but may otherwise need maintenance dilations.

SURGICAL MANAGEMENT

- Vaginoplasty
  - The individual anatomic situation will dictate whether neovagina construction or augmentation of the caliber of the vaginal canal is required.
  - Skin or mucosal grafts, nongenital pedicled flaps (bowel), and local tissue flaps may be incorporated in the vaginal reconstruction.
  - Choice of donor tissue may be based upon surgeon experience, patient expectations and preferences, donor tissue availability, harvest site morbidity and scarring, and donor tissue properties.
- Monsplasty and labioplasty
  - Inferomedial rotation of mons tissue in bladder exstrophy or cloacal exstrophy
    - Addresses soft tissue asymmetry
    - Allows for concomitant midline abdominal scar revision, with or without umbilicoplasty if desired, and removal of non–hair-bearing midline tissue
    - Melds with labia majora to create greater privacy for the clitoris, labia minora, and vaginal vestibule
    - Supports concomitant revision of asymmetric or mobile labia minora tissue and/or vaginoplasty
  - Mobilization of tissue flaps to allow cosmetic and functional coverage of glans clitoris if overexposed after prior feminizing genitoplasty
- Reduction labioplasty
  - Excision or reconfiguration of physically bothersome hypertrophic labia minora

Preoperative Planning

- Review of prior operative notes in individuals with prior pelvic reconstructive procedures.
- A thorough pelvic examination with or without cystoscopy and vaginoscopy is often helpful in surgical planning and patient preparation and counseling.
  - Offer anesthesia or sedation due to the invasive and physically or emotionally uncomfortable nature of the examination.
- Schedule one or more detailed consultations with patient to review all surgical options in the context of individual anatomy and goals.

- Surgical scheduling with consideration of menstrual cycle
  - Avoid menses on day of surgery and for first postoperative week when vaginal stent or mold is used.
  - Continuous menstrual suppression may be considered perioperatively if cycles predictably unpredictable.
- Mechanical bowel preparation in patients with anorectal anomaly and in those who will have bowel vaginoplasty. Enema advised in other vaginal cases.

Positioning

- Sequential compression devices in place prior to positioning
- Position in dorsal lithotomy with all pressure points carefully padded (**FIG 2**).
  - Adequate padding on bed and/or protective barrier on sacral bony prominence, if present
  - Gentle support of atypical lumbosacral anatomy, if present
  - Attention to limited range of motion at hip or lower extremity with some diagnoses
- Standard to low dorsal lithotomy is preferred.
  - Minimizes stress on the spine and nerves in those with pre-existing pathology.

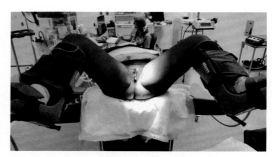

FIG 2 • Dorsal lithotomy positioning. This depicts the highest and widest positioning recommended. Position should accommodate either two surgeons between legs or one surgeon assisting patient's hip. Functional status and hip joint flexibility need to be considered for some diagnoses.

- Acute neurologic change may occur with more exaggerated or prolonged lithotomy.
  - Allows participation of cosurgeon from step stool at patient's hip.

TECHNIQUES

■ Augmentation of Caliber of Vaginal Canal: Vaginoplasty and Introitoplasty

- This technique is not neovagina or vaginal replacement but rather augmentation of the existing vaginal canal caliber or circumference (**TECH FIG 1**).
  - Introital, distal, or mid vaginal stenosis
  - Globally narrow but patent vaginal canal
  - Angulation of vaginal canal at introitus
    - Anteriorly positioned and narrow introitus relative to axis of vaginal canal after having undergone exstrophy repair techniques without deep mobilization of the urogenital complex
    - Laterally positioned and angulated introitus in vaginal duplication of cloacal exstrophy

- Remarkably increases vaginal caliber but cannot increase vaginal length due to presence of uterus.
  - Relevant to exstrophy where cervix may sit more distally even when well supported.

Enlargement of the Vaginal Canal Caliber

- Radial incisions made at 3:00 and 9:00 with electrocautery (**TECH FIG 2**).
  - Lateral location of incisions least likely to injure urethra, bladder base, or rectum.
  - Incisions sequentially deepened to expand vaginal caliber without compromising support.
  - Desired caliber for penetrative intercourse: two fingers, spread to 2.5 to 3 fingerbreadths.
- For tight stenosis or atresia or with anterior introitus/angulated canal, the authors prefer oral (buccal) mucosa free graft.

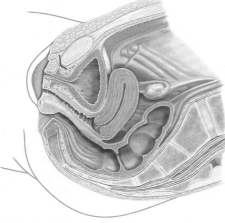

TECH FIG 1 • Narrow vaginal caliber can be augmented with graft techniques. The relationship between the posterior vaginal wall and rectum may be closer than natural relationship in setting of prior reconstruction.

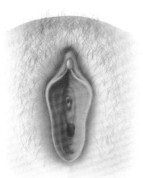 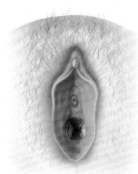

TECH FIG 2 • Perineal approach to augmentation procedures. Incisions at 3 and 9 o'clock minimize risk of injury to urethra and rectum, more of a concern in complex anomalies. The incisions are extended cranially into healthy proximal vagina so that even and adequate caliber established.

- For isolated introital stenosis, a local perineal skin flap can be utilized, alone or in combination with free graft, if it does not deform or compromise surrounding anatomy.

Resurfacing With Native Tissues: Buccal Mucosa

- Grafts are harvested from one or both cheeks, depending upon amount of substrate required.
- Graft is defatted and meshed by hand with strokes of scalpel. Alternatively, it may be intermittently temporarily folded and incised with fine scissors (**TECH FIG 3A**).
- Triangular defects will be created bilaterally by the radial incisions.

- The rectangular meshed buccal graft is cut obliquely into two triangles.
- 4-0 Vicryl suture is preplaced in apex of graft and advanced to apex of the triangular incision.
- The meshed graft is expanded to fill the defect and quilted into the dissected bed with resorbable suture (**TECH FIG 3B,C**). With the introitus and labia at rest, vagina appears normal, not gaping.
- Insert vaginal mold (**TECH FIG 3D**).
- An inflatable vaginal mold with central drainage port is not currently commercially available, but the concept elements are ideally applied to employed substitute.
  - Graft stability without undue pressure on urethra; sterile; impermeable; central drainage port for mucus and blood

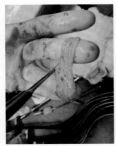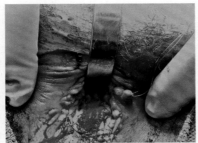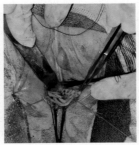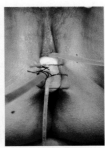

TECH FIG 3 • **A.** Harvested buccal tissue has been defatted and hand meshed to cover wider defect. For use in bilateral defects, it is divided obliquely into two triangular grafts to advance into defect. **B,C.** Two uses of buccal for augmentation procedures. **B.** Triangular grafts quilted in place bilaterally. Note that native vaginal mucosa remains along posterior wall. **C.** Young adult with deferred repair of urogenital sinus. The vagina was mobilized toward the perineum and spatulated. Buccal mucosa is being inset to bridge to gap and to improve introital caliber. **D.** Vaginal mold carefully inserted. Labia sutured across to prevent expulsion.

■ Neovagina Construction

Perineal Dissection

- Perineal dissection of rectovesical space to create adequate vaginal vault.
- In the expected region of a vaginal opening, there may be a short pouch of supple tissue or flat, firm granular tissue.
- Selection of skin incisions allows the vestibular tissue to be incorporated as local flaps to minimize risk of introital stenosis (**TECH FIG 4**).

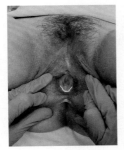

TECH FIG 4 • Vaginal agenesis. Incisions avoid infringing upon adjacent anatomy and can preserve tissue to advance into the neovagina. Tissue in this region is not uniformly good quality, however.

- After elevation of flaps and initial electrocautery, the remainder of the dissection occurs bluntly with judicious use of cautery.
  - Care is taken to maintain awareness of urinary tract and rectum during dissection.
- Desired caliber for penetrative intercourse: two fingers, spread to 2.5 to 3 fingerbreadths and at least 8 cm depth. Deep dissection will push peritoneum away but not enter it.

Graft Substrates and Techniques

- After the neovaginal bed has been dissected to allow adequate depth and caliber and a natural axis, the skin or mucosal graft is harvested and prepared.
- Historically, the McIndoe skin graft vaginoplasty was the preferred approach.
  - Harvest classically is a split-thickness graft from the buttocks, although full-thickness grafts have been described.
  - Graft is sewn over a vaginal mold with dermal side facing outward. The mold and form are inserted into the neovaginal cavity and held in place for 1 week to allow graft to take.
  - Contracture, lack of natural lubrication, and visible harvest site are the primary liabilities.

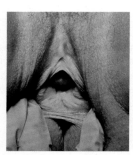

TECH FIG 5 • Healed buccal mucosa neovagina in case of vaginal agenesis. Note the pliable but not lax introitus and nice match to surrounding tissues.

- Oral (buccal) mucosa free graft is a newer concept for neovagina.
  - It has excellent take and histologic characteristics more similar to vaginal mucosa than skin[1] (**TECH FIG 5**).
  - Neovagina creation and more extensive defects will require maximal harvest from both cheeks.[2]
  - Graft is inset to line the cavity with interrupted resorbable sutures.
  - Vaginal mold carefully inserted and secured by sutures across labia.
  - Oral care: Chlorhexidine mouthwash and frequent cheek exercises to prevent harvest site contracture during secondary healing.
  - Strict bed rest with log rolling and HOB less than 30 degrees for 6 to 7 days with vaginal mold in place, along with Foley catheter.
- Peritoneal flap neovagina
  - Laparoscopic Davydov procedure[3] involves multiple peritoneal flaps mobilized and pulled through to the perineum to create a neovaginal scaffold.
    - Subsequent epithelialization by squamous metaplasia to have vaginal properties.
  - Single peritoneal flap modification[4] involves laparoscopically raising a 10 × 10 cm supravesical peritoneal flap, leaving an intact pedicle infraumbilically.

- The flap is pulled through to the perineum and tubularized over a mold.
- The apex of the neovagina is created laparoscopically with a purse-string suture.
- The pelvic peritoneum is run closed transversely.
- Stenting is required continually for 3 months until epithelialized, and then nightly until consistently having penetrative intercourse.

Pedicled Flap Techniques

Sigmoid Colon and Ileum

- Bowel vaginoplasty principles
  - Segment of small or large bowel is harvested on its mesentery and pulled through the dissected rectovesical space for anastomosis at the perineum.
- A 12- to 15-cm segment of sigmoid colon is isolated on a branch of the inferior mesenteric artery via open or laparoscopic abdominal approach. The distal most branches may be ligated to allow more mobility of the mesentery and sigmoid segment[5] (**TECH FIG 6A**).
- The segment is maintained isoperistaltic. The sigmoid is reconstituted.
- The segment is pulled through to the perineum and secured with interrupted anastomosis of resorbable sutures.
- The apex of the neovagina is oversewn in two layers and fixed to the sacral promontory to minimize prolapse.
- Monti principle
  - Described in small series, with limited follow-up, for sigmoid and ileum.
  - Bowel segment is isolated and opened and retubularized longitudinally.
    - Sigmoid Monti: An 8- to 10-cm segment of ileum is opened near anterior mesentery, such that mesentery forms a cap at apex. This configuration most favorable to allow vagina to reach perineum and to support apex of neovagina[6] (**TECH FIG 6B,C**).
    - Ileal Monti: 12-cm segment of ileum opened on antimesenteric border. Two segments may be combined end to end.[7]

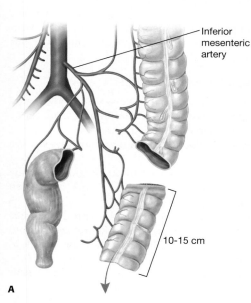

Inferior mesenteric artery

10-15 cm

A

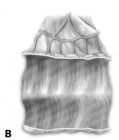

B

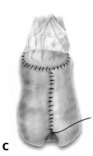

C

TECH FIG 6 • **A.** Harvest of sigmoid colon for vaginoplasty. Knowledge of vascular supply to colon is essential. Maintaining isoperistaltic orientation may support mucus efflux. Support of the apex minimizes global prolapse, but redundancy may also result in prolapse. **B.** In sigmoid Monti construction, the isolated 8- to 10-cm segment of sigmoid is unfurled to its longest by opening close to the mesenteric border. **C.** The sigmoid is then retubularized in the opposite plane to create the neovagina. The neovagina is then pulled down through the neovaginal bed created via perineal and abdominal dissection.

- Neovagina caliber based upon length of bowel segment harvested. Length of neovagina determined by circumference of bowel segment. Sigmoid has advantage in that regard.
- Advantages over nonreconfigured sigmoid or ileum are the length of segment required and the more mobile and less obtrusive mesentery.
- Postoperative stenting is recommended with ileal Monti to maintain caliber while the neovaginal cavity heals.[7] A dilation program then ensues.
- A petroleum jelly gauze roll splint may be left for 24 to 48 hours after sigmoid neovagina. Longer-term stenting is not required with sigmoid neovagina, likely due to bulk of the tissue and natural interior caliber, but dilation of the introitus may be advantageous to prevent stenosis.
- Both segments provide self-lubrication, but the mucus from colonic neovagina may be more problematic in terms of quantity and odor, particularly if redundant segment or introital stenosis.
- Prolapse is uncommon if the bowel segment is designed to limit redundancy and if well supported. Redundant tissue may be excised, and dilations are advisable while healing.
- Diversion colitis related to isolation of the colonic segment from the remainder of the GI tract may result in pain, bleeding, and discharge. Primary gastrointestinal conditions, including malignancy, may also afflict the segment.

Pudendal Thigh (Singapore) Flaps

- This is a fasciocutaneous axial sensate flap based on posterior labial vessels and terminal branches of the pudendal nerve[8,9] (**TECH FIG 7A,B**).
- Donor area usually has not been involved in previous urogenital and lower abdominal wall reconstructions.
- Donor site closes in a primary manner and hides parallel to the labia majora in the groin/leg sulcus.
- Does not need postoperative stenting or routine dilation.
- Sensation is from the local neural plexus.
- Vagina will be lined with epithelium. Desquamation leads to secretion of sebaceous material. When used to create a total neovagina, lubrication is required for penetrative sexual activity.
- Flap is designed lateral to the labia majora, raised distal to proximal including the deep fascia.
  - Rotation into an expanded vaginal canal or introitus occurs most naturally at the 4 and 8 o'clock positions (rather than 3 and 9 o'clock vaginal incisions) with minimal tension on the point of rotation (**TECH FIG 7C**).
  - Inset with resorbable suture.
  - Close donor in layers, also with resorbable suture material. No need for drains.
- For total vaginal reconstruction, bilateral flaps can be raised, 15 × 6 cm, and sewn to each other with epithelial side lining the tube, which becomes the neovaginal canal. The neovagina is then situated into the dissected space between bladder and rectum and suspended well to the most superior point to maintain length and prevent prolapse. Drainage is recommended in this situation.

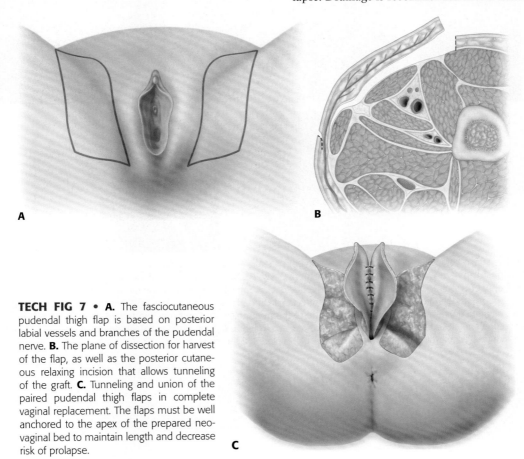

TECH FIG 7 • A. The fasciocutaneous pudendal thigh flap is based on posterior labial vessels and branches of the pudendal nerve. **B.** The plane of dissection for harvest of the flap, as well as the posterior cutaneous relaxing incision that allows tunneling of the graft. **C.** Tunneling and union of the paired pudendal thigh flaps in complete vaginal replacement. The flaps must be well anchored to the apex of the prepared neovaginal bed to maintain length and decrease risk of prolapse.

TECHNIQUES

■ Monsplasty and Labioplasty

- Surgeon must determine well in advance of planned procedure whether the mons tissue is adequate for rotational flaps or whether tissue expansion is required.
- Goals:
  - Remove midline shiny hairless skin, revising adjacent midline surgical scar
  - Rotate hair-bearing tissue to midline
  - Create a natural contour of mons and labia majora to allow the clitoris, labia minora and vaginal vestibule to enjoy less overt exposure.
    - Interestingly, the inferomedial rotation to cover the genitalia in females is opposite of the goal in males of evening up the pubic hairline and tissue while visually increasing penile stature through upward rotation of tissues.
- Pubic hair can be clipped but not shaved prior to marking the hair-bearing rotational flaps.
- If vaginoplasty will be performed as well, it will be completed prior to the monsplasty and labioplasty.
- Rotation flaps are marked with relaxing incisions (**TECH FIG 8A**). Midline scar excision and umbilicoplasty incisions are planned as well, if part of the requested procedure.

- The labia minora may require advancement or partial excision for improved cosmesis or patient comfort/hygiene (**TECH FIG 8B**).
  - Planning occurs along with the monsplasty but the actual labial work is easier to visualize prior to recreating the mons.
- A semilunar incision creates a non–hair-bearing skin flap just cranial to the labial complex. This is previously operated tissue (**TECH FIG 8C**).
  - Resultant flap will be turned down to become the underside of the mons-labial confluence and will form part of a hood for clitoral unit.
- The semilunar flap is turned down and rolled to deepen the "hood" or to line the anterior fusion of the labia majora and mons (**TECH FIG 8D**).
- The hair-bearing mons flaps are rotated toward the midline and sutured to each other in layers with resorbable sutures. The inferior or caudal edge of the flaps is sutured to the "hood"/ledge with resorbable suture (**TECH FIG 8E**).
  - Expanded flaps require postoperative drains for 4 to 6 days until the flap is well seated.

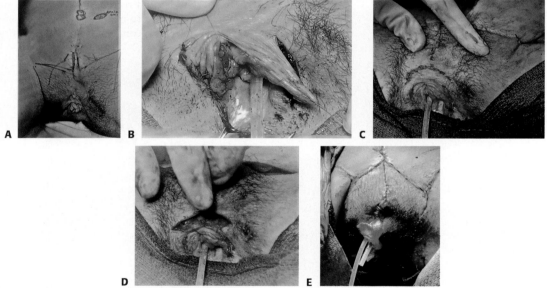

TECH FIG 8 • The surgical steps are depicted from two different patients. **A.** Exposed urethra and genital tissues to be better concealed with monsplasty. Rotational flaps are marked in preparation for monsplasty. **B.** Advancement of mobile or anteriorly mounded labia minora for improved concealment of clitoris and urethra after childhood repair of exstrophy. **C.** Semilunar incision is raised from previously operated midline hairless tissue. Tissue expanders have been removed and midline closure preplanned with staples. This hairless flap will be turned down to conceal the more intimate anatomy and to line the underside of the monsplasty. **D.** Semilunar flap turned down. Note that the flap has been trimmed in the midline and closed vertically to conceal the upper labia minora. **E.** Final appearance after monsplasty flaps rotated and approximated. Scar revision, umbilicoplasty and vaginoplasty were also completed in this patient.

■ Reduction Labioplasty

- ■ Goal is to restore comfort rather than to address cosmetic misgivings (**TECH FIG 9**). Reassurance regarding wide spectrum of "normal" is central.
- ■ Defer any intervention until adequate time for adjustments has occurred, as well as development one or more years beyond menses. Potential to "regrow" bulk if development incomplete.
- ■ For whichever is used of the three techniques described below, adhere to the following:
  - ■ Place traction sutures in the tips of the labia minora to gauge tissue to be excised.
  - ■ Mark inner and outer surface of labia minora.
  - ■ Mark both sides for symmetry prior to revising either labia.
  - ■ Perform a two-layer closure.

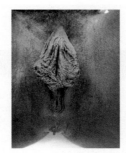

TECH FIG 9 • Marked, physically bothersome hypertrophy of the labia minora is seen with the labia at rest.

Simple Excision and Closure

- ■ This method offers easiest recovery and least chance to redevelop bulk. There is no potential for flap dehiscence.
  - ■ Greater risk of exposing clitoris or creating irregularity anteriorly, due to more difficulty blending into the naturally folded clitoral hood contour (**TECH FIG 10A**).
- ■ Skin is incised sharply and dartos divided with electrocautery.
- ■ Dartos is run longitudinally with resorbable suture.
- ■ Skin is also closed with continuous resorbable suture.
- ■ Suture line is anterior and may result in more friction during healing but this is not generally symptomatic (**TECH FIG 10B,C**).

Wedge Excision With Advancement

- ■ This method is more prone to postoperative edema and discomfort, more prone to redevelop bulk, and more prone to dehiscence without layered closure.
- ■ Wedge excision and advancement is a full-thickness resection of the central portion of the hypertrophied labia.
- ■ The apex of the flap will advance to the bottom of the wedge incision (**TECH FIG 11A**).
- ■ First layer closure with running resorbable suture begins in corner of wedge incision, gradually anchoring the flap.
- ■ Skin closure is hidden on lateral and medial surfaces of the labia minora. Longer lasting resorbable suture is used on the cutaneous layer at the apex of the flap (**TECH FIG 11B,C**).

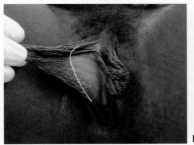
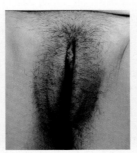
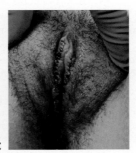

TECH FIG 10 • **A.** Retracted labia marked for simple excision. Care must be taken to taper onto the clitoral hood to avoid cranial irregularity and to avoid exposing glans clitoris. **B.** Labia at rest after simple excision. **C.** Immediate postoperative appearance with labia spread. The anterior suture line is not typically irritating, as it is concealed by the labia majora.

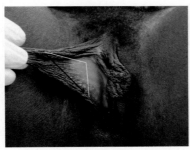
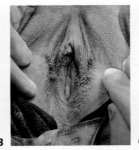
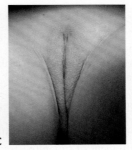

TECH FIG 11 • **A.** Retracted labia marked for wedge resection and advancement. The running closure of the dartos begins in the apex and progresses down to the tip of the flap. Longer lasting resorbable sutures are recommended at the tip. **B.** Postoperative appearance in a different patient. Note that the suture line is anterior with simple excision but here is hidden in the inner and outer labial surfaces. **C.** The appearance is similar at rest to simple excision.

Hybrid Approach

- Useful in cases in which the labia minora are globally enlarged with posterior insertion.
- Offers benefits of hidden suture line and natural blending with clitoral hood, with a less extensive flap recession than the wedge excision (**TECH FIG 12**).
- Rationale for two-layer closure, regardless of technique:
  - Finlike rather than flat contour of labia
  - Hemostasis, decreased risk of hematoma. Insurance against dehiscence in advancement cases.

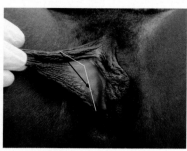

TECH FIG 12 • Retracted labia marked for hybrid excision with partial advancement and partial simple closure. Again, the running closure of the dartos begins in the apex and progresses down to the tip of the flap. In this approach, the flap is shorter so the posterior aspect of the closure will be simple two-layer closure.

PEARLS AND PITFALLS

Patient readiness	■ Older teens may profess readiness for vaginal reconstruction with immediate goal of ease of tampon use and desire to prepare for future sexual activity, but they may primarily desire to "get it over with." ■ Unless imminently prepared for sexual activity and willing to accept support, they may lack the emotional maturity for the procedure and to adhere to a postoperative dilation program.
Operative preparation	■ A strong understanding of pelvic anatomy and potential congenital or postsurgical variations is relevant when dissecting space for neovagina or widening the vaginal canal. ■ Injury to the urethra, bladder, or rectum significantly changes the operative experience and potentially long-term functionality.
Hemostasis	■ Address vault bleeding with packing rather than blind coagulation in deep cavity. ■ Remain alert to adjacent pelvic structures.
Progression of postoperative therapies	■ Even with a highly motivated and mature patient, frequent office visits are recommended early postoperatively. ■ Provider reinforces or redirects patient regarding adequacy of axis and depth of daily use of dilators.

Patient selection for reduction labioplasty	■ Reduction of prominent labia minora for cosmetic purposes is strongly discouraged.
	■ Reassure about normal variations in prominence of labia minora in girls and women.
	■ For physical bother due to bulky tissue and friction/irritation from clothing:
	  ■ Instruct in trial of manually tucking redundant tissue in after bathing and toileting.
	  ■ Instruct in application of bland ointment nightly to manage irritation. Ointment in daytime may increase bother.
	■ Defer surgical management until estrogenization and maturation of tissues is secure.
	  ■ Surprising "regrowth" of tissues may occur if maturation in early evolution.

Labioplasty and perineal care	■ Dehiscence of labial flaps can result in prolonged healing, unfavorable cosmetic result, or asymmetry.
	  ■ Two-layer closure of the labioplasty, particularly at the tip of the labia, reduces risk of separation.
	  ■ Moist perineal environment and oral or topical antibiotic use increase risk of candidal infection and healing concerns. Nystatin powder to groin creases may be protective.

POSTOPERATIVE CARE

- Vaginal packing and vaginal stents/molds
  - Inflatable and solid forms have been utilized. None currently commercially available.
  - Not required for pudendal thigh flaps.
  - Required for approximately 7 days for graft take with skin or oral mucosa.
  - Required all day and night for 3 months in peritoneal flaps due to requirement of squamous metaplasia.
- Mouth care after buccal mucosa harvest
  - Donor site heals by secondary intention and forms fibrinoid plaque within 2 days.

  - Chlorhexidine mouthwash rinses several times daily.
  - Mouth exercises minimize likelihood of function-limiting donor contraction. Open wide. Puff check. Mindful manual massage of site by tongue.
- Home dilation program: as described above for each technique. Frequent visits to reinforce technique and improve compliance.
- Activity restrictions
  - Avoid lifting, straddle stance or activity, squatting, or kneeling with perineal pressure for 3 to 4 weeks. Driving restrictions based upon approach.
  - No tampon use or sexual activity until adequate healing determined by surgeon.

OUTCOMES

- A paucity of data exists regarding objective short- and long-term surgical outcomes as well as validated patient-reported outcomes.
  - Female Sexual Function Inventory scores compared favorably to controls in large peritoneal flap series.[4]
  - Long-term results after sigmoid vaginoplasty report high level of success and patient satisfaction.[5,10]
    - However, decreased sexual function with abnormal depression indices may occur highlighting importance of pre- and postoperative counseling and support.[11]
  - Tissue quality and match and adequacy of vaginal caliber are very good after buccal mucosa vaginoplasty.[1,2]
- Sexual activity is allowed by successful maintenance dilations. If pregnancy is achieved, consultation with maternal fetal medicine and caesarean delivery is recommended in neovagina, regardless of type.

COMPLICATIONS

- Injury to surrounding structures: urethra, bladder base/ureter, or rectum may occur with dissection of the neovaginal cavity
- Vaginal contracture or stricture
- Introital stenosis
- Prolapse of pedicled tissues
- Bothersome discharge (sigmoid)
- Secondary changes within donor substrate (eg, chronic inflammation, inflammatory bowel, malignancy)
- Unsatisfactory cosmetic or functional result

REFERENCES

1. DaJusta D, Granberg C, Baker LA. Vaginoplasty with autologous buccal mucosa graft: a close histologic match. *J Urol.* 2011;185:e103.
2. Nambiar A, Arevalo MK, Grimsby G, et al. *Autologous buccal mucosa vaginoplasty in 22 patients with congenital adrenal hyperplasia.* Presented at the Pediatric Urology Fall Congress, Montreal, Canada, September 2017.
3. Fedele L, Frontino G, Ciappina N, et al. Creation of a neovagina by Davydov's laparoscopic modified technique in patients with Rokitansky syndrome. *Am J Obstet Gynecol.* 2010;202:33.e1-33.e6.
4. Zhao X, Ma J, Wang Y, et al. Laparoscopic vaginoplasty using a single peritoneal flap: 10 years of experience in the creation of neovagina inpatients with Mayer-Rokitansky-Kuster-Hauser syndrome. *Fertil Steril.* 2015;104:241-247.
5. Nowier A, Esmat M, Hamza RT. Surgical and functional outcomes of sigmoid vaginoplasty among patients with variants of disorders of sex development. *Int Braz J Urol.* 2012;38:380-388.
6. Garcia-Roig M, Castellan M, Gonzalez J, et al. Sigmoid vaginoplasty with a modified single Monti tube: a pediatric case series. *J Urol.* 2014;191:1537-1542.
7. Trombetta C, Liguoria G, Siracusano S, et al. Transverse retubularized ileal vaginoplasty: a new application of the Monti principle—preliminary report. *Eur Urol.* 2005;48:1018-1024.
8. Joseph VT. Pudendal-thigh flap vaginoplasty in the reconstruction of genital anomalies. *J Pediatr Surg.* 1997;32:62-65.
9. Monstrey S, Blondeel P, VanLanduyt K, et al. The versatility of the pudendal thigh flap used as an island flap. *Plast Reconstr Surg.* 2001;107:719-725.
10. Kim SK, Park JW, Lim KR, Lee KC. Is rectosigmoid vaginoplasty still useful? *Arch Plast Surg.* 2017;44:48-52.
11. Djordjevic M, Bizic M, Kojovic V, et al. Sigmoid vaginoplasty and its impact on psychosocial and sexual life in patients with vaginal agenesis. *J Urol.* 2016;195:e791.

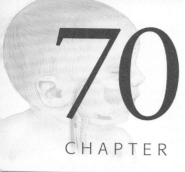

70

CHAPTER

Ambiguous Genitalia

Deborah L. Jacobson and Elizabeth B. Yerkes

DEFINITION

- Individuals born with ambiguous genitalia have external genitalia that are not fully typical male or female in appearance. Others have developmental differences that are not externally apparent but may impact future function or well-being. These groups have some degree of discordance between genetic, gonadal, and phenotypic sexual characteristics.
- Medical nomenclature used over the decades was well intentioned but has been viewed as pejorative. Accordingly, nomenclature with multiple subterminologies has evolved with the goal of correcting this situation.
  - Hermaphroditism, pseudohermaphroditism, intersex state/disorder, and disorders of sex development (DSD) have been used to describe the state of having ambiguous or nontypical genitalia with or without chromosomal or gonadal anomaly.
  - Even the most recent nomenclature, which originated from a consensus of experts, affected individuals, and advocates, is not uniformly accepted by the community. "Disorder" is not widely embraced as a desired description.
- Whereas genital ambiguity and differences of sex development have historically been considered pathologic and in need of surgical correction, contemporary viewpoints acknowledge many phenotypic variations on the continuum of human genital development.
- The authors understand that surgical reconstruction of ambiguous genitalia is a controversial topic and do not presuppose that surgical intervention is necessary for, or would be preferred by, any given individual.
- This chapter will cover the technical aspects of genital reconstruction; however, surgical management should only be undertaken after extensive counseling and shared decision-making. Longitudinal multidisciplinary care for the individual and family is strongly encouraged.
- This chapter will focus on feminizing genital procedures and the diagnoses that could involve decision-making for these types of procedures.

ANATOMY

- Clitoris
  - The corpora cavernosa (erectile bodies) of the clitoris originate proximally as paired crura, swell medially to form the clitoral bulbs, and unite distally.
  - The paired cavernosa support a glans covered by a prepuce of labia minora. MRI imaging studies performed by O'Connell et al demonstrate that the glans lies caudal to the corporal bodies, leading to a natural hairpin curve.[1]

- Autonomic input is via the paired cavernous nerves, which originate from the vaginal plexus at the 10 and 2 o'clock positions along the vagina and course dorsally along the proximal urethra.[2] The nerves travel with the cavernous arteries and enter the clitoral bodies under the pubic arch.
- Somatic supply is via the paired dorsal nerves of the clitoris, which originate from the pudendal nerves, run dorsolaterally along the crura and ischiopubic rami at approximately the 11 and 1 o'clock positions, and enter the glans at the corona. The nerves branch, fanning out along the clitoral bodies dorsally and laterally. Nerves are absent in the dorsal midline and deficient ventrally.
- The cavernous arteries originate from the internal pudendal artery, travel with the cavernous nerves, and enter the clitoral body under the pubic arch. Dissection between the crura at the pubic arch should be avoided.
- Variations from typical clitoral anatomy should be expected in patients with virilization of female genital tissue.
- Labia
  - The labia majora embryologically correspond to the male scrotum. They are separated by the vulvar cleft, which contains the labia minora and clitoris. Together the structures conceal the vestibule.
  - The labia minora and urethral plate correspond to the male anterior urethra. The labia join superiorly to frame the glans clitoris as the clitoral hood.
- Vagina
  - The vagina consists of a rugated mucous membrane fixed to a bilayered muscular invagination. It is suspended from the levator ani ventrally, the rectovaginal septum dorsally, and the cervix apically.
  - Arterial supply is via uterine, vaginal, and internal pudendal branches coursing along the anterolateral surface of the vagina.
  - Innervation originates anterolaterally via autonomic branches of the uterovaginal plexus and somatic branches of the pudendal nerve.
  - The ureters pass adjacent to the lateral margins of the vagina and insert into the base of the urinary bladder.

PATHOGENESIS

- Cloacal development
  - The cloacal membrane folds with differential embryonic growth beginning in week 4, and the cloaca partitioned into anterior (urogenital sinus—UG sinus) and posterior (hindgut) compartments with the descent of the urorectal septum.

- Disruption of normal cloacal development can lead to persistent cloaca or UG sinus anomalies.
- Development of the external genitalia
  - Fetal androgenization leads to elongation of the genital tubercle, fusion of the urethral folds, and fusion of the labioscrotal folds.
- Development of the abdominal wall
  - Failure of mesodermal ingrowth or premature rupture of the cloacal membrane leads to bladder or cloacal exstrophy.
- Development of the UG sinus
  - Caudal paramesonephric (Müllerian) duct deficiencies may lead to agenesis of the proximal vagina and variable anatomy of the uterus/fallopian tubes (Mayer-Rokitansky-Küster-Hauser syndrome).
  - Lateral paramesonephric (Müllerian) fusion anomalies may lead to uterus didelphys, bicornuate uterus, or unicornuate uterus.
  - Deficiency of the distal UG sinus may lead to vaginal atresia.
  - Incomplete vaginal canalization may lead to an imperforate hymen or transverse vaginal septum.

NATURAL HISTORY

- The natural history of an individual in this population, or the population as a whole, is not entirely known.
- For androgenized individuals, it is unclear what the prenatal hormonal milieu (both in terms of absolute androgen levels and the response of developing genital/nervous tissues) portends for future gender identity or sexuality.
- For virilized females (such as patients with congenital adrenal hyperplasia) in whom medical control is irregular, continued irreversible changes may occur in the genital tissues.
- The psychosocial outcomes of early vs delayed surgery remain unclear, as does the definition and likelihood of surgical success.

PATIENT HISTORY AND PHYSICAL FINDINGS

- Antenatal course: complications, history of prematurity, and other anomalies
- Evidence of maternal exposure to endogenous or exogenous androgen
  - Severe acne, abnormal hair growth, clitoral enlargement, or Cushingoid appearance
  - Drugs, virilizing tumors, or adrenal disorders
- Family history:
  - Known chromosomal anomalies
  - Fetal/neonatal demise
  - Genital ambiguity or urologic anomalies
  - Infertility or consanguinity
- Physical examination
  - General: overall appearance, dysmorphic features, and general infant well-being
  - Spine: gross deformity or neurocutaneous marks
    - Anomalous findings may indicate genetic syndromes or fetal exposures.
    - Tethered cord or occult spinal cord anomalies are common with select diagnoses.
  - Abdomen: marked distention, hernias, suprapubic masses, and wall abnormalities

- May indicate bladder outlet obstruction, hydrometrocolpos, or urinary ascites
- Perineum
  - Labioscrotal folds: prominence, rugation, pigmentation, and presence of gonads
  - Clitorophallic structure: dorsal stretched length, glans width, and corporal consistency
  - Perineal orifices: number, location, and patency
  - Gonads: presence by palpation, location, and consistency
    - Palpable gonadal tissue suggests presence of at least some ipsilateral testicular tissue

IMAGING AND SPECIALIZED EXAMINATION

- Modalities are employed selectively based upon clinical findings and the active differential diagnosis.
- Ultrasonography: Evaluation of the adrenals, kidneys, ureters, bladder, Müllerian structures, and gonads
  - Dilation of genital ducts or duplications or unclear anatomy may lead to additional radiographic or operative investigations.
- Genitography: Delineation of internal genitourinary anatomy
  - A Foley catheter or occlusive nipple is used to occlude the UG sinus orifice.
  - Retrograde administration of contrast material defines the proximal anatomy including sinus length and level of confluence.
  - The vaginal confluence may be missed if the system is not well distended.
- Voiding cystourethrography (VCUG)
  - The catheter may be advanced for VCUG after genitogram if indicated or if the sinus is not opacified. Vesicoureteral reflux and bladder anatomy is assessed during filling, at bladder capacity, during voiding, and after voiding is complete.
  - VCUG alone may not opacify the vagina, so it is less useful study for assessing the UG sinus.
- Endoscopy: Direct visualization of patient anatomy
  - Because general anesthesia is required, endoscopy may be performed at the time of definitive reconstruction unless additional anatomic evaluation is required for surgical decision-making.
- MRI: Delineation of pelvic anatomy and associated spinal anomalies
  - MRI often requires anesthesia in young children and would therefore be considered when other imaging studies are inconclusive.
- Diagnostic laparoscopy: very selectively used in infancy if additional information required
  - Laparoscopy is utilized to clarify internal anatomy and gonadal characteristics.
  - Gonadal biopsy may be necessary in select cases.

DIFFERENTIAL DIAGNOSIS

This list includes only conditions in which patients could potentially be candidates for feminizing procedures.

- Differences in gonadal differentiation
  - Pure gonadal dysgenesis
  - Mixed gonadal dysgenesis
  - Ovotesticular DSD (previously "true hermaphroditism")
- Differences in androgenization
  - Adrenal sources

- Congenital adrenal hyperplasia (in 46 XX patients)
- 21-Hydroxylase deficiency
- 11β-Hydroxylase deficiency
- 3β-Hydroxysteroid dehydrogenase deficiency
- 17β-Hydroxysteroid dehydrogenase deficiency (late virilization in 46 XY phenotypic female)
- Androgen-secreting tumor
- Maternal sources
  - Drugs
  - Androgen-secreting tumor
  - Placental sources
- Placental aromatase deficiency
- Androgen receptor dysfunction
  - Variations in activity of androgen receptor in various tissues (46 XY patients)
  - Complete androgen insensitivity syndrome (external genitalia phenotypically female, lacking Müllerian structures due to intact MIS)
  - Partial androgen insensitivity (diverse external phenotype, degree of virilization at puberty and innate gender identity not predictable)
- Differences in embryonic development
  - Persistent cloaca
  - Exstrophy-epispadias and cloacal exstrophy
  - Müllerian anomalies
    - Müllerian agenesis (Mayer-Rokitansky-Küster-Hauser syndrome)
    - Vaginal atresia
    - Fusion anomalies
    - Vaginal duplication
    - Uterine duplication
    - Vaginal septum variations
    - Urogenital sinus anomalies
      - High vaginal confluence
      - Low vaginal confluence

NONOPERATIVE MANAGEMENT

- Create a multidisciplinary team incorporating experienced pediatric urologists/pediatric surgeons/pediatric gynecologists, endocrinologists, psychiatrists/psychologists, geneticists, and nurses/social support members to work with the parents and child to guide patient care. Consider formal ethics consultations when appropriate.
  - There is a broad spectrum of "normal" female external genitalia. Referring providers, parents, and patients may be reassured by education on range of "normal." Appearance and future functionality are important to consider in the pediatric patient if surgery is requested.
  - The timing and indications for feminizing genital reconstruction are currently controversial, and there may be long-term consequences of both action and inaction in this arena.
  - Performing feminizing surgery in prepubertal children precludes autonomous self-determination in surgical decision-making and may lead to regret.
- Consider the psychosocial consequences of genital ambiguity, and provide appropriate counseling for patient and parent.
  - Patients deserve long-term psychological support, with or without surgical intervention.
  - Extended support networks may be found both within the hospital and in the patient's own community.

- Discuss patient reproductive potential, optimizing patient sexual development and fertility when possible. Administration of androgens or estrogens may be recommended in longer term, depending on the underlying anatomy and function.
- Consider the potential for gonadal malignancy, which varies significantly with gonadal histology and patient pathophysiology. Whenever possible, gonadal preservation should be considered.

SURGICAL MANAGEMENT
Preoperative Planning

- Diagnostic laboratory evaluation may include karyotype, serum electrolytes, 17-hydroxyprogesterone, testosterone, luteinizing hormone, and follicle-stimulating hormone levels. Additional adrenal and sex hormone testing is used more selectively but is essential to make a diagnosis in some cases.
- A thorough examination under anesthesia should be completed, including inspection of external genitalia, palpation for gonads, cystoscopy, vaginoscopy (if applicable), and genitography.
- Consider the need for gonadal biopsy or gonadectomy at the time of intervention, along with possible gonad cryopreservation.
- Patients undergoing vaginoplasty require bowel preparation (enema vs polyethylene glycol solution) prior to surgical intervention.

Positioning

- Isolated genitoplasty with or without repair of a low UG sinus is generally performed in frog-leg (infants, young children) or dorsal lithotomy (older patients) position with padding of all pressure points.
- For reconstruction of a high UG sinus, most patients will require both prone and supine positioning, so total lower body preparation is utilized. This preparation may be advantageous in infants and young children for sterility of the field, whether high or low confluence.
  - Ensure there are no IVs in lower extremities.
  - A single-shot caudal block is reasonable in eligible patients, but a continuous caudal catheter is not utilized intraoperatively.
  - After endoscopy and catheter placement, keep the catheters sterile and move the patient up the table for second prep. Prep the lower body circumferentially from the xiphoid to the toes.
  - Place feet and legs in a stockinette.
  - Drape to allow for lower body repositioning from supine to prone within the drape (**FIG 1**).
  - Position the patient with stacked towels under the pelvis. Initial prone vs supine positioning will depend upon the planned procedures.

Approach

- Primary components of the feminizing genitoplasty include the following:
  - Clitoral degloving
  - Elevation of the urethral plate and mobilization of the common UG sinus
  - Clitoral reduction
  - Urogenital sinus reconstruction and vaginoplasty
  - Creation of a clitoral hood and labioplasty

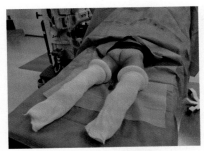

FIG 1 • Prone view of circumferential body preparation from the xyphoid to the toes. The child is toweled out and "passed through" a drape to allow transitions from supine to prone within the drape. The hips will be elevated on stacked towels.

- Several clitoral reduction techniques are utilized in contemporary feminizing genitoplasty.
  - Each is performed with attention to clitoral nerve sparing.
- The timing of reconstruction elements is controversial.
  - "Early" single-stage reconstruction of the genitalia and UG sinus is performed with the goal of no additional procedures and no memory of the recovery. Additionally, the excess UG sinus tissue and genital skin can be redistributed as needed if the procedure is completed in a single stage. Despite these potential advantages, the smaller caliber of the infant vagina may increase the risk of vaginal stenosis and the likelihood of secondary procedures. Routine postoperative vaginal dilations are not recommended in this age group.
  - "Late" reconstruction preserves autonomous self-determination and allows the full advantage of virgin planes and tissues.
    - There may be limited options for positioning older patients.
    - Vaginal dilations will be required postoperatively, whether by medical grade dilators or sexual activity, so emotional maturity and commitment to outcomes are essential.
  - A staged reconstruction, by deferring either genitoplasty or vaginoplasty, precommits to two operative events and limits the redistribution of healthy tissues. The second stage may involve previously operated tissues.
- The operative approach varies based on:
  - The surgical components to be included
  - The level of vaginal confluence in the UG sinus ("high" vs "low")
  - The degree of virilization

Feminizing Genitoplasty: Examination

- If repair of the UG sinus (urethroplasty and vaginoplasty) will occur:
  - Examination under anesthesia and endoscopy is performed in the dorsal lithotomy position to define UG sinus anatomy and denote the relative positions of the urethra and vagina.
  - A Fogarty catheter is inserted into the vagina and clamped. A Foley catheter is inserted into the bladder and periodically drained.
- Alternatively, a Councill tip Foley catheter may be introduced into the vagina over a wire after emptying the bladder. Once the confluence of urethra and vagina is identified surgically, the catheter is redirected to the bladder.
- A sponge may be placed into the rectum to allow for intraoperative palpation of the anterior rectal wall.
- If repair of the UG sinus will *not* occur:
  - Examination under anesthesia is performed.
  - A Foley catheter is inserted into the bladder and periodically drained.

Contemporary Nerve Sparing Clitoral Degloving

- Blunt lysis of adhesions between the glans clitoris and inner prepuce is performed.
- A retraction suture is placed through the dorsal midline of the glans (**TECH FIG 1A**).
- The skin is retracted to expose the inner prepuce. A dorsal degloving incision is made more proximally than a standard circumcising incision to preserve preputial tissue for glans coverage as the inner layer of the clitoral hood (**TECH FIG 1B**).
- Placement of the ventral degloving incision varies with the degree of virilization and intended procedure.
- When the UG sinus meatus is found on the glans clitoris, the ventral degloving incision is immediately beneath the corona.
- When the UG sinus meatus is located proximal to the glans clitoris, the ventral degloving incision begins immediately proximal to the orifice and extends distally to flank the urethral plate (**TECH FIG 1C**).
- The clitoris is sharply degloved to the base, preserving the dartos with the skin and leaving Buck fascia and the underlying neurovascular bundle undisturbed (**TECH FIG 1D**).
  - The suspensory ligament will be encountered dorsally and should be left in situ proximally to support the proximal clitoral body and the glans after clitoral reduction.

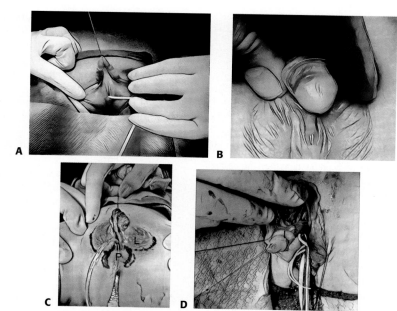

TECH FIG 1 • A. A traction suture placed through the dorsum of the glans clitoris facilitates visualization of the urethral plate. **B.** The clitoral degloving incision is more proximal than is typical for circumcision to allow for creation of the inner layer of a clitoral hood. The *blue line* delineates the typical circumcising incision, and the *green line* delineates the preferred degloving incision. **C.** When the urethra is proximal, the ventral degloving incision flanks the urethral plate. A posteriorly based omega-shaped perineal flap is created on the perineum at the time of the dorsal and ventral degloving incisions. The labia majora will ultimately be moved posteriorly to flank the perineal flap after it has been advanced into the vagina. "P" denotes a posteriorly based flap and "L" denotes the labia majora. **D.** Preservation of the paired dorsal neurovascular bundles beneath Buck fascia. "I" represents the inner prepuce, which becomes the inner layer of the clitoral hood. The dorsal overlaid lines represent the neurovascular tissue.

Elevation of the Urethral Plate and Mobilization of the Common UG Sinus

- Terminology: If the orifice of the UG sinus is on the clitoral body, a "urethral plate" consisting of a mucosal strip and its underlying spongiosum extends along the ventral clitoral body from the UG sinus orifice to the glans. "UG sinus" refers to the intact common channel.
- The urethral plate/common UG sinus is elevated off the ventrum of the clitoral body, leaving the tunica albuginea intact.
- The point of distal division varies based on the degree of virilization and whether reconstruction of the UG sinus is planned.
  - If UG sinus reconstruction is planned, the urethral plate or common UG sinus is divided along the distal clitoral body and fully mobilized (**TECH FIG 2**). If the UG sinus orifice is in the glans, the UG sinus is transected distally rather than dissected out of the glans.

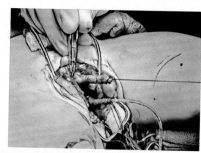

TECH FIG 2 • The prepuce is fully mobilized away from the clitoral body. Note that the inner layer of the clitoral hood is partially covering the glans in this photograph. The UG sinus is also mobilized. A catheter is in place, and multiple traction sutures assist with mobilization.

  - If UG sinus reconstruction is deferred, the urethral plate is elevated and ultimately partially resected to allow recession of the glans.

Clitoral Reduction

- Historical feminizing genitoplasty procedures included clitorectomy and clitoral recession procedures, each of which resulted in dysfunction. Contemporary approaches emphasize both cosmesis and function. The dorsal neurovascular tissue is preserved in each approach.

- Conservation of clitoral tissue and its neural innervation is of paramount importance for the preservation of genital sensitivity.[3]
- Two main techniques allow debulking of the hypertrophied corpora cavernosa with preservation of the glans clitoris on its neurovascular pedicle.

- In both techniques, Buck fascia is incised ventrally, exposing the tunica albuginea.
- In the description coined nerve-sparing ventral clitoroplasty (NSVC),[3] the dorsal neurovascular bundle is elevated off the tunica albuginea along the length of the clitoral body and left in continuity with the glans (**TECH FIG 3A**). Use of papaverine minimizes vascular spasm that may compromise the glans clitoris.
  - The erectile bodies are dismembered from the glans and transected 1.5 to 2 cm from the bifurcation.
  - The tunica albuginea is oversewn to allow for clitoral erection.
  - The glans is reseated with care to avoid kinking of the neurovascular bundle.
  - Glans support and proximal engorgement are afforded.
- The alternative nerve-sparing approach, as preferred by the authors, differs in that the dorsal tunica albuginea is preserved along with the neurovascular bundle (**TECH FIG 3B**).
  - The intact tunica albuginea protects the neurovascular tissue without adding problematic bulk.
  - Parallel incisions are created along the ventrum of the clitoral body and the erectile tissue.

- The erectile tissue is bluntly dissected and ligated proximally, preserving the shell of tunica albuginea dorsally and laterally.
- The glans is approximated to the corporal stump. The intact dorsal tissue gently bows into the subcutaneous tissue[4] (**TECH FIG 3C**).
- Corporal-sparing clitoroplasty has been proposed as a means of preserving the corporal bodies to allow for potential reversal of feminizing procedures and phalloplasty in the future.[5]
  - After the clitoris is degloved, the glans and neurovascular tissue are elevated off the clitoral body as a unit.
  - The plane between the corpora is sharply dissected, allowing separation of the hemicorpora.
  - The tunica albuginea of each hemicorpora is oversewn with absorbable sutures to create independent bodies.
  - The hemicorpora are now rotated inferolaterally into dartos pouches fashioned within the labia majora.
- The glans clitoris is rarely reduced in size. Concealment can be accomplished without glans reduction.
- If reduction is deemed necessary, wedge resection from the ventrum is favored. Innervation is denser dorsally.[6]

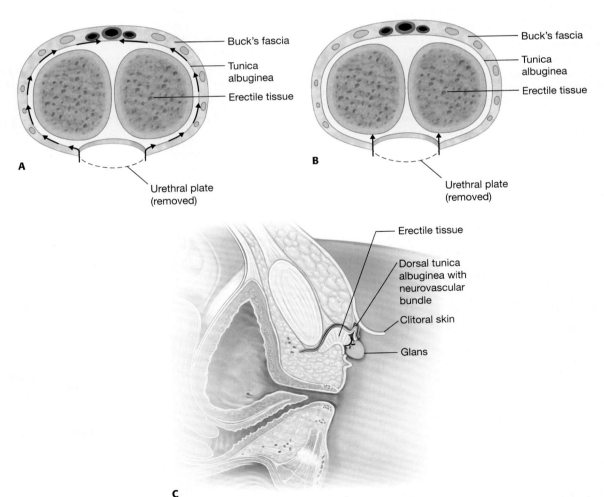

A. Buck's fascia
Tunica albuginea
Erectile tissue
Urethral plate (removed)

B. Buck's fascia
Tunica albuginea
Erectile tissue
Urethral plate (removed)

C. Erectile tissue
Dorsal tunica albuginea with neurovascular bundle
Clitoral skin
Glans

TECH FIG 3 • **A.** Buck fascia and the neurovascular tissue are mobilized off the clitoral bodies and preserved. Full-thickness resection of the clitoral bodies is performed. **B.** Dissection proceeds ventrally into the corpora. Spongy erectile tissue is excised and ligated proximally, but the shell of tunica albuginea and the neurovascular tissue are both preserved. **C.** Sagittal view of the glans clitoris seated on debulked clitoral bodies. Note that the neurovascular tissue is preserved and not kinked.

◼ Urogenital Sinus Reconstruction and Vaginoplasty

Creation of a Perineal Flap

- If UG sinus mobilization is planned for urethroplasty and vaginoplasty, a posteriorly based omega-shaped perineal flap is created on the perineum at the time of the dorsal and ventral degloving incisions (see **TECH FIG 1C**).
- Raising a perineal flap exposes the bulbar portion of the UG sinus and allows dissection between the UG sinus and rectum.
- The flap will ultimately be advanced into the vagina to increase the distal vaginal caliber. Advancing the flap reduces the risk of stenosis.
- Flap vaginoplasty without partial mobilization of the UG sinus enlarges the UG sinus, but the urethral meatus remains recessed, or hypospadiac.
- Overzealous advancement of the perineal flap may result in dehiscence, ischemia, or an unnatural slope of the perineal body. Additionally, this tissue will typically be hair-bearing and lacks mucosal properties.

Total and Partial Urogenital Mobilization (TUM and PUM) (**TECH FIG 4A**)

- Mobilization of the common UG sinus brings the genitourinary complex toward the perineum,[7,8] facilitating either flap vaginoplasty or pull-through vaginoplasty.
- Multiple stay sutures are placed around the common UG sinus orifice to facilitate a traumatic retraction. The common UG sinus is dissected as a unit proximally, including partial dissection under the pubis (**TECH FIG 4B**).

- The posterior perineal attachments are sharply divided, dropping the rectum away from the bulbar section of the UG sinus. As posterior dissection continues, the peritoneum is bluntly pushed away from the posterior wall of the UG sinus.
- If this degree of anterior and posterior mobilization is not sufficient to access the confluence, additional dissection occurs anteriorly, dividing the pubourethral ligament. This step differentiates PUM from TUM.[8] TUM bears the potential risk of disturbing pelvic support and continence mechanisms.
- The sinus is further mobilized toward the perineum, and the vaginal balloon catheter is palpated.
- If the confluence is still high, the patient is placed prone and the vagina is separated from the common UG sinus.
  - The common UG sinus is opened over the distal vagina near the confluence, where the vagina is relatively underdeveloped. The posterior wall incision can be extended proximally and distally until the urethral meatus is seen. If a Councill tip Foley was placed into the vagina, the catheter is redirected up the urethra into the bladder.
  - Meticulous sharp dissection creates a plane between the anterior wall of the vagina and the urethra and bladder base. Multiple traction sutures are placed on the vagina (**TECH FIG 4C**).
  - Following adequate vaginal mobilization, the common UG sinus becomes the urethra with a running closure of absorbable suture over the Foley catheter.

Use of the Excess Mobilized Common UG Sinus

- Best use determined by the distance for the vagina to reach the perineum.

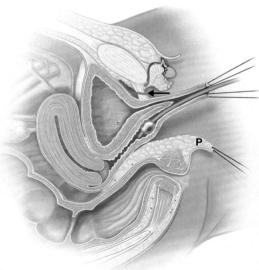
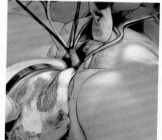
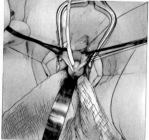

TECH FIG 4 • Urogenital mobilization, sagittal view. A posteriorly based perineal flap (*P*) has been mobilized to facilitate posterior exposure and for incorporation to vagina, if needed. **A.** In total urogenital mobilization (TUM), the UG sinus is mobilized as a unit both between the vagina and rectum and anteriorly under the pubis. The supportive pubourethral ligament (*black arrow*) are taken down for this extensive mobilization. In partial urogenital mobilization (PUM), the anterior dissection stops short of dividing the pubourethral ligaments. **B.** A catheter is in place in the UG sinus and multiple traction sutures facilitate dissection. **C.** The vagina has reached the perineum and is spatulated posteriorly to allow advancement of a perineal flap.

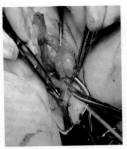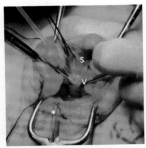

TECH FIG 5 • The mobilized UG sinus may be opened anteriorly **(A)** so that the excess sinus may be incorporated into the vagina. Patient A had an ASTRA. If the sinus is opened posteriorly **(B)**, the excess sinus creates a mucosa-lined vestibule. Patient B had partial urogenital mobilization. Note the open sinus (*S*), the frondular hymenlike tissue at the vaginal opening (*V*) and the posteriorly based perineal flap. The vagina will be spatulated further posteriorly to reach normal caliber. The flap will be advanced to complete the posterior wall of vagina.

- If the vagina remains high, the urogenital sinus can be used to complete the vaginal wall.
    - The common UG sinus can be incised anteriorly and the tissue is everted and advanced to become the anterior vaginal wall as a Passerini-type flap[9] **(TECH FIG 5A)**.
    - The excess UG sinus tissue can be used in a variety of ways to augment the vagina.[9,10]
    - The patient is then turned supine and the perineal flap is advanced posteriorly if needed.
- If the vagina has reached the perineum, the patient is turned supine.
    - The common UG sinus is incised posteriorly, and the redundant sinus tissue is used to line the vaginal vestibule **(TECH FIG 5B)**.
    - The posterior vaginal wall is spatulated to accept the perineal flap.
- Labioplasty is completed.

Comparison of Surgical Options for Vaginoplasty Based on Level of Confluence

Low Vaginal Confluence (TECH FIG 6)

- If a low vaginal confluence is present, partial urogenital mobilization (PUM) is completed (see above).
- The mobilized sinus is opened posteriorly to expose the urethra and vagina.

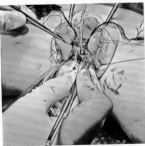

TECH FIG 6 • Completion of vaginoplasty after PUM. Note separate urethral (*U*) and vaginal (*V*) openings. The posteriorly based perineal flap (*asterisk*) allows a wider vaginal caliber. Silk traction sutures are holding the excess UG sinus, which will line the vestibule with a robust mucosa. The labia majora will be advanced posteriorly to flank the perineal flap.

- The vagina is incised posteriorly to increase the caliber, and the perineal flap is advanced into the vagina with interrupted absorbable sutures.
- Labioplasty is completed.

High Vaginal Confluence

- If a high vaginal confluence is present, prone positioning will optimize visualization for a vaginal pull-through procedure.
- Either a classic pull-through or TUM with pull-through may be used.
    - In the classic pull-through, the UG sinus is not mobilized. It is opened posteriorly in the midline, extending the incision into the normal-caliber vagina. The vagina is dissected off the urethra or bladder base and mobilized toward the perineum.
    - In TUM, the UG sinus has been fully mobilized (see above), and if the vagina has not reached the perineum, the UG sinus is opened over the confluence to expose the vaginal lumen and proximal urethra. Keeping the UG sinus tissue intact allows more flexibility for use of excess tissue.[9,10]
- Stay sutures are placed along the incised margin of the vagina to facilitate retraction.
- A malleable retractor is placed and elevated toward the rectum to optimize exposure.
- The investing structures are dissected off the vagina along the posterior and lateral walls.
- Once the posterior wall is exposed, the retractor is placed in the vaginal lumen to facilitate exposure of the junction of the vagina with the common UG sinus.
- The mucosa of the anterior vagina is incised transversely and additional traction sutures are placed.
- The anterior plane is dissected sharply; it is very thin distally and care must be taken to avoid entering the urethra or urinary bladder. Dissection continues anteriorly and posteriorly until the vagina can reach the perineum with or without local flaps.
- Following adequate vaginal mobilization, the common UG sinus is reconstituted as the urethra via multilayer closure over the Foley catheter.
- Regional flaps can be mobilized to help the vagina reach the perineum.
    - If TUM was employed, the excess common UG sinus may be incised anteriorly to allow eversion of the flap and incorporation as the anterior vaginal wall (Passerini-type flap).
    - The patient is rotated supine and the perineal flap is affixed to the vagina with interrupted absorbable sutures.
- One can imagine how the advantages provided by alternating between the posterior prone approach and the supine anterior view are unrealistic in teens and adults. Even if the urogenital sinus work can be completed prone, clitoroplasty and labioplasty should only be attempted supine or in lithotomy.

Anterior Sagittal Transrectal Approach

- Anterior sagittal transrectal approach (ASTRA) is a newer alternative approach for pull-through vaginoplasty in the setting of a high confluence.[11]
- Aside from the transrectal exposure of the UG sinus, the dissection of the vagina off the common UG sinus and subsequent urethroplasty is similar to a TUM.

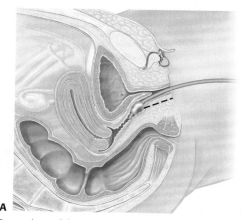 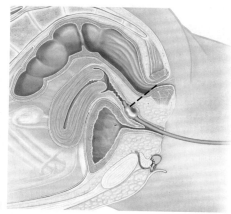

TECH FIG 7 • Comparison of the approach to the vagina for urogenital mobilization (perineal; **A**) vs ASTRA (transanorectal; **B**).

- Exposure of the posterior wall of the vagina is afforded by a full-thickness sagittal incision of the anterior wall of the anus and rectum; the surgeon's view and the access to the vagina are thereby more direct. There is a trade-off between this enhanced exposure and the potential morbidity of opening the rectum. The procedure can be safely completed without colostomy, but some opine that this additional risk is not justified (**TECH FIG 7**).
- Suitability for the ASTRA approach is determined at the time catheter placement by transrectal palpation of the vaginal catheter balloon (greater than 3 cm from the anus).
- Perioperative preparation includes the following:
  - Preoperative mechanical bowel preparation.
  - Triple antibiotic therapy or equivalent for 72 hours.
  - Diet held until evidence of bowel function.
- The procedure begins in prone position, and the rectum is opened (**TECH FIG 8A**).
- Clitoroplasty and dissection of the distal UG sinus are deferred.
- Without otherwise mobilizing the UG sinus first, the vagina is opened posteriorly (**TECH FIG 8B**) and dissected off the common UG sinus, similar to that described for TUM, and the UG sinus is closed as the urethra.

- The perineal skin is then incised to the level of the UG sinus orifice, and the posterior wall of the UG sinus is dissected (**TECH FIG 8C**).
- The procedure otherwise differs from TUM in that the anterior wall of the UG sinus is only mobilized under the pubis if additional sinus tissue will be needed to complete the vaginal wall.
- Otherwise the posterior wall of the sinus is opened, exposing healthy mucosa to line the vestibule.
- The rectum is closed and the anterior sphincter complex is reconstituted. The perineal body is closed in layers and sutured directly to the spatulated posterior vaginal wall.
- The patient is rotated prone for clitoroplasty and labioplasty.
- Because the cutaneous incision extends from anus to common UG sinus orifice, there is no midline posteriorly based flap.
  - This has not generally been required, but a flap could be raised from each side if necessary.
  - In either case, closure of the deep perineal tissues and a two-layer skin closure are recommended.

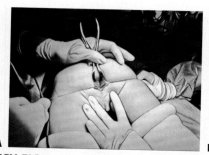 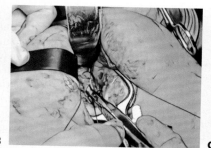 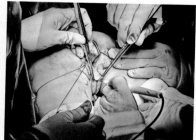

TECH FIG 8 • **A.** Full-thickness incision of the anterior anus and rectal wall. Nasal speculum in rectum. Catheter will be redirected to urethra. **B.** UG sinus opened to expose vaginal catheter. **C.** Skin is being incised in the midline toward the UG sinus meatus. Note that there is no midline posteriorly based perineal flap.

■ Creation of a Clitoral Hood and Labioplasty

- The remaining dorsal clitoral skin is incised in the midline to approximately 1.5 cm from the base, creating the Byars flaps that will be fashioned into the clitoral hood and labia minora (**TECH FIG 9A**).
- The intact 1.5 cm of clitoral skin is plicated with interrupted absorbable dermal sutures to provide contour to the clitoral hood.
- This outer layer of the clitoral hood is sutured to the inner layer of the hood reserved at the time of initial clitoral degloving.
- The paired Byars flaps are tapered and tucked next to the urethral plate, creating a fin of tissue similar to labia minora. The medial border of each flap is sutured to the urethral plate or mucosa-lined vestibule with interrupted absorbable sutures.

- If UG sinus reconstruction with vaginoplasty has been completed, the labia majora will also be addressed (**TECH FIG 9B,C**).
  - If the labia majora are anteriorly positioned, they are mobilized and advanced posteriorly to flank the perineal flap (if used).
  - Full-thickness debulking at the apex may improve appearance, although rugations of the androgenized tissue may persist. Care should be taken with fibrofatty debulking, as this may result in devascularization or asymmetry.
- A cleft is preserved between the labia minora and the labia majora by excising a dog-ear of skin anteriorly. Closure is via interrupted absorbable sutures.
- A two-layer closure at the apex of each labium will minimize the risk of dehiscence.

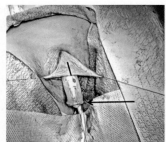

A

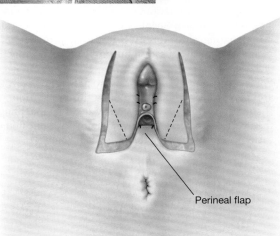

Perineal flap

B

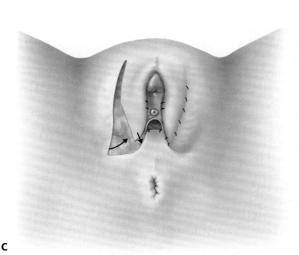

C

TECH FIG 9 • **A.** Fashioning clitoral hood and labia minora from clitoral skin. The clitoral skin is incised to create Byars flaps (*black line*). The incision stops about 1.5 cm short of the base to create the outer hood. Note that the initial clitoral skin incision allowed sufficient skin to form the inner layer of the hood (*black arrow*). **B.** Byars flaps are draped around the glans clitoris as the clitoral hood and labia minora. Dermal sutures provide contour to the outer layer of the clitoral hood. The labia minora are trimmed (*dotted lines*) for labial configuration and sutured to vestibular tissue. Dog ears of clitoral body skin are trimmed anteriorly to allow provide a grooved contour between the labia minora and majora. Two-layer closure of the inferior apices will minimize the risk of labial dehiscence. **C.** Completion of labioplasty after clitoral reduction and vaginoplasty with a posteriorly based perineal flap. Full-thickness debulking at the apices of the labia majora may be undertaken to reduce the loose skin folds. Rugation will persist to some degree. The labia majora are advanced posteriorly to flank the perineal flap, with a two-layer closure at the apices.

PEARLS AND PITFALLS

Preoperative decision-making	■ Multidisciplinary guidance is essential prior to performing irreversible genital surgery, and operative interventions should only be undertaken after extensive counseling. ■ The impact of deferring intervention until the age of consent is not fully understood.
Positioning	■ Coordinate with the anesthesia team to ensure upper body IV access, avoidance of continuous caudal catheterization in setting of total lower body preparation, and communication regarding multiple anticipated position changes. ■ Create a broad sterile field with total lower body preparation and strategic use of surgical drapes to facilitate genitoplasty and UG sinus reconstruction in younger children. ■ Adolescents and young adults should be placed in dorsal lithotomy position. The exposure for high dorsal dissection is much more limited in this population.
Labioplasty	■ Two-layer closure of the apices of Byars and labia majora flaps will minimize the risk of labial dehiscence as postoperative edema ensues.
Inadequate surgical preparation	■ Inadequate familiarity with patient anatomy can lead to rectal injury during posterior dissection of the UG sinus or can lead to neurovascular injuries of the clitoris and urinary tract. ■ A collaborative mentality is strongly recommended when complex anatomy may place patients beyond an individual surgeon's expertise.

POSTOPERATIVE CARE

■ A Penrose drain is placed in the vagina after vaginoplasty and removed in 24 to 48 hours.

■ An indwelling urethral catheter is left to drainage for several days postoperatively. Catheters may be left in place for up to 2 weeks depending on the nature of the UGS, the degree of urethral reconstruction, or other patient factors.

■ Care should be taken to secure the catheter so it does not compromise the integrity of the labial flaps.

■ Ointment and bulky fluff compression dressings are applied to the perineum and left in place for 2 or 3 days. Dressings are removed prior to discharge.

■ Perineal mobility is minimized in the early postoperative period.

■ In infants, a mermaid wrap around the knees is appropriate. Foam or a thick gauze roll between knees and ankles prevents pressure damage.

■ Older individuals should be instructed to avoid straddling, squatting, kneeling, or Valsalva to minimize perineal engorgement.

■ Short-duration, plain water tub soaks are begun approximately 3 days postoperatively, except in ASTRA.

■ Bacitracin ointment is applied to the perineum for 3 days postoperatively, after which use of bland ointment is recommended.

■ Care is taken to avoid moisture trapping beneath the ointment with consequent skin maceration or dehiscence.

OUTCOMES

■ Historic outcomes evaluations revealed substantial patient dissatisfaction with genital appearance and the need for repeated surgical intervention.[12,13]

■ Creation of an adult-caliber vaginal introitus in infancy is neither feasible nor desired.

■ Under ideal circumstances, creation of a supple introitus during infant vaginoplasty will allow for passive or active vaginal dilations at the age of sexual maturity. There is a reasonable probability of introital revision, and this should be emphasized in preoperative counseling.

■ Retrospective cohort studies have described impairment in clitoral sensitivity among patients undergoing feminizing genitoplasty[13,14] and demonstrated a linear correlation between diminished sensation and sexual dysfunction.[15]

■ As surgical technique has improved, prospective cohort studies reveal more favorable cosmetic outcomes following feminizing genital surgery[5,16,17] (**FIG 2**).

■ Retrospective evaluation of clitoral sensation and perfusion reveals improvement in functional outcomes following nerve-sparing clitoroplasty[18]; however, prospective assessments of clitoral sensation and overall sexual function are lacking.

■ Further prospective studies are also needed to assess surgical and psychosocial outcomes among this population.

■ If surgery is done during infancy, there is a significant lag time between surgery and sexual maturity. Educated modifications in technique are therefore challenging.

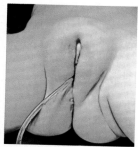

FIG 2 • Immediate postoperative result after a pull-through vaginoplasty via ASTRA in a child with completely fused labia majora and a high UG sinus. Creation of clitoral hood includes contouring dermal plication sutures. The labia majora did not require posterior mobilization in this child. Due to the ASTRA approach, there are perineal body sutures rather than a posteriorly based perineal flap.

COMPLICATIONS

- Clitoral ischemia with loss of tissue
- Dehiscence
- Vaginal stenosis
- Diminished clitoral sensation, impaired sexual function
- Unsatisfactory cosmetic outcome
- Patient regret

REFERENCES

1. O'Connell HE, DeLancey JOL. Clitoral anatomy in nulliparous, healthy, premenopausal volunteers using unenhanced magnetic resonance imaging. *J Urol*. 2005;173:2060-2063.
2. Puppo V. Anatomy and physiology of the clitoris, vestibular bulbs, and labia minora with a review of the female orgasm and the prevention of female sexual dysfunction. *Clin Anat*. 2013;26:134-152.
3. Poppas DP, Hochsztein AA, Baergen RN, et al. Nerve sparing ventral clitoroplasty preserves dorsal nerves in congenital adrenal hyperplasia. *J Urol*. 2007;178:1802-1806.
4. Leslie JA, Cain MP, Rink RC. Feminizing genital reconstruction in congenital adrenal hyperplasia. *Indian J Urol*. 2009;25:17-26.
5. Pippi Salle JL, Braga LP, Macedo N, et al. Corporeal sparing dismembered clitoroplasty: an alternative technique for feminizing genitoplasty. *J Urol*. 2007;178:1796-1800.
6. Baskin LS, Erol A, Li YW, et al. Anatomical studies of the human clitoris. *J Urol*. 1999;162:1015-1020.
7. Pena A. Total urogenital mobilization—an easier way to repair cloacas. *J Pediatr Surg*. 1997;32:267-268.
8. Rink RC, Metcalfe PD, Kaefer M, et al. Partial urogenital mobilization: a limited proximal dissection. *J Pediatr Urol*. 2006;2:351-356.
9. Rink RC, Metcalfe PD, Cain MP, et al. Use of the mobilized sinus with total urogenital mobilization. *J Urol*. 2006;176:2205-2211.
10. Gosalbez R, Castellan M, Ibrahim E, et al. New concepts in feminizing genitoplasty—is the Fortunoff flap obsolete? *J Urol*. 2005;174:2350-2353.
11. Salle JLP, Lorenzo AJ, Jesus LE, et al. Surgical treatment of high urogenital sinuses using the anterior sagittal transrectal approach: a useful strategy to optimize exposure and outcomes. *J Urol*. 2012;187:1024-1031.
12. Creighton SM, Minto CL, Steele SJ. Objective cosmetic and anatomical outcomes at adolescence of feminising surgery for ambiguous genitalia done in childhood. *Lancet*. 2001;358:124-125.
13. Minto CL, Liao L-M, Woodhouse CRJ, et al. The effect of clitoral surgery on sexual outcome in individuals who have intersex conditions with ambiguous genitalia: a cross-sectional study. *Lancet*. 2003;361:1252-1257.
14. Lesma A, Bocciardi A, Corti S, et al. Sexual function in adult life following Passerini-Glazel feminizing genitoplasty in patients with congenital adrenal hyperplasia. *J Urol*. 2014;191:206-211.
15. Crouch NS, Liao LM, Woodhouse CRJ, et al. Sexual function and genital sensitivity following feminizing genitoplasty for congenital adrenal hyperplasia. *J Urol*. 2008;179:634-638.
16. Braga LHP, Lorenzo AJ, Tatsuo ES, et al. Prospective evaluation of feminizing genitoplasty using partial urogenital sinus mobilization for congenital adrenal hyperplasia. *J Urol*. 2006;176:2199-2204.
17. Nihoul-Fékété C, Thibaud E, Lortat-Jacob S, et al. Long-term surgical results and patient satisfaction with male pseudohermaphroditism or true hermaphroditism: a cohort of 63 patients. *J Urol*. 2006;175:1878-1884.
18. Yang J, Felsen D, Poppas DP. Nerve sparing ventral clitoroplasty: analysis of clitoral sensitivity and viability. *J Urol*. 2007;178:1598-1601.

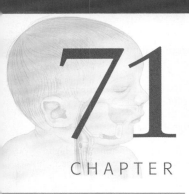

71

CHAPTER

Section XIX: Emergency Department Lacerations
Facial Laceration Emergency Room Closure Techniques

Christina Marie Pasick and Peter J. Taub

DEFINITION

- Facial soft tissue injuries are commonly encountered in the emergency room. Common etiologies are motor vehicle collisions, animal bites, sports and job-related injuries, and interpersonal violence.
- These injuries are often complex and may have significant impact on the patient's facial form and function.
- Plastic surgeons are often consulted by the emergency room physician or requested by the patients themselves for facial injuries ranging from simple lacerations to complex craniofacial trauma.

ANATOMY

- Facial aesthetic subunits should be considered when planning reconstruction so that incisions lie within or along the border of the involved subunit (**FIG 1**).
- Lacerations deep to the superficial musculoaponeurotic system (SMAS) risk injury to the facial nerve branches. See Table 1 for physical exam findings in injured facial nerve branches.
  - Blunt injuries to the face may cause a temporary neuropraxia to the nerve that does not require immediate operative measures but instead should be observed for 3 weeks.

- Extensive branching and cross-innervation of the branches of the facial nerve is present medial to the lateral canthus (**FIG 2**). As a general rule, lacerations of the nerve medial to the lateral canthus do not require repair. However, lacerations to the marginal mandibular nerve medial to the lateral canthus of the eye should be repaired, as there is not adequate crossover for functional recovery of the depressor muscles following medial injury to the marginal mandibular nerve. The temporal branch is another facial nerve branch with minimal crossover, but this nerve will most likely have innervated its target muscles (frontalis) should a laceration occur medial to the lateral canthus.
- The sensory nerves of the face can be utilized as guidelines for local anesthesia nerve blocks. Suspicion for nerve laceration should be elevated when lacerations are present in these regions.
- Knowledge of the location of the major arteries of the face can raise suspicion for lacerated vessels in deep wounds in these locations (**FIG 3**).
- The parotid duct or Stensen duct lies in the line drawn between the tragus and the middle of the upper lip. Stensen duct empties into the mouth at the buccal mucosa overlying the second maxillary molar.

PATHOGENESIS

- The mechanism of injury (ie, motor vehicle collision) can help to gauge the force involved in creating the injury and help determine if additional radiographic studies are necessary.
  - Suspect a larger area of tissue injury when dealing with a crush wound as opposed to a simple laceration.
- Human bites should all be treated as contaminated wounds, and the need for careful irrigation and prophylactic antibiotics apply.

FIG 1 • The facial aesthetic subunits. Scars are more inconspicuous when planned within or along these lines.

Table 1 The Physical Exam Findings Behind Injuries of the Facial Nerve Branches

Facial Nerve Branch Injured	Weakness Observed on Physical Exam
Temporal branch	Inability to elevate eyebrow
Zygomatic branch	Inability to close eye
Buccal branch	Inability to elevate upper lip
Marginal mandibular branch	Inability to evert lower lip
Cervical branch	Inability to activate platysma

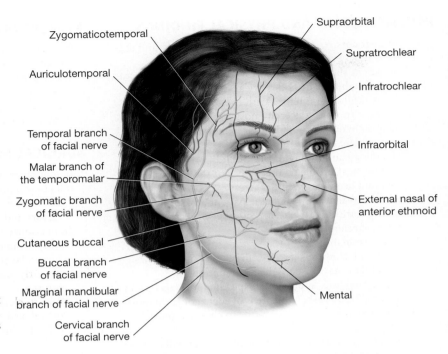

FIG 2 • The branches of the facial nerve: temporal, zygomatic, buccal, marginal mandibular, cervical. Extensive branching and cross-innervation is present medial to the lateral canthus (*marked line*). As a rule, lacerations of the nerve medial to the lateral canthus do not require repair.

- Organisms often found in human mouths include *Eikenella*, *Staphylococcus*, *Streptococcus viridans*, and *Bacteriodes*.[1]
- If the initial injury is not treated and the patient presents with a developed infection, inpatient therapy with IV antibiotics is often warranted, with a low threshold for OR debridement and washout.
- Dog bites are the most common type of animal bite in the emergency room and are often contaminated with various bacteria, including *Pasteurella multocida*, *Bacteroides*, *S viridans*, and *Capnocytophaga*.[1]
  - Infection rates are not as high as seen in cat bites due to lower bacterial levels and the open avulsion-type injury

seen in dog attacks rather than the deep puncture injury in cat bites that can trap bacteria. These open wounds facilitate irrigation.
- Crush component of dog bites often results in substance loss and requires debridement and reconstruction of avulsed tissue.[2]
- High incidence in the pediatric population.[3]
- Cat bites should always be considered heavily contaminated wounds, as the nature of the long and narrow cat teeth lead to deeply penetrating wounds with a very narrow orifice, resulting in seeding of bacteria into deep structures.
  - Organisms often found include *Pasteurella multocida* and *Bartonella henselae*.

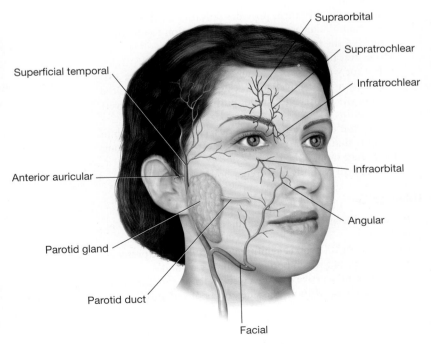

FIG 3 • The major arteries of the face. These arteries arise from the external carotid system (in *red*) and the internal carotid system (in *green*). Path of the parotid duct or Stensen duct. Lacerations in this line should be evaluated for laceration of the parotid duct system.

PATIENT HISTORY AND PHYSICAL FINDINGS

- Trauma patients require a primary trauma survey and secondary trauma evaluation immediately.
  - The patient should be assessed for more serious intracranial, ophthalmologic, and cervical spine injuries.
  - Suspect skull base fracture with the following signs: raccoon eyes (periorbital ecchymosis), battle sign (postauricular ecchymosis), otorrhea, or hemotympanum.
- Take a complete history.
  - The etiology and timing of the wound
  - Other medical problems that may put the patient at risk for wound healing difficulties
  - Medications that may make the patient a bleeding risk
  - Smoking status
  - Tetanus vaccination history
- Physical examination
  - Remove all clothing, jewelry, dried blood, and foreign material that may obscure the examination.
  - Use a systematic approach, inspecting for lacerations, avulsions, "road rash," and areas of edema or ecchymosis.
  - Palpate wounds for bony step-offs to clue into underlying fracture.
    - To rule out Le Fort fracture, depress the maxilla bilaterally with your thumbs to feel for mobility. If mobile, proceed to grasp the maxillary teeth with one hand while holding the nasal spine in place with the other hand. Movement of the dental alveolus points toward a Le Fort I fracture, whereas movement of the nasal bridge points toward a Le Fort II or III fracture.
  - Check for involvement of deeper structures: muscle, nerve, artery, bone, joint.
    - Especially in bite wounds with fangs, the deeper structures may be injured.
    - Irrigation of the base of the wound provides more thorough visualization.
  - Sensory test for nerve involvement:
    - V1 ophthalmic branch: provides sensation to the forehead
    - V2 maxillary branch: provides sensation to the cheek
    - V3 mandibular branch: provides sensation to the lower third of the face/chin
  - Motor test for facial nerve involvement:
    - Test for weakness in the facial nerve (cranial nerve VII) quickly and effectively by asking the patient to raise the eyebrows, close eyes, smile, puff out cheeks, and evert lower lips.
  - Assess for crepitus (subcutaneous emphysema) in bite wounds that would indicate an infection forming along the deeper fascial planes.
  - Examine all wounds for foreign body contaminants.

IMAGING

- If facial fractures are suspected, a CT scan should be performed.
- Plain x-ray or CT scan is helpful in determining the presence and location of foreign bodies within the wound.
- Ultrasound may prove as a quick and reliable tool for locating foreign body without the side effects of radiation.

NONOPERATIVE MANAGEMENT

- Nonoperative, or nonsurgical, management may occur in cases with very superficial and noncontaminated lesions, where washout, debridement, and closure are not necessary.
- Small wounds may have a preferred aesthetic outcome when allowed to close secondarily.

SURGICAL MANAGEMENT

- It is important to emphasize to the patient that any full-thickness injury to the skin will result in a scar.
  - The type of scar that forms can be dependent on multiple factors and is largely based on genetic predisposition.
- To maximize the chance of forming a fine-lined scar:
  - Most wounds require irrigation and debridement and closure in layers.
  - An early and tension-free closure of lacerations is a main priority.
  - Aim to close the wound in the direction of Langer lines, the relaxed skin tension lines of the face (**FIG 4**).
    - Find Langer lines in younger patients by asking them to animate their faces; the resultant skin folds simulate Langer lines.
- Delaying closure beyond 8 hours may increase the risk of infection of the wound bed and compromise aesthetic results, as swelling obscures anatomical landmarks.[4]

Preoperative Planning

- Use emergency room anesthesia: create a comfortable environment for the surgeon and the patient.

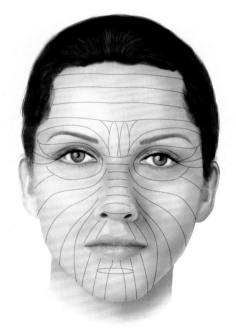

FIG 4 • Relaxed skin tension lines are ideal vectors for final scar placement.

- Topical anesthetic
  - Eutectic mixture of local anesthetics (EMLA) cream, composed of a mixture of 2.5% prilocaine and 2.5% lidocaine, is widely present in the emergency room—its effect is directly dependent on the time the cream has been on the skin.
    - Place cream on skin and cover with a Tegaderm (3M, St. Paul, MN) or other occlusive dressing for at least 45 minutes.
    - This often will need to be supplemented with local injected anesthesia but is a useful start for pediatric cases in which there is high anxiety associated with the local anesthesia.
- Local injected anesthetics
  - Lidocaine: most commonly used form of anesthesia in the ED. Maximum safe dose is 4.5 mg/kg. Effect usually lasts for 2 hours.
  - Epinephrine 1:100 000 may be added to the lidocaine solution to prolong the duration of its effect (to 4 hours) and reduce the amount of local anesthesia needed by reducing its diffusion away from the wound.
    - When epinephrine is added to lidocaine, the maximum safe dose is raised to 7 mg/kg.
    - Epinephrine takes about 7 to 15 minutes to take effect.
    - It was previously believed that epinephrine should not be used around end arteries such as the nose and stellate lacerations but is now accepted as safe practice.
  - Bicarbonate may be added to local anesthesia in the awake patient to reduce the burning pain on injection by raising the pH of the acidic lidocaine solution.
    - Bicarbonate also increases the effectiveness of the local anesthetic by favoring the nonionized form of the molecule, which passes through the cell membrane more easily.
    - Add 1 cc of 1 mEq/mL bicarbonate for every 9 cc of local anesthetic.
  - Bupivacaine: a longer-acting anesthetic, which may be added to the solution per the surgeon's discretion
    - Max safe dose: 2.5 mg/kg. Effect usually lasts 4 hours. When epinephrine is added, max safe dose is raised to 3 mg/kg, and the effect is prolonged to 8 hours.
  - Improve comfort on injection: warm the local anesthetic solution, use a higher-gauge (smaller caliber) needle, inject through wound instead of through skin
- Nerve blocks
  - For large lacerations in a single nerve distribution, nerve blocks can be effective and reduce the tissue distortion, which results when a large amount of local anesthetic is given as a field block.
- Conscious sedation
  - Beneficial for pediatric patients who are uncooperative, making repair of facial lacerations difficult.
  - Helps to make the repair safer and reduces emotional trauma to the patient.[5]
  - This requires continuous monitoring of vital signs, requiring a nurse to be present throughout.
  - For pediatric cases, a combination of ketamine and versed are commonly used.
    - Ketamine: analgesic and amnestic agent
      - Pediatric dosing: 6 to 10 mg/kg PO once, 30 minutes prior to procedure; or 0.5 to 2 mg/kg IV once at start of procedure
    - Versed: sedative-hypnotic and amnestic agent
      - Pediatric dosing: 0.25 to 0.5 mg/kg PO or IM 15 minutes prior to procedure; or 0.05 to 0.1 mg/kg IV 3 minutes prior to procedure
- Irrigation
  - Thoroughly irrigate all wounds to remove blood, foreign body debris, and bacteria.
  - Use of a pressured irrigation system is helpful if available in the ED.
  - May use 1-L bottle of normal saline with holes punched in the lid with an 18-gauge needle as a make-shift pressurized system.
- Debridement
  - Trimming of jagged skin edges with a 15-blade for optimal cosmetic closure.
  - Debridement of devitalized skin and tissue will reduce contamination and facilitate healing.
  - Be mindful of the location of your debridement, as heavy debridement in the critical areas in the face (eyelid, nose) may lead to significant disfigurement.
- Hemostasis
  - Use pressure, suture ligature such as Vicryl 4-0 (Ethicon, Somerville, NJ), Surgicel (Ethicon, Somerville, NJ), silver nitrate, thrombin, or fibrin. Electrocautery is now often available in the ED.
  - Because of extensive collateralization of vessels in the head and neck, even major vessels such as the facial artery may be ligated if bleeding is uncontrolled.
  - If bleeding is significant, you may extend the laceration to achieve visualization of the bleeding vessel.
  - Do not blindly clamp tissues as this risks injury to nearby nerves and other structures.
  - If the bleeding vessel cannot be clearly visualized, the wound should be packed, pressure applied, and the patient should be brought to the operating room promptly.

Positioning

- Prior to beginning any procedure in the emergency room, ensure you have a well-lit and adequate space.
- Head of bed should be elevated on a pillow for head and neck lacerations.
- Pediatric cases may require "papoosing" of the child by nursing staff and may require that a family member present throughout the procedure.

Approach

- Wounds may be closed with sutures, staples, skin tape, or wound adhesive.
- Suture choice:
  - Absorbable for all deeper layers and for mucosa and pediatric epidermis
  - Nonabsorbable for suture ligation of large vessels and for epidermal approximation
  - Nonbraided (monofilament) material best for contaminated wounds

Table 2 Appropriate Suture Choice for Specific Facial Laceration Locations

Location	Suture Material[a]	Suture Size	Suture Half-life	Removal
Scalp				
Galea	Vicryl/PDS	2-0	2–3 wk/4 wk	Absorbable
Skin	Prolene or staples	3-0	Permanent	7–14 d
	Or chromic gut		2 wk	Absorbable
General face				
Muscle	Vicryl/PDS	3-0 or 4-0	2–3 wk/4 wk	Absorbable
Deep dermal	Monocryl	4-0 or 5-0	1–2 wk	Absorbable
Epidermis	Nylon or Prolene	5-0 or 6-0	Permanent	5 d
Eyelids				
Orbicularis	Vicryl	6-0	2–3 wk	Absorbable
Skin	Nylon	6-0	Permanent	3–5 d
Ear				
Cartilage/skin	Nylon or Prolene	5-0 or 6-0	Permanent	5 d
Nose				
Cartilage	PDS/clear nylon	4-0	4 wk/permanent	Absorbable/permanent
Skin	Nylon or Prolene	5-0 or 6-0	Permanent	3–5 d
Lip				
Muscle	Vicryl/PDS	3-0 or 4-0	2–3 wk/4 wk	Absorbable
Mucosa	Chromic gut	3-0 or 4-0	2 wk	Absorbable
Vermilion border	Nylon or Prolene	6-0	Permanent	5 d
Intraoral mucosa	Chromic or Vicryl Rapide	3-0 or 4-0	2 wk	Absorbable
Pediatric skin	Fast absorbing plain gut	6-0 or 6-0	5 d	Absorbable

[a]All suture materials refer to those supplied by Ethicon, Inc. (Somerville, NJ).

- Taper/round needle ideal for muscle, fascia, mucosa
- Cutting needle ideal for skin
- Common emergency department suture choices available are as follows:
  - Muscle: Vicryl 4-0, Monocryl 4-0, PDS 4-0 (Ethicon, Somerville, NJ)
  - Skin:
    - Buried deep dermal layer: Monocryl 4-0 or 5-0
    - Superficial subcuticular layer: nylon/Prolene 5-0 or 6-0 (Ethicon, Somerville, NJ)
  - Mucosa: simple chromic/Vicryl Rapide 3-0 or 4-0 (Ethicon, Somerville, NJ)
  - Pediatrics: simple fast absorbing plain gut 5-0 or 6-0
- Proper suture choice for specific anatomic locations of the face is imperative for maximizing healing and minimizing scar formation (Table 2).

General Laceration Closure Techniques

- Simple interrupted: standard for closing all layers. Allows for optimal tissue reapproximation, especially in wounds with uneven lengths. Recommended for buried deep dermal and epidermal closure (**TECH FIG 1A**).
- Simple running: quicker means of closing epidermis in wounds with long length. Optimal for use in wounds where both sides evenly line up and there is no apparent "dog ear."
  - Disadvantages:
    - Not as precise as simple interrupted stitch
    - Unintentional breakage of the suture will lead to separation of the entire wound
    - Need to remove entire suture length if infection develops postrepair
- Vertical mattress: optimal for eversion of skin edges, yet is widely known as the most ischemic suture method and may result in skin ischemia if placed too tightly.

- Horizontal mattress: particularly useful in thick glabrous skin.
  - Similar to the vertical mattress counterpart in that it is effective in everting skin but risks development of skin ischemia.
- Staples: optimal for fast and effective closure of scalp wounds. May be used in very contaminated wounds that need to be closed loosely.
- Adhesive skin tape: beneficial for very superficial and small wounds closed with minimal tension[6,7]
  - Brief and painless procedure
  - Difficult to exactly approximate edges and maintain eversion of epidermis
  - Resulting scar similar to suture repair[7,8]
  - Best for upper third of the face as this area is of least skin tension
- Dermabond: may be used for clean wounds closed with minimal or no tension.

TECHNIQUES

Over and over sutures
(interrupted and continuous)

Subcuticular sutures
(interrupted and continuous)

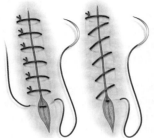
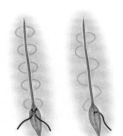

Horizontal mattress sutures
(interrupted and continuous)

Vertical mattress sutures
(interrupted and continuous)

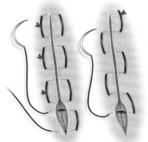
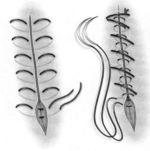
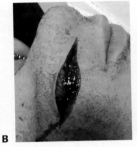
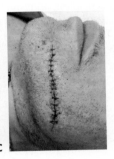

A   **B**   **C**

TECH FIG 1 • A. Suture closure techniques. **B,C.** Ideal closure for reapproximation of edges is simple interrupted suture.

- In crush injuries where the extent of the damage is unclear, tissues can be loosely reapproximated.
- If flap is avulsed, it should be tacked down where it lies, so that the closure is tension free. If there is undue tension on the flap, chance of necrosis is high.
- Epidermis should be everted at the edges, as eversion will flatten out to create a flat scar. Skin that is not everted at closure may produce a concave-shaped scar.

- Deeper wounds that cannot be closed can be packed with normal saline wet-to-dry dressings or iodoform gauze packing strips. Exposed bone or neurovascular structures can be covered first with Xeroform.
- Burns and abrasions can be treated with Adaptic gauze and bacitracin or with silver sulfadiazine.

■ Scalp Lacerations

- Two-layered closure:
  - Galea layer: use 2-0 Vicryl or PDS (Ethicon, Somerville, NJ) for tension-bearing layer.
  - Skin: use full-thickness continuous suture with 3-0 Prolene (Ethicon, Somerville, NJ) or staples.
    - Alternatively, can use 3-0 chromic as this does not requires suture removal

- Scalp defects fewer than 3 cm can usually be closed primarily.
  - Galea scoring may be necessary to gain laxity for closure.
- Attempt to prevent hair from being entangled in the sutures.
- May use Penrose drainage for first 24 to 48 hours (**TECH FIG 2**).

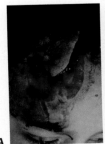
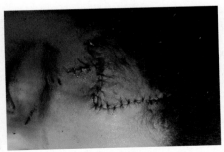

A   **B**

TECH FIG 2 • A. Laceration and partial avulsion of the forehead and anterior scalp. **B.** Galea layer reapproximated with Vicryl 2-0 (Ethicon, Somerville, NJ) and skin closed with interrupted nylon sutures.

■ Eyelid Lacerations

- First complete a full exam +/– ophthalmology consult to rule out ocular injury and lacrimal duct injury.
  - Jones I: instill fluorescein dye in the eye, wait 5 minutes, check for drainage through ipsilateral nare.[9]
    - Absence of fluorescein indicates nonfunctioning lacrimal system, and Jones II is performed.
  - Jones II: irrigate residual fluorescein dye in the nasolacrimal system with saline and watch for reflux from the canaliculi or presence of fluorescein dye in the wound. Either finding indicates damage to lacrimal duct system.
- Proper alignment of all layers minimizes risk of lid notching, ectropion, and functional deficit.
- Three layered closure of conjunctiva, tarsus, and skin
  - Orbicularis and tarsus: 6-0 Vicryl (Ethicon, Somerville, NJ).
    - Skin: 6-0 fast absorbing gut suture or 6-0 nylon.
    - Keep all knots directed away from the cornea.
- If lid margin is involved, approximate the gray line and tarsal plate with everting vertical mattress suture to prevent notching of the eyelid (**TECH FIG 3**).
  - Depth of suture: through skin and half way through tarsus
- Partial-thickness defects involving less than 50% of eyelid length can be closed with local advancement flaps. Involvement greater than 50% requires a skin graft harvested from the contralateral eyelid for a tension-free closure.[9]
- Full-thickness defects involving less than 33% of the upper lid and 50% of the lower lid can be closed primarily.
- More significant eyelid defects require flaps for closure.

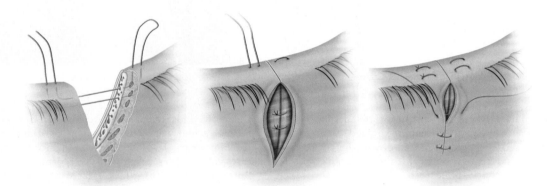

TECH FIG 3 • Laceration of the eyelid margin requires everting vertical mattress suture into the tarsus to realign lid margin and prevent notching of the eyelid. After the eyelid margin is realigned, the remainder of the laceration can be reapproximated.

■ Ear Lacerations

- Irrigate ear lacerations thoroughly to prevent possible chondritis.
- Debride skin conservatively to avoid cartilage exposure after closure.
- As long as the skin is still adherent to the cartilage, approximating only the skin in suture bites is sufficient for realignment of the cartilage. Use 5-0 or 6-0 Prolene (Ethicon, Somerville, NJ).
- Large defects with exposed cartilage should be covered with Xeroform petrolatum gauze dressing (Covidien, Mansfield, MA) with frequent dressing changes until reconstruction is completed.

- Avulsion injuries: should be promptly debrided, and small avulsion fragments less than 1.5 cm in width can be reattached as a composite graft in the first 12 hours. Large avulsions/amputation may require intraoperative microvascular replantation.
  - Venous congestion is a common problem following microvascular arterial anastomosis; postoperative leech therapy is commonly employed.
- Dress ear laceration with Xeroform gauze (Covidien, Mansfield, MA) and fluffed gauze in a pressure dressing with circumferential head wrap to avoid hematoma formation (**TECH FIG 4**).

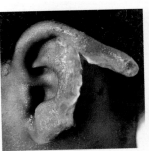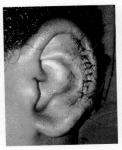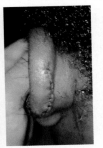

TECH FIG 4 • A. Laceration of the ear through cartilage, with partially avulsed helical rim flap. **B,C** Irrigated and closed with interrupted nylon sutures anteriorly and interrupted chromic sutures posteriorly.

■ Nasal Lacerations

- Nasal hemostasis may need to be achieved with either anterior or posterior nasal packing layered cottonoid or Xeroform gauze (Covidien, Mansfield, MA).
- Septal nasal hematomas must be ruled out. If visualization of the septum is not clear, slide your small finger into each nostril for palpation of a bulging hematoma.
  - If septal hematoma is present, this should be drained under direct vision with an no. 11 blade.
- Unlike ear lacerations, reapproximating the skin does not necessarily reapproximate the underlying cartilages, and lacerations should be addressed separately.

- Use 4-0 Vicryl (Ethicon, Somerville, NJ) or clear nylon suture for cartilage reapproximation.
- Use nylon or 5-0 or 6-0 Prolene (Ethicon, Somerville, NJ) for skin closure.
- The traditional view of resecting an entire subunit of the nose if greater than 50% is compromised has been challenged in favor of retaining all native healthy tissue.
- Defects of tissue may be repaired in the operating room with local flaps such as the dorsal nasal, nasolabial, and paramedian forehead flap.[10]

■ Lip Lacerations

- By taking care to align the "white roll" of the vermilion border, the outcome will be the most cosmetic. Differences in alignment of the white roll as small as 1 mm can be noticeable to the human eye at conversational distance.
- Align the white roll (vermillion-cutaneous junction), philtral columns, and cupids bow before any injection with anesthetic to avoid distortion of these landmarks by the added volume of the anesthetic (**TECH FIG 5**).
  - You may mark these by tattooing with methylene blue.
- Primary closure can be accomplished when less than 30% of the lip is involved in the defect.[9]
  - Defects in the central upper lip may distort the anatomy of the philtral columns. The defect should be closed with the available lip tissue and may be corrected later.
- Closure of each layer of the laceration is necessary to maintain appropriate thickness of the lip throughout the laceration.

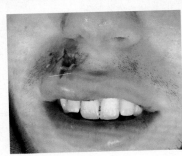

TECH FIG 5 • A demonstration of a lip laceration through the cutaneous-vermillion border. The first stitch for optimal reapproximation is at the level of the white roll (*white line*).

- Muscle: 3-0 or 4-0 Vicryl (Ethicon, Somerville, NJ)
- Epithelialized skin and white roll stitch: 6-0 nylon/Prolene (Ethicon, Somerville, NJ)
- Mucosa (lip surface): 3-0, 4-0 chromic suture

■ Facial Nerve Injury

- Any laceration in the path of the branches of the facial nerve should be explored for laceration of nerve (see **FIG 2**).
- Deep lacerations through the parotid gland are at high risk of nerve injury (**TECH FIG 6**).

- Repair of the lacerated nerve should take place as soon as possible and within 72 hours of injury.
- Repair delayed after 72 hours is difficult secondary to inability to stimulate the distal end of the nerve due to depletion of neurotransmitters at the motor end plates and contraction of the cut segment of nerve.

TECHNIQUES

- In the operating room and under magnification vision, the ends of the nerve should be trimmed and coapted tension free with 9-0 or 10-0 nylon epineural sutures.
- If repair cannot be completed without tension, consider nerve grafting or placement of a nerve conduit.

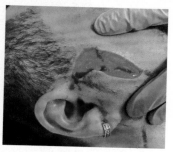

TECH FIG 6 • Laceration of preauricular region of the face, deep through parotid gland and lacerating the main trunk of the facial nerve as well as the parotid duct.

■ Parotid Duct Injury

- Evaluate a parotic duct injury by cannulating the intraoral segment with a 22-gauge Angiocath, and inject 1 cc of hydrogen peroxide, methylene blue, or milk into the duct. Blue dye (caution: messy!), milk, or foaming of hydrogen peroxide in the wound indicates a ductal injury.

- If the laceration appears to only involve gland tissue, the lacerated gland can be oversewn.
- Repair lacerated duct over a stent (red rubber catheter) using 7-0 nylon.
- Keep stent in place for 5 days with prophylactic antibiotics (**TECH FIG 7**).

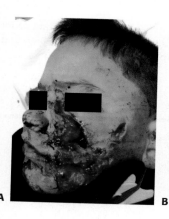
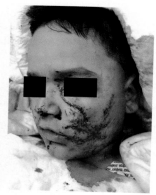

TECH FIG 7 • **A.** Unrestrained child in motor vehicle collision with multiple significant lacerations and significant loss of tissue. Extensive debridement in the ED revealed multiple pieces of glass in the wound. **B.** After thorough irrigation, the wound was closed in layered interrupted fashion.

PEARLS AND PITFALLS

Preoperative planning	■ Treat all bite wounds as contaminated wounds with thorough irrigation, debridement, and antibiotics. ■ Small wounds may heal as well or better if left to heal secondarily. ■ Always consider facial aesthetic lines when planning closure for optimal scar placement. ■ Be aware that crush injuries can produce larger areas of damage than initially appreciated.
Irrigation	■ Thoroughly irrigate all wounds; you can never overirrigate.
Debridement	■ Debridement of devitalized skin will reduce contamination and improve healing.
Closure	■ Be mindful of proper suture choice for each anatomic location. ■ Alignment of skin edges is optimal with simple interrupted suture. ■ Align critical regions (ie, the white roll of the vermillion border or the eyelid margin) first to minimize distortion of these regions.
Final outcome	■ In addition to factors such as timing, technique, and suture material, healing has a large genetic component.

POSTOPERATIVE CARE

- One dose of IV antibiotics should be given in ED for all facial lacerations.
- If wound is grossly contaminated or patient is diabetic, send the patient home on an oral outpatient antibiotic regimen with MRSA coverage (clindamycin or Bactrim).
- Rarely, acute wounds will require IV antibiotic treatment.
- Subacute and severely contaminated wounds may require admission for IV antibiotics.
- Bite wounds should be treated as contaminated wounds in the acute setting and require anaerobic coverage.
  - First-line treatment for bite wound is Augmentin (875 mg PO bid × 7 days for adults, and 45 kg/d PO bid × 7 days for pediatric dosing).
  - IV therapy for bite wounds: first line is Unasyn (Pfizer, Inc., New York, NY) 1.5 g IV q6h.
- All wounds should be given care instructions for daily cleaning and bacitracin application TID until sutures are removed
- Tetanus prone wounds: greater than 6 hours old, contaminated or in contact with soil, puncture wounds, animal or human bites, largely devitalized, infected.[3]
  - Incompletely immunized or uncertain: full tetanus vaccine (if moderate- to high-risk wound, also give tetanus immunoglobulin)
  - Greater than 10 years since immunization: give tetanus toxoid (if high risk, give tetanus immunoglobulin)
  - Five to ten years since immunization: if moderate to high risk, give toxoid.
  - If less than 5 years since immunization: no need for booster

OUTCOMES

- In general, the high vascularity of the face results in good healing with a low infection and dehiscence rate.
- Final scar maturation is completed by 1 year postoperatively, and as aesthetic appearance is always a concern to patients, maximizing aesthetic outcome should always be a priority

COMPLICATIONS

- Infection
  - Dog bite infection rates around 5% to 8% after ED washout[3,11] (**FIG 5**).
  - No change in incidence of dog bite infection rate between closure and nonclosure of wounds; therefore, approximation of tissues is recommended.[12]
- Hematoma
  - Auricular hematomas should be drained promptly through incisions in skin, and a compressive bolster dressing should be placed to prevent reaccumulation.

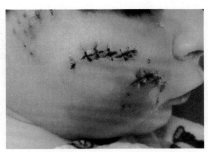

FIG 5 • Child presenting with cellulitis and abscess of the right cheek 48 hours after ED closure of dog bite wounds.

- Sialocele
  - Unidentified laceration of the parotid gland or parotid duct may result in delayed accumulation of saliva, presenting as swelling and tenderness of one cheek. Treatment involves compressive dressing, and if drainage is required, perform I&D through intraoral route.
- Chondritis
  - Delayed onset of pain after ear laceration warrants prompt evaluation for chondritis. Cartilage is poorly vascularized, and infection requires IV antibiotic therapy.

REFERENCES

1. Ball V, Younggren B. Emergency management of difficult wounds: part I. *Emerg Med Clin North Am.* 2007;25(1):101-121.
2. Gurunluoglu R, et al. Retrospective analysis of facial dog bite injuries at a Level I trauma center in the Denver metro area. *J Trauma Acute Care Surg.* 2014;76(5):1294-1300.
3. Toure G, Angoulangouli G, Meningaud J. Epidemiology and classification of dog bite injuries to the face: a prospective study of 108 patients. *J Plast Reconstr Aesthet Surg.* 2015;68(5):654-658.
4. Aceta A, Casati P. Soft tissue injuries of the face: early aesthetic reconstruction in polytrauma patients. *Ann Ital Chir.* 2008;79:415-417.
5. Bar-Meir E, et al. Nitrous oxide administered by the plastic surgeon for repair of facial lacerations in children in the emergency room. *Plast Reconstr Surg.* 2006;117:1571-1575.
6. Goktas N, et al. Comparison of tissue adhesive and suturing in the repair of lacerations in the emergency department. *Eur J Emerg Med.* 2002;9:155-158.
7. Hyunhjoo K, Kim J, Choi J, Jung W. The usefulness of Leukosan SkinLink for simple facial laceration repair in the emergency department. *Arch Plast Surg.* 2015;42:431-437.
8. Simon H, et al. Long-term appearance of lacerations repaired using a tissue adhesive. *Pediatrics.* 1997;99(2):193-195.
9. Kretlow J, McKnight A, Izaddoost S. Facial soft tissue trauma. *Semin Plast Surg.* 2010;24(4):348-356.
10. Huang A, Wong M. Acute nasal reconstruction with forehead flap after dog bite. *Ann Plast Surg.* 2013;70:401-405.
11. Cheng H, Hsu Y, Chao-l W. Does primary closure for dog bite wounds increase the incidence of wound infection? A meta-analysis of randomized controlled trials. *J Plast Reconstr Aesthet Surg.* 2014;67(10):1448-1450.
12. Paschos N, et al. Primary closure versus non-closure of dog bite wounds. A randomized controlled trial. *Injury.* 2014;45:237-240.

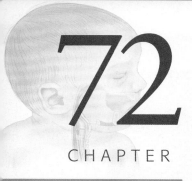

Section XX: Craniofacial Prosthetics

Craniofacial Anaplastology: Prosthetic Osseointegration

Chad A. Purnell, Rosemary Seelaus, and Pravin K. Patel

DEFINITION

- Anaplastology derives from the Greek *ana* to make again, anew, upon *plastos*—something made, formed, molded *logy*—the study of art and science of restoring a malformed or absent part of the human body through artificial means.
- Prosthetic derives from Greek *prósthesis*, addition, application, attachment as an artificial device that replaces a missing body part that may be lost through trauma, disease, or congenital conditions.
- Prosthetic and autologous reconstructive techniques are complementary, and in many circumstances, both are required to achieve an optimal aesthetic outcome in the reconstruction of craniofacial defects.[1] Prosthetic reconstruction can result in significantly improved quality of life for patients when conventional reconstruction reaches its limits.[1,2]
- Although autologous techniques remain the standard for long-term stable nasal and ear reconstruction, it frequently requires multistage surgical procedures with difficulty in achieving consistency of outcome and patient acceptability. Though the prosthetic approach can achieve consistency in outcome with minimal surgical intervention, it requires a lifetime of maintenance[4,5] (Table 1). Each approach must be considered by having the patient and family involved in the discussion. However, in some instances such as orbital exenteration, ocular and periorbital prosthesis is the only option for the patient as no autogenous alternatives exist.[3]
- Facial prosthetics can be either adhesive retained or fixed to osseointegrated implants. Other means of retention have been described but are less ideal. Due to disadvantages of skin reactions and less secure fixation with adhesives, implant-retained prostheses are most commonly used and result in the higher patient satisfaction.[1,4]
- *Osseointegration* derives from the Greek *osteon*, bone, and the Latin *integrare*, to make whole. The term refers to the direct structural and functional connection between living bone and the surface of a load-bearing implant.[5] Osseointegrated implants may retain a prosthesis through magnets or through a bar-and-clip mechanism (**FIG 1**).

ANATOMY

- The placement of osseointegrated implants into the craniofacial skeleton requires an understanding of the bony buttresses of the face (**FIG 2**). These areas of greater bony strength provide adequate bone stock for implant placement.
- The patient-specific anatomy for cranial bone thickness and the mastoid region must be taken into consideration for placement of temporal bone osseointegrated implants and implants for bone conducting hearing amplification.
- Orbital prostheses are retained by the thickened bony rim of the orbit. Nasal prostheses are retained by the thickened bony rim of the pyriform aperture.

PATIENT HISTORY AND PHYSICAL FINDINGS

- Because of the extensive deformity whether of congenital, traumatic, or from tumor ablation, a multidisciplinary team tailored to the patient's needs will help in achieving the patient's goals with an understanding of what can and what cannot be achieved by surgical autologous and prosthetic approaches. The team ideally consists of a craniofacial surgeon, an anaplastologist, a psychologist, and in the case of auricular reconstruction and bone anchored implants, an audiologist and otolaryngologist are included. The psychologist plays a critical role in providing the supportive voice for the patient during the decision-making process and in the accepting of the outcome with their own expectations, which may not be technically achievable. Communication and educating the patient and family is critical.
- A history of the patient should be collected, with particular focus on the area to be reconstructed. History of pathology leading to tissue loss, prior reconstructive attempts and donor sites, and pathology that contributes to wound healing should all be elicited. This importantly includes a history of tobacco use, corticosteroid use, and radiation therapy.
- This examination should fully assess soft tissue quality and vascularity of the area to be reconstructed. Areas targeted for placement of implants must have stable and adequate soft tissue coverage.

Table 1 Comparison of Autologous vs Prosthetic Techniques for Facial Reconstruction

Autologous	Prosthetic
Often complex, multistage surgery	Minimal surgery
Reconstruction requires minimal maintenance once complete	Significant, lifetime maintenance
Can be higher risk for comorbid patients	Safer in patients with comorbidities
Wide range of reconstructive outcomes	Typically provides near-exact replication of anatomic structure
Own tissues used, late complications rare	Creates prosthetic-tissue interface, late complications more common

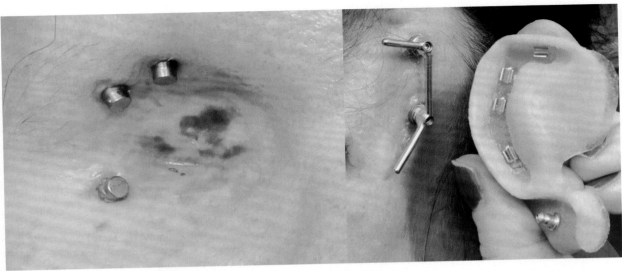

FIG 1 • Magnet (*left*) and bar-and-clip (*right*) attachment methods for prostheses.

- Bone in areas for potential osseointegrated implant placement should be assessed for quality and areas of potential bone loss. This assessment is best done through skeletal imaging.
- The patient should be evaluated to determine the appropriateness of practical prosthetic use. This includes an evaluation of manual dexterity (to don/doff prosthesis), general personal hygiene, social support, history of compliance with medical treatment, and access to anaplastology services.

IMAGING

- Conventional 2D photography and 3D soft tissue imaging is ideal not only for documentation but for virtual design and planning of prosthetic implants.

- For straightforward placement of osseointegrated implants in the temporal/mastoid region in patients with normal bony anatomy, imaging may not be necessary. However, imaging is frequently necessary for symmetrical anatomical restoration and for virtual planning of the implants. CT or CBCT imaging is essential to evaluate bone depth and density, which may be abnormal. Areas of prior bony resection or reconstruction are evaluated carefully for residual bone. Bone quality is of paramount importance after radiation therapy, and abnormal anatomy in craniofacial syndromes should be noted.
- Preoperative 3D planning software that integrates the soft tissue and the underlying skeletal anatomy allows the simulated placement of screws into bone to determine ideal vectors and locations of placement (**FIG 3**). These technologies can be merged with intraoperative stereotactic guidance for particularly challenging cases to ensure optimal placement.[6] At our center, we prefer to use a computer-generated guide for precise implant placement[7] (**FIG 4**).

SURGICAL MANAGEMENT

Preoperative Planning

- The number of implants to be placed should be decided with an anaplastologist to ensure adequate fixation. This decision will be affected by the location of the prosthesis

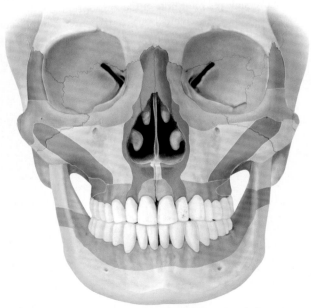

FIG 2 • The craniofacial buttresses (shown in color) are areas of increased bony strength in the facial skeleton, which are the safest locations for implant placement.

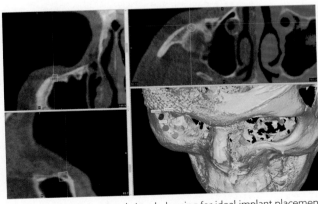

FIG 3 • Three-dimensional virtual planning for ideal implant placement.

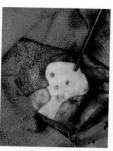

FIG 4 • Custom 3D printed drill guide for precise implant placement.

as well as the type of fixation (magnet vs bar-and-clip). Magnet fixation may require additional implants to be placed.

- The anaplastologist, with the craniofacial surgeon, will prepare a template of the area to be reconstructed with implant locations designated to guide surgical placement. In the case of the ear, this template is usually made from the position of the contralateral ear and centered around the external auditory meatus or tragus if present.
- The implant depth is often decided prior to implant placement but can be decided intraoperatively based on clinical assessment of bone depth and density. Most craniofacial implant systems come in 3 and 4 mm depths.

Positioning

- Standard supine positioning with a head drape and general endotracheal anesthesia is used for most implant placements. For uncomplicated implant placement, some surgeons may prefer local anesthesia with sedation.
- Hair in the operative area is trimmed in a limited fashion.
- If surgical drapes will obscure visualization of a contralateral normal structure, marking should be performed prior to draping to ensure symmetry.

Approach

- A one- or two-stage technique can be utilized for implant placement. In a one-stage technique, the implant is positioned and an abutment is immediately placed through the skin. The one-stage approach is appropriate in a majority of scenarios.
- In a two-stage technique, skin is reclosed over implants capped with a cover screw. The implants are then allowed to integrate into bone (approximately 3 months). Exposure of implants and abutment placement occurs at a later stage. A two-stage approach is generally indicated if bone is irradiated or of poor quality, in children, or in the orbital or maxillary region.[8,9] We typically favor a more conservative two-stage approach for many of our patients rather than early loading of the implant. Osseointegration and healing time may range from 3 to 9 months depending on patient comorbidities and bone quality. This is typically based on intraoperative assessment.

■ General Technique of Implant Placement

- Using the template created by anaplastology, the sites for implant placement are marked utilizing a needle dipped in methylene blue buried through skin and into bone.
- After a skin flap is raised (see specific anatomic areas for skin flap design), the skin is thinned to an ideal thickness of 2 to 3 mm (**TECH FIG 1A**). The skin flap is depilated through thinning or electrocautery of hair follicles or prior laser treatment. Periosteum is elevated (**TECH FIG 1B**).

- The sites for implant placement are identified. A guide drill with depth stop is used to drill a pilot hole in the correct vector (**TECH FIG 1C**). If the 3-mm depth stop results in complete drilling through bone, the 3-mm depth stop widening bit should be used and a 3-mm depth implant placed. If significant bone remains with the 3-mm depth stop, the 4-mm depth stop and implant can be used.
- A wider drill bit with countersink is used to widen and countersink the pilot hole at the appropriate depth.
- Outer table particulate bone is harvested and placed within the depth of the cranial bone at the dural interface when it is drilled full thickness.

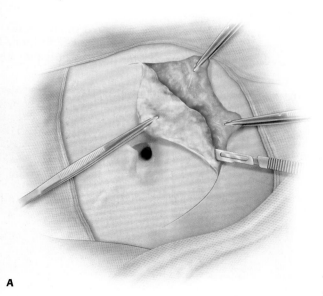

A

TECH FIG 1 • **A.** Skin flap is thinned to an ideal thickness of approximately 3 mm.

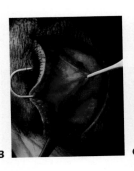

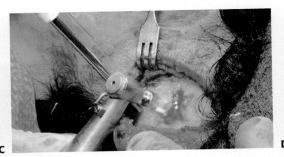

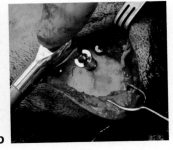

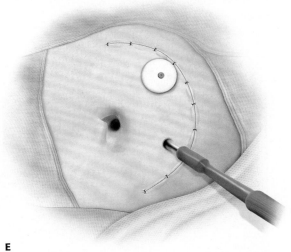

TECH FIG 1 (Continued) • **B.** Periosteum elevated. **C.** Drill with depth stop at predetermined implant locations. **D.** The implant is tightened with a torque wrench. **E.** Biopsy Punch used to perforate skin at location of implants in one-stage technique.

- Implants are placed into the holes with a handpiece set at slow speed of 2000 rpm at 25 N-cm handpiece. The torque of 25 N-cm can be increased depending on the density of the bone.
- Tighten implant with torque device by the hand to recommended torque level of the implant system (**TECH FIG 1D**).
- At this point, if a one-stage technique is planned, a biopsy punch is used to make skin holes directly over each implant (**TECH FIG 1E**).

- Healing or standard abutments are placed into each implant in the one-stage technique.
- If a two-stage technique is used, cover screws are placed over each implant and skin is closed.
- The skin incision is closed in layers, including the periosteum.

Implants for Auricular Prostheses

- A skin flap is designed in the proposed area of implant placement by avoiding pre-existing scars if possible. Typically, this is an anteriorly based single flap encompassing the area of all implants. Implants are ideally placed 2 cm from proposed or actual external auditory meatus, at least 1 cm apart from each other, with at least one implant above and one below the meatus. Incision is planned 1 to 2 cm posterior to the implants (**TECH FIG 2A**).

- Two implants are usually adequate for fixation of a bar-and-clip prosthesis. These are placed within the confines of the planned ear prosthesis, with positions above, below, and posterior to the external auditory meatus[10] (**TECH FIG 2B,C**).
- If an anchor for a bone-anchored hearing aid is to be placed, this is placed posterior to the planned auricular prosthesis into the temporal bone. If a magnetic-type implant is planned, it is 30 mm in diameter and thus must be located further from the ear.

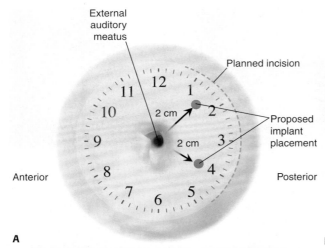

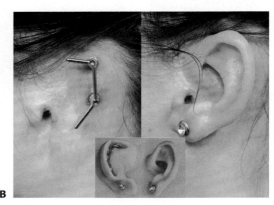

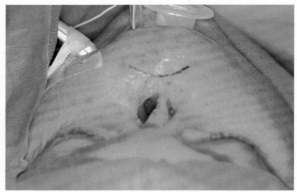

TECH FIG 2 • A. Skin flap design for auricular prosthesis. Incision planned 1 to 2 cm posterior to planned implants, which are placed 2 cm from external auditory meatus, at 2 and 4 o'clock position, or 8 and 10 o'clock position. **B.** Auricular prosthesis. (*Left*) Contralateral native ear. (*Right*) Prosthetic reconstruction. **C.** (*Left*) Bar-and-clip mechanism of implant attachment. (*Right*) Prosthetic in place. (*Inset*) Prosthesis showing clips for attachment.

■ Implants for Nasal Prostheses

- Ideally, at least three implants are utilized for fixation of a nasal prosthetic.
- Incisions are designed to be hidden by the eventual prosthesis, and flaps are raised anteriorly and posteriorly (**TECH FIG 3A**).

- Good-quality bone is limited around the nasal cavity. The frontal process of the maxilla (medial buttress) or premaxilla are sources of reasonable bone for fixation. The radix can also be used (**TECH FIG 3B**).
- Correlation with dental anatomy is essential to avoid the maxillary tooth roots if placing implants into the premaxilla.

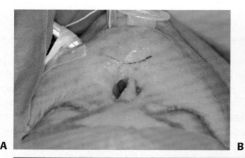

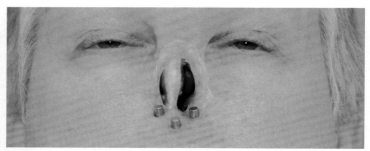

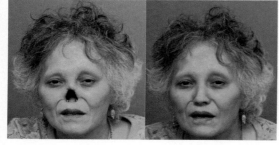

TECH FIG 3 • A. Curvilinear incision used to access premaxilla for nasal implant placement. This incision will be completely hidden by the prosthesis. **B.** Implant locations for nasal prosthesis. **C.** (*Left*) Implants in place for magnet-retained nasal prosthesis. (*Right*) Prosthesis in place.

▪ Implants for Orbital Prostheses

- Typically, three to five implants are adequate for fixation of an orbital prosthesis. Extra implants are often placed as it is assumed that an implant will be lost at some point.
- Incision is made at the orbital rim, under the area of the planned prosthesis. Flaps are raised in both directions from the incision, with the majority of the dissection deep to the rim (**TECH FIG 4A**).

- Implant location is generally designed in the superolateral orbital rim, if present, due to thicker bone in this area and for consideration of prosthetic appearance. If the lateral orbital rim is unavailable, the inferior and superior rims are selected for implant placement. The medial orbital bone is thin and of limited utility for fixation (**TECH FIG 4B**).
- Longer length implants should be used if possible given higher rates of implant loss in the orbit.

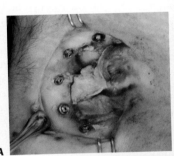
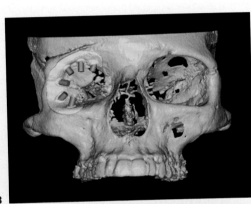
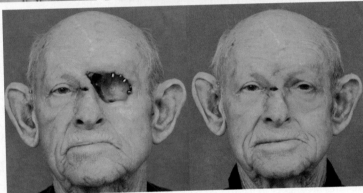

TECH FIG 4 • A. Orbital exposure for implant placement. Note rim incision and subperiosteal dissection into orbit. **B.** Surgical planning for orbital implant placement. Lateral orbital rim is the location for the majority of implants. Multiple implants placed due to higher instability of orbital implants. **C.** (*Left*) Orbital exenteration defect with implants in place. (*Right*) Defect with prosthesis in place.

PEARLS AND PITFALLS

Communication/education	▪ Educating the patient and family is critical to a successful outcome for the patient and for the treating team. Patients need to understand of the details of the steps involved to achieving the desired outcome. Expectations are best managed from the beginning. The psychologist and nurse are critical to this dialogue.
Implant vector	▪ Implants should be placed to full depth and ideally perpendicular to both bone and soft tissue. ▪ The guide drill must be used completely down to the depth stop to ensure proper seating.
Soft tissue contour	▪ Soft tissue should be thinned in a gentle taper around the implant area to avoid a step-off.
Hair at site of implants	▪ If hair remains after surgery, this can be treated with a laser depilation at a later time.
Postoperative maintenance	▪ It is critical that patients with the support of their family establish a daily routine for the management of the peri-implant soft tissue and care of the prosthesis. Failure to provide adequate care will lead to loss of implant.
Follow-up	▪ Patients with prostheses should be followed frequently at a minimum of an annual visit to assess the peri-implant tissue and the quality of the prosthesis. It is important for the team to assess its own outcomes and understand the patient's satisfaction or dissatisfaction with the treatment.

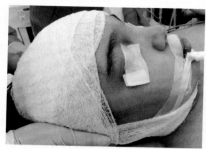

FIG 5 • Head wrap dressing used postoperatively after auricular implant placement.

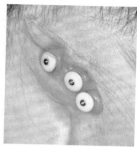

FIG 6 • Exuberant granulation tissue reaction around abutments.

POSTOPERATIVE CARE

- The area of reconstruction is covered with a pressure dressing and then a head wrap dressing (**FIG 5**), which is left in place for a period of 2 to 3 days. After this point, abutment site care is initiated and showering is permitted.
- The abutment site is cleaned daily with mild soap and a soft bristle brush to prevent crusting or buildup. Peri-implant hair should be trimmed and ideally removed permanently.
- If a one-stage technique is utilized, healing abutments are left in place for 10 to 12 weeks until the final abutment is positioned. In a two-stage technique, a period of 12 or more weeks is allowed for osseointegration. Once the final abutment is in place, the prosthesis fabrication can begin.

OUTCOMES

- Craniofacial implant–anchored prosthetics are well tolerated and have a long history of success. A majority of patients are able to wear their prosthesis for greater than 12 hours/d.[1,11,12] Implant anchoring tends to improve patient-reported quality of life overall.
- Implant failure rates are low in nonirradiated patients, with failure rates of 5% to 20% in nonirradiated sites in long-term studies.[7,11,13,14]
- Failure rates are higher in irradiated patients.[15] Large studies have shown failure rates of 23% to 54% over time in irradiated fields.[7,13,14,16,17] Studies are mixed on whether high-dose radiation increases implant failure rates over low-dose radiation.
- The role of hyperbaric oxygen (HBO) on implant survival in irradiated fields is as of yet unclear.[15] Some studies suggest that HBO used after implant placement may decrease failure in irradiated bone,[13,17] whereas others have seen no differences in outcomes.[16]
- Prostheses themselves have a limited life. Many studies cite a 2- to 5-year life span.[18] However, prostheses may last significantly less time depending on the patient's tolerance of discoloration or level of activity with prosthetics in place due to tearing or damage.[19]

COMPLICATIONS

- The most common complication with osseointegrated implants are soft tissue–related reactions due to inflammation.[15,20,21] Reactions are typically graded on a scale of 1 to 4 (Holgers scale). One is slight local erythema. Two is erythematous and slightly moist, 3 is moist with granulation tissue, and 4 is infection.[21] Rates of reactions overall range from 3% to 26%, with grade 1 reactions being by far the most common.[9,14,21] Device removal due to infection is extremely rare. The vast majority of skin reactions can be treated with medication. In cases of exuberant granulation tissue, local tissue around the abutment can be removed surgically (**FIG 6**). Aggressive thinning of peri-implant soft tissues at the time of placement in order to eliminate skin mobility around the implant is the best way of limiting peri-implant soft tissue reaction.

- Implant failure can occur early because of inadequate osseointegration with poor bone quality and can occur late due to chronic soft tissue infection affecting the peri-implant bone interface.

- During drilling for auricular implants, occasionally the dura of the middle cranial fossa or the sigmoid sinus will be exposed or perforated. In these cases, if bone stock is good, the implant can be placed as normal and the leak will seal. If the bone stock is poor, the leak should be sealed with pericranial tissue followed by autogenous particulate bone harvested from the same operative field and packed densely into the defect with fibrin sealant. The implant should be relocated.

REFERENCES

1. Chang TL, Garrett N, Roumanas E, Beumer J III. Treatment satisfaction with facial prostheses. *J Prosthet Dent.* 2005;94:275-280.
2. Nemli SK, Aydin C, Yilmaz H, et al. Quality of life of patients with implant-retained maxillofacial prostheses: a prospective and retrospective study. *J Prosthet Dent.* 2013;109:44-52.
3. Greig AV, Jones S, Haylock C, et al. Reconstruction of the exenterated orbit with osseointegrated implants. *J Plast Reconstr Aesthet Surg.* 2010;63:1656-1665.
4. Thiele OC, Brom J, Dunsche A, et al. The current state of facial prosthetics—a multicenter analysis. *J Craniomaxillofac Surg.* 2015;43:1038-1041.
5. Albrektsson T, Branemark PI, Hansson HA, Lindstrom J. Osseointegrated titanium implants. Requirements for ensuring a long-lasting, direct bone-to-implant anchorage in man. *Acta Orthop Scand.* 1981;52:155-170.
6. Meltzer NE, Garcia JR, Byrne PJ, Boahene DK. Image-guided titanium implantation for craniofacial prosthetics. *Arch Facial Plast Surg.* 2009;11:58-61.
7. Cohen M, Reisberg D, Patel P, et al. Facial rehabilitation with implant-retained prostheses: a 16-year perspective. *Plast Reconstr Surg.* 2009;124:1-2.
8. Habal MB, Davilla E. Facial rehabilitation by the application of osseointegrated craniofacial implants. *J Craniofac Surg.* 1998;9:388-393.
9. Sinn DP, Bedrossian E, Vest AK. Craniofacial implant surgery. *Oral Maxillofac Surg Clin North Am.* 2011;23:321-335, vi-vii.
10. Lundgren S, Moy PK, Beumer J III, Lewis S. Surgical considerations for endosseous implants in the craniofacial region: a 3-year report. *Int J Oral Maxillofac Surg.* 1993;22:272-277.

11. Westin T, Tjellstrom A, Hammerlid E, et al. Long-term study of quality and safety of osseointegration for the retention of auricular prostheses. *Otolaryngol Head Neck Surg.* 1999;121:133-143.

12. Han K, Son D. Osseointegrated alloplastic ear reconstruction with the implant-carrying plate system in children. *Plast Reconstr Surg.* 2002;109:496-503.

13. Granstrom G. Osseointegration in irradiated cancer patients: an analysis with respect to implant failures. *J Oral Maxillofac Surg.* 2005;63:579-585.

14. Karakoca S, Aydin C, Yilmaz H, Bal BT. Survival rates and periimplant soft tissue evaluation of extraoral implants over a mean follow-up period of three years. *J Prosthet Dent.* 2008;100:458-464.

15. Abu-Serriah MM, McGowan DA, Moos KF, Bagg J. Extra-oral craniofacial endosseous implants and radiotherapy. *Int J Oral Maxillofac Surg.* 2003;32:585-592.

16. Toljanic JA, Eckert SE, Roumanas E, et al. Osseointegrated craniofacial implants in the rehabilitation of orbital defects: an update of a retrospective experience in the United States. *J Prosthet Dent.* 2005;94:177-182.

17. Granstrom G, Tjellstrom A, Branemark PI. Osseointegrated implants in irradiated bone: a case-controlled study using adjunctive hyperbaric oxygen therapy. *J Oral Maxillofac Surg.* 1999;57:493-499.

18. Wilkes GH, Wolfaardt JF. Osseointegrated alloplastic versus autogenous ear reconstruction: criteria for treatment selection. *Plast Reconstr Surg.* 1994;93:967-979.

19. Karakoca S, Aydin C, Yilmaz H, Bal BT. Retrospective study of treatment outcomes with implant-retained extraoral prostheses: survival rates and prosthetic complications. *J Prosthet Dent.* 2010;103:118-126.

20. Balik A, Ozdemir-Karatas M, Peker K, et al. Soft tissue response and survival of extraoral implants: a long-term follow-up. *J Oral Implantol.* 2016;42:41-45.

21. Holgers KM, Tjellstrom A, Bjursten LM, Erlandsson BE. Soft tissue reactions around percutaneous implants: a clinical study of soft tissue conditions around skin-penetrating titanium implants for bone-anchored hearing aids. *Am J Otol.* 1988;9:56-59.

73
CHAPTER

Section XXI: Conjoined Twins

Conjoined Twin Separation

Michael R. Bykowski, Joseph E. Losee, and Lorelei Grunwaldt

DEFINITION

- Conjoined twins are individuals who are physically connected by their anatomy and share one or more organs. The site of fusion and orientation of the twins characterize the different types of conjoined twins. Although some conjoined twins can live functional lives, surgical separation is often performed for religious beliefs, cultural beliefs, parental wishes, and/or to promote survival of one or both twins.
- Conjoined twin separation is the procedure of surgically dividing the conjoined twins, allocation and reconstruction of shared organs, and soft tissue coverage. The challenge of the complex anatomy and physiology requires comprehensive preoperative planning and coordination by a multidisciplinary team often lead by the plastic surgeon.
- Because there is great variability of fusion patterns of conjoined twins, surgical management cannot be reliably predicted and is not amendable to treatment within fixed protocols. As such, this chapter discusses the general key principles for planning and executing separation of conjoined twins.

ANATOMY

- The detailed anatomy of conjoined twins is dependent on each set of twins. In general, however, the larger the connecting bridge between twins, the more complex its contents.
- The tissues of conjoined twins are normal but the anatomy is not. The anatomy is always abnormal but not in a reliably predictable manner. Nonetheless, there are general patterns to the anatomy based on the fusion type. The anatomical arrangements may be such that one twin may be incapable of independent existence.
- Classification is based on terminology according to the most prominent site of connection plus the suffix "pagus," which is the Greek word meaning "that which is fixed".[1] Some forms are described below:
  - Thoracopagus (40 cases; **FIG 1A**): junction primarily at the chest with varying amount of fusion of the heart, pericardium, and diaphragm.
  - Omphalopagus (34 cases; **FIG 1B**): joined at the abdomen and often have fusion of the liver and gastrointestinal (GI) tracts.
  - Pygopagus (18 cases; **FIG 1C**): connection at the sacrum/perineum and commonly face away from each other. May have fusion of the terminal spinal cord and associated meninges.
  - Ischiopagus (6 cases; **FIG 1D**): connected at the pelvic level. Each twin may have a normal leg and a common fused leg (ischiopagus tripus) or each has two normal legs

(ischiopagus tetrapus). Often have fusion of distal small intestine/large intestine and genitourinary system.
  - Craniopagus (2 cases; **FIG 1E**): fusion of the skull and meninges. (The separation of craniopagus twins is often driven by the neurosurgical team and is not discussed in detail in this chapter.)

PATHOGENESIS

- Conjoined twins are monozygotic, monoamniotic, and monochorionic.
- There are two leading theories for the pathogenesis of conjoined twin formation.[2]
  - Failure of separation of the embryonic plate approximately 15 to 17 days of gestation
  - Union of two separate embryonic discs

NATURAL HISTORY

- Conjoined twinning occurs in 1.5 per 100 000 births.[3]
- Other congenital anomalies that are not related to conjoining frequently occur and impact survival with cardiac abnormalities occurring in greater than 60%.[4]

PATIENT HISTORY AND PHYSICAL FINDINGS

- The minimal diagnostic criterion is the fusion of some portion of monozygotic twins.
- The main physical finding—ie, the site at which the twins are connected—provides insight to the internal anatomy. Predictable patterns of fusion occur and are associated with shared organs and organ abnormalities (see **FIG 1**).

IMAGING

- From the time of prenatal diagnosis to the time of surgical separation, imaging is the most important aspect of conjoined twin management.
- Prenatal and postnatal imaging evaluations are critical for predicting prognosis, obstetrical planning, medical management, and ultimately surgical separation.
- Conjoined twins can be first diagnosed by prenatal ultrasound by the 12th week of gestation.[5]
  - Specific diagnostic ultrasound findings include fixed position of the twin bodies on repeated examinations over time, lack of a separating membrane between the twins, and an inability to visualize a separation between the fetal bodies and skin contours.
- Once the presence of conjoined twins is diagnosed prenatally, further imaging is crucial to delineate the anatomy and

extent of shared organs; both of which are important for obstetrical purposes and prognosis.

- Due to the high incidence of cardiac abnormalities, fetal echocardiography is the most important prenatal evaluation.
  - All conjoined twins (irrespective of the site of connection, but especially for those with a ventral union pattern)[4] should undergo fetal echocardiography.
  - The degree of cardiac fusion and the severity of associated cardiac anomalies can help predict the postnatal viability and thus provide information for parental counseling.
- Prenatal computed tomography (CT) is useful to delineate the anatomic arrangement of the twins, primarily bony anatomy.

- Magnetic resonance imaging (MRI) is the best modality to provide the most detailed imaging of the fetuses as well as their associated anomalies and extent of union.
  - Ultrafast T2-weighted MRI sequences eliminate the need for maternal sedation and allow precise anatomical assessment of fetal organs avoiding the artifact due to fetal movement.
- Once the fetuses are determined to be viable and subsequently survive birth and the neonatal period, elective surgery can be planned with a team approach and with repeat postnatal imaging (discussed in detail below under "Preoperative Planning").

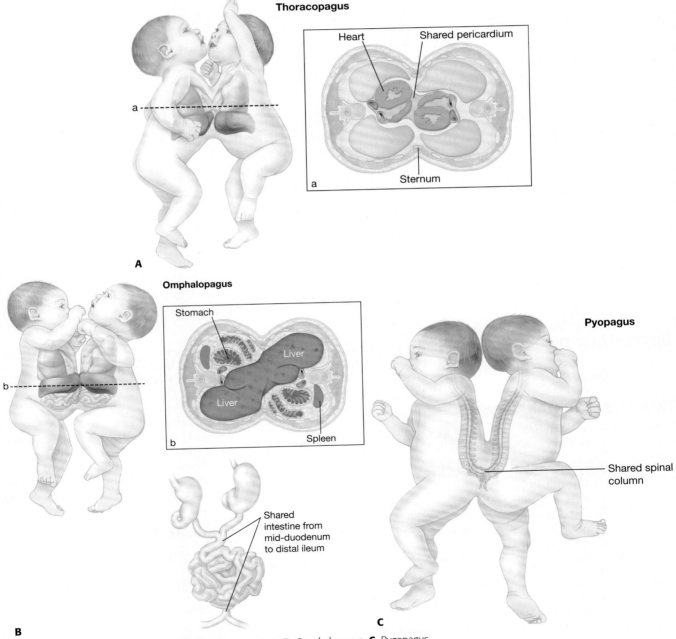

FIG 1 • Five most common classifications. **A.** Thoracopagus. **B.** Omphalopagus. **C.** Pygopagus.

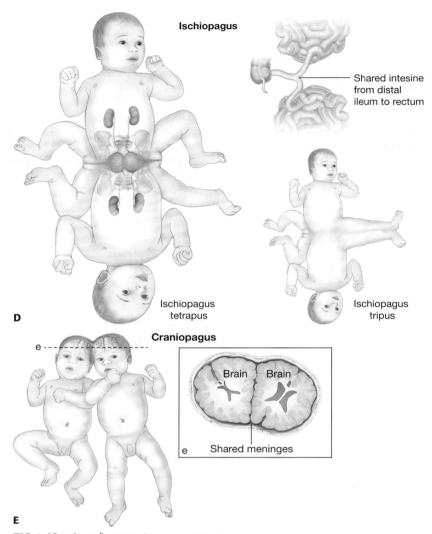

FIG 1 (Continued) • **D.** Ischiopagus. **E.** Craniopagus.

DIFFERENTIAL DIAGNOSIS

- Teratoma
- Lymphatic malformation

NONOPERATIVE MANAGEMENT

- In determining operative vs nonoperative management of conjoined twins, a pragmatic approach is necessary to balance:
  - What is technically feasible by the health care team.
  - The parental wishes.
  - The likely outcome for the children with or without separation. (The issue of parental consent is beyond the scope of this chapter.) The technical feasibility and prognosis are issues that depend on each other and are dictated by which organs are connected and the extent of their connections.
- An extreme example demonstrating successful nonoperative management of a set of conjoined twins is the famous Eng and Chang Bunker. These twins—born in Siam in 1811—gained notoriety while traveling with the Barnum & Bailey Circus under the exhibition name "Siamese Twins." Despite their abdominal connection, Eng and Chang married sisters, fathered 22 children, and lived together for 63 years.
- Separation of conjoined twins is contraindicated in the following circumstances:
  - Thoracopagus twins with complex cardiac fusion
  - Craniopagus twins with extensive cerebral fusion
  - Separation that would result in physical disability, which is unacceptable to the parents. This is often associated with shared organ systems with compromise of one or both twins when the organ system is removed from one twin (often seen in parapagus, extensive ischiopagus, and craniopagus).

SURGICAL MANAGEMENT

- The discussion of this chapter focuses on elective separation, but the management of conjoined twins can be characterized as three distinct groups:
  - Nonoperative
  - Emergency separation
  - Elective separation
- The objective of the operation is to separate the conjoined twins while adequately allocating each individual with

organs for survival and to obtain soft tissue coverage over the resulting defect. In general, the anatomy of the junction and the shared organs and structures dictate the technical details of the procedure.

- A multidisciplinary approach is required along with frequent planning meetings, involving all of the staff necessary before, during, and after surgical separation.
  - The staff should include nursing, neonatologists, pediatricians, critical care physicians, anesthesiologists, and a variety of surgical specialists. Because a critical factor in conjoined separation is soft tissue coverage, the plastic surgeon is often the team leader and coordinates all activity.
- Elective separation should be delayed until at least 2 months of age if possible.[6] The timing of separation varies widely from 2 months to 2 years of age. The critical factor is to allow time for extensive preoperative planning and simultaneous medical optimization.
  - Occasionally, conjoined twins require mechanical ventilation to preserve respiratory functioning toward the end of tissue expansion of the abdomen or thorax, as there may be decreased tidal volume from external compression.[7]
- Due to the varied anatomy of conjoined twins, it is usually not possible to follow a predetermined protocol for surgical separation. In general, the main steps of the procedure are as follows:
  - Exposure of shared organs
  - Division, allocation, and reconstruction of shared organs
  - Identification and ligation of cross-circulation
  - Abdominal wall reconstruction and wound closure with rotational flaps, previously expanded tissues, and skin substitute materials

Preoperative Planning

- Although the health care team is large and multidisciplinary, it must be clear that there is a lead surgeon who is in charge and makes the final decisions on preoperative evaluations and treatment.
- Conjoined twin separation is technically challenging due to the various organs that can be fused. The most important factor for successful separation is preoperative planning through postnatal multimodal imaging modalities.
- Postnatal imaging is the keystone of preoperative planning to, firstly, assess operability and, secondly, to understand the shared anatomy and help with surgical planning.
- Three features are key to determining survival and thus should be a focus of preoperative planning:
  - Major vascular connections
    - CT angiogram: this modality is necessary to visualize vascular connections.
  - Management of the body wall closure: without adequate soft tissue coverage, the patient is at risk for exposure of viscera, evisceration, and sepsis. CT imaging allows sufficient assessment of the anticipated soft tissue deficiency and can help determine reconstructive options. If closure is too tight, cardiac and pulmonary functioning can be compromised. Therefore, additional soft tissue coverage needs to be created or temporizing measures must be employed.
    - Tissue expansion.
    - Mesh or dermal substitutes.
    - Rotational flaps can be used as an adjunct to tissue expansion and skin substitutes.

- Performance of both hearts after separation: cardiovascular performance after separation is not predictable given potential changes in cardiac functioning and changes in circulation.
- Even with extensive postnatal imaging, close monitoring and treatment in the intensive care unit is necessary.
- Because congenital anomalies (unrelated to conjoined twinning) are common,[3] all patients regardless of the form of conjoined twin should undergo cranial ultrasound, abdominal ultrasound, CT, and MRI. Three-dimensional models can be created to aid in surgical planning.
- As stated above, each type of union is associated with specific structural abnormalities, so preoperative evaluation and planning will vary.
- Each organ system should be preoperatively evaluated in a systematic manner.
  - Cardiovascular system: due to the high rate of cardiac abnormalities in all forms of conjoined twins, all twins should undergo postnatal echocardiography to characterize cardiac anomalies. Thoracopagus twins should undergo electrocardiographic-gated cardiac CT or cardiac MRI for detailed assessment of cardiac anatomy.
  - Respiratory system: CT is performed to demonstrate the anatomy of the lungs and airways. Parapagus twins often have abnormalities of the tracheobronchial tree. Although the respiratory systems in thoracopagus and omphalopagus twins develop separately, there may be associated abnormalities (eg, hypoplastic lobes secondary to diaphragmatic hernia or asymmetric chest union).
  - Hepatobiliary tree: the number of gallbladders, liver, and pancreas should be known. Furthermore, liver vascularity and hepatic venous drainage for each twin must be ascertained. The liver is fused in all parapagus twins, most thoracopagus and omphalopagus twins, and less frequently in ischiopagus twins. Cross-sectional imaging will demonstrate the degree of fusion and visualize the intrahepatic vessels. MRI or CT scan with contrast injected into one twin can help to delineate the plane of liver separation. Overall, 25% of thoracopagus twins share a biliary system. Magnetic resonance cholangiopancreatography (MRCP) provides a detailed assessment of biliary anatomy.
  - GI system: the length of the alimentary tract should be evaluated. Though laparoscopy or upper GI contrast studies have been used to evaluate bowel distribution, much of the anatomy can be determined and managed during the separation procedure by the general surgeons. The lower GI tract is shared most often in ischiopagus twins (70% of cases) and in 25% of pygopagus twins. Pygopagus twins often have varying degrees of rectal fusion and common anuses. Contrast enema along with MRI will demonstrate complex anorectal abnormalities.
  - Urinary tract: imaging studies are performed to assess the number, reflux status, and anatomy of the kidneys, ureters, urinary bladders, and urethras. Cystograms can identify small fistulae not revealed by cross-sectional imaging. In 15% of pygopagus cases, the bladder is shared. Half of ischiopagus twins share pelvic organs.
  - Genital system: in pygopagus and ischiopagus twins, vaginoscopy is mandatory to assess vaginal and cervical anatomy. MRI can demonstrate the number of uteri, ovaries, vaginas, and testes.

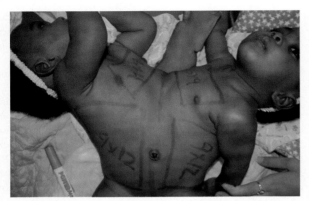

FIG 2 • Markings prior to chest and abdominal tissue expander placement and subsequent removal due to restrictive lung disease.

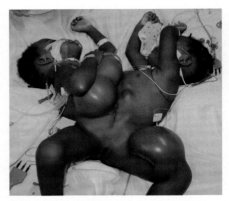

FIG 4 • Tissue expanders removed for the chest of one twin but maintained in the other. A tissue expander is placed on the left extremity.

- ■ Central nervous system: the nature and extent of spinal cord fusion is assessed in pygopagus, ischiopagus, and parapagus twins with spinal MRI.
- ■ Integumentary system: the soft tissue deficiency that will occur following separation can be estimated with CT scan. This information can be used to plan for the number of and placement of tissue expanders. Vascular territories of the skin can be mapped by intravenous fluorescein dye.
- ■ Musculoskeletal system: CT scan provides detailed assessment of bony anatomy, which is especially useful to determine pelvic and spinal bony anatomy in cases of caudal union. MR angiography can be used as an adjunct to determine blood supply when vascularized muscle flaps are planned—eg, when a shared limb will be used for wound closure.
- ■ The primary goal of the plastic surgeon is to provide coverage overlying the newly created defect following separation.
- ■ Tissue expanders have been placed intraperitoneally and in subcutaneous positions throughout the bodies of conjoined twins.
  - ■ The size of the defect following separation can be extensive and require multiple strategies in addition to tissue expanders, including meshes or dermal substitutes.
    - • Tissue expansion overlying the abdomen/thorax can compress the compliant chest wall and immature respiratory muscles of young children, leading to restrictive lung disease[7] (**FIGS 2** and **3**). As such, tissue expanders should be minimized around the thorax (**FIG 4**).

- ■ When plausible, expanders should be placed near the pelvic ring so that counter pressure is provided to optimize tissue expansion. Caution must be taken to avoid expanding too rapidly to avoid skin ischemia and expander exposure.
- ■ Due to the thin subcutaneous layer in infants, smooth wall tissue expanders are used. Textured implants tend to minimize capsule formation, which can promote thinning of the skin.
  - • Distant ports are used rather than integrated ports. The reason is that the thin skin overlying the expander is more prone to breakdown from repeated injections during the expansion process.
- ■ Tissue expansion using pneumoperitoneum is an alternative. Sterile air is injected (500–1500 cc) every 3 days to expand abdominal circumference.[8] Ischiopagus tripus twins present with an accessory hip joint and lower extremity, giving a tripod, or "tripus" configuration. As discussed below in "Techniques," the tripus (**FIG 5**) can provide additional coverage by filleting it open for maximal use of the skin, subcutaneous tissues, and muscle.

Positioning

- ■ Positioning will depend on how the twins are conjoined. Due to the potential for a long duration of surgery, the twins must be well padded to prevent the development of decubitus wounds.

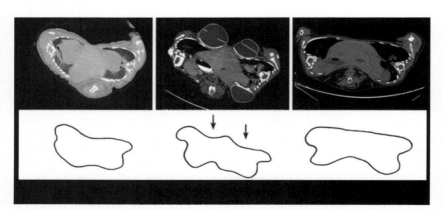

FIG 3 • **Top row.** CT cross-section view through ischiopagus twins with and without tissue expanders. **Bottom row.** Lind drawing of chest cavity showing deformation of anterior chest wall with tissue expanders in place. (*Left*) Preoperative chest CT scan. (*Center*) Chest scan with tissue expanders inflated and resultant chest deformation. (*Right*) Chest scan 6 months after tissue expander removal and resolution of clinical respiratory symptoms.

Positioning must allow adequate exposure to the planned line of separation.

If a posterior approach is favored, position the patient supine initially. Once intubated and venous access secured,

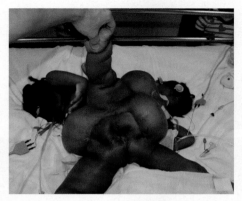

FIG 5 • Posterior view of the conjoined twins that demonstrates the tripus (after bones removed), which will be used for the abdominal wall reconstruction.

the twins can be turned prone. This maneuver can be cumbersome. Circumferential sterile surgical preparation is often required.

An important consideration is that a separate room is prepared and staffed for once the separation is completed. One twin will be transferred from the initial operating room to the other room while final reconstruction and wound closure is performed for each. After separation, each individual should have its own anesthesia team, surgical team, surgical staff, and operating room.

A staff member is assigned to communicate ongoing progress of the surgery and coordinates patient transfers.

Approach

An anterior approach is most often performed.

Depending on the conjoined twin anatomy, some surgeons favor a posterior approach.

■ Separation of Ischiopagus Conjoined Twins

Outline and Order of Procedures

Anterior incision extending from the chest to perineum.

Anterior pelvic osteotomy and "booking open" of fused pelvic ring.

Ligation and reimplantation of twin no. 1's left ureter.

Transabdominal liver separation.

Separation of two ileums from the single channel into the colon.

Posterior pelvic osteotomy with excision of the extranumerary hip joint of the tripus.

Fillet of the tripus to create two musculocutaneous flaps.

Repair of ventral abdominal wall and pelvic floor defects with allograft, tissue expanded advancement flaps, and musculocutaneous flaps for each twin.

Initial Steps

Plan the skin incision to provide optimal exposure of the shared internal organs to facilitate equal allocation and reconstruction of organs. Special attention is paid to the pelvic region where the most complex connection occurs between the gastrointestinal and genitourinary tracts.

Markings: while the twins are supine, mark the most cephalad point at the junction between the twins. Extend the marking inferiorly along the midline (in line with the umbilicus) toward the pelvis. The marking continues to the left of twin no. 1's labia majora, which was preoperatively determined to go with twin no. 1 (**TECH FIG 1A**).

Sharply incise the ventral surface along the midline through the skin between the tissue expanders (**TECH FIG 1B**).

Continue the incision deep through subcutaneous tissue with electrocautery to enter the abdominal cavity. Continue dissection inferiorly to the pelvic region to directly expose the anterior aspect of the pelvic ring.

TECHNIQUES

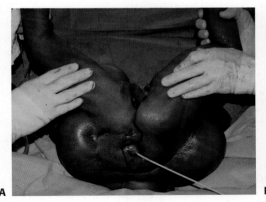

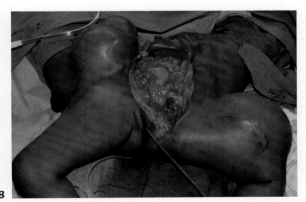

A   **B**

TECH FIG 1 • **A.** Inferior view of the twins demonstrating the markings about the perineum. **B.** The ventral incision is performed along the midline to provide adequate exposure of internal anatomy.

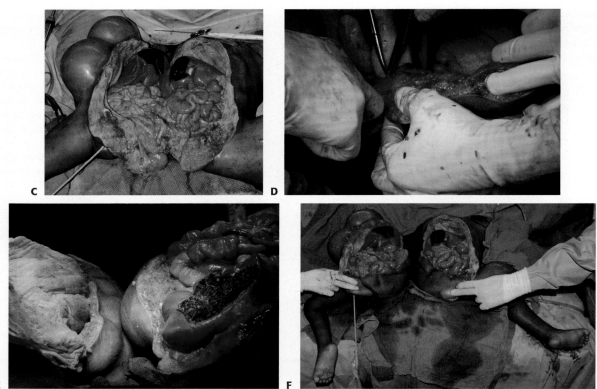

TECH FIG 1 (Continued) • **C.** The conjoined livers are exposed and separated with electrocautery and ligation of small venous branches that traverse the isthmus. **D.** The small soft tissue bridge is the only connection of the twins. **E.** These soft tissues are separated, and the twins are entirely separate. **F.** The tripus of each twin is rotated medially and laterally and tacked down to be used for pelvic reconstruction.

Note: it is known from preoperative imaging that the pubic symphysis is near-normal and midline.

- The urologists dissect, identify, and retract the ureters and bladders to prepare for safe division of the anterior pelvic ring at the pubic symphysis.
- In conjunction with the orthopedic surgeon, the pubic symphysis is visualized and divided using a combination of electrocautery and an osteotome. This maneuver allows the pelvis to "book" open.
- With this exposure, dissection is carried posteriorly toward the rectum, which appears to have two blood supplies, one from each twin.
- With focus moved more proximally, it is ascertained that each twin has an entire length of small bowel to near the distal end where there is a common channel of small bowel that leads into a single colon.
- Attention is directed to the anterior chest where dissection is carried down deep between the chest cavities of both twins. Dissection is continued along this plane to the posterior aspect of the twins toward the operating table.
- The connected livers are now adequately exposed, which are fused at the midline for a broad segment encompassing an approximately 8-cm span. The shared liver is separated with electrocautery and ligation of small venous branches that traverse the isthmus with 3-0 Vicryl sutures (**TECH FIG 1C**).
- Once the liver is divided, each twin's liver, stomach, and proximal small bowel can be easily retracted to the right and to the left to identify the four kidneys in the retroperitoneum.

- A Balfour retractor is placed to give adequate exposure.
- Attention is then turned to separate the small bowel. At the level of the Meckel diverticulum, an EndoGIA stapler is fired across twin no. 2's small bowel who will later undergo creation of an end ileostomy.
- Twin no. 1's small bowel, colon, and colonic mesentery are separated from twin no. 2's small bowel. A bulldog clamp is used to assess the vascularity of the colon, which is determined to have two separate active blood supplies. The colonic blood supply of twin no. 2 is divided because she will not have a colonic conduit.
- Of note, because twin no. 1 had more of the perineum, it was preoperatively decided to leave the rectum with twin no. 1.
- The colon is retracted laterally to allow the urology team to proceed. The balloon in each bladder is palpated to determine its location in the shared pelvis. Twin no. 2's left ureter, which connects to the contralateral twin's bladder, is ligated with 3-0 Vicryl at the ureterovesical junction.
- Dissection is performed to create definition between the bladders.
- Dissection is continued to isolate the uterus, fallopian tubes, and ovaries of each twin with their respective pedicles. This dissection further delineates the plane of cleavage for the twins.
- The previously ligated ureter of twin no. 2 is tunneled through the mesentery, spatulated, and closed to the neohiatus of the bladder. Good efflux of urine is confirmed, and the bladder is irrigated easily.

- After genitourinary reconstruction, attention is turned to the bony pelvis as it is still connected at the posterior aspect along with the extranumerary hip joint of the tripus.
- From preoperative evaluation, the iliac vessels are known to feed the conjoined connection within the single nonfunctional tripus.
- Using an abdominal retractor, the organs of each twin are retracted laterally to provide access to their medial shared hip structures and components.
- The aortas are palpated, and the iliac vessels of each child are identified and followed, which lead to either side of the hip joint. With the help of the orthopedic surgeon, osteotomies are created on either side of the hip joint, which is then is excised.
- The distal portion of the femur was previously removed in a separate procedure due to concerns with pressure necrosis on adjacent tissue expanded skin. The proximal femur is then directly visualized and is grabbed with a towel clip. The proximal femur is skeletonized with electrocautery and removed in continuity.
- After the removal of the hip joint and the proximal femur, further dissection of the iliac vessels is performed as they course into the tripus internally. The dissection of the iliac vessels is performed cautiously with a handheld Doppler device until each set of iliac vessels is traced into the tripus. The tripus is then split longitudinally to create two individual musculocutaneous axial pattern flaps.
- At this point, a small soft tissue bridge only connects the twins (**TECH FIG 1D**). These soft tissues are separated, and the twins are entirely separate (**TECH FIG 1E**).
- The tripus of each twin is rotated medially and laterally and tacked down to be used for pelvic reconstruction (**TECH FIG 1F**).
- A patient bed is brought into the operating room, and twin no. 2 is transferred to the adjacent operating room where further reconstruction is completed.

Twin no. 2

- The procedure begins with the inset of the tripus, which is on the posterolateral right side of her lower body. The hemitripus is reflected as a musculocutaneous flap from lateral to medial at the inferior aspect of her ventral wound recreating her pelvic floor. The hemitripus is inset into the inferior edge of the wound initially into layers closing the deep soft tissues with 2-0 Vicryl (Ethicon, Inc., Somerville, NJ) in interrupted buried fashion followed by a single closure utilizing 3-0 Monocryl (Ethicon, Inc., Somerville, NJ) in an interrupted buried deep dermal fashion.
- The left upper leg expander, left chest wall tissue expander, and right upper chest wall tissue expander are removed to create the left leg inferiorly based advancement flap. This flap is elevated in the subfascial plane while also harvesting the capsule. The composite tissues are advanced centrally toward the ventral defect.
- On the left lower lateral abdomen, a wide-based rotation flap is created from removal of its tissue expander,

which is rotated medially. Similarly, on the right upper posterior chest, the tissue expander is removed to create a wide-based rotation flap, which is based superiorly and rotated centrally.
- A large sheath of extra thick AlloDerm is used to close the fascial defect of the ventral body. The AlloDerm is inset to the surrounding fascia and body wall utilizing 2-0 PDS (Ethicon, Inc., Somerville, NJ) in a horizontal mattress fashion.
- On the inferior aspect of the ventral defect, the tripus remnant is used to recreate the pelvic floor by suturing muscular elements of the tripus to the surrounding remnants of the muscular pelvic girdle.
- The advancement flaps are closed in layers utilizing 2-0 Vicryl in an interrupted buried fashion within the deep tissues followed by skin closure utilizing 4-0 plain gut in a simple running fashion.
- The ventral defect is decreased in size using a no. 1 Maxon (Ethicon, Inc., Somerville, NJ) suture along the periphery of the closure to create a purse-string effect.
- The general surgeons re-entered the case to create a left-sided ostomy by incising the AlloDerm. The end ileostomy is brought through the left abdominal wall.
- A negative suction-assisted closure device is placed on the skin defect area directly atop the AlloDerm.
- The patient is transferred to the intensive care unit. Over the oncoming weeks, the vacuum-assisted suction device is used to promote formation of granulation tissue (**TECH FIG 2**).

Twin no. 1

- As with twin no. 2, the split tripus is used as an axial-based musculocutaneous flap for pelvic floor reconstruction. A large piece of 16 × 20-cm AlloDerm is sewn across the abdominal wall to act as a barrier and also to act as a substitute for the anterior rectus sheath.
- The four tissue expanders were removed. The expanders from the anterior chest and the lateral chest wall are used as advancement flaps.

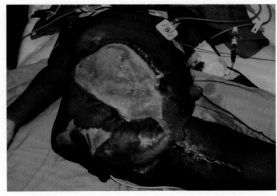

TECH FIG 2 • Postoperative photograph of twin no. 2 showing healing of soft tissue defect.

- Back cuts are made along the lateral abdominal wall into the right axilla and also into the left axilla in the left lateral chest wall. These flaps are advanced into the middle and are sutured to each other.
- A large central defect remains that measures 10 × 15 cm where the AlloDerm is exposed. A negative suction-assisted closure device is placed atop of the exposed AlloDerm.
- The patient is transferred to the intensive care unit. Over the oncoming weeks, the vacuum-assisted suction device is used to promote formation of granulation tissue (**TECH FIG 3**).

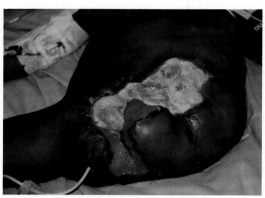

TECH FIG 3 • Postoperative photograph of twin no. 1 showing healing of soft tissue defect.

PEARLS AND PITFALLS

Preoperative imaging	■ Images obtained without anesthesia can be suboptimal. CT scans under general anesthesia allow suspension of respiration to minimize artifact. ■ An additional benefit is that the anesthesia team has an opportunity to assess how each twin behaves hemodynamically while under general anesthesia.
Abdominal closure	■ Primary closure of the abdomen should be completed under no tension, as tension can lead to cardiopulmonary insufficiency and death. ■ A combination of techniques should be used to obtain tension-free closure, including tissue expanders, pneumoperitoneum, dermal replacement materials, and/or meshes (as a temporary measure).
Abdominal tissue expansion	■ Use of tissue expanders overlying the abdomen can be used to achieve skin expansion and coverage of moderately sized soft tissue defects. However, additional measures are often required such as rotational flaps and/or dermal replacement materials. ■ Tissue expanders should be placed near the pelvic ring to provide counter pressure to optimize soft tissue expansion.
Thorax tissue expanders	■ Circumferential placement of thorax expanders can lead to restrictive lung disease. This problem is especially true in younger patients with more compliant chest walls and immature respiratory muscles. ■ Restriction of respiratory mechanics is more pronounced in twins who are joined at the chest, which results in compressive forces on three of the four sides of the chest wall.
Pressure relief	■ A pressure relieving bed is critical to reduce decubitus ulcer development. ■ Pressure relief is paramount, especially with use of posterior tissue expanders, to avoid soft tissue necrosis and expander exposure.
Tripus fillet procedure	■ The third leg in ischiopagus tripus twins is deformed and nonfunctional and can even induce pressure necrosis to adjacent soft tissues undergoing expansion. ■ The filleted tripus can be separated to create musculocutaneous flaps for each twin for abdominal and/or pelvic floor reconstruction.

POSTOPERATIVE CARE

- Planning of postoperative care occurs in the preoperative period. Meticulous supportive care in the intensive care unit is mandatory. The acute physiological changes occur after separation, especially when cardiac separation is performed and/or extensive cross-circulation is present prior to separation.
  - Cardiovascular instability should be anticipated.
- In most cases, elective paralysis and mechanical ventilation is necessary for 24 to 48 hours for cardiopulmonary stabilization.

- Aside from critical care support, attention should be focused to promote wound healing.
  - Nutrition must continue to be optimized postoperatively.
    - Parenteral and enteral feeding should be considered.
  - Focus should be to reduce the risk of health care–associated infection with the strict use of gowns and gloves to decrease exposure to hospital pathogens.
  - Pressure-relieving beds are required for wound healing and to prevent development of decubitus ulcers.
  - Extremity immobilization can promote flap healing and can prevent accidental trauma induced by the moving infants.

OUTCOMES

- Patient outcomes depend on the extent and complexity of the connection of the conjoined twins.[9,10]
  - Omphalopagus twins typically have the least extensive connection and have the highest survival rates.
  - Due to complex cardiac connections and abnormalities, thoracopagus twins have the lowest survival rates, with the exception of craniofacial anomalies.[10]

COMPLICATIONS

- Tight closure of the abdomen or thoracic cavities can lead to cardiopulmonary insufficiency, which can lead to abdominal compartment syndrome, restrictive lung disease, or a cardiac low-output state.
- Wound healing complications are common postoperatively.
  - Tissue necrosis can occur with high-tension closure, especially due to unpredictable blood supply of soft tissues.
  - With inadequate soft tissue coverage or subsequent breakdown, abdominal viscera can be exposed.

REFERENCES

1. Spencer R. Anatomic description of conjoined twins: a plea for standardized terminology. *J Pediatr Surg.* 1996;31(7):941-944.
2. Spencer R. Conjoined twins: theoretical embryologic basis. *Teratology.* 1992;45(6):591-602.
3. Mutchinick OM, et al. Conjoined twins: a worldwide collaborative epidemiological study of the International Clearinghouse for Birth Defects Surveillance and Research. *Am J Med Genet C Semin Med Genet.* 2011;157C(4):274-287.
4. McMahon CJ, Spencer R. Congenital heart defects in conjoined twins: outcome after surgical separation of thoracopagus. *Pediatr Cardiol.* 2006;27(1):1-12.
5. Chen CP, et al. Conjoined twins detected in the first trimester: a review. *Taiwan J Obstet Gynecol.* 2011;50(4):424-431.
6. Kiely EM, Spitz L. Planning the operation. *Semin Pediatr Surg.* 2015;24(5):221-223.
7. Losee JE, et al. Induced restrictive lung disease secondary to tissue expansion in ischiopagus conjoined twins. *Plast Reconstr Surg.* 2009;123(4):1378-1383.
8. Qazi AQ, et al. Separation of xiphi-omphalo-ischiopagus tetrapus twins with favorable internal anatomy. *J Pediatr Surg.* 2002;37(5):E9.
9. Jackson OA, Low DW, Larossa D. Conjoined twin separation: lessons learned. *Plast Reconstr Surg.* 2012;129(4):956-963.
10. Tannuri AC, et al. Conjoined twins: twenty years' experience at a reference center in Brazil. *Clinics (Sao Paulo).* 2013;68(3):371-377.

Index

Note: Page numbers followed by the letter "*f*" refer to figures; those followed by the letter "*t*" refer to tables; and those followed by the letter "*b*" refer to boxes.

A

Abbe flap, 58–59, 58*f*–59*f*
Abdominal compartment syndrome, 437
Abdominal wall
  anatomy, 436, 437*f*
  complications, 442
  definition, 436, 436*f*
  imaging, 438, 438*f*
  merits and demerits, 441*b*
  natural history, 437–438, 438*f*
  outcomes, 442
  pathogenesis, 436–437
  patient history and physical findings, 438
  postoperative care, 441–442
  surgical management, 438, 439*t*
Abdominoplasty, umbilical stenosis after, 446, 446*f*
Acellular dermal allograft, 62, 62*f*
Acellular dermal matrix (ADM), 104
Active Movement Scale, 355
ADM (acellular dermal matrix), 104
Adrenaline
  furlow palatoplasty, 70
  hard palate incisions, 82
Airway assessment, 24
Airway compromise, 73, 88
Airway contracture, 172, 172*f*–173*f*
Airway obstruction, 80, 96, 100
  palatal fistula, 110
  two-flap palatoplasty, 95
  velopharyngeal insufficiency, 119
Alar base, 35, 37
  anatomy, 12
  elevation, 16
  on lateral lip element, 14*f*–15*f*, 15
  repositioning of, 18, 19*f*
Alar cartilage, 23
Allografts, 175
Alopecia, 209
Alveolar bone, 22
Alveolar cleft, 102
Ambiguous genitalia
  anatomy, 468
  complications, 479
  definition, 468
  differential diagnosis, 469–470
  examination, 469
  imaging, 469
  merits and demerits, 478*b*
  natural history, 469
  nonoperative management, 470
  outcomes, 472*f*, 478
  pathogenesis, 468–469
  patient history and physical findings, 469
  postoperative care, 478
  surgical management
    approach, 470–471

  patient position, 470, 471*f*
  preoperative planning, 470
Ankyloglossia, 97
Anophthalmic orbit. *See* Microphthalmos
Anophthalmos, 283
Antegrade masseter-to-facial nerve transfer, 334–335, 335*f*
Anterior sagittal transrectal approach (ASTRA), 475–476, 476*f*
Apgar score, 68
Aponeurotic ptosis, 256
Aspiration, 301
ASTRA (anterior sagittal transrectal approach), 475–476, 476*f*
Aural atresia, 222*f*
Auricular prosthesis implants, 493, 494*f*

B

Bacitracin ointment, 478
BAHA (bone-anchored hearing aid), 222, 222*f*
Bicarbonate, 483
Bilateral cleft lip
  adhesion, 39–40, 39*f*–40*f*
  nasal deformity, 121*t*
  repair
    anatomy, 43
    definition, 43
    diagnosis, 44
    imaging, 44
    incisions, 46, 46*f*–47*f*
    lip fusion, 43
    markings, 45, 45*f*
    merits and demerits, 48*b*
    nonoperative management, 44, 44*f*
    outcomes, 48–49, 49*f*
    pathogenesis, 43
    patient history and physical findings, 43, 43*f*
    postoperative care, 48
    reconstruction, 46–47, 47*f*
    surgical management, 44, 45*f*
    variations in technique, 47, 48*f*
Bilateral complete cleft palate, two-flap palatoplasty, 94, 94*f*
Bilateral V-Y gluteal myocutaneous flaps, 194, 194*f*
Bilobed flap, 233, 233*f*–234*f*
Biobrane double-layer dressing, 175
Bipolar diathermy, 85
Bleeding, 80, 95
  NLDO, 281
  palatal fistula, 110
  velopharyngeal insufficiency, 119
Blepharoptosis, 255
Bolster sutures
  constricted ear, 236, 236*f*
  cryptotia, 240

prominent ears, 245, 245*f*
Stahl ear, 230, 230*f*
Bone-anchored hearing aid (BAHA), 222, 222*f*
Branchial cleft sinuses and cysts
  anatomy, 304, 304*f*, 305*t*
  complications, 310
  definition, 304
  differential diagnosis, 306
  endoscopic management, 308, 309*f*
  excision, 309
  imaging, 305, 306*f*
  merits and demerits, 310*b*
  nonoperative management, 306
  outcomes, 310
  pathogenesis, 304
  patient history and physical findings, 304–305
  postoperative care, 310
  surgical management
    approach, 306
    patient position, 306
    preoperative planning, 306
Branchial fistula
  type 1, 306–308, 307*f*
  type 2, 308, 308*f*
Branchio-oto-renal syndrome, 305
Breast contractures
  definition, 189
  merits and demerits, 190*b*
  natural history, 189
  pathogenesis, 189
  patient history and physical findings, 189
  postoperative care, 190
  surgical management, 189
    approach, 189, 189*f*, 190*f*
    patient position, 189
    preoperative planning, 189
Buccal mucosa graft, for redo hypospadias repair, 454–455
Buccal myomucosal flap, 106–107, 106*f*
Buccal sulcus incision, 37, 39
Bupivacaine
  emergency room anesthesia, 483
  furlow palatoplasty, 70
Buried sutures technique, 267, 267*f*
Burn injury
  anatomy, 211
  complications, 215
  definition, 211
  imaging, 212
  merits and demerits, 214*b*
  natural history, 211–212
  outcomes, 215
  pathogenesis, 211
  patient history and physical findings, 212
  postoperative care, 215
  surgical management, 212

Burn scar contractures, 173, 173f
Burned hand reconstruction
  anatomy, 178
  complications, 182
  contracture release with full-thickness skin
      grafting, 180–181, 181f
  definition, 178
  imaging, 178
  merits and demerits, 181b
  natural history, 178
  pathogenesis, 178
  patient history and physical findings, 178
  postoperative care, 182
  surgical management, 178–179
    patient position, 179
    preoperative planning, 179
Byars flaps, 453, 453f–454f

C
C flap
  inset of, 19
  on medial lip element, 14–15, 14f–15f
Canalicular injury, 281
Cannula use, 217
Canthopexy
  anatomy, 269, 269f
  complications, 274
  definition, 269
  imaging, 270
  merits and demerits, 274b
  natural history, 269
  nonoperative management, 270
  outcomes, 274
  pathogenesis, 269
  patient history and physical findings,
      269–270
  postoperative care, 274
  surgical management, 270–274
    approach, 270–274
    patient position, 270
    preoperative planning, 270
Carbon dioxide lasers, 206
Cardiovascular system, conjoined twins, 501
Cartilage turnover and rotation methods,
    Stahl ear, 227
Cat bites, 481
Caudal septum, 38f
CEA (cultured epithelial autograft), 175
Central nervous system, conjoined twins,
    502
Cheilion, 135
Chest wound closure, microtia, auricular
    reconstruction for, 224
Chondritis, 241, 246, 489
Chordee correction
  corporal body grafting, 453, 453f
  deep transverse incisions of tunica albu-
      ginea, 452
  dorsal plication, 450, 450f
  urethra and glanuloplasty tubularization,
      454
  urethral plate defect, bridging of, 453,
      453f–454f
  urethral plate division, 452
Circular excision and purse-string closure,
    167–168, 167f
Circumvertical skin reduction, 395, 395f
Claw hand, 178

Cleft lip
  anatomy, 2
  complications, 11
  definition, 2
  differential diagnosis, 2
  dissection
    lateral nasolabial element, 9
    medial lip element, 8, 8f
    nasal structures, 8–9
  etiology, 2
  lateral lip element elevation, 5, 6f
  lateral nasolabial element
    matching nasolabial lengths, 6–8, 8f
    nasal sill, 6, 7f
    Nordhoff point, 6, 7f
  lip closure
    cutaneous approximation, 10
    muscle repair, 9–10, 9f
  medial nasolabial element
    measurements and interpositional
        triangle, 4, 5f
    vermilion, Cupid's bow, and nose,
        3–4, 4f
  merits and demerits, 10b
  outcomes, 11, 11f
  pathogenesis, 2
  patient history and physical findings, 2
  postoperative care, 11
  surgical management, 2–3
    approach, 3
    patient position, 3
    preoperative planning, 3
  suture techniques, 10
Cleft lip adhesion
  bilateral, 39–40, 39f–40f
  unilateral
    completion, 39, 39f
    incision and dissection, 37, 38f
    markings, 37, 37f
    suturing, 37–39, 38f
Cleft lip repair. See also Bilateral cleft lip
    repair
Cleft palate repair
  Sommerlad palatoplasty
    anatomy, 81
    approach, surgical management, 82, 82f
    complications, 88
    definition, 81
    imaging, 81
    incisions and dissection, 82–83, 82f–83f
    merits and demerits, 88t
    nasal layer, 84–85, 85f–86f, 87
    nasal layer elevation, 83–84, 83f
    oral layer, 84, 84f
    outcomes, 88
    patient history and physical findings, 81
    patient position, 82
    postoperative care, 88
    preoperative planning, 81–82
    von Langenbeck incisions, 84, 84f
  two-flap palatoplasty (See Two-flap pala-
      toplasty)
  von Langenbeck palatoplasty (See Von
      Langenbeck palatoplasty)
Clitoral degloving, 471, 472f
Clitoral hood, creation of, 477, 477f
Clitoral reduction, 472–473, 473f
Clitoris, 468

Cloacal membrane, 468
Closure, lip. See Lip closure
CMN. See Congenital melanocytic nevi
    (CMN)
Coleman technique, 56
Coloboma, 126f
Colorado needle, 28
Columella, 12, 23
Combination technique, 394
Commissuroplasty, 135
  and skin closure, 138, 139f
Complete cleft, 12, 32f–34f, 74
Computed tomography (CT), 499
Congenital glaucoma, 277
Congenital melanocytic nevi (CMN)
  complications, 149
  definition, 141
  dermabrasion and curettage, 143
  differential diagnosis, 141–142
    classification, 141–142
    nevus distribution, 142, 142f
  imaging, 141
  laser, 143
  malignancy risk, 141
  natural history, 141
  nevus excision with expanded flap recon-
      struction
    approach, 146, 146f
    closure, 148, 148f
    excision, 147f, 149b
    incision, 146b, 146f–147f
    merits and demerits, 149t
    patient position, 145
    postoperative care, 149
    preoperative planning, 145
    suturing, 148, 148f
  nonoperative management, 143
  outcomes, 149
  pathogenesis, 141
  patient history and physical findings,
      142–143
  surgical management, 143
  tissue expander placement
    approach, 144
    merits and demerits, 145t
    patient position, 144
    postoperative care, 145, 145f
    preoperative planning, 143–144
    technique, 144b
Congenital midline nasal mass
  anatomy, 150, 150f
  complications, 157
  definition, 150
  differential diagnosis, 152
  endoscopic excision of intranasal glioma,
      156, 156f
  imaging, 151, 152f
  medial orbit composite unit translocation,
      155–156, 155f
  merits and demerits, 157t
  natural history, 151
  outcomes, 157
  pathogenesis, 150–151
  patient history and physical findings, 151,
      151f
  postoperative care, 157
  surgical management
    approach, 152, 153f

patient position, 152
preoperative planning, 152
transcranial NDSC resection
bandeau/frontal bone repair, 154
completion, 154
cranial base repair and seal, 154, 155f
incisions, dissection, and craniotomy, 153, 154f
keystone osteotomy and dermal sinus excision, 153–154, 154f
nasal approach/frozen biopsy, 153–154, 153f
Congenital ptosis, 159
anatomy, 255, 255f
complications, 262
definition, 255
differential diagnosis, 256
imaging, 256
merits and demerits, 262b
natural history, 256
nonoperative management, 256
outcomes, 262
pathogenesis, 255–256
patient history and physical findings, 256
postoperative care, 262
surgical management, 256–262
approach, 257–262
patient position, 257
preoperative planning, 257
Congenital vaginal atresia. See Vaginal agenesis
Conjoined twin
anatomy, 498
complications, 507
definition, 498
differential diagnosis, 500
imaging, 498–499
merits and demerits, 506b
natural history, 498
nonoperative management, 500
outcomes, 507
pathogenesis, 498
patient history and physical findings, 498
postoperative care, 506
separation of ischiopagus, 503–506, 503f–504f
surgical management, 500–503
approach, 503
patient position, 502–503
preoperative planning, 501–502, 502f–503f
Conjunctivitis, 277
Conjunctivomullerectomy, 260, 261f
Constricted ear
anatomy, 232
complications, 237
definition, 232, 232f
markings, 233, 233f–234f
merits and demerits, 236b
nonoperative management, 232–233
outcomes, 236, 237f
patient history and physical findings, 232
postoperative care, 236
rib cartilage
harvest, 234, 234f
splitting, 234, 235f
skin tunnel creation, 234, 235f
surgical management

approach, 233–236
patient position, 233
preoperative planning, 233, 233f
Contracture release, 172, 180–181, 181f
Corneal neurotization
anatomy, 348
complications, 352–353
definition, 348
diagnostic studies, 348
differential diagnosis, 348–349
imaging, 348
merits and demerits, 352b
natural history, 348
nonoperative management, 349
outcomes, 352
pathogenesis, 348
patient history and physical findings, 348
postoperative care, 352
surgical management, 349
patient position, 349, 349f
preoperative planning, 349
Corporal body graft, 453, 453f
Corporal-sparing clitoroplasty, 473
Cranial base repair and seal, 154, 155f
Craniofacial anaplastology
anatomy, 490, 491f
auricular prosthesis implants, 493, 494f
complications, 496
definition, 490
imaging, 492f
implant placement, 492–493, 492f–493f
merits and demerits, 495b
nasal prosthesis implants, 494, 494f
orbital prosthesis implants, 495, 495f
outcomes, 496, 496f
patient history and physical findings, 490–491
postoperative care, 496, 496f
surgical management
approach, 492
patient position, 492
preoperative planning, 491–492
Craniofacial anatomy, 158
Craniopagus, 498
Craniotomy, congenital midline nasal mass, 153, 154f
Cross face nerve graft, 342, 342f
anatomy, 319, 319f
complications, 324
definition, 319
imaging, 320
merits and demerits, 324b
natural history, 319–320
outcomes, 324
patient history and physical findings, 320
postoperative care, 324
surgical management
approach, 320
patient position, 320, 320f
preoperative planning, 320
Cryptotia
anatomy, 238
complications, 241
definition, 238
differential diagnosis, 238
merits and demerits, 240b
nonoperative management, 238

outcomes, 240–241, 241f
pathogenesis, 238
patient history and physical findings, 238, 238f
postoperative care, 240
surgical management
patient position, 238–240
preoperative planning, 238
Cultured epithelial autograft (CEA), 175
Cupid's bow, 3–4, 4f, 9f
anatomy, 12
deformities, 51b, 51f
asymmetry more than 2 mm high, 53, 53f–54f
mismatch of 1 to 2 mm, 52, 52f
Customized chest wall implants, 386, 386f
Cutaneous lip, 2
Cutaneous scar modifications, 139, 139f
Cutler-beard, eyelid coloboma, 252–253, 252f–253f
Cysts, branchial cleft sinuses and
anatomy, 304, 304f, 305t
complications, 310
definition, 304
differential diagnosis, 306
endoscopic management, 308, 309f
excision, 309
imaging, 305, 306f
merits and demerits, 310b
nonoperative management, 306
outcomes, 310
pathogenesis, 304
patient history and physical findings, 304–305
postoperative care, 310
surgical management
approach, 306
patient position, 306
preoperative planning, 306

D
Dacryocystorhinostomy (DCR), 277–278
Dacryoscintigraphy, 277
DCR (dacryocystorhinostomy), 277–278
De novo umbilicoplasty without midline incision, 445, 445f
Debridement, pressure injury, 193b, 198, 198f–199f
Debulking, sacrococcygeal teratoma, 425, 426f
Deep pars marginalis, 22
Deep transverse incisions of tunica albuginea (DTITA), 452
Dehiscence, 41
Delayed hard palate repair
anatomy, 64
definition, 64
hard palate repair, 65–66, 66f
imaging and diagnosis, 64
merits and demerits, 67b
outcomes, 67
pathogenesis, 64
soft palate repair, 65, 65f
surgical management, 64
Depressor alae nasi, 2
Dermabrasion, and curettage, 143
Dermal sinus excision, 153–154, 154f
Dermoid cysts, 151

Diagnostic laparoscopy, ambiguous genitalia, 469
Diazepam, 89
Distal hypospadias repair, tubularized incised plate urethroplasty for anesthesia, 449
initial approach, 449, 449*f*
Dog bites, 481
Dorsal plication, correction of chordee with, 450, 450*f*
Double-opposing Z-plasty, 68
Drawbridge effect, 82
Dry eye, 277
DTITA (deep transverse incisions of tunica albuginea), 452
Dura
and myofascial closure, 416, 416*f*, 421
skin closure, 416, 416*f*
Dynamic sphincter pharyngoplasty
dissection, 115, 116*f*
markings, 115, 116*f*
surgical management, 113
Dysesthesia, prominent ears, 246

E
Ear cartilage exposure, cryptotia, 240
Ear lacerations, 486, 487*f*
Ehrlich approach, prune belly, 429
Elbow reconstruction. *See also* Neonatal brachial plexus palsy (NBPP)
complications, 374
elbow release, 365–366, 366*f*–367*f*
outcomes, 374
postoperative care, 373
restoration of elbow flexion
free functioning gracilis transfer, 369, 369*f*
latissimus dorsi transfer, 368–369, 368*f*
steindler flexorplasty, 367–368, 367*f*
Elbow splints, 41
EMLA (Eutectic mixture of local anesthetics) cream, 483
Encephalocele, 151
Endoscopy
ambiguous genitalia, 469
Poland syndrome, 386, 386*f*
Epiblepharon
anatomy, 263
complications, 268
definition, 263
merits and demerits, 268*b*
nonoperative management, 264
outcomes, 268
with outlining markings, 264*f*
pathogenesis, 263
patient history and physical findings, 263, 263*f*
postoperative care, 267–268
surgical management
approach, 264–267
patient position, 264
preoperative planning, 264
Epinephrine, 37, 39
bilateral cleft lip repair, 44
emergency room anesthesia, 483
eyelid coloboma, 249
nasal tip hemangioma, 294

neck contracture, 187
secondary deformities, of lip and nose, 51, 54
Eustachian tubes, 64
Eutectic mixture of local anesthetics (EMLA) cream, 483
Everting sutures, 267, 267*f*
External dacryocystorhinostomy, 280, 280*f*
Extubation, 100
Eye contracture, 172, 172*f*–173*f*
Eyelid(s)
anatomy, 183
definition, 183
merits and demerits, 185*b*
nonoperative management, 183
pathogenesis, 183
patient history and physical findings, 183
surgical management, 183–184
lower lid, 183
patient position, 184
preoperative planning, 184
upper lid, 183
Eyelid coloboma
anatomy, 248
complications, 253
definition, 248
differential diagnosis, 249
merits and demerits, 253*b*
natural history, 248
nonoperative management, 249
outcomes, 253
pathogenesis, 248
patient history and physical findings, 248, 248*f*
postoperative care, 253
surgical management, 249–253
approach, 249–253
patient position, 249
preoperative planning, 249
Eyelid ectropion/entropion, 277
Eyelid lacerations, 486, 486*f*

F
Facial artery musculomucosal flap, 107, 107*f*, 110
Facial laceration
emergency room closure techniques, facial soft tissue injury
anatomy, 480, 480*t*, 480*f*–481*f*
approach, surgical management, 483–484
complications, 489, 489*f*
definition, 480
merits and demerits, 488*b*
nonoperative management, 482
outcomes, 489
pathogenesis, 480–481
patient history and physical findings, 482
patient position, 483
preoperative planning, 482–483
postoperative care, 489
surgical management, 482–484, 482*f*
locations, 484*t*
Facial nerve
anatomy, 338, 339*f*
injury, 487–488, 488*f*

Facial paralysis
anatomy, 339*f*
causes, 338*t*
definition, 338
pathogenesis of, 338
Facial reanimation. *See* Pediatric facial reanimation
Facial reconstruction, autologous *vs.* prosthetic techniques for, 490*t*
Facial soft tissue injury
anatomy, 480, 480*t*, 480*f*–481*f*
complications, 489, 489*f*
definition, 480
merits and demerits, 488*b*
nonoperative management, 482
outcomes, 489
pathogenesis, 480–481
patient history and physical findings, 482
postoperative care, 489
surgical management, 482–484, 482*f*
approach, 483–484
patient position, 483
preoperative planning, 482–483
Fascial closure techniques, 439–441
delayed fascial approximation anticipated, 440, 440*f*
fascial approximation anticipated, 439–440, 440*f*
negative pressure wound therapy, 440–441, 441*f*
Fasciocutaneous grotting flap transposition, 235, 235*f*
Fat grafting
anatomy, 216
complications, 219
definition, 216
differential diagnosis, 216
imaging, 216
merits and demerits, 219*b*
natural history, 216
outcomes, 219
pathogenesis, 216
patient history and physical findings, 216
postoperative care, 219
surgical management, 216–217
approach, 217
patient position, 217
preoperative planning, 217
Feminizing genitoplasty, 471
Femoral bone marrow margin, 379, 379*f*
Femoral vessels, 378, 378*f*
Fiberoptic nasendoscopy, 96
Fistula, 73, 88, 95, 102. *See also* Palatal fistula
intentional, 102
Pittsburgh fistula classification, 102
unintentional, 102
Flap elevation, 321, 321*f*
Flap necrosis, 80, 95
Forearm reconstruction. *See also* Neonatal brachial plexus palsy (NBPP)
biceps rerouting, 370, 370*f*
complications, 374
outcomes, 374
postoperative care, 373
PT release/rerouting, 370, 371*f*

Fractional CO2 laser
    anesthesia, 213
    application, 213–214, 214f
    wound care, 214
Free tissue transfer, palatal fistula, 109, 109f
Frontalis suspension
    brow sutures, 257, 258f
    markings and eyelid sutures, 257, 258f
Frozen biopsy, 153–154, 153f
Full-thickness skin grafts, 175, 180–181,
        181f
    harvesting of, 177
Functional burn reconstruction
    airway, eyes and lips, 172, 172f–173f
    anatomy, 171
    burn scar contractures, 173, 173f
    contracture release, 172
    definition, 171
    imaging, 172
    merits and demerits, 174t
    natural history, 171
    nonoperative management, 172
    pathogenesis, 171
    patient history and physical findings, 171
    surgical management, 172
Furlow palatoplasty
    anatomy, 68
    closure, 72
    complications, 73
    definition, 68, 68f–69f
    hard palate, 70
    imaging, 69
    merits and demerits, 73t
    nasal layer, 71
    oral layer, 70
    outcomes, 73
    palatal fistula conversion by, 105
    patient history and physical findings, 68–69
    postoperative care, 73
    surgical management
        approach, 69
        patient position, 69
        preoperative planning, 69
    velopharyngeal insufficiency
        dissection, 114, 115f
        markings, 114, 114f
        surgical management, 113
    Z-plasty with intravelar veloplasty, 72–73

G

Gastroschisis
    complications, 435
    definition, 432
    diagnostic studies, 432
    differential diagnosis, 432
    imaging, 432
    merits and demerits, 435b
    patient history and physical findings, 432,
        433f
    postoperative care, 435
    repair
        closure, 434, 434f
        delayed closure with silo placement,
            434, 434f
        immediate reduction, 434
    surgical management
        patient position, 433
        preoperative planning, 432–433

Genital system, conjoined twins, 501
Genitography, 469
GILLS score, 97
Gingivobuccal sulcus incision, 16
Glanuloplasty, 454
Glioma, 151
Gluteal muscles, bilateral V-to-Y
        advancement of, 194, 194f
Gluteus maximus myocutaneous flap, 194,
        194f
Gracilis muscle
    anatomy, 339, 339f
    harvest, 344–345, 345f
    inset, 345, 346f
Graft harvest, 322, 322f
Graft passage and completion, 323, 323f
Greater palatine artery, 77
Greater palatine vessels isolation, 91–92, 92f
Gynecomastia
    anatomy, 389, 389f–390f
    complications, 397
    definition, 389
    differential diagnosis, 391
    imaging, 391
    merits and demerits, 396b
    natural history, 390, 390f
    nonoperative management, 391
    outcomes, 396, 397f
    pathogenesis, 389–390
    patient history and physical findings,
        390–391
    postoperative care, 396
    surgical management, 391–392
        approach, 392
        patient position, 392
        preoperative planning, 391

H

Halitosis, palatal fistula, 110
Hard palate repair, 65–66, 66f
Hearing, 24
Hemangioma(s), 165–166
Hemangioma resection of, nasal tip heman-
        gioma, 296, 296f
Hematoma
    auricular, 489
    to prevent reaccumulation of, 302f
Hemifacial microsomia, 135
Hemitransfixion incision, 301
Hemostasis, emergency room anesthesia,
        483
Hepatobiliary tree, conjoined twins, 501
Heterotopic ossification (HO), 171
Horner syndrome, 256, 355
Human bites, 480
Hypernasal speech, 113
Hypertelorism, 151
Hypertrophic scars, 171, 212
Hypervascularity, 158
Hypogastric plexiform tumor, 161, 162f
Hypoplasia, 23
Hypoplastic medial/lateral lip element,
        56–57, 56f–57f
Hypospadias
    anatomy, 447
    complications, 456
    definition, 447
    imaging, 447

merits and demerits, 455b
nonoperative management, 448
outcomes, 456
pathogenesis, 447
patient history and physical findings, 447
postoperative care, 455–456
prevalence of, 447
repair, algorithm for, 449f
surgical management, 448
    approach, 448, 449f
    patient position, 448
    preoperative planning, 448

I

Incomplete clefts, 12
Inflatable orbital expanders, 288, 289f
Infraorbital nerve, 46
Infraorbital rim, 130f
Injectable fillers, 287
Inner preputial inlay graft, 451, 452f
Inner preputial skin flap, 453, 454f
Integumentary system, conjoined twins, 502
Intense pulsed light (IPL) device, 208, 208f
Internal/endoscopic dacryocystorhinostomy,
        279, 279f
Intranasal glioma
    endoscopic excision of, 156, 156f
    pathogenesis, 151
Intravelar veloplasty, Z-plasty with,
        72–73
Introitoplasty, 460–461, 460f, 461f
Inverted-T excision, 61–62, 62f
IPL (intense pulsed light) device, 208, 208f
Ischial pressure injury, 193, 199, 199f
    debridement with gluteal rotation flap,
        194, 194f
    V-Y advancement flap for, 193, 193f
Ischiopagus conjoined twins, 498,
        503–506, 503f–504f. See also
        Conjoined twins

J

Joseph Periosteal Elevator, 105
Juvenile breast hypertrophy
    anatomy, 398, 399f
    complications, 406
    definition, 398
    differential diagnosis, 399
    imaging, 399
    merits and demerits, 405b
    natural history, 398
    nonoperative management, 400
    outcomes, 406
    pathogenesis, 398
    patient history and physical findings,
        398–399
    postoperative care, 406
    surgical management, 400–402
        patient position, 401–402, 401f
        preoperative planning, 400–401,
            400f–401f

K

Kaposiform hemangioendothelioma, 165
Ketamine, 483
Keystone osteotomy, 153–154, 154f
Kidney ureter bladder radiograph (KUB),
        428

L

L flap
on lateral lip element, 14f–15f, 15
suturing, 16
Labia, 468
Labial mucosal flap, palatal fistula, 106, 106f
Labioplasty, 459, 464, 464f, 477, 477f
Laceration closure techniques, 484–485, 485f
Lacrimal sump syndrome, 282
Laser burn scar revision. *See* Burn injury
Laser handpiece, 208f
Laser treatment, of vascular lesions, 208, 208f
Lateral canthoplasty, 270f–271f, 271–273
creation, 271–273, 272f
suturing, 273, 273f
Lateral lip elements
anatomy, 12
hypoplastic, 56–57, 56f–57f
Millard/Mohler modifications
alar base and L flap, 14, 14f–15f
dissection, 15–16, 16f
markings, 13, 14f–15f
Lateral mucosa fullness, 54, 55f
Lateral nasolabial element
matching nasolabial lengths, 6–8, 8f
nasal sill, 6, 7f
Nordhoff point, 6, 7f
Lateral tarsal strip. *See* Lateral canthoplasty
Latham device, 36
Latissimus dorsi muscle transfer, 368–369, 368f, 385–386, 385f
Lenticular excision and linear closure, 166b
Levator resection, congenital ptosis, 259, 259f–260f
Levator veli palatini (LVP), 78, 93
Levobupivacaine
furlow palatoplasty, 70
hard palate incisions, 82
Lidocaine, 271, 483
Limited preauricular approach, 327, 328f
Lip adhesion
anatomy, 35
bilateral cleft lip adhesion, 39–40, 39f–40f
complications, 41
definition, 35
merits and demerits, 41b
nonoperative management, 36
outcomes, 41
patient history and physical findings, 35–36
postoperative care, 41
premaxillary setback, 40–41, 40f
surgical management, 36–41
approach, 36–41
patient position, 36
preoperative planning, 36
unilateral cleft lip adhesion
completion, 39, 39f
incision and dissection, 37, 38f
markings, 37, 37f
suturing, 37–39, 38f
Lip closure
cutaneous approximation, 10
Millard/Mohler modifications, 18–19, 19f
muscle repair, 9–10, 9f

Lip contracture, 172, 172f–173f
Lip element
lateral, Millard/Mohler modifications
alar base and L flap, 14, 14f–15f
anatomy, 12
dissection, 15–16, 16f
markings, 13, 14f–15f
medial, Millard/Mohler modifications
anatomy, 12
C flap and M flap, 14, 14f–15f
dissection, 8, 8f, 15, 16f
markings, 13, 14f–15f
Lip lacerations, 487, 487f
Lip lengthening, skin flap for, 29–30, 29f
Lip pits, 60–62
acellular dermal allograft, 62, 62f
inverted-T excision, 61–62, 62f
split lip advancement technique, 61, 61f
transverse elliptical excision, 60, 61f
vertical elliptical wedge excision, 60, 61f
LipiVage, 218, 218f
Lip-nose adhesion, 37
Liposuction, 393, 393f
LLC (lower lateral cartilage), 10, 120
Lower extremity, rotationplasty of
anatomy, 376, 376f
complications, 382
definition, 376
imaging, 376
merits and demerits, 381b
outcomes, 381–382
patient history and physical findings, 376
postoperative care, 381, 381f
surgical management, 377
approach, 377, 377f
patient position, 377
preoperative planning, 377
Lower lateral cartilage (LLC), 10, 120
Lower lateral cartilage reconstruction, 296
Lower lid reconstruction, eyelids, 184
Lumenis UltraPulse fractional CO2 laser, 214f
LVP (levator veli palatini), 78, 93
Lymphatic malformations (LM), 204–205

M

M flap, on medial lip element, 14–15, 14f–15f
Macrocystic lymphatic malformation, 166, 205
Macrostomia, 135
Macrostomia repair, Tessier 7
anatomy, 135, 135f
complications, 140
cutaneous scar modifications, 139, 139f
definition, 135
imaging, 136
merits and demerits, 139t
natural history, 135
outcomes, 140
pathogenesis, 135
patient history and physical findings, 135–136
postoperative care, 140
surgical management, 136
approach, 136
patient position, 136
preoperative planning, 136

vermilion-shifted commissuroplasty with optional cutaneous Z-plasty
commissuroplasty and skin closure, 138, 139f
design, 137, 138f
dissection and orbicularis repair, 137–138, 138f
markings, 137, 137f
Magnetic resonance imaging (MRI), 499
Malignant peripheral nerve sheath tumors (MPNST), 158–159
Mallet scale, 355
Mandibular distraction osteogenesis, 97
Marcaine, palatal fistula, 104
Marcus Gunn jaw-winking ptosis, 256
Margin reflex distance (MRD), 256
Masseter for innervation, of free muscle flap
anatomy, 325, 325f
complications, 329
definition, 325
imaging, 326
merits and demerits, 328b
outcomes, 328–329
pathogenesis, 325
patient history and physical findings, 325–326
postoperative care, 328
surgical management
approach, 326
patient position, 326, 326f
preoperative planning, 326
Masseter-to-facial nerve transfer
anatomy, 330–331, 330f
antegrade, with distal, selective, facial nerve branch transection, 334–335, 335f
complications, 337
with cross face nerve grafts, 336, 336f
definition, 330
with fascia lata grafts, 336
imaging, 331
merits and demerits, 336b
outcomes, 337
pathogenesis, 331
patient history and physical findings, 331
postoperative care, 336–337
retrograde, 332–333, 332f, 333f, 334f
surgical management
approach, 332
patient position, 331–332, 331f
preoperative planning, 331
Mattress sutures placement, in prominent ears, 244, 245f
Maxilla, anatomy, 12, 13f
Mechanical ptosis, 256
Medial inframalleolar perforator flap, 200, 201f
Medial lip element
anatomy, 12
dissection, 6f, 8
hypoplastic, 56–57, 56f–57f
Millard/Mohler modifications
C flap and M flap, 14, 14f–15f
dissection, 15, 16f
markings, 13, 14f–15f
Medial nasolabial element
measurements and interpositional triangle, 4, 5f
vermilion, Cupid's bow, and nose, 3–4, 4f

Medial orbit composite unit translocation, 155–156, 155f
Meningocele, 151
Meningoencephalocele, 151
Mental nerve neurofibromatosis, 162, 163f
Meticulous hemostasis, 180
Microform clefts, 12
Microphthalmos
  anatomy, 283
  complications, 291
  definition, 283
  diagnostic studies, 284
  imaging, 284
  merits and demerits, 290b
  natural history, 283, 284f
  nonoperative management, 284–285, 284f–287f
  outcomes, 291
  pathogenesis, 283
  patient history and physical findings, 283–284
  surgical management, 286
Microtia, auricular reconstruction for
  anatomy, 221, 221f, 222f
  anesthesia, 223
  complications, 225f, 226
  definition, 221
  framework, 221f, 222f, 223–224
  graft harvest, 223
  markings, 223
  merits and demerits, 225b
  outcomes, 224f, 226
  pathogenesis, 221
  patient history and physical findings, 221–222
  patient transfer, 224
  postoperative care, 225
  second stage, 225, 225f
  surgical management, 222–223, 222f, 223f
  variable presentation of, 221f
Midface rotation advancement, 127, 133f
Midshaft hypospadias repair
  inner preputial inlay graft, 451, 452f
  transverse preputial island flap, 451
Minor clefts, 12
Mixed dentation stage, 32f
MMC. See Myelomeningocele (MMC)
Modified Hotz technique, markings and incisions, 266, 266f, 267f
Modified Sistrunk procedure
  hyoid and tongue base dissection, 313–315, 314f
  modifications, 315, 315f
  neck and wound incision preparation, 313, 313f
  thyroglossal cyst and tract exposure, 313, 314f
  wound closure, 315, 315f
Mohler back cut, 14–15, 14f–15f
Monfort approach, prune belly, 429–430, 430f
Monsplasty, 459, 464, 464f
Motor nerve branch, 333, 333f
MPNST (malignant peripheral nerve sheath tumors), 158–159
MRD (margin reflex distance), 256
MRI (magnetic resonance imaging), 499

Mucosa
  closure, Millard/Mohler modifications, 16–17, 17f–18f
  deformities, 54–58
  repair, 51
  Z-plasty, 57
Mucosal flaps, 65
Mulliken technique, 45
Muscles, 2
  repair during lip closure, 9–10
Muscular dehiscence, 51
Musculoskeletal system, conjoined twins, 502
Mustardé's radiated suture techniques, 243f
Myelomeningocele (MMC)
  postnatal repair
    anatomy, 413, 413f
    definition, 413
    merits and demerits, 417b
    natural history, 413
    pathogenesis, 413
    patient history and physical findings, 413–414, 414f
    postoperative care, 417
    surgical management, 414, 415f
  prenatal repair
    anatomy, 418, 418f
    definition, 418
    evaluation, 418, 419t
    merits and demerits, 421b
    natural history, 418
    pathogenesis, 418
    postoperative care, 422
    surgical management, 418–419

N
NAM (nasoalveolar molding), 12–13, 24, 36
Nanophthalmos, 283
Nasal air emission, 113
Nasal conformers, 41
Nasal dermoid sinus cyst (NDSC)
  anatomy, 150
  definition, 150
  natural history, 151
  patient history and physical findings, 151
  transcranial NDSC resection
    bandeau/frontal bone repair, 154
    completion, 154
    cranial base repair and seal, 154, 155f
    incisions, dissection, and craniotomy, 153, 154f
    keystone osteotomy and dermal sinus excision, 153–154, 154f
    nasal approach/frozen biopsy, 153–154, 153f
Nasal dissection, Millard/Mohler modifications, 17–18, 18f
Nasal floor closure, 16, 17f–18f
Nasal lacerations, 487
Nasal layer, two-flap palatoplasty
  closure, 93
  mucoperiosteum dissection, 92–93, 93f
Nasal mucosa, von Langenbeck palatoplasty
  closure, 78, 78f
  dissection, 77
Nasal prosthesis implants, 494, 494f

Nasal septal hematoma
  anatomy, 299, 299f–300f
  complications, 303
  definition, 299
  differential diagnosis, 300
  imaging, 300
  merits and demerits, 303b
  natural history, 300
  nonoperative management
  outcomes, 303
  pathogenesis, 299
  patient history and physical findings, 300
  postoperative care, 303
  surgical management, 301
    approach, 301
    patient position, 301
    preoperative planning, 301
Nasal sill, 6
Nasal structures, dissection, 8–9
Nasal subunit approach, 295, 295f
Nasal tip, 23
Nasal tip hemangioma
  anatomy, 293
  complications, 298
  definition, 293
  differential diagnosis, 294
  imaging, 294
  merits and demerits, 297b
  natural history, 293
  nonoperative management, 294, 294f
  outcomes, 298, 298f
  pathogenesis, 293
  patient history and physical findings, 293–294, 293f
  postoperative care, 297
  surgical management, 294–297
    approach, 294–297
    patient position, 294
    preoperative planning, 294
Nasendoscopy, 113
Nasoalveolar molding (NAM), 12–13, 24, 36
Nasolabial element
  lateral
    dissection, 8f, 9
    repair, 6–8, 7f, 8f
  medial, repair, 3–4, 4f, 5f
Nasolacrimal duct obstruction (NLDO)
  anatomy, 276, 276f
  complications
    intraoperative, 281
    postoperative, 281–282
  definition, 276
  differential diagnosis, 277
  imaging, 277
  merits and demerits, 281b
  outcomes, 281
  pathogenesis, 276
  patient history and physical findings, 276–277
  postoperative care, 281
  surgical management, 277–278, 278f
    patient position, 278
    preoperative planning, 278
Nasolacrimal stents, 279–280
Nasopharyngoscopy, 103
NBPP. See Neonatal brachial plexus palsy (NBPP)

NCM (neurocutaneous melanosis), 141
NDSC. *See* Nasal dermoid sinus cyst (NDSC)
Neck contracture
  anatomy, 186
  complications, 188
  definition, 186
  imaging, 186
  incision for, 187f
  merits and demerits, 188b
  natural history and progression, 186
  nonoperative management, 186
  outcomes, 188
  pathogenesis, 186
  patient history and physical findings, 186
  postoperative care, 188
  surgical management, 186–187
    patient position, 187
    preoperative planning, 187
Neonatal brachial plexus palsy (NBPP)
  anatomy, 354, 354f, 364
  complications, 363, 374
  definition, 354, 364
  diagnostic studies, 356
  differential diagnosis, 356
  imaging, 356, 364, 365f
  merits and demerits, 362b, 372b
  natural history, 355
  nonoperative management, 356, 364
  outcomes, 362–363, 374
  pathogenesis, 354–355, 364
  patient history and physical findings, 355, 364
  postoperative care, 362
    elbow reconstruction, 373
    forearm reconstruction, 373
    wrist/fingers reconstruction, 373–374
  surgical management, 356, 364–365
    approach, 357, 365
    patient position, 357, 357f, 365
    preoperative planning, 356–357, 365
Neophiltrum, 46
Neovagina construction
  graft substrates and techniques, 461–462, 461f
  pedicled flap techniques
    pudendal thigh flaps, 463, 463f
    sigmoid colon, 462–463, 462f–463f
    perineal dissection, 460f, 461
Nerve branch, 333, 334f
Nerve grafting, neuroma resection with, 359, 359f
Nerve mobilization, 322, 322f
Nerve to masseter
  anatomy, 338–339, 339f
  identification, 342, 343f
Nerve transfer
  accessory to suprascapular, 360, 360f
  intercostal to musculocutaneous, 361, 361f
  radial to axillary, 361–362, 362f
  ulnar to musculocutaneous, 360, 360f
Nerve-sparing ventral clitoroplasty (NSVC), 473
Neurocutaneous melanosis (NCM), 141
Neurofibromatosis (NF)
  anatomy, 158, 159f
  breast and chest wall plexiform, 162, 162f

definition, 158
differential diagnosis, 159
hypogastric plexiform tumor, 161, 162f
imaging, 159
inferior orbital nerve tumor, 161, 161f
left orbital and mental nerve, 162, 163f
merits and demerits, 163t
natural history, 158–159
nonoperative management, 159
orbital, 158
pathogenesis, 158
patient history and physical findings, 159
plexiform, 158
postoperative care, 164
principles, 161
surgical management, 159–160
  approach, 160, 160f
  patient position, 160
  preoperative planning, 160
Neuroma resection, with nerve grafting, 359, 359f
Nevus excision with expanded flap reconstruction
  approach, 146, 146f
  closure, 148, 148f
  excision, 147f, 149b
  incision, 146b, 146f–147f
  merits and demerits, 149t
  patient position, 145
  postoperative care, 149
  preoperative planning, 145
  suturing, 148, 148f
NLDO. *See* Nasolacrimal duct obstruction (NLDO)
Noordhoff's vermilion flap technique, 30, 30f
Nordhoff point, 6, 7f
Nose, 3–4, 4f
  anatomy, 2, 12, 13f
  repair, Salyer unilateral cleft lip/nose repair, 24
Nose deformity. *See* Salyer unilateral cleft lip/nose repair
Nostril apex elevation, 19, 20f
Nostril correction, 123
Nostril floor, 19, 19f
NSVC (nerve-sparing ventral clitoroplasty), 473

O
Obstructive sleep apnea, palatal fistula, 110
Occlusion, 34f
Omphalocele
  complications, 435
  definition, 432
  diagnostic studies, 432
  differential diagnosis, 432
  imaging, 432
  merits and demerits, 435b
  patient history and physical findings, 432, 433f
  postoperative care, 435
  surgical management
    patient position, 433
    preoperative planning, 433
Omphalopagus, 498

Open abdomen. *See* Abdominal wall
Open cleft lip rhinoplasty
  incision and dissection, 122, 122f
  shape correction, 122–123, 122f
Open tip rhinoplasty approach, 295, 295f
Oral mucosa, 17, 17f–18f
  two-flap palatoplasty
    closure, 93–94
    oral mucoperiosteal flaps elevation, 91, 91f
  von Langenbeck palatoplasty
    closure, 79, 79f
    dissection, 77
    oral mucoperiosteal flaps elevation, 76, 76f
Oral propranolol, 206
Orbicularis
  epair, 137–138, 138f
  oris, 2, 12, 18, 22, 27, 35, 53
Orbital nerve neurofibromatosis, 162, 163f
  inferior, 161, 161f
Orbital prosthesis implants, 495, 495f
Orbital tissue injury, 281
Orofacial clefting, 23, 74, 89
Osseointegration, 490, 491f
Osteotomies, 379, 379f
Otoplasty grid, 243f

P
Palatal fistula
  anatomy, 102, 102f
  buccal myomucosal flap, 106–107, 106f
  complications, 110
  conversion by Furlow palatoplasty, 105
  definition, 102
  differential diagnosis, 103
  excision and reapproximation, 104
  facial artery musculomucosal flap, 107, 107f
  free tissue transfer, 109, 109f
  imaging, 103
  labial mucosal flap, 106, 106f
  lateral relaxing incisions and rerepair
    Pittsburgh type II fistula, 104–105
    Pittsburgh type III fistula, 105
    Pittsburgh type IV fistula, 105
    preparation, 104, 105f
  merits and demerits, 110t
  natural history, 102
  nonoperative management, 103
  outcomes, 110
  pathogenesis, 102
  patient history and physical findings, 102–103
  posterior pharyngeal flap, 105
  postoperative care, 110
  premaxillary turnover flap, 108–109, 109f
  surgical management, 103–104
    approach, 104
    patient position, 104
    preoperative planning, 104
  tongue flap, 108, 108f
Palate repair, delayed hard. *See* Delayed hard palate repair
Palatopharyngeal disproportion, 112

Palatoplasty, 33f
  Sommerlad palatoplasty
    anatomy, 81
    approach, surgical management, 82, 82f
    complications, 88
    definition, 81
    hard palate, 82–84, 82f–83f
    imaging, 81
    merits and demerits, 88t
    nasal layer, 84–85, 85f–86f, 87
    oral layer, 84, 84f
    outcomes, 88
    patient history and physical findings, 81
    patient position, 82
    postoperative care, 88
    preoperative planning, 81–82
  two-flap palatoplasty (See Two-flap
    palatoplasty)
  von Langenbeck palatoplasty (See Von
    Langenbeck palatoplasty)
Palatoplasty, furlow. See Furlow palatoplasty
Palmar burns, 178
Parotid duct injury, 488, 488f
Pars alaris, 2
Pars marginalis muscle, 22
Pars superficialis, 22
Partial urogenital mobilization (PUM), 474,
  474f
PAS (projected adult size), 141, 142t
PDL. See Pulsed dye laser (PDL)
Pectus carinatum
  complications, 412
  definition, 407
  diagnosis studies, 407
  differential diagnosis, 407
  imaging, 407
  open ravitch procedure for, 411
  outcomes, 411–412
  patient history and physical findings, 407
  postoperative care, 411
  surgical management, 408
Pectus excavatum
  complications, 412
  definition, 407
  diagnosis studies, 407
  differential diagnosis, 407
  imaging, 407
  minimally invasive approach for
    closure, 408
    endoscopic bar placement, 408, 409f
    positioning and incision, 408
  open ravitch procedure for
    abnormal ribs exposure and resection,
      409–410, 410f
    closure, 411
    positioning and incisions, 409, 410f
    sternal closure, 410–411
  outcomes, 411–412
  patient history and physical findings, 407
  postoperative care, 411
  surgical management, 408
Pediatric facial reanimation
  anatomy
    facial nerve, 338, 339f
    gracilis muscle, 339, 339f
    nerve to masseter, 338–339, 339f
  complications, 347
  definition, 338, 338t

  imaging, 340
  merits and demerits, 346b
  nonoperative management, 340
  outcomes, 347, 347f
  patient history and physical findings,
    339–340, 339f
  postoperative care, 346–347
  surgical management, 340–341
    approach, 341, 341f
    patient position, 341
    preoperative planning, 340–341
Periareolar skin reduction, 394–395, 394f
Perineum, 469
Peroneal nerve, 378, 378f
Pharyngeal flap
  pharyngoplasty, 113
  posterior
    dissection, 116–117, 117f
    markings, 116, 117f
  stenting of reconstructed ports, 118
Pharyngeal wall augmentation, 113
Pharyngoplasty, dynamic sphincter. See
  Dynamic sphincter pharyngoplasty
Phenylephrine test, congenital ptosis, 256
Philtral column, 12
Philtrum, 4
Pierre Robin sequence (PRS)
  anatomy, 96, 96f
  complications, 100
  definition, 96
  imaging, 96
  merits and demerits, 100t
  natural history, 96
  nonoperative management, 96–97
  outcomes, 100
  pathogenesis, 96
  patient history and physical findings, 96
  postoperative care, 100
  subperiosteal release, mouth floor
    incision, 98, 98f
    tongue and lip flaps, 97, 97f
    tongue closure and tensioning, 98–99,
      99f
    tongue suspension suture placement,
      98, 99f
  surgical management
    approach, 97
    patient position, 97
    preoperative planning, 97
Piriform aperture incision, 15
Pitkin solution, 176
Pittsburgh fistula classification, 102, 102f,
  104
  type I fistula, 103
  type II fistula, 103–105
  type III fistula, 103, 105
  type IV fistula, 103, 105
  type V fistula, 103
  type VI and VII fistula, 104
Placode dissection, 415, 415f
Placode release, 420, 420f
Plexiform neurofibromatosis, 158
  breast, 162, 162f
  chest wall, 162, 162f
Pocket dissection, microtia, auricular reconstruction for, 223
Poland syndrome
  anatomy, 383, 383f

  complications, 387
  definition, 383
  differential diagnosis, 384
  imaging, 384
  merits and demerits, 387b
  natural history, 383–384
  nonoperative management, 384
  outcomes, 387, 387f
  pathogenesis, 383
  patient history and physical findings, 384
  postoperative care, 387
  surgical management, 384–385
    approach, 385
    patient position, 385
    preoperative planning, 384–385, 385f
Polysomnogram, 96
Port creation, 217, 218f
Port-wine stain (PWS), 204–207
Postadjuvant antiangiogenesis therapy, 209
Postpalatoplasty, 112
Post-traumatic deformity, auricular recon-
    struction for
  anatomy, 221, 221f, 222f
  anesthesia, 223
  auricular framework, 221f, 222f, 223–224
  complications, 225f, 226
  definition, 221
  graft harvest, 223
  markings, 223
  merits and demerits, 225b
  outcomes, 224f, 226
  pathogenesis, 221
  patient history and physical findings,
    221–222
  patient transfer, 224
  postoperative care, 225
  second stage, 225, 225f
  surgical management, 222–223, 222f,
    223f
Premaxillary turnover flap, 108–109, 109f
Pressure injury
  anatomy, 196
  complications, 195, 203
  definition, 192, 196
  diagnostic studies, 192
  imaging, 192, 197
  merits and demerits, 195b, 203b
  natural history, 192, 196–197
  nonoperative management, 192–193, 197
  outcomes, 195, 203
  pathogenesis, 192, 196
  patient history and physical findings, 192,
    197
  postoperative care, 195, 203
  surgical management, 193–194, 197–198
    approach, 198
    patient position, 193–194, 198
    preoperative planning, 193, 197–198
Presurgical infant orthopedics (PSIO), 35–36
Prilocaine, 206
Projected adult size (PAS), 141, 142t
Prominent ears
  anatomy, 242, 242f
  complications, 246
  definition, 242
  differential diagnosis, 242
  merits and demerits, 245b
  nonoperative management, 242

Prominent ears (*Continued*)
outcomes, 244f–245f, 246
pathogenesis, 242
patient history and physical findings, 242
postoperative care, 246
surgical management, 242–243
approach, 243, 243f
patient position, 243, 243f
prediction of projection reduction, 242–243
preoperative planning, 242, 242f–243f
Propeller flap, 202, 202f
Proximal hypospadias repair, 452, 452f
PRS. *See* Pierre Robin sequence (PRS)
Prune belly
complications, 431
definition, 428, 428f
diagnostic studies, 428
differential diagnosis, 428
imaging, 428
merits and demerits, 431b
patient history and physical findings, 428
postoperative care, 431
surgical management, 429, 429f
Pseudoptosis, 256
PSIO (presurgical infant orthopedics), 35–36
Ptosis, congenital, 159
Pulsatile exophthalmos, 163f
Pulsed dye laser (PDL), 207, 207t
anesthesia, 213
application, 213, 213f
wound care, 213
PUM (partial urogenital mobilization), 474, 474f
"Pumpkin-teeth" flaps, 444, 444f–445f
Punctum, 126f
Puregraft, 218, 218f
PWS (port-wine stain), 204–207
Pygopagus, 498
Pyogenic granuloma, 165

R
Radiographic fistulograms, 103
Recipient site preparation, 343–344, 343f
Red lip, 2
Redo hypospadias repair, buccal mucosa graft for, 454–455
Reduction labioplasty
hybrid approach, 466, 466f
simple excision and closure, 465, 465f
wedge excision with advancement, 465, 465f
Respiratory system, conjoined twins, 501
Retrograde masseter-to-facial nerve transfer, 332–333, 332f, 333f, 334f
Rhinoplasty, secondary cleft. *See* Secondary cleft rhinoplasty
Rigid spherical orbital implants, 287, 287f–290f
Rigotomy, 217
Ring-Adair-Elwyn (RAE) tube, 44, 45f
Robin sequence, 73, 81
Rose-Thompson effect, 4, 5f
Rotationplasty, of lower extremity
anatomy, 376, 376f
complications, 382
definition, 376

imaging, 376
merits and demerits, 381b
outcomes, 381–382
patient history and physical findings, 376
postoperative care, 381, 381f
surgical management, 377
approach, 377, 377f
patient position, 377
preoperative planning, 377
Rotation/reconstruction, distal limb, 379, 380f
Rotterdam/extended L rhinotomy approach, 296

S
Sacral pressure injury, 193, 199, 199f
Sacrococcygeal teratoma (SCT), 425
anatomy, 423
complications, 427
debulking, 425, 426f
definition, 423
differential diagnosis, 423
imaging, 423, 423f–424f
merits and demerits, 427b
outcomes, 427
pathogenesis, 423
postoperative care, 427
surgical management, 424, 424f
Salyer unilateral cleft lip/nose repair
anatomy
abnormal cleft lip/nose, 22–23
normal upper lip, 22
anterior palate, Abyholm closure of, 30, 31f
complications, 32
definition, 22
differential diagnosis, 24
imaging, 24
lateral lip element elevation, 27
marking, 25–27, 26f–29f
medial lip incision, 27
merits and demerits, 32t
muscle repair, 24
natural history, 23
nonoperative management, 24
Noordhoff's vermilion flap technique, 30, 30f
nose repair, 24
outcomes, 32, 32f–34f
pathogenesis, 23
patient history and physical findings, 24
postoperative care, 32
skin flap for lip lengthening, 29–30, 29f
surgical management, 24–25
approach, 25
patient position, 25
preoperative planning, 24–25
Scalp lacerations, 485, 485f
Scarring
of lip, 41
of ostium, 282
Sciatic nerve, 378, 378f
Scoliosis, 158
SCT. *See* Sacrococcygeal teratoma (SCT)
Secondary cleft rhinoplasty
anatomy, 120
complications, 124
definition, 120

dorsal correction, 123
imaging, 121
merits and demerits, 124b
nasal framework correction, 123
nostril correction, 123
open cleft lip rhinoplasty
incision and dissection, 122, 122f
shape correction, 122–123, 122f
outcomes, 124
patient history and physical findings, 120–121, 120t, 121t
postoperative care, 124
surgical management, 121
approach, 121
patient position, 121
preoperative planning, 121
tip and ala, reshaping, 123
Secondary deformities, of lip and nose
Abbe flap, 58–59, 58f–59f
anatomy, 50
complications, 63
Cupid's bow, 51b, 51f
asymmetry more than 2 mm high, 53, 53f–54f
mismatch of 1 to 2 mm, 52, 52f
definition, 50
lip pits, 60–62
acellular dermal allograft, 62, 62f
inverted-T excision, 61–62, 62f
split lip advancement technique, 61, 61f
transverse elliptical excision, 60, 61f
vertical elliptical wedge excision, 60, 61f
merits and demerits, 62b
outcomes, 63
pathogenesis, 50
patient history and physical findings, 50
postoperative care, 63
surgical management
approach, 50–51
patient position, 50
preoperative planning, 50
vermilion and mucosa, 54–58
hypoplastic medial/lateral lip element, 56–57, 56f–57f
lateral mucosa fullness, 54, 55f
notch in free edge, 57–58, 57f
red line malalignment, 54
Septum, 23
anatomy, 12, 13f
reconstruction, 301–302, 302f
Short scar periareolar inferior pedicle (SPAIR) technique, 401
closure, 404–405, 405f
flap creation, 402, 403f
incisions, 402, 402f
shaping, 402, 403f
skin plication, 404, 404f
Sialocele, 489
Siamese twins, 500
Skin closure, 297, 297f
prune belly, 430, 430f
Stahl ear, 230
Skin flap dissection
cryptotia, 240
prominent ears, 244
Skin flap transposition, cryptotia, 240

Skin grafts harvest
    advantages, 175
    anatomy, 175
    definition, 175
    full-thickness skin grafts, 175
        harvesting of, 177
    merits and demerits, 177t
    natural history, 175
    postoperative care, 177
    prognosis, 175
    split-thickness skin grafts, 175–177, 176f, 177f
    surgical management, 175
Skin necrosis, 241
Skin release and mobilization, 415, 415f, 421
Skin resection, 297, 297f
Skull base fracture, 281
SLAT (split lip advancement technique), 61, 61f
SMAS flap, 321, 321f, 332–333
Soft palate repair, 65, 65f
Sommerlad palatoplasty
    anatomy, 81
    complications, 88
    definition, 81
    hard palate
        incisions and dissection, 82–83, 82f–83f
        nasal layer elevation, 83–84, 83f
        von Langenbeck incisions, 84, 84f
    imaging, 81
    merits and demerits, 88t
    nasal layer, 84, 85f
        closure, 87, 87f
        muscle dissection, 85, 85f–86f
    oral layer, 84, 84f
    outcomes, 88
    patient history and physical findings, 81
    postoperative care, 88
    surgical management
        approach, 82, 82f
        patient position, 82
        preoperative planning, 81–82
Speech problems, 88
Speech therapy, velopharyngeal insufficiency, 113
Sphenoid greater wing, 158
Sphincter pharyngoplasty, dynamic. See Dynamic sphincter pharyngoplasty
Split lip advancement technique (SLAT), 61, 61f
Split-thickness skin grafts, 175
    harvesting of, 176–177, 176f, 177f
Stahl ear
    anatomy, 227, 227f
    complications, 231
    definition, 227
    excision and suturing, 229, 229f–230f
    merits and demerits, 230b
    nonoperative management, 227
    outcomes, 231, 231f
    pathogenesis, 227
    patient history and physical findings, 227
    postoperative care, 231
    preoperative assessment, 228f
    surgical management, 227–231, 228f
        approach, 227–231, 228f–229f
        patient position, 227
        preoperative planning, 227, 228f

Stair-step incisions, 317–318, 317f
Standard preauricular approach, 326–327, 327f
Stapedial artery, 135
Steindler flexorplasty, 367–368, 367f
Stenstrom-type anterior scoring, 243
Steri-Strips, 41
Straightline cleft palate repair. See Sommerlad palatoplasty
Stryker-Leibinger, 28
Sturge-Weber syndrome (SWS), 205
Subcision cannula, 217, 218f
Submucous cleft palate, 68
    velopharyngeal insufficiency, 112
Sural nerve harvest
    anatomy, 317
    coaptation, 352, 352f
    complications, 318
    definition, 317
    dissection, 351, 351f
    identification, 350, 350f
    imaging, 317
    merits and demerits, 318b
    outcomes, 318
    patient history and physical findings, 317
    postoperative care, 318
    surgical management
        approach, 317
        patient position, 317
        preoperative planning, 317
    tunneling, 350–352, 350f, 351f
Suture closure techniques, 485f
Syndromic cleft palate, 75

T
Tanzer constricted ear classification, 232f
Tarsomarginal graft, eyelid coloboma, 251–252, 251f
Tendon stripper, harvest with, 318
Tensor veli palatini (TVP), 93
Tenzel semicircular flap, eyelid coloboma, 250–251, 250f–251f
Teratogen exposure, 2
Tessier 3 and 4 clefts
    anatomy, 125, 126f
    complications, 134
    definition, 125, 125f
    dissection and facial flap elevation, 129–130, 129f–130f
    eyelid correction, 130, 130f
    facial musculature repositioning, 131, 131f–132f
    imaging, 126, 127f
    incisions, 128, 128f
    markings, 128, 128f
    merits and demerits, 132t
    outcomes, 132–133, 133f
    patient history and physical findings, 125
    postoperative care, 132
    surgical management, 126–127
        approach, 126
        patient position, 127
        preoperative planning, 127
Tessier 7—macrostomia repair
    anatomy, 135, 135f
    complications, 140
    cutaneous scar modifications, 139, 139f
    definition, 135

imaging, 136
    merits and demerits, 139t
    natural history, 135
    outcomes, 140
    pathogenesis, 135
    patient history and physical findings, 135–136
    postoperative care, 140
    surgical management, 136
        approach, 136
        patient position, 136
        preoperative planning, 136
    vermilion-shifted commissuroplasty with optional cutaneous Z-plasty
        commissuroplasty and skin closure, 138, 139f
        design, 137, 138f
        dissection and orbicularis repair, 137–138, 138f
        markings, 137, 137f
TGDC. See Thyroglossal duct cysts (TGDC)
Thoracopagus, 498
Thumb reconstruction
    surgical management, 178–179
    Z-plasty, 179–180, 179f–180f
Thyroglossal duct cysts (TGDC)
    anatomy, 311, 311f
    complications, 316
    definition, 311
    differential diagnosis, 311
    exposure of, 313, 314f
    imaging, 311, 312f
    merits and demerits, 315b
    natural history, 311
    nonoperative management, 311–312
    outcomes, 316
    pathogenesis, 311, 312f
    patient history and physical findings, 311
    postoperative care, 316
    surgical management
        patient position, 312
        preoperative planning, 312
Tibial nerve, 378
TIP (tubularized incised plate) urethroplasty, 450–451, 450f–451f
Tissue expander placement
    approach, 144
    merits and demerits, 145t
    patient position, 144
    postoperative care, 145, 145f
    preoperative planning, 143–144
    technique, 144b
Tissue expansion with implants, 385
Tongue flap (anteriorly based), 108, 108f
Tongue-lip adhesion. See Pierre Robin sequence (PRS)
Topical antibiotics, 209
Topical liposomal lidocaine, 206
Topical tetracaine, 249, 252, 264, 267, 271
Topical timolol, 206
Toronto Test Score, 355
Total urogenital mobilization (TUM), 474, 474f
TPIF (transverse preputial island flap), 451
Transcanalicular diode laser, 278
TransCyte double-layer dressing, 175
Transverse elliptical excision, lip pits, 60, 61f
Transverse mucosal resection, 168, 168f

Transverse preputial island flap (TPIF), 451
Traumatic ptosis, 256
Trichiasis, 277
Trochanteric pressure injury, 199, 199f
Tubularization, 454
Tubularized incised plate (TIP) urethroplasty, 450–451, 450f–451f
Tunica vaginis flap, 454
TVP (tensor veli palatini), 93
Two-flap palatoplasty
    anatomy, 89
    bilateral complete cleft palate, 94, 94f
    complications, 95
    definition, 89
    differential diagnosis, 89–90
    merits and demerits, 94t
    natural history, 89
    nonoperative management, 90
    outcomes, 95
    pathogenesis, 89
    patient history and physical findings, 89
    postoperative care, 95
    surgical management, 90
        approach, 90
        patient position, 90
        preoperative planning, 90
    for unilateral complete cleft palate
        greater palatine vessels isolation, 91–92, 92f
        markings, 91, 91f
        nasal closure, 93
        nasal mucoperiosteum dissection, 92–93, 93f
        oral closure, 93–94
        oral mucoperiosteal flaps elevation, 91, 91f
        velar musculature dissection and reconstruction, 93

U

Umbilical stenosis, after abdominoplasty, 446, 446f
Umbilicoplasty
    anatomy, 443, 443f–444f
    complications, 446
    definition, 443
    merits and demerits, 446b
    midline incision, 444–445, 444f–445f
    outcomes, 446
    patient history and physical findings, 443
    postoperative care, 446
    surgical management, 444
Umbilicus, 443
Unilateral cleft lip
    adhesion
        completion, 39, 39f
        incision and dissection, 37, 38f
        markings, 37, 37f
        suturing, 37–39, 38f
    nasal deformity, 121t
Unilateral cleft lip repair
    anatomy, 12, 13f
    clefting degree, 12
    complications, 21
    definition, 12
    imaging, 12
    merits and demerits, 20t
    Millard/Mohler modifications

incisions, 15
    lateral lip dissection, 15–16, 16f
    lip closure, 18–19, 19f
    markings, 13–15, 14f–15f
    medial lip dissection, 15, 16f
    mucosa closure, 16–17, 17f–18f
    nasal dissection, 17–18, 18f
    nasal refinement, 19–20, 20f
    outcomes, 21
    patient history and physical findings, 12
    postoperative care, 21
    surgical management, 12–13
        approach, 13
        patient position, 13
        preoperative planning, 13
Unilateral complete cleft palate, two-flap palatoplasty
    greater palatine vessels isolation, 91–92, 92f
    markings, 91, 91f
    nasal closure, 93
    nasal mucoperiosteum dissection, 92–93, 93f
    oral closure, 93–94
    oral mucoperiosteal flaps elevation, 91, 91f
    velar musculature dissection and reconstruction, 93
Upper eyelid, anatomy of, 255f
Upper lateral cartilage, 120
Upper lid reconstruction, eyelids, 184, 184f–185f
Upper lip, 12, 13f, 22
Urethral plate defect, bridging of, 453, 453f–454f
Urethral plate elevation, 472, 472f
Urinary tract, conjoined twins, 501
Urogenital sinus mobilization, 472, 472f
    perineal flap creation, 474, 474f
    reconstruction, 472, 472f
    TUM and PUM, 474, 474f
    use, 474–475, 475f

V

Vagina, 468
Vaginal agenesis, 458
Vaginal canal caliber, 460–461, 460f, 461f
Vaginal reconstruction
    anatomy, 458, 459f
    complications, 467
    definition, 458
    imaging, 459
    merits and demerits, 466b
    natural history, 458
    nonoperative management, 459
    outcomes, 467
    pathogenesis, 458
    patient history and physical findings, 458–459
    postoperative care, 466
    surgical management, 459–460, 460f
Vaginoplasty, 459–461, 460f, 461f
    anterior sagittal transrectal approach, 475–476, 476f
    high vaginal confluence, 475
    low vaginal confluence, 475, 475f
Van der Woude syndrome, 24
Vascular anomalies

anatomy, 165
    circular excision and purse-string closure, 167–168, 167f
    complications, 169
    definition, 165
    differential diagnosis, 165
    imaging, 165
    lenticular excision and linear closure, 166b
    merits and demerits, 169b
    natural history, 165
    nonoperative management, 165
    outcomes, 169
    patient history and physical findings, 165
    postoperative care, 169
    suction-assisted lipectomy, 168–169, 169f
    surgical management, 165–166
        approach, 166
        patient position, 166
        preoperative planning, 166
    transverse mucosal resection and linear closure, 168, 168f
Vascular lesions
    anatomy, 204
    complications, 209
    definition, 204
    imaging, 205–206
    laser treatment, 208, 208f
    merits and demerits, 209b
    natural history, 204
    nonoperative management, 206
    outcomes, 209
    pathogenesis, 204
    patient history and physical findings, 204–205, 205f
    postoperative care, 209
    surgical management, 206–208
        approach, 207–208, 207t, 208f
        patient position, 206–207
        preoperative planning, 206
Vascular malformations, 204
Vaseline gauze packing, 302
VCUG (voiding cystourethrography), 428, 469
Veau classification, of cleft palate, 74, 74f
Veau clefts, 102
Velar musculature, 78
    dissection and reconstruction, in two-flap palatoplasty, 93
Velopharyngeal dysfunction (VPD), 103
Velopharyngeal incompetence (VPI), 64
Velopharyngeal insufficiency (VPI)
    anatomy, 112
    complications, 119
    definition, 112
    diagnosis, 113
    differential diagnosis, 113
    dynamic sphincter pharyngoplasty
        dissection, 115, 116f
        markings, 115, 116f
    Furlow palatoplasty/double-opposing Z-plasty
        dissection, 114, 115f
        markings, 114, 114f
    imaging, 113
    merits and demerits, 118b
    natural history, 112
    nonoperative management, 113

outcomes, 119
pathogenesis, 112
patient history and physical findings, 113
posterior pharyngeal flap
    dissection, 116–117, 117f
    markings, 116, 117f
postoperative care, 118–119
surgical management, 113–114
    approach, 113
    patient position, 114
    preoperative planning, 114
Veloplasty, Z-plasty with, 72–73
Venous malformations (VM), 204–205
Vermilion, 3–4, 4f, 46
    abnormalities of, 54–58
        hypoplastic medial/lateral lip element,
            56–57, 56f–57f
        lateral mucosa fullness, 54, 55f
        notch in free edge, 57–58, 57f
        red line malalignment, 54
Vermilion flap, 137
Vermilion-shifted commissuroplasty
    commissuroplasty and skin closure, 138,
        139f
    design, 137, 138f
    dissection and orbicularis repair, 137–138,
        138f
    markings, 137, 137f
Vertical elliptical wedge excision, lip pits,
    60, 61f
Vestibular web obliterating suture, 20, 20f
Video fluoroscopy, 103
Virginal breast hypertrophy. See Juvenile
    breast hypertrophy
Voiding cystourethrography (VCUG), 428,
    469
Vomer bone, 65
Vomer flap, 64
Von Langenbeck palatoplasty
    anatomy, 74, 74f
    complications, 80
    definition, 74

differential diagnosis, 75
elevation of oral mucoperiosteal flaps,
    76
greater palatine vessels isolation, 77
markings, 76, 76f
merits and demerits, 79t
muscle and intravelar veloplasty
    dissection, 78
nasal mucosa
    closure, 78, 78f
    dissection, 77
natural history, 74–75
nonoperative management, 75
oral mucoperiosteal flaps elevation, 76,
    76f
oral mucosa
    closure, 79, 79f
    dissection, 77
outcomes, 79–80
pathogenesis, 74
patient history and physical findings, 75
postoperative care, 79
surgical management, 75
    approach, 75
    patient position, 75
    preoperative planning, 75
VPD (velopharyngeal dysfunction), 103
VPI (velopharyngeal incompetence), 64
Vulvar reconstruction
    anatomy, 458, 459f
    complications, 467
    definition, 458
    imaging, 459
    merits and demerits, 466b
    natural history, 458
    nonoperative management, 459
    outcomes, 467
    pathogenesis, 458
    patient history and physical findings,
        458–459
    postoperative care, 466
    surgical management, 459–460, 460f

V-Y advancement flap
    gluteal muscles of, bilateral, 194, 194f
    for ischial pressure injury, 193, 193f

W
Warwick-James elevator, 82
Wedge skin excision, Stahl ear, 227,
    229f–230f
Would closure, prominent ears, 245
Wound closure
    constricted ear, 236, 236f
    cryptotia, 240
    microtia, auricular reconstruction for,
        223–224
    thyroglossal duct cysts, 315, 315f
W-plasty, cutaneous scar, 139
Wrist/fingers reconstruction. See also
        Neonatal brachial plexus palsy (NBPP)
    complications, 374
    FCU to ECRB tendon transfer, 371–372,
        371f
    finger flexion, free functioning gracilis
        transfer for, 372, 372f
    outcomes, 374
    postoperative care, 373–374

Y
Y-V medial canthopexy, 274, 274f

Z
Z-plasty. See also Furlow palatoplasty
    cryptotia, 239, 239f
    cutaneous scar, 139
    double-opposing
        dissection, 114, 115f
        markings, 114, 114f
        surgical management, 113
    with intravelar veloplasty, 72–73
    optional cutaneous, 137–138, 137f, 138f,
        139f
    oral and nasal layers, 68f–69f
    thumb reconstruction, 179–180, 179f–180f